Pregnancy and Childbirth:
A Woman-Centered Approach

Pregnancy and Childbirth: A Woman-Centered Approach

Editor: Katie Beckett

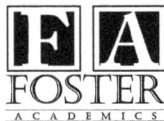

FA FOSTER
ACADEMICS

www.fosteracademics.com

www.fosteracademics.com

FA
FOSTER
ACADEMICS

Cataloging-in-Publication Data

Pregnancy and childbirth : a woman-centered approach / edited by Katie Beckett.
    p. cm.
Includes bibliographical references and index.
ISBN 978-1-63242-668-0
1. Pregnancy. 2. Childbirth. 3. Women--Health and hygiene.
4. Women--Medical examinations. 5. Obstetrics. I. Beckett, Katie.
RG551 .P74 2019
618.2--dc23

Foster Academics,
118-35 Queens Blvd., Suite 400,
Forest Hills, NY 11375, USA

ISBN 978-1-63242-668-0 (Hardback)

Contents

Preface..IX

Chapter 1 **Previous Early Antenatal Service Utilization Improves Timely Booking**................................ 1
Tadesse Belayneh, Mulat Adefris and Gashaw Andargie

Chapter 2 **Pregnant Women in Louisiana Are Not Meeting Dietary Seafood Recommendations**..8
M. L. Drewery, A. V. Gaitán, C. Thaxton, W. Xu and C. J. Lammi-Keefe

Chapter 3 **Paradox of Modern Pregnancy: A Phenomenological Study of Women's Lived Experiences from Assisted Pregnancy**..17
Fahimeh Ranjbar, Mohammad-Mehdi Akhondi, Leili Borimnejad, Saeed-Reza Ghaffari and Zahra Behboodi-Moghadam

Chapter 4 **Implementation of the International Association of Diabetes and Pregnancy Study Groups Criteria: Not Always a Cause for Concern**..25
Pooja Sibartie and Julie Quinlivan

Chapter 5 **Perinatal Risks Associated with Early Vanishing Twin Syndrome following Transfer of Cleavage- or Blastocyst-Stage Embryos**..30
Nigel Pereira, Katherine P. Pryor, Allison C. Petrini, Jovana P. Lekovich, Jaclyn Stahl, Rony T. Elias and Steven D. Spandorfer

Chapter 6 **Mild Anemia and Pregnancy Outcome in a Swiss Collective**................................36
Gabriela Bencaiova and Christian Breymann

Chapter 7 **Postpartum Visit Attendance Increases the Use of Modern Contraceptives**...43
Saba W. Masho, Susan Cha, RaShel Charles, Elizabeth McGee, Nicole Karjane, Linda Hines and Susan G. Kornstein

Chapter 8 **A New Model for Providing Cell-Free DNA and Risk Assessment for Chromosome Abnormalities in a Public Hospital Setting**..50
Robert Wallerstein, Andrea Jelks and Matthew J. Garabedian

Chapter 9 **Can Obstetric Risk Factors Predict Fetal Acidaemia at Birth? A Retrospective Case-Control Study**...56
Habiba Kapaya, Roslyn Williams, Grace Elton and Dilly Anumba

Chapter 10 **Determinants and Outcomes of Emergency Caesarean Section following Failed Instrumental Delivery**..64
Sian McDonnell and Edwin Chandraharan

Chapter 11   Predictors of Perinatal Mortality Associated with Placenta Previa and Placental Abruption: An Experience from a Low Income Country...70
Yifru Berhan

Chapter 12   Clinical Presentation of Preeclampsia and the Diagnostic Value of Proteins and their Methylation Products as Biomarkers in Pregnant Women with Preeclampsia and Their Newborns...80
Maria Portelli and Byron Baron

Chapter 13   Physiologic Course of Female Reproductive Function: A Molecular Look into the Prologue of Life...103
Joselyn Rojas, Mervin Chávez-Castillo, Luis Carlos Olivar, María Calvo, José Mejías, Milagros Rojas, Jessenia Morillo and Valmore Bermúdez

Chapter 14   Reference Ranges of Amniotic Fluid Index in Late Third Trimester of Pregnancy: What Should the Optimal Interval between Two Ultrasound Examinations be?...124
Shripad Hebbar, Lavanya Rai, Prashant Adiga and Shyamala Guruvare

Chapter 15   Prevalence and Factors Associated with Teenage Pregnancy, Northeast Ethiopia, 2017...131
Yohannes Ayanaw Habitu , Anteneh Yalew and Telake Azale Bisetegn

Chapter 16   Naegele Forceps Delivery and Association between Morbidity and the Number of Forceps Traction Applications...138
Naoki Matsumoto, Toshifumi Takenaka, Nobuyuki Ikeda, Satoshi Yazaki and Yuichi Sato

Chapter 17   Utilization of Antenatal Care Services in Dalit Communities...145
Mamata Sherpa Awasthi, Kiran Raj Awasthi, Harish Singh Thapa, Bhuvan Saud, Sarita Pradhan and Roshani Agrawal Khatry

Chapter 18   Maternal Morbidity in Women with Placenta Previa Managed with Prediction of Morbidly Adherent Placenta by Ultrasonography...153
Midori Fujisaki, Seishi Furukawa, Yohei Maki, Masanao Oohashi, Koutarou Doi and Hiroshi Sameshima

Chapter 19   A Qualitative Study to Examine Perceptions and Barriers to Appropriate Gestational Weight Gain among Participants in the Special Supplemental Nutrition Program for Women Infants and Children Program...158
Loan Pham Kim, Maria Koleilat and Shannon E.Whaley

Chapter 20   Frequency, Risk Factors, and Adverse Fetomaternal Outcomes of Placenta Previa...167
Elizabeth Eliet Senkoro, Amasha H. Mwanamsangu, Fransisca Seraphin Chuwa, Sia Emmanuel Msuya, Oresta PeterMnali, Benjamin G. Brown and Michael Johnson Mahande

Chapter 21   Mode of Delivery according to Leisure Time Physical Activity before and during Pregnancy: A Multicenter Cohort Study of Low-Risk Women...174
Emilie Nor Nielsen, Per Kragh Andersen, Hanne Kristine Hegaard and Mette Juhl

Chapter 22   **Determinants of Malaria Prevention and Treatment Seeking Behaviours of Pregnant Undergraduates Resident in University Hostels**..182
Anthonia Ukamaka Chinweuba, Noreen Ebelechukwu Agbapuonwu,
JaneLovena Enuma Onyiapat, Chidimma Egbichi Israel,
Clementine Ifeyinwa Ilo and Joyce Chinenye Arinze

Chapter 23   **Discordance in Couples Pregnancy Intentions and Breastfeeding Duration: Results from the National Survey of Family Growth 2011–2013**...191
Jordyn T. Wallenborn , Gregory Chambers, Elizabeth P. Lowery and Saba W. Masho

Chapter 24   **Factors Associated with Successful Trial of Labor after Cesarean Section**..198
Aram Thapsamuthdechakorn, Ratanaporn Sekararithi and Theera Tongsong

Chapter 25   **Scoping Review on Maternal Health among Immigrant and Refugee Women in Canada: Prenatal, Intrapartum and Postnatal Care**...203
N. Khanlou, N. Haque, A. Skinner, A. Mantini and C. Kurtz Landy

Chapter 26   **Patient Preferences and Experiences in Hyperemesis Gravidarum Treatment**...217
Relin van Vliet, Marieke Bink, Julian Polman, Amaran Suntharan, Iris Grooten,
Sandra E. Zwolsman, Tessa J. Roseboom and Rebecca C. Painter

Chapter 27   **Improved Value of Individual Prenatal Care for the Interdisciplinary Team**.......................225
Ella Damiano and Regan Theiler

Permissions

List of Contributors

Index

Preface

This book was inspired by the evolution of our times; to answer the curiosity of inquisitive minds. Many developments have occurred across the globe in the recent past which has transformed the progress in the field.

The time during which one or more offspring develops inside a woman's body is known as pregnancy. The state of pregnancy can occur by sexual intercourse or assisted reproductive technology. The birth of a child usually occurs after nine months, i.e., 40 weeks from the last menstrual period. Childbirth is the ending of a pregnancy by one or more child leaving a woman's uterus by vaginal passage or Caesarean section. Vaginal delivery is the most common way of childbirth. Three stages of labor, namely the shortening and opening of the cervix, descent and birth of the baby, and the delivery of the placenta are involved in it. This book explores all the important aspects of pregnancy and childbirth in the present day scenario. It includes some of the vital pieces of work being conducted across the world, on various topics related to pregnancy and childbirth. Those in search of information to further their knowledge will be greatly assisted by this book.

This book was developed from a mere concept to drafts to chapters and finally compiled together as a complete text to benefit the readers across all nations. To ensure the quality of the content we instilled two significant steps in our procedure. The first was to appoint an editorial team that would verify the data and statistics provided in the book and also select the most appropriate and valuable contributions from the plentiful contributions we received from authors worldwide. The next step was to appoint an expert of the topic as the Editor-in-Chief, who would head the project and finally make the necessary amendments and modifications to make the text reader-friendly. I was then commissioned to examine all the material to present the topics in the most comprehensible and productive format.

I would like to take this opportunity to thank all the contributing authors who were supportive enough to contribute their time and knowledge to this project. I also wish to convey my regards to my family who have been extremely supportive during the entire project.

Editor

Previous Early Antenatal Service Utilization Improves Timely Booking: Cross-Sectional Study at University of Gondar Hospital, Northwest Ethiopia

Tadesse Belayneh,[1] Mulat Adefris,[2] and Gashaw Andargie[3]

[1] Department of Medical Anesthesiology, College of Medicine and Health Sciences, University of Gondar, Kebele 16, P.O. Box 196, Gondar, Ethiopia
[2] Department of Gynecology and Obstetrics, College of Medicine and Health Sciences, University of Gondar, P.O. Box 196, Gondar, Ethiopia
[3] Institute of Public Health, College of Medicine and Health Sciences, University of Gondar, P.O. Box 196, Gondar, Ethiopia

Correspondence should be addressed to Tadesse Belayneh; tadbel20@gmail.com

Academic Editor: R. L. Deter

Background. Early booking of antenatal care (ANC) is regarded as a cornerstone of maternal and neonatal health care. However, existing evidence from developing countries indicate that lots of pregnant woman begin ANC booking lately. *Objective.* It was aimed to assess timing of ANC booking and associated factors among pregnant women attending ANC clinic at University of Gondar Hospital, 2013. *Methods.* An institution based cross-sectional study design was used to collect data with a face-to-face interview technique. Bivariate and multivariate analysis was used to identify associated factors for early ANC visit using SPSS version 20. *Results.* From total women (N = 369) interviewed, 47.4% were timely booked. Mothers with younger age (AOR = 3.83, 95% CI: 1.89, 10.53), formal education (AOR = 1.06, 95% CI: 1.03, −7.61), previous early ANC visit (AOR = 2.39, 95% CI: 2.23, 9.86), and perceived ANC visit per pregnancy of four and greater were significantly associated with early ANC visit. *Conclusions.* Although late booking is a problem in this study, previous early utilization of ANC visit favors current timely booking. This indicates that the importance of early booking was appropriately addressed from previous visits. Counseling of timely booking during ANC visit should be strengthened. Moreover, empowering through education is also recommended.

1. Introduction

World Health Organization (WHO) with a fifth Millennium Development Goal has planned to reduce maternal deaths by three-quarters by the year 2015 [1]. Antenatal care, a care given to pregnant women, is widely used for prevention, early diagnosis, and treatment of general medical- and pregnancy-related complications [2].

Early ANC booking and regular follow-up of services usually provides opportunities for delivering health information and interventions (i.e., via early detection of modifiable preexisting medical conditions like Heart disease, Diabetes Mellitus, Hypertensive disorders, HIV/AIDS, and severe anemia) that can significantly enhance the health of the mother and fetus [3–9]. On the contrary, opportunities to provide information and other interventions pertaining to their reproductive health and the health of their unborn child are missed when a woman initiates ANC in late time of her pregnancy [10, 11].

The new World Health Organization ANC model states that every pregnant woman is at risk of complications and recommends early an ANC visit, of which the first should be during the first trimester. The visit is used to classify pregnant women into two groups based on previous history of pregnancy, current pregnancy state, and general medical conditions. Those eligible to receive routine ANC (basic component) and those who need special care on average account for 25% of all pregnant women initiating ANC [12]. Low ANC coverage, few visits, and late booking are common problems throughout Sub-Saharan Africa posing difficulty in accomplishing the WHO recommendation [13, 14].

According to the Ethiopian Demographic and Health Survey 2011 report, only 11.2% of women had an ANC visit before their fourth month of pregnancy, almost twofold increase from 6 percent in the 2005 EDHS. In urban settings where the health services are physically accessible relative to rural areas, 31.0% of mothers seek the service before four months of gestation and 23.1% did not attend at all. The figure for rural women is much worse than this; that is, 7.7% sought ANC before 16 weeks and 63.1% did not attend ANC at all. In Ethiopia, ANC services are provided free of payment at the governmental health facilities [15]. A similar study done in Addis Ababa showed a 40.0% of first trimester booking with a recommended period [16]. Likewise, study finding in Nairobi, Kenya indicated that 85% of women initiated visits later than the first trimester [17]. These trends have been also noted in other Sub-Saharan African countries [18, 19].

Utilization of health services is a complex behavioral phenomenon. Empirical studies of preventive and curative services have often found out that the use of health services is related to the availability, quality, cost of services, social structure, health beliefs, and personal characteristics of the users [20–22]. Reviewed literatures showed that maternal age, marital status, maternal education, occupation, ethnicity, religion, family income, residence, parity, history of abortion, child birth outcome, experience of service utilization, pregnancy-related complications, wanted or unwanted pregnancy, and influence of the husband were predictors that either positively or negatively influence timing of ANC booking (Figure 1) [23–26].

Studies on the prevalence of early ANC visit and associated factors are scanty in Ethiopia and unavailable in the study area. Therefore, this study aimed at giving information about the prevalence of early ANC visit and associated factors in order to help improve the health of mothers and their fetus among pregnant women attending ANC at the University of Gondar Hospital, Northwest Ethiopia.

2. Methods

Hospital-based cross-sectional study was conducted from January 1 to February 28, 2013, at the University of Gondar Hospital. The Hospital is a 500-bed capacity teaching hospital founded in Amhara region, Northwest Ethiopia. Medical, gynecologic and obstetrics, pediatrics, and surgical patients are served by the Hospital at outpatient and inpatient levels. It serves for more than 5 million populations in area. According to EDHS 2011, 59.1% of women in Amhara region did not attend ANC at all [15].

The sample size ($N = 369$) was calculated using single population proportion formula based on the following assumptions: taking 40% prevalence on early timing of the first ANC visit at 12 weeks from a study conducted in Addis

Ababa [16], 95% confidence interval, and a 5% margin of error.

Study subjects were recruited for the study at ANC service when they appear to begin the service or return for ANC follow-up. Every second case that was willing to participate during the study period was taken until the required sample size was obtained.

Data were collected using a pretested structured questionnaire via trained female nurses who were not from the same facility. Pretesting was conducted outside the study area. Data collectors interviewed pregnant women waiting after they completed their daily visits. The purpose of data collection and the importance of the study as well as the significance of true information were enlightened in order to maximize the response rate and to generate reliable data.

All responses to the questionnaires were coded, entered, and analyzed using SPSS version 20.0.

Variables with P value of up to 0.2 in bivariate analysis were entered into the multivariate model. The binary logistic regression method was employed and variables with a P value of <0.05 were considered as significantly associated with the early ANC visit. The early ANC visit is considered if pregnant women started their first ANC visit within the first 12 weeks of gestation. P value and 95% confidence interval were used to check the statistical significance. The odds ratio was utilized to determine the strength of association between independent variables and ANC booking. Ethical clearance was obtained from the Institutional Review Board of University of Gondar and an official permission letter was secured from the University of Gondar Hospital Clinical Director. Participants were communicated individually about the purpose of the study and verbal informed consent was taken before the interview. The right of participants to withdraw from the study at any time, without any precondition, was kept and disclosed to respondents. The name of participants was not taken for reasons of confidentiality.

3. Results

3.1. Sociodemographic Characteristics of the Study Participants. All pregnant mothers ($N = 369$) who attended the service responded to the interview (100%). The mean age of the participants was 24.9 years (±4.1 years). One hundred and forty-two (38.5%) of the participants had secondary school level education and 124 (33.6%) were employed. Almost all 366 (99.2%) participants were married (Table 1).

3.2. Timing of Initial ANC Visit. Out of 369 pregnant mothers included in this study, 174 (47.2%) pregnant mothers started their first ANC visit early (CI 1.48–1.58, with mean of 1.52), while the remaining 195 (52.8%) pregnant mothers started ANC late in either second or third trimester. In both cases, the timing of the first ANC booking ranges from 1 month to 8 months of gestation. Similarly, the mean month of initiation of ANC was 4.4 months (SD = 1.4), and the median duration was 5 months.

3.3. Obstetric Characteristics of the Participants. As shown in Table 2, among 170 respondents who had a history of

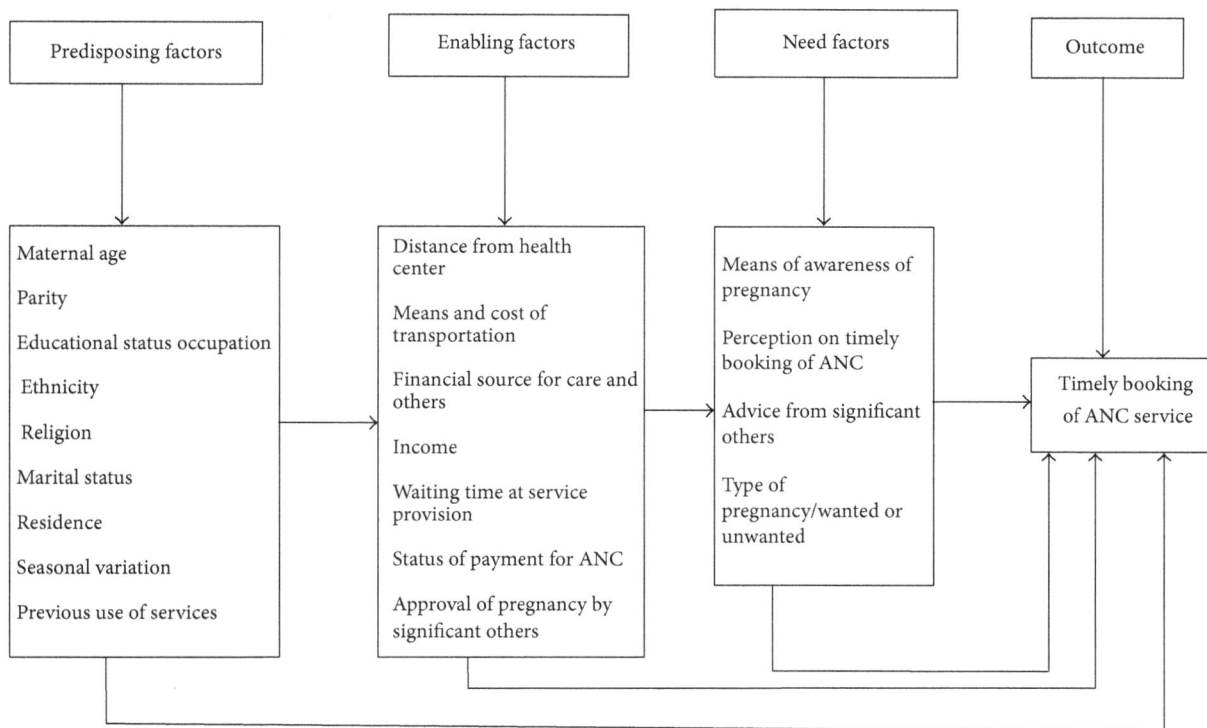

FIGURE 1: Conceptual framework for timely use of ANC (adapted from Anderson 1995).

pregnancy, 131 (77.1%) of them visited ANC. Of those who visited ANC, 62 (47.3%) of them booked within 12 weeks of pregnancy, while the remaining 69 (52.7%) participants booked after 12 weeks of gestation. The current pregnancy was planned and wanted in the majority (90.0%) of the women.

Regarding to perception of correct time of ANC booking, 256 (69.4%) mother perceived within 12 weeks of gestation, while 113 (30.6%) were after 12 weeks of gestation. Of those who correctly perceived the recommended time, 122 (70.1%) booked early in the current pregnancy.

232 (62.9%) of women perceived that four and more ANC visits were necessary. On the contrary, 137 (37.1%) of them perceived that less than four ANC visits were sufficient throughout the whole pregnancy period (Table 2).

3.4. Factors Associated with Early Booking of ANC Visit. The analysis was done using bivariate and multivariate binary logistic regression. The model fitness was checked with Hosmer and Lemeshow test. Results from multivariate analysis indicated that pregnant mothers of younger age, having a higher educational level, previous late booking practice, history of abortion, and the perception of ANC visit per pregnancy, were significantly associated with the early ANC visit. However, the number of children alive, mode of pervious delivery, planned pregnancy, place of ANC visit, pregnancy-related complications in the current pregnancy, history of abortion, having less than five children, and means of approving pregnancy were not significantly associated with the early ANC visit. Accordingly, pregnant mothers at younger age were 3.83 times more likely to book earlier

compared to older ones (AOR = 3.89, 95% CI: 1.89, 10.53). Similarly, those having formal education were 1.06 times more likely to book earlier compared to those who cannot read and write (AOR = 1.06, 95% CI: 1.03, −7.61). Those women who booked early in previous pregnancy were 2.39 times more likely to book earlier compared to those who booked lately (AOR = 2.39, 95% CI: 2.23, 9.86). Moreover, those who attended four and greater ANC visits per pregnancy (AOR = 1.39, 95% CI: 1.89, 7.53) were more likely to book earlier compared to their counterparts (Table 3).

4. Discussion

Antenatal care is more beneficial in preventing adverse pregnancy outcomes when received early in pregnancy and continued until delivery [27–29]. Early detection of problems in pregnancy leads to timely referrals for women in high-risk categories or with complications; this is particularly true in Ethiopia, where three-quarters of the population lives in rural areas and where physical barriers pose a challenge to providing health care [15].

According to this study, nearly half (47.4%) of the respondents started their ANC within the recommended time and the rest (52.6%) booked late. This result is low compared to the recommendation of WHO which states that each and every pregnant woman should start the first ANC within the first trimester of pregnancy [12]. On the contrary, the finding was high compared to the National EDHS report (11.0%, 2011), ANC coverage in Addis Ababa (40.0%, 2008), Debre Berhan (26.2%, 2012), Hadiya Zone (8.7%, 2010), and (12.5%,

TABLE 1: Sociodemographic characteristics of pregnant mothers by time of booking, University of Gondar Hospital, Northwest Ethiopia, 2013 ($N = 369$).

Variables	Frequency (%)
Age	
15–19	24 (6.5%)
20–24	153 (41.5%)
25–29	135 (36.6%)
30–34	46 (12.5%)
35–40	11 (3.0%)
Marital status	
Married	366 (99.2%)
Single	3 (0.8%)
Educational status	
No formal education	72 (19.5%)
Primary (1–8)	74 (20.1%)
Secondary (9–12)	142 (38.5%)
Above secondary	81 (22.0%)
Ethnicity	
Amhara	354 (95.9%)
Tigre	15 (4.1%)
Religion	
Christianity#	320 (86.7%)
Muslim	49 (13.3%)
Occupation	
Employed	124 (33.6%)
Nonemployed	245 (66.4%)

Christianity# = orthodox + protestant + catholic.

TABLE 2: Obstetric characteristics of pregnant women by time of booking, University of Gondar Hospital, Northwest Ethiopia, 2013.

Variables	Total (%)
Number of children alive ($N = 168$)	
1-2 children	120 (74.4%)
>2 children	48 (25.6%)
Had ANC visit for last pregnancy ($N = 170$)	
Yes	131 (77.1%)
No	39 (22.9%)
Previous ANC first visit ($N = 131$)	
Booked early (≤4 months)	62 (47.3%)
Booked lately (>4 months)	69 (52.7%)
State of current pregnancy ($N = 369$)	
Planned	332 (90.0%)
Unplanned	37 (10.0%)
History of abortion ($N = 369$)	
Yes	94 (25.5%)
No	275 (74.5%)
History of death of child ($N = 369$)	
Yes	38 (10.3%)
No	331 (89.7%)
Perceptions on timing of first visit ($N = 369$)	
Early (≤12 weeks)	256 (69.4%)
Lately (>12 weeks)	113 (30.6%)
Perceived number of ANC visits per pregnancy ($N = 369$)	
<4 times	137 (37.1%)
≥4 times	232 (62.9%)
Mode of previous delivery ($N = 166$)	
Spontaneous vaginal delivery	143 (86.1%)
C-section	23 (13.9%)

2009) Yem Southern Ethiopia [15, 16, 30–32]. This gap might be because of differences in the study population; that is, this study included urban residents, whereas the others (Debre Berhan, Hadiya, and Yem) in both urban and rural residents. Moreover, this can be influenced by the fact that the study used hospital based setting and therefore they were more likely to attend ANC earlier than the general population. Time gap might also be the other reason. This finding suggests that physical and financial accessibilities of the service alone cannot ensure proper utilization of available service. The result was also higher compared to other African countries, South Western Nigeria (29%, 2008), Tanzania (19%, 2000), Lao People's Democratic Republic (28%, 2010), and (17.4%, 2006) rural Western Kenya [13, 33–35]. However, this result is remarkably lower than the findings from developed and some developing countries, where the vast majority of pregnant women present early for ANC [36, 37].

In the current study, women having formal education were more likely to initiate ANC visit earlier than their counterparts (AOR 1.06, 95% CI: 1.03–7.6) which is similar to a study conducted elsewhere in the developing countries [1, 38, 39]. This could be explained by the fact that women with secondary school or higher education were more likely to be employed have more income than their counterparts. The rationale is that by educating girls especially of secondary school or higher level, they are equipped not only with the

right tools to make proper health care decisions, but also with skills that enhance their future financial independence, thereby elevating their status in the communities where they live [38, 39].

The proportion of respondents who have had their first visit within the recommended time in the preceding pregnancy was 47.3%, while 56.9% of these pregnant women who booked ANC within the recommended time in the previous pregnancy were booked within the current pregnancy. Accordingly, those who visited ANC earlier in former pregnancy were more likely to book earlier for their current pregnancy (AOR = 2.39, 95% CI: 2.23, 9.86), showing that past experience of early ANC service utilization demonstrated timely booking in the current visit. This depicted that women were appropriately informed on time of booking from counseling and health education sessions during previous pregnancies. The result of this study is in contradiction with Addis Ababa's finding which showed that previous ANC utilization did not improve timely booking [16].

The result of this study showed that good perception of the initial ANC visit was a factor for an early ANC visit.

TABLE 3: Factors affecting booking of first ANC visit, University of Gondar Hospital, Northwest Ethiopia, 2013 ($N = 369$).

Variables	Time at first visit		Crude OR (95% CI)	Adjusted OR (95% CI)
	Timely booked n (%)	Lately booked n (%)		
Educational status				
Cannot read and write	33 (19.0)	39 (20.0)	1	1
Formal education	141 (81.0)	156 (80.0)	3.16* (1.03–8.64)	1.06* (1.03–7.61)
Age				
16–30	167 (95.9)	168 (86.2)	2.33* (1.09–11.91)	3.83* (1.89–10.53)
31–45	7 (4.1)	27 (13.8)	1	1
Previous ANC first time visit ($n = 131$)				
Before and at 12 weeks	33 (56.9)	26 (35.6)	2.01* (1.12–4.04)	2.39* (2.23–9.86)
After 12 weeks	25 (43.1)	47 (64.4)	1	1
History of abortion				
Yes	41 (11.1)	53 (27.2)	1	1
No	133 (36.0)	142 (72.8)	1.01* (2.44–5.84)	1.21* (2.17–7.94)
Perceived sufficient number of ANC visits/pregnancy				
Less than 4 times	43 (24.7)	61 (31.3)	1	1
More than 4 times	131 (75.3)	134 (68.7)	1.18* (1.99–4.26)	1.39* (1.89–7.53)
Occupation				
Employed	42 (24.1)	82 (42.1)	1	1
Nonemployed	132 (75.9)	113 (57.9)	3.12# (1.23–12.3)	2.28 (0.71–10.2)#
Had ANC visit for last pregnancy ($n = 170$)				
Yes	54 (80.6)	77 (74.8)	0.71 (0.33–1.51)#	4.67 (1.34–16.27)#
No	13 (19.4)	26 (25.2)	1	1
State of current pregnancy ($N = 369$)				
Planned	154 (85.5)	178 (91.3)	1.36 (0.69–2.69)#	4.37 (0.79–24.11)#
Unplanned	20 (11.5)	17 (8.7)	1	1

*Significant and #nonsignificant from the multivariate logistic regression.

Women who perceived initiation of ANC visit in the first trimester were more likely to make four or more visits than those who initiated care in the second and third trimesters. This finding was supported by studies done in Addis Ababa [16] and Niger Delta, Nigeria, which showed that the major reason for the late ANC visit was a misconception about the early ANC visit [40].

The current study also showed that age was associated with early booking. Women less than 30 years old were more likely to book for ANC earlier than older women. This finding was similar to those of studies done in Addis Ababa (Ethiopia), Nigeria, Kenya, and India [6, 16, 23, 24]. This might be because young women at their first pregnancy are more careful about their pregnancy and therefore require institutional care more than older women. In addition, younger women tend to be more educated than older ones [2].

It was reported by different researchers that previous obstetric complications such as stillbirth, abortion, eclampsia, intrauterine fetal death, and cesarean section have no influence on gestational age at booking [21, 22]. Similarly, the current study showed that those women who had no history of abortion were more likely to book earlier than women with abortion history.

5. Limitations of the Study

As this is a cross-sectional study, the associations observed may not be causal enough, and since this study is institution based it may not be generalisable. Additionally, it only includes the urban clients who have more access to services and information.

6. Conclusions and Recommendations

In conclusion, even though the ANC services are available freely to all women, late booking continues to be a problem in the study setting. Maternal education, previous history of early booking, age, and perception on frequency of ANC visit per pregnancy were significantly associated with the early ANC visit. As per the findings of this study, awareness creation and strengthening on the importance of the early

ANC visit need to be emphasized at the time of service provision. Empowering mothers through education is also recommended.

Conflict of Interests

The authors declare that there is no conflict of interests regarding the publication of this paper.

Authors' Contribution

Tadesse Belayneh designed the study, analyzed the data, and drafted the paper. Mulat Adeferese and Gashaw Andargie participated in designing the study and drafting the paper. All authors read and approved the final paper.

Acknowledgments

The authors are grateful to the pregnant women who participated in this study. They thank also the University of Gondar for the funding.

References

[1] C. Abou-Zahr and T. Wardlaw, *Maternal Mortality in 2000: Estimates Developed by WHO, UNICEF, UNFPA*, World Health Organization, Geneva, Switzerland, 2004.

[2] K. Beeckman, F. Louckx, and K. Putman, "Predisposing, enabling and pregnancy-related determinants of late initiation of prenatal care," *Maternal and Child Health Journal*, vol. 15, no. 7, pp. 1067–1075, 2011.

[3] K. T. Barnhart, B. Casanova, M. D. Sammel, K. Timbers, K. Chung, and J. L. Kulp, "Prediction of location of a symptomatic early gestation based solely on clinical presentation," *Obstetrics and Gynecology*, vol. 112, no. 6, pp. 1319–1326, 2008.

[4] "Antenatal care, routine care for pregnant women, clinical guideline," 2009, http://www.nice.org.uk/nicemedia/live/11947/40145/4 0145.

[5] E. Kirk, G. Condous, and T. Bourne, "The non-surgical management of ectopic pregnancy," *Ultrasound in Obstetrics and Gynecology*, vol. 27, no. 1, pp. 91–100, 2006.

[6] A. Oladokun, R. E. Oladokun, I. Morhason-Bello, A. F. Bello, and B. Adedokun, "Proximate predictors of early antenatal registration among Nigerian pregnant women," *Annals of African Medicine*, vol. 9, no. 4, pp. 222–225, 2010.

[7] S. Riskin-Mashiah, G. Younes, A. Damti, and R. Auslender, "First-trimester fasting hyperglycemia and adverse pregnancy outcomes," *Diabetes Care*, vol. 32, no. 9, pp. 1639–1643, 2009.

[8] S. Bryan, "Current challenges in the assessment and management of patients with bleeding in early pregnancy," *Emergency Medicine*, vol. 15, no. 3, pp. 219–222, 2003.

[9] D. Watson-Jones, B. Gumodoka, H. Weiss et al., "Syphilis in pregnancy in Tanzania. II. The effectiveness of antenatal syphilis screening and single-dose benzathine penicillin treatment for the prevention of adverse pregnancy outcomes," *The Journal of Infectious Diseases*, vol. 186, no. 7, pp. 948–957, 2002.

[10] M. King, R. Mhlanga, and H. De Pinho, "The context of maternal and child health. South African Health Review," Health Systems Trust, Durban, South Africa, 2006.

[11] *All Parliamentary Groups on Population, Development and Reproductive Health. The Return of the Population Growth Factor—Its Impact Upon the MDGs*, 2007.

[12] J. Villar and P. Bergsj, *Randomized Trial; Manual for the Implementation of New Model*, World Health Organization, Geneva, Switzerland, 2002.

[13] D. A. Adekanle and A. I. Isawumi, "Late antenatal care booking and its predictors among pregnant women in South Western Nigeria," *Online Journal of Health and Allied Sciences*, vol. 7, no. 1, article 4, 2008.

[14] W. Delva, E. Yard, S. Luchters et al., "A Safe Motherhood project in Kenya: assessment of antenatal attendance, service provision and implications for PMTCT," *Tropical Medicine & International Health*, vol. 15, no. 5, pp. 584–591, 2010.

[15] CSA and ICF International, "Ethiopia Demographic and Health Survey 2011. Addis Ababa, Ethiopia and Calverton, Md, USA," Central Statistical Agency and ICF International, 2012.

[16] A. Tariku, Y. Melkamu, and Z. Kebede, "Previous utilization of service does not improve timely booking in antenatal care: cross sectional study on timing of antenatal care booking at public health facilities in Addis Ababa," *Ethiopian Journal of Health Development*, vol. 24, no. 3, pp. 226–233, 2010.

[17] M. Magadi, "Maternal and child health," in *APHRC. Population and Health Dynamics in Nairobi's Informal Settlements*, African Population and Health Research Center, Nairobi, Kenya, 2002.

[18] N. Abrahams, R. Jewkes, and Z. Mvo, "Health care-seeking practices of pregnant women and the role of the midwife in Cape town, South Africa," *Journal of Midwifery and Women's Health*, vol. 46, no. 4, pp. 240–247, 2001.

[19] L. Myer and A. Harrison, "Why do womn seek antenatal care late? Perspectives from rural South Africa," *Journal of Midwifery & Women's Health*, vol. 48, no. 4, pp. 268–272, 2003.

[20] P. Low, J. Paterson, T. Wouldes, S. Carter, M. Williams, and T. Percival, "Factors affecting antenatal care attendance by mothers of Pacific infants living in New Zealand," *The New Zealand Medical Journal*, vol. 118, no. 1216, Article ID U1489, 2005.

[21] M. A. Okunlola, O. A. Ayinde, K. M. Owonikoko, and A. O. Omigbodun, "Factors influencing gestational age at antenatal booking at the University College Hospital, Ibadan, Nigeria," *Journal of Obstetrics and Gynaecology*, vol. 26, no. 3, pp. 195–197, 2006.

[22] L. T. T. Trinh and G. Rubin, "Late entry to antenatal care in New South Wales, Australia," *Reproductive Health*, vol. 3, article 8, 2006.

[23] M. A. Magadi, N. J. Madise, and R. N. Rodrigues, "Frequency and timing of antenatal care in Kenya: explaining the variations between women of different communities," *Social Science & Medicine*, vol. 51, no. 4, pp. 551–561, 2000.

[24] K. Navaneetham and A. Dharmalingam, "Utilization of maternal health care services in Southern India," *Social Science and Medicine*, vol. 55, no. 10, pp. 1849–1869, 2002.

[25] N. Chandiok, B. Dhillon, I. Kambo et al., "Determinants of ANC utilization in rural areas of India," *The Journal of Obstetrics and Gynecology of India*, vol. 56, no. 1, pp. 47–52, 2006.

[26] Y. Mekonnen and A. Mekonnen, *Utilization of Maternal Health Care Services in Ethiopia*, ORC Macro, Calverton, Md, USA, 2002.

[27] B. Fekede and A. G Mariam, "Antenatal care services utilization and factors associated in Jimma Town (South West Ethiopia)," *Ethiopian Medical Journal*, vol. 45, no. 2, pp. 123–133, 2007.

Previous Early Antenatal Service Utilization Improves Timely Booking: Cross-Sectional Study...

7

[28] WHO and UNICEF, *Antenatal Care in Developing Countries: Promises, Achievements and Missed Opportunities: An Analysis of Trends, Levels and Differentials, 1990–2001*, WHO, Genevea, Switzerland, 2003.

[29] F. Mugisha, K. Bocar, H. Dong, G. Chepng'eno, and R. Sauerborn, "The two faces of enhancing utilization of health-care services: determinants of patient initiation and retention in rural Burkina Faso," *Bulletin of the World Health Organization*, vol. 82, no. 8, pp. 572–579, 2004.

[30] M. Amtatachew, D. Bitew, and D. N. Koye, "Prevalence and determinants of early antenatal care visit among pregnant women attending antenatal care in Debre Berhan Health Institutions, Central Ethiopia," *African Journal of Reproductive Health*, vol. 17, no. 4, pp. 130–136, 2013.

[31] B. Tewodros, A. G. Mariam, and Y. Dibaba, "Factors affecting antenatal care utilization in Yem Special Woreda, Southwestern Ethiopia," *Ethiopian Journal of Health Sciences*, vol. 19, no. 1, pp. 45–51, 2009.

[32] A. Zeine, W. Mirkuzie, and O. Shimeles, "Facors influencing antenatal care service utilization in Hadya zone," *Ethiopian Journal of Health Sciences*, vol. 20, no. 2, pp. 75–82, 2010.

[33] K. Gross, S. Alba, T. R. Glass, J. A. Schellenberg, and B. Obrist, "Timing of antenatal care for adolescent and adult pregnant women in south-eastern Tanzania," *BMC Pregnancy and Childbirth*, vol. 12, article 16, 2012.

[34] C. Manithip, A. Sihavong, K. Edin, R. Wahlstrom, and H. Wessel, "Factors associated with antenatal care utilization among rural women in Lao People's Democratic Republic," *Maternal and Child Health Journal*, vol. 15, no. 8, pp. 1356–1362, 2011.

[35] A. M. van Eijk, H. M. Bles, F. Odhiambo et al., "Use of antenatal services and delivery care among women in rural western Kenya: a community based survey," *Reproductive Health*, vol. 3, article 2, 2006.

[36] A. Yoong and T. Chard, "The effectiveness of current antenatal care," in *Progress in Obstetrics and Gynecology*, vol. 12, pp. 3–18, Churchill Livingstone, Edinburgh, Scotland, 1996.

[37] A. O. Omigbodun, "Preconception and antenatal care," in *Comprehensive Obstetrics in the Tropics*, E. Y. Kwawukume and E. E. Emuveyan, Eds., chapter 2, pp. 7–14, Asante and Hittscher, Accra, Ghana, 2002.

[38] V. Filippi, C. Ronsmans, O. M. Campbell et al., "Maternal health in poor countries: the broader context and a call for action," *Lancet*, vol. 368, no. 9546, pp. 1535–1541, 2006.

[39] C. Grown, G. R. Gupta, and R. Pande, "Taking action to improve women's health through gender equality and women's empowerment," *The Lancet*, vol. 365, no. 9458, pp. 541–543, 2005.

[40] P. N. Ebeigbe, E. P. Ndidi, G. O. Igberase, and I. G. Oseremen, "Reasons given by pregnant women for late initiation of antenatal care in the Niger delta, Nigeria," *Ghana Medical Journal*, vol. 44, no. 2, pp. 47–51, 2010.

Pregnant Women in Louisiana Are Not Meeting Dietary Seafood Recommendations

M. L. Drewery,[1] A. V. Gaitán,[1] C. Thaxton,[1] W. Xu,[2] and C. J. Lammi-Keefe[1,2]

[1]Louisiana State University, Baton Rouge, LA 70803, USA
[2]Louisiana State University AgCenter, Baton Rouge, LA 70803, USA

Correspondence should be addressed to M. L. Drewery; merrittdrewery@gmail.com

Academic Editor: Ellinor Olander

Background. The 2015–2020 Dietary Guidelines for Americans recommend that pregnant women and women of childbearing ages consume 8–12 oz. of seafood per week. Fish are the major dietary source of omega-3 long chain polyunsaturated fatty acids, which have benefits for the mother and fetus. *Methods.* In this observational study, we investigated dietary habits of pregnant women in Baton Rouge, Louisiana, USA, to determine if they achieve recommended seafood intake. A print survey, which included commonly consumed foods from protein sources (beef, chicken, pork, and fish), was completed by pregnant women at a single-day hospital convention for expecting families in October 2015. Women ($n = 221$) chose from six predefined responses to answer how frequently they were consuming each food. *Results.* Chicken was consumed most frequently (75% of women), followed by beef (71%), pork (65%), and fish (22%), respectively. Consumption frequency for the most consumed fish (catfish, once per month) was similar to or lower than that of the least consumed beef, chicken, and pork foods. Consumption frequency for the most consumed chicken and beef foods was at least once per week. *Conclusion.* Our data indicate that pregnant women in Louisiana often consume protein sources other than fish and likely fail to meet dietary seafood recommendations.

1. Introduction

Optimal fetal development and infant outcome depend on availability of specific nutrients during the preconceptual and gestational periods, including the omega-3 long chain polyunsaturated fatty acids (LCPUFAs), docosahexaenoic acid (DHA), and eicosapentaenoic acid (EPA) [1, 2].

In response to maternal omega-3 LCPUFA intake during pregnancy, infants have improved performance on cognitive and developmental tests [3–5], accelerated maturation of the visual and autonomic nervous systems [6–8], and leaner body composition [9, 10].

Health benefits of omega-3 LCPUFA intake in pregnancy may also extend to the mother. The relationship between dietary omega-3 LCPUFA intake and maternal mental health conditions (depressive disorders during and after pregnancy) has been examined. There is evidence that omega-3 LCPUFA intake may benefit women with preexisting depressive illnesses [11–14]. These findings are complemented by observational studies which point to an association between

low dietary omega-3 LCPUFA intake, especially DHA, and increased risk of depressive disorders during and following pregnancy [15, 16].

There is evidence that omega-3 LCPUFAs also positively affect general pregnancy outcome. Omega-3 LCPUFAs prolong pregnancy duration, reducing the risk of birth before 34 gestational weeks by 31% in normal and 61% in high-risk pregnancies [17, 18]. Increasing pregnancy duration has implications for decreasing incidence of preterm birth and intrauterine growth retardation [19].

These measurable and documented benefits of omega-3 LCPUFA underscore the recommendations of the 2015–2020 Dietary Guidelines for Americans [20] that pregnant women and women of childbearing ages consume 8–12 oz., or two to three 4 oz. servings, of seafood per week, as cold water marine fish are the major dietary source of omega-3 LCPUFAs (Table 1) [21]. In general, fish are regarded as good dietary sources of omega-3 LCPUFAs; however, fatty acid content depends on variety, geographical location, method of farming/harvesting, and other factors [21].

TABLE 1: DHA and EPA content of major dietary sources of omega-3 LCPUFA[1,2].

	DHA, mg/4 oz.	EPA, mg/4 oz.	Number of 4 oz. servings to provide 250 mg DHA + EPA[3]	Oz. to provide 250 mg DHA + EPA
Bass				
Sea	492	183	0.37	1.48
Striped	663	192	0.29	1.17
Catfish				
Farmed	64	19	3.02	12.10
Wild	265	147	0.61	2.43
Cod				
Atlantic	136	72	1.20	4.81
Pacific	109	39	1.69	6.76
Herring				
Atlantic	977	804	0.14	0.56
Pacific	781	1099	0.13	0.53
Flounder	123	155	0.90	3.61
Salmon				
Atlantic, farmed	1251	977	0.11	0.45
Atlantic, wild	1264	364	0.15	0.61
Pink	377	207	0.43	1.71
Sockeye	1797	395	0.11	0.46
Tilapia	97	5	2.44	9.74
Trout	599	229	0.30	1.21
Tuna				
Bluefin	1009	321	0.19	0.75
Light, canned in water	223	32	0.98	3.93
Yellowfin	100	13	2.21	8.82
White, canned in water	713	264	0.26	1.02

[1] Adapted from the USDA National Nutrient Database for Standard Reference, Release 27 [21]; DHA: docosahexaenoic acid; EPA: eicosapentaenoic acid; LCPUFA: long chain polyunsaturated fatty acid.
[2] Nutrient values are estimates and depend on species of fish, total fat content of fish, geographical location, method of raising/harvesting, and cooking. All values are for raw portions and, as such, are overestimates after cooking is considered [21].
[3] Number of servings (4 oz.) were calculated to meet 250 mg of omega-3 LCPUFA per day, as recommended for pregnant women by the Dietary Guidelines for Americans (2015–2020) [20].

These recommendations translate to approximately 250 mg omega-3 LCPUFAs per day and are in line with the recommendation of 200 mg DHA per day set forth by an international panel of experts in an earlier consensus statement [22].

The Food and Drug Administration and Environmental Protection Agency further specify that servings should be from a variety of fish that have low levels of methylmercury [23]. Nearly all fish contain trace amounts of methylmercury; however, larger fish with longer lifespans have greater accumulations of the neurotoxin [24]. As methylmercury crosses the placenta, it accumulates in the fetus at higher concentrations than those in the mother [25, 26]. Fetal exposure to excess amounts of methylmercury in utero, when the brain is especially vulnerable to environmental insults, can negatively affect brain and nervous system development [27]. Tilefish from the Gulf of Mexico, shark, swordfish, and king mackerel contain high levels of methylmercury [21, 23]; thus, pregnant women and women of childbearing ages are advised to avoid these fish [23].

During pregnancy, the fetus relies on maternal intake and placental transfer of nutrients to meet developmental demands. Although prenatal vitamins and other vitamins/supplements are marketed to pregnant women, they may not contain omega-3 LCPUFAs or women may not consume them at all or with any regularity [28]. Thus, low fish intake during pregnancy could result in low fetal accumulation of DHA and EPA.

Previous estimates of dietary omega-3 LCPUFA intake point to low consumption by pregnant women and women of childbearing ages. In a small sample ($n = 21$) of pregnant women in Baton Rouge, Louisiana, USA, data from our laboratory [28] indicate the average dietary intake of DHA is 72 mg per day, which translates to 95% of pregnant women not meeting the recommendation of 200 mg DHA per day [22]. When supplement intake was taken into consideration,

62% of pregnant women still failed to meet the recommended DHA intake. In an earlier study, we reported that nonpregnant women of childbearing ages (n = 183; average age: 20 years; age range: 18–28 years) consumed an average of 66 mg DHA per day, which included both dietary and supplemental sources of DHA [29].

Given the role of omega-3 LCPUFAs in infant development, pregnancy outcome, and maternal health, it is important to assess if pregnant women are adhering to the dietary recommendation to include seafood in their diets and, if not, what foods they are choosing to consume instead. Therefore, the aim of the study was to investigate the dietary habits of pregnant women in Baton Rouge, Louisiana, USA. Specifically, we evaluated their consumption of various dietary protein sources.

Geographically, Baton Rouge is located directly on the Mississippi River and approximately 157 miles north of the Gulf of Mexico. As Louisiana is a coastal state and fish are an intricate part of the regional culture and cuisine [30], we hypothesized that pregnant women in the Greater Baton Rouge area would meet the recommended seafood intake for pregnant women and women of childbearing ages.

2. Materials and Methods

2.1. Study Overview. For this observational study, we approached women at an event held for expecting women and their partners at a hospital in Baton Rouge, Louisiana. The free, single-day event was held in October 2015. Women were approached and invited to complete a survey about their dietary habits during pregnancy and respond to a demographic questionnaire; the survey and questionnaire were provided as separate documents. All pregnant women who visited the research booth at the event were invited to participate; the only inclusion criterion was current pregnancy and there was no selection bias. Our efforts resulted in 221 completed surveys and questionnaires; the responses from each were separated at the time of completion.

Compensation for study completion was entry into a raffle for free baby books and other materials for expecting families. Women provided their first name and telephone number on a separate piece of paper; this paper was not attached to the survey or questionnaire. When a name was drawn in the raffle, the woman was contacted by a call or text and returned to the booth to pick up her raffle prize. All contact information was destroyed at the conclusion of the convention.

The survey included a statement that completion of the survey constituted consent to participate and participation were voluntary. All procedures involving human subjects were approved by The Louisiana State University AgCenter and Woman's Hospital Institutional Review Boards.

Contact and demographic information were not attached to the survey and, as such, responses were anonymous. The women were allowed to complete their survey and the questionnaire and provide their contact information on an individual clipboard standing away from the table at which the researchers were stationed.

2.2. Survey and Demographic Questionnaire. The survey was designed to be completed by participants in approximately 5 minutes with minimal input or direction from the researchers. Women were instructed to complete the survey in accordance with their usual dietary habits during pregnancy. The survey has not been previously validated and was developed as a tool to provide preliminary, descriptive data that provides a direction and foundation upon which to build for future research.

The survey contained four sections ("protein sources"), labeled and ordered as follows: "Beef," "Chicken," "Fish," and "Pork." Each section included a list of foods commonly consumed for that respective protein source; these foods were subjectively chosen by the researchers.

"Beef" included, in order, "Steak," "Hamburger," "Stew meat," "Brisket," and "Roast." "Chicken" included, in order, "Wings," "Breast," and "Legs." "Fish" included, in order, "Canned tuna," "Tuna steak," "Tilapia," "Salmon," "Cod," "Catfish," "Swordfish," "Trout," "Bass," "Flounder," and "Herring." "Pork" included, in order, "Chop," "Tenderloin," and "Roast."

More specific information about the foods and food preparation was not sought. For example, "Steak" could include any cut of steak, "Salmon" could include any species of salmon, and "Wings" could include any preparation and/or cooking style of chicken wings.

Each question had six predefined responses to assess how frequently the women were consuming each: "Never," "Once/week," "2-2+/week," "Once/month," "2-3/month," and "4-4+/month." The majority of women checked only one box per food; however, if multiple or none of the boxes were checked, that data point was entered as missing.

As the primary focus of our study was fish consumption by pregnant women, we constructed our survey to include a variety of fish, including those that are poor and good sources of omega-3 LCPUFAs and those that are indigenous and nonnative to the area (canned tuna, tuna steak, tilapia, salmon, cod, catfish, swordfish, trout, bass, flounder, and herring).

The demographic questionnaire, included as a separate document, included questions about participant age, ethnicity, education level, and if she was a first-time mother. All documents were provided in print.

2.3. Interpretation of Results. Our survey did not indicate the size of a serving. Rather, we asked how often the women consumed each food and assumed portion sizes for each. In speculating whether pregnant women are meeting the omega-3 LCPUFA recommendations by dietary fish intake, we assumed each serving to be 4 oz.

This assumption was based on a table in the 2015–2020 Dietary Guidelines for Americans [20]. Nutritional aspects of common seafood varieties were provided for 4 oz. portions of each. Although the guidelines specify that pregnant women should "consume 8 to 12 oz. of seafood per week from a variety of sources", a serving size is not defined. However, The Food and Drug Administration and Environmental Protection

TABLE 2: Demographics of the survey population.

	% of women, $n = 221$
Age, years	
<20	3.2
20–25	29.0
26–30	37.3
31–35	23.0
36–40	6.9
No answer	0.5
Education	
Some high school	3.2
High school graduate	6.5
Some college	23.5
2-year degree	8.8
4-year degree	29.0
Graduate degree	28.6
No answer	0.5
Ethnicity	
African American	20.3
Caucasian	71.4
Hispanic	2.3
American Indian	0.5
Asian	4.6
Multiracial	0.5
No answer	0.5
First-time mom	
Yes	78.5
No	21.5
No answer	1.4

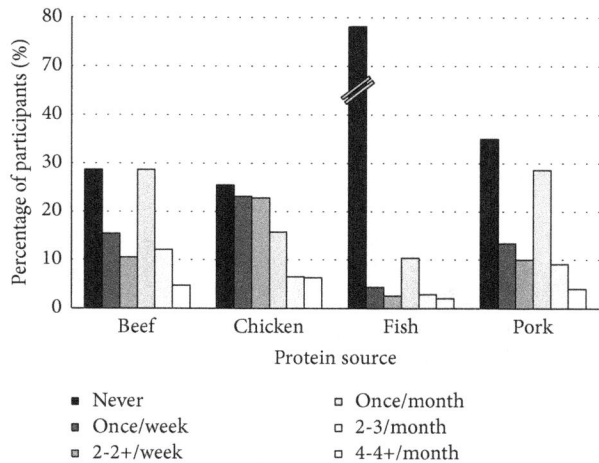

FIGURE 1: Consumption rate and frequency of protein sources by pregnant women.

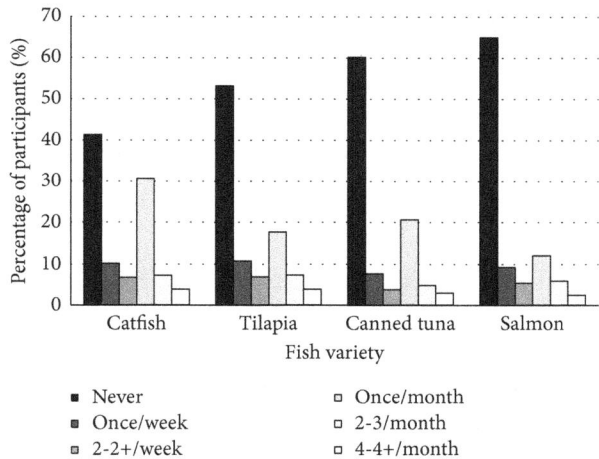

FIGURE 2: Consumption rate and frequency of the more consumed fish varieties by pregnant women.

Agency specify that the recommended 8–12 oz. translates to two to three servings of fish per week [23].

3. Results

3.1. Population Demographics. Demographic data ($n = 221$) for our survey population are provided in Table 2. The majority of the women in our population were Caucasian (71%), 26–30 years old (37%), and had completed some college (24%), a 4-year college degree (29%), or a graduate degree (29%). African American was the second most common ethnicity (20%) and 20–25 years of age was the second most common age range (29%). First-time mothers comprised the majority of our population (79%).

3.2. Response Rate. Of the women approached (estimated 250–275), 221 completed the survey. The average response rate for each food was 92%. Women responded to the frequency with which they ate stew meat least often (i.e., did not answer the question; 88% response rate) and chicken breast most often (96% response rate).

3.3. Consumption Habits of Pregnant Women: Fish. Twenty-two percent of women reported consuming fish, when consumption of all individual varieties was averaged (Figure 1). Catfish was consumed by a majority of the population, 59% of women. Tilapia, canned tuna, and salmon were consumed by 47, 40, and 35% of women, respectively. Swordfish, herring, and flounder were consumed by less than 3% of women.

The most common consumption frequency for catfish, tilapia, canned tuna, and salmon was once per month, followed by once per week. Consumption rate and frequency for each fish variety are presented in Figures 2 and 3.

3.4. Consumption Habits of Pregnant Women: Beef, Chicken, and Pork. Consumption rate for beef, chicken, and pork, when all foods were averaged within protein source, was 71, 74, and 65%, respectively. Hamburger, chicken breast, and pork chops were the most consumed foods for each protein source, with 90, 92, and 63% of women reporting that they

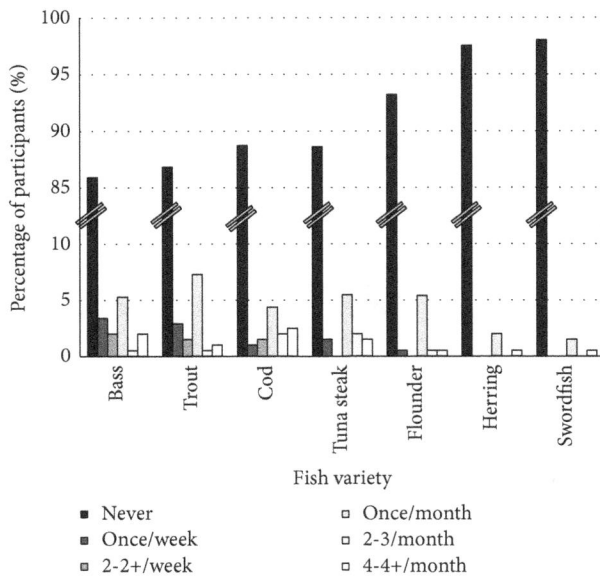

FIGURE 3: Consumption rate and frequency of the less consumed fish varieties by pregnant women.

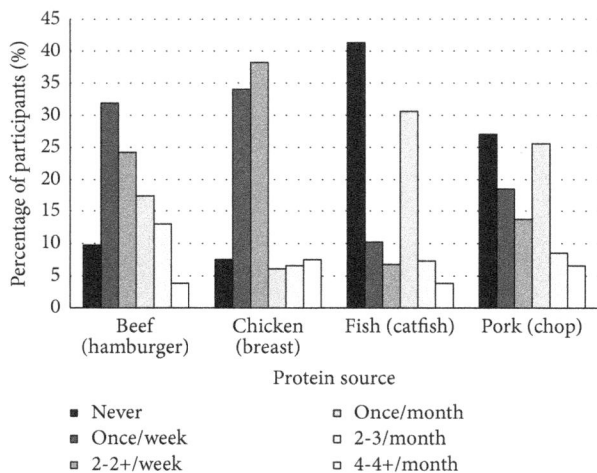

FIGURE 4: Consumption rate and frequency of the most consumed foods for each protein source by pregnant women.

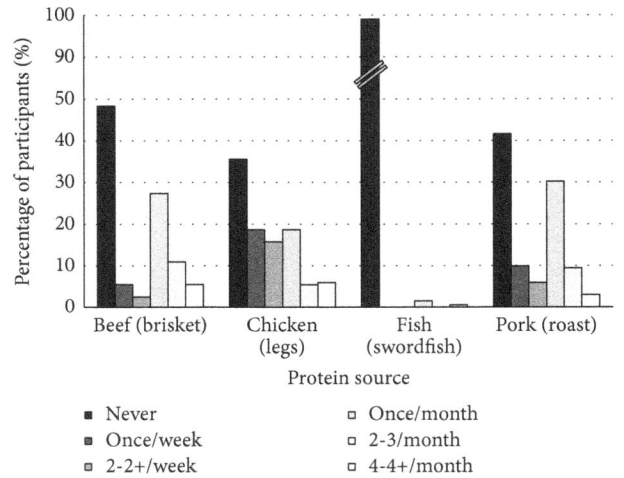

FIGURE 5: Consumption rate and frequency of the least consumed foods for each protein source by pregnant women.

4. Discussion

4.1. Achieving Dietary Omega-3 LCPUFA Recommendations for Pregnant Women. The two most commonly consumed fish varieties by our population (catfish and tilapia) have significantly lower concentrations of omega-3 LCPUFAs than the varieties which were rarely consumed (Table 1) [21]. Of particular interest is the finding that canned tuna, which is widely available, is inexpensive, has a long shelf life, and is amenable to easy preparation [31], was not consumed by more women or more frequently. Salmon, a similar variety to canned tuna in terms of preparation and favorable omega-3 LCPUFA content [21], was also consumed at a low frequency.

To meet the recommendation of an average intake of 250 mg omega-3 LCPUFA per day [20], one would have to consume 12 oz. of farmed catfish or 9.7 oz. of tilapia every day (Table 1) [21]. This equates to approximately 21 servings of farmed catfish or 17 servings of tilapia per week, assuming a 4 oz. serving size. As the women in our population reported consuming catfish, tilapia, and canned tuna (the three most consumed varieties) each at a frequency of once per month, they are likely to not be achieving recommended intakes of omega-3 LCPUFAs.

Dietary incorporation of canned white tuna and/or salmon at a frequency of twice per week would satisfy recommended levels of omega-3 LCPUFA intake, exclusive of intake of other varieties (Table 1) [21].

4.2. Intake of Fish Known to Have High Methylmercury Content. The Food and Drug Administration and Environmental Protection Agency advise pregnant women and women of childbearing ages to avoid consumption of tilefish from the Gulf of Mexico, shark, swordfish, and king mackerel due to their high methylmercury content [23]. In our population, three women (1.4%) reported consumption of swordfish at a frequency of once per month and one (0.5%) indicated she consumed swordfish at least four times per month. The other varieties were not included in our survey. These data may

consume each, respectively. Brisket, chicken legs, and pork roast were the least consumed foods for each protein source, with 52, 65, and 58% of women reporting that they consume each, respectively.

Women most commonly reported intake of the most consumed beef (hamburger) and chicken foods (chicken breast) at a frequency of once or at least twice per week. A consumption frequency of once per month was the most common response for the least popular beef, chicken, and pork foods (brisket, chicken legs, and pork roast, resp.). The most popular pork food (pork chops) was most often consumed at a frequency of once per month. Consumption rate and frequency of consumption for the most and least consumed foods, grouped by protein source, are presented in Figures 4 and 5, respectively.

point to a need to further emphasize the recommendation that pregnant women and women of childbearing ages should avoid fish known to contain high levels of methylmercury [23].

4.3. Comparison of Dietary Intake of Fish and Other Protein Sources. In the current study, consumption rate of beef, chicken, and pork was at least threefold higher than that of fish. The most consumed fish varieties were consumed at a frequency that was similar to or less than that of the least consumed beef, chicken, and pork foods. Clearly, when choosing a protein source, pregnant women are opting to consume beef, chicken, and/or pork in favor of fish.

4.4. Comparison with Previous Findings and International Differences in Dietary Seafood Habits. Our data is in line with that of a previous investigation [32] in which it was reported that 89% of pregnant women in Massachusetts, USA, consume less than 3 fish meals per month and the average canned tuna consumption is 2 servings per month. Similarly, pregnant women in Ontario, Canada [33], were reported to consume 0.7 fish meals per week, which equates to less than 3 fish meals per month. These findings are also similar to those for pregnant women in southwestern Quebec, Canada, where the women consumed 3.6 fish meals per month [34].

There is a stark difference in dietary seafood habits of pregnant women between the North American countries of the United States and Canada and that of other regions.

A large, observational study [35] found that 88% of pregnant women in the United Kingdom consumed at least 8 seafood meals per month. Pregnant Norwegian women, on average, consumed approximately 45 seafood meals per month [36] and 77% of pregnant women living on the Faroe Islands consumed at least 12 seafood meals per month [37].

A comparison of two studies assessing pregnant women in Denmark [38] and Netherlands [39] revealed that 22% of the Danish population consumed at least 560 g of fish per month (equivalent to 4.9 servings) versus 56% of the Dutch population. These results are in agreement with those in a different Danish population [40], where the average fish consumption for pregnant women was 3.9 meals per month. Pregnant Swedish women were reported to consume 6.7 fish/shellfish meals per month, with less than 1% of women reporting they never consumed fish at all [41].

In Spanish populations, 86% of pregnant women reported consuming at least 12 seafood meals per months [42] and 61% of pregnant women ate canned tuna at a minimal frequency of 4 times per month [43]. Findings from a Taiwanese study indicate 99% of pregnant women in Taipei consumed fish during pregnancy at an average rate of 11 meals per month [44].

Although those North American populations outlined above [32–34], along with the population in the current study, all live within 160 miles of the coast or a major body of water, it is apparent that pregnant women in these locations eat less seafood than their European and East Asian counterparts. The international difference in fish and seafood consumption

is likely fueled by the typical Western diet that is characteristic of North America, as supported by our current observation that pregnant women in Baton Rouge, Louisiana, USA, have a strong preference for hamburger or chicken breast.

Given the wide availability of seafood in coastal regions [45], one may expect pregnant women living in inland locations in North America to have even lower seafood intakes than those reported in the current and previous studies. It is important to note, as well, that our population is well educated, with 90% having completed some college. Thus, even pregnant women who are educated are not consuming recommended amounts of fish.

The international disparity in seafood intake reflects the findings of a 2010 study, which qualitatively determined knowledge and behavior of pregnant women ($n = 22$) in Northeastern USA with regard to fish consumption [46]. The researchers found that while a fair amount of pregnant women (46%) was aware that fish contained a potential toxic contaminant (methylmercury), less knew that fish contained DHA (36%) or a function of DHA during pregnancy (23%). Furthermore, none of the women (0%) had been advised to consume fish during pregnancy.

Two studies [32, 34] from 2003 and 2004 found that women from Northeastern USA and Canada more often maintained or reduced fish intake after becoming pregnant rather than increasing it. The decreased consumption after becoming pregnant was calculated to be 1.4 servings per month [34]. The authors speculated that this effect was a result of national mercury advisories in the early 2000s which recommended pregnant women limit consumption of certain fish [32]. These findings contrast those of the aforementioned study in Taiwan [44], conducted in 2006, where the percentage of women who consumed fish increased from 95 to 99% upon becoming pregnant. Thus, our data may suggest that, in 2015, pregnant women in North America may remain uncomfortable incorporating fish as a dietary protein source and opt for chicken, beef, or pork foods instead.

It is important to note that, for each study outlined above, dietary data were collected from and reported in a variety of ways. For comparison with our results, we converted the data to servings per month by assuming a serving was 4 oz., if the data were reported as g consumed per unit of time. We note that dietary data were collected by various methods (food frequency questionnaires, 24-hour dietary recalls) but assumed each method to be equal. These data manipulations could affect the precision of our comparisons.

4.5. Future Research Direction. Future studies should assess whether pregnant women and women of childbearing ages have knowledge of the dietary recommendations for seafood consumption. These efforts should aim to elucidate if (1) there are specific groups of pregnant women who are less likely to meet dietary fish recommendations and (2) why these women fail to meet those recommendations.

Replication of the current survey across different geographic areas would also provide insight into the effect of coastal versus inland location on fish intake and dietary protein preferences.

4.6. Study Limitations. Our survey was conducted in a convenience sample and since the survey and demographic questionnaires were not connected, we are unable to examine potential group differences or correlations between demographic parameters and responses.

We assumed values for portion sizes. Although this assumption does not affect our observations of dietary habits, it does affect the precision of our calculations in regard to whether pregnant women are meeting omega-3 LCPUFA recommendations or not. Furthermore, we did not consider how foods were prepared. Certain cooking styles are related to differences in the fatty acid content of the resulting product [21]. This, too, affects calculations of omega-3 LCPUFA intake.

The characteristics of our study population differ from those published by the United States Census Bureau [47] for Baton Rouge, Louisiana. The population of Baton Rouge are African Americans (55%) or Caucasians (39%) who have completed high school (26%) or some college (23%). The overall population of Louisiana is more similar to that of our study population; 63% Caucasian or 32% African Americans who have completed high school (26%), some college (23%), or a 4-year college degree (19%).

It is important to note that educational attainment data from the United States Census Bureau data reflects that of the population aged 25 years and older, without specificity to gender. Approximately 32% of our population was aged 25 years or less. Additionally, the ethnic breakdowns provided by the United States Census Bureau data reflect that of the entire population in that region without regard to age, gender, or pregnancy status. These discrepancies make it difficult to draw conclusions on the generalizability of our data.

5. Conclusion

These data reveal that pregnant women in Baton Rouge, Louisiana, USA, are not meeting dietary recommendations for seafood consumption and, therefore, likely do not consume adequate amounts of omega-3 LCPUFAs for optimal maternal health, fetal development, and infant outcome. These data also reveal the protein sources and specific foods that pregnant women are consuming in lieu of fish.

The apparent deficit in omega-3 LCPUFA intake has major implications during and after pregnancy and should be addressed with intensified efforts to provide nutrition and lifestyle education to pregnant women and women of childbearing ages.

Although our data indicate pregnant women, in general, do not meet dietary seafood recommendations, future research will help us better understand the habits of pregnant women, directing us in our development of targeted education efforts which emphasize the importance of consumption of fish low in methylmercury during pregnancy.

Competing Interests

There are no competing interests regarding the publication of this paper.

Acknowledgments

The authors would like to acknowledge Woman's Hospital for allowing them to conduct their survey and the women who participated. Funding was received from Louisiana State University and Louisiana State University Agricultural Center to support the graduate students collecting data and preparing the paper.

References

[1] M. Neuringer, G. J. Anderson, and W. E. Connor, "The essentiality of n-3 fatty acids for the development and function of the retina and brain," *Annual Review of Nutrition*, vol. 8, pp. 517–541, 1988.

[2] B. Koletzko, C. Agostoni, S. E. Carlson et al., "Long chain polyunsaturated fatty acids (LC-PUFA) and perinatal development," *Acta Paediatrica*, vol. 90, no. 4, pp. 460–464, 2001.

[3] I. B. Helland, L. Smith, K. Saarem, O. D. Saugstad, and C. A. Drevon, "Maternal supplementation with very-long-chain n-3 fatty acids during pregnancy and lactation augments children's IQ at 4 years of age," *Pediatrics*, vol. 111, no. 1, pp. e39–e44, 2003.

[4] M. P. Judge, O. Harel, and C. J. Lammi-Keefe, "Maternal consumption of a docosahexaenoic acid-containing functional food during pregnancy: benefit for infant performance on problem-solving but not on recognition memory tasks at age 9 mo," *The American Journal of Clinical Nutrition*, vol. 85, no. 6, pp. 1572–1577, 2007.

[5] J. A. Dunstan, K. Simmer, G. Dixon, and S. L. Prescott, "Cognitive assessment of children at age 2.5 years after maternal fish oil supplementation in pregnancy: a randomised controlled trial," *Archives of Disease in Childhood: Fetal and Neonatal Edition*, vol. 93, no. 1, pp. F45–F50, 2008.

[6] M. P. Judge, O. Harel, and C. J. Lammi-Keefe, "A docosahexaenoic acid-functional food during pregnancy benefits infant visual acuity at four but not six months of age," *Lipids*, vol. 42, no. 2, pp. 117–122, 2007.

[7] S. M. Innis and R. W. Friesen, "Essential omega-3 fatty acids in pregnant women and early visual acuity maturation in term infants," *American Journal of Clinical Nutrition*, vol. 87, pp. 548–557, 2008.

[8] K. M. Gustafson, J. Colombo, and S. E. Carlson, "Docosahexaenoic acid and cognitive function: is the link mediated by the autonomic nervous system?" *Prostaglandins Leukotrienes and Essential Fatty Acids*, vol. 79, no. 3–5, pp. 135–140, 2008.

[9] R. L. Bergmann, K. E. Bergmann, E. Haschke-Becher et al., "Does maternal docosahexaenoic acid supplementation during pregnancy and lactation lower BMI in late infancy?" *Journal of Perinatal Medicine*, vol. 35, no. 4, pp. 295–300, 2007.

[10] A. B. Courville, O. Harel, and C. J. Lammi-Keefe, "Consumption of a DHA-containing functional food during pregnancy is associated with lower infant ponderal index and cord plasma insulin concentration," *British Journal of Nutrition*, vol. 106, no. 2, pp. 208–212, 2011.

[11] A. M. Llorente, C. L. Jensen, R. G. Voigt, J. K. Fraley, M. C. Berretta, and W. C. Heird, "Effect of maternal docosahexaenoic acid supplementation on postpartum depression and information processing," *American Journal of Obstetrics & Gynecology*, vol. 188, no. 5, pp. 1348–1353, 2003.

[12] M. P. Freeman, M. Davis, P. Sinha, K. L. Wisner, J. R. Hibbeln, and A. J. Gelenberg, "Omega-3 fatty acids and supportive psychotherapy for perinatal depression: A Randomized Placebo-Controlled Study," *Journal of Affective Disorders*, vol. 110, no. 1-2, pp. 142–148, 2008.

[13] K.-P. Su, S.-Y. Huang, T.-H. Chiu et al., "Omega-3 fatty acids for major depressive disorder during pregnancy: results from a randomized, double-blind, placebo-controlled trial," *Journal of Clinical Psychiatry*, vol. 69, no. 4, pp. 644–651, 2008.

[14] B. Doornbos, S. A. van Goor, D. A. J. Dijck-Brouwer, A. Schaafsma, J. Korf, and F. A. J. Muskiet, "Supplementation of a low dose of DHA or DHA + AA does not prevent peripartum depressive symptoms in a small population based sample," *Progress in Neuro-Psychopharmacology and Biological Psychiatry*, vol. 33, no. 1, pp. 49–52, 2009.

[15] J. A. Golding, C. A. Steer, P. A. Emmett, J. M. B. Davis, and J. R. C. Hibbeln, "High levels of depressive symptoms in pregnancy with low omega-3 fatty acid intake from fish," *Epidemiology*, vol. 20, no. 4, pp. 598–603, 2009.

[16] A.-M. Rees, M.-P. Austin, and G. B. Parker, "Omega-3 fatty acids as a treatment for perinatal depression: randomized double-blind placebo-controlled trial," *Australian & New Zealand Journal of Psychiatry*, vol. 42, no. 3, pp. 199–205, 2008.

[17] H. Szajewska, A. Horvath, and B. Koletzko, "Effect of omega-3 long-chain polyunsaturated fatty acid supplementation of women with low-risk pregnancies on pregnancy outcomes and growth measures at birth: a meta-analysis of randomized controlled trials," *American Journal of Clinical Nutrition*, vol. 83, no. 6, pp. 1337–1344, 2006.

[18] A. Horvath, B. Koletzko, and H. Szajewska, "Effect of supplementation of women in high-risk pregnancies with long-chain polyunsaturated fatty acids on pregnancy outcomes and growth measures at birth: a meta-analysis of randomized controlled trials," *British Journal of Nutrition*, vol. 98, no. 2, pp. 253–259, 2007.

[19] J. M. Coletta, S. J. Bell, and A. S. Roman, "Omega-3 fatty acids and pregnancy," *Reviews in Obstetrics and Gynecology*, vol. 3, pp. 163–171, 2010.

[20] US Department of Agriculture and US Department of Health and Human Services, *2015–2020 Dietary Guidelines for Americans*, 8th edition, 2015, http://health.gov/dietaryguidelines/2015/guidelines/.

[21] U.S. Department of Agriculture, Agricultural Research Service, and Nutrient Data Laboratory, *USDA National Nutrient Database for Standard Reference*, 2010, http://www.ars.usda.gov/ba/bhnrc/ndl.

[22] B. Koletzko, E. Lien, C. Agostoni et al., "The roles of long-chain polyunsaturated fatty acids in pregnancy, lactation and infancy: review of current knowledge and consensus recommendations," *Journal of Perinatal Medicine*, vol. 36, no. 1, pp. 5–14, 2008.

[23] Environmental Protection Agency—Food and Drug Administration, "Fish: what pregnant women and parents should know," 2015, http://www.fda.gov/Food/FoodborneIllnessContaminants/Metals/ucm393070.htm.

[24] T. W. Clarkson, "Mercury: major issues in environmental health," *Environmental Health Perspectives*, vol. 100, pp. 31–38, 1993.

[25] B. H. Choi, L. W. Lapham, L. Amin-Zaki, and T. Saleem, "Abnormal neuronal migration, deranged cerebral cortical organization, and diffuse white matter astrocytosis of human fetal brain: a major effect of methylmercury poisoning in utero," *Journal of Neuropathology & Experimental Neurology*, vol. 37, no. 6, pp. 719–733, 1978.

[26] T. W. Clarkson, "The toxicology of mercury," *Critical Reviews in Clinical Laboratory Sciences*, vol. 34, no. 4, pp. 369–403, 1997.

[27] B. J. Koos and L. D. Longo, "Mercury toxicity in the pregnant woman, fetus, and newborn infant. A review," *American Journal of Obstetrics and Gynecology*, vol. 126, no. 3, pp. 390–409, 1976.

[28] A. Gaitán, M. Drewery, R. Pinkston et al., *Docosahexaenoic Acid Status in Pregnancy Is Lower in African-Americans Compared to Caucasians and Hispanics: Difference in Fatty Acid Metabolism*, American Oil Chemists' Society, Salt Lake City, Utah, USA, 2016.

[29] A. V. Gaitán, C. L. Childress, C. A. Thaxton et al., *Risk Factors for Age-Related Macular Degeneration (AMD) Appear Early in Life Among Female College-Aged Students*, American Oil Chemists' Society, Orlando, Fla, USA, 2015.

[30] J. H. Diaz, "Is fish consumption safe?" *The Journal of the Louisiana State Medical Society*, vol. 156, no. 1, pp. 42–49, 2004.

[31] A. D. Liese, K. E. Weis, D. Pluto, E. Smith, and A. Lawson, "Food store types, availability, and cost of foods in a rural environment," *Journal of the American Dietetic Association*, vol. 107, no. 11, pp. 1916–1923, 2007.

[32] E. Oken, K. P. Kleinman, W. E. Berland, S. R. Simon, J. W. Rich-Edwards, and M. W. Gillman, "Decline in fish consumption among pregnant women after a national mercury advisory," *Obstetrics and Gynecology*, vol. 102, no. 2, pp. 346–351, 2003.

[33] J. Denomme, K. D. Stark, and B. J. Holub, "Directly quantitated dietary (n-3) fatty acid intakes of pregnant canadian women are lower than current dietary recommendations," *The Journal of Nutrition*, vol. 135, no. 2, pp. 206–211, 2005.

[34] J. Morrissette, L. Takser, G. St-Amour, A. Smargiassi, J. Lafond, and D. Mergler, "Temporal variation of blood and hair mercury levels in pregnancy in relation to fish consumption history in a population living along the St. Lawrence River," *Environmental Research*, vol. 95, no. 3, pp. 363–374, 2004.

[35] J. R. Hibbeln, J. M. Davis, C. Steer et al., "Maternal seafood consumption in pregnancy and neurodevelopmental outcomes in childhood (ALSPAC study): An Observational Cohort Study," *The Lancet*, vol. 369, no. 9561, pp. 578–585, 2007.

[36] A. L. Brantsæter, M. Haugen, Y. Thomassen et al., "Exploration of biomarkers for total fish intake in pregnant Norwegian women," *Public Health Nutrition*, vol. 13, no. 1, pp. 54–62, 2010.

[37] S. F. Olsen, P. Grandjean, P. Weihe, and T. Videro, "Frequency of seafood intake in pregnancy as a determinant of birth weight: evidence for a dose dependent relationship," *Journal of Epidemiology and Community Health*, vol. 47, no. 6, pp. 436–440, 1993.

[38] T. I. Halldorsson, H. M. Meltzer, I. Thorsdottir, V. Knudsen, and S. F. Olsen, "Is high consumption of fatty fish during pregnancy a risk factor for fetal growth retardation? A study of 44,824 Danish pregnant women," *American Journal of Epidemiology*, vol. 166, no. 6, pp. 687–696, 2007.

[39] D. H. M. Heppe, E. A. P. Steegers, S. Timmermans et al., "Maternal fish consumption, fetal growth and the risks of neonatal complications: the Generation R Study," *British Journal of Nutrition*, vol. 105, no. 6, pp. 938–949, 2011.

[40] S. F. Olsen and N. J. Secher, "Low consumption of seafood in early pregnancy as a risk factor for preterm delivery: Prospective Cohort Study," *British Medical Journal*, vol. 324, no. 7335, pp. 447–450, 2002.

[41] K. A. Björnberg, M. Vahter, K. Petersson-Grawé et al., "Methyl mercury and inorganic mercury in Swedish pregnant women and in cord blood: influence of fish consumption," *Environmental Health Perspectives*, vol. 111, no. 4, pp. 637–641, 2003.

[42] M. A. Mendez, E. Plana, M. Guxens et al., "Seafood consumption in pregnancy and infant size at birth: results from a prospective Spanish cohort," *Journal of Epidemiology and Community Health*, vol. 64, no. 3, pp. 216–222, 2010.

[43] R. Ramón, F. Ballester, X. Aguinagalde et al., "Fish consumption during pregnancy, prenatal mercury exposure, and anthropometric measures at birth in a prospective mother-infant cohort study in Spain," *American Journal of Clinical Nutrition*, vol. 90, no. 4, pp. 1047–1055, 2009.

[44] C.-S. Hsu, P.-L. Liu, L.-C. Chien, S.-Y. Chou, and B.-C. Han, "Mercury concentration and fish consumption in Taiwanese pregnant women," *BJOG: An International Journal of Obstetrics and Gynaecology*, vol. 114, no. 1, pp. 81–85, 2007.

[45] R. E. Martin, G. J. Flick, and L. A. Granata, "A history of the seafood industry," in *The Seafood Industry: Species, Products, Processing, and Safety*, pp. 1–16, 1990.

[46] A. Bloomingdale, L. B. Guthrie, S. Price et al., "A qualitative study of fish consumption during pregnancy," *The American Journal of Clinical Nutrition*, vol. 92, no. 5, pp. 1234–1240, 2010.

[47] United States Census Bureau, "American Community Survey," 2010–2014, https://www.census.gov/programs-surveys/acs/.

3

Paradox of Modern Pregnancy: A Phenomenological Study of Women's Lived Experiences from Assisted Pregnancy

Fahimeh Ranjbar,[1] **Mohammad-Mehdi Akhondi,**[2] **Leili Borimnejad,**[3] **Saeed-Reza Ghaffari,**[2] **and Zahra Behboodi-Moghadam**[1]

[1]School of Nursing & Midwifery, Tehran University of Medical Sciences, Tehran 1419733171, Iran
[2]Reproductive Biotechnology Research Center, Avicenna Research Institute, ACECR, Tehran 196151177, Iran
[3]School of Nursing and Midwifery, Iran University of Medical Sciences, Tehran 1996713883, Iran

Correspondence should be addressed to Zahra Behboodi-Moghadam; behboodi@tums.ac.ir

Academic Editor: Fabio Facchinetti

The purpose of our study was describing the meaning of pregnancy through Assisted Reproductive Technologies (ARTs). A qualitative design with hermeneutic phenomenology approach was selected to carry out the research. Semistructured in-depth interviews were conducted with 12 women who experienced assisted pregnancy. Three themes emerged from women's experience including finding peace in life, paradoxical feelings, and struggling to realize a dream. We concluded that pregnancy is the beginning of a new and hard struggle for women with fertility problems. The findings of our study resulted in helpful implications for the health care professionals managing assisted pregnancies.

1. Introduction

Infertility treatment has quite many physiological and psychological effects on people and getting pregnant does not necessarily mean an end to these problems [1]. Treatment via Assisted Reproductive Technologies (ARTs) is quite an emotionally and physically difficult process [2]. The specific stressors associated with this treatment are beyond the positive pregnancy test [3]. Couples who become pregnant after ARTs cannot easily overcome the negative feelings related to infertility and are different in a number of personality dimensions and affective reactions toward pregnant women having become pregnant naturally [4, 5]. In pregnancies resulting from ARTs, women sometimes experience new stresses, uncertainty or fear about pregnancy [6]. Signs of increased anxiety are found more in mothers and spouses who have experienced high infertility stress. Those couples who become pregnant through ARTs are more anxious in the early stages of pregnancy than those who conceive naturally. These couples are more fretful about pregnancy loss [7]. With each failure and even success a feeling of not

becoming a mother will bother them again [2]. Although these techniques are known as medical technology, sociocultural norms are considered a very important factor in its acceptance. Sociocultural norms may act as a barrier or even cause later problems [8]. Understanding the context and complexity of such pregnancy is so important for the health care professionals working with these women [9]. As more families are seeking pregnancy using assisted reproductive techniques, more research is needed to explore the concept of assisted pregnancy [10]. ARTs have become increasingly popular in Iran because of high prevalence of infertility. More than 20% of Iranian couples experience infertility during their reproductive life. Currently, more than 75 clinics provide ARTs in all types [8, 11, 12]. Despite the fact that a considerable body of literature has focused on infertility in qualitative researches in Iran [13–17], less is known about the sociocultural problems and the need of Iranian women who have experienced assisted pregnancy. The purpose of our study was to explore how women make sense of assisted pregnancy in Iranian culture and context.

2. Method and Material

Qualitative research has been deemed as a valuable tool for collecting and analyzing data in complex health and social issues [18]. Hermeneutic phenomenological method as described by van Manen was employed for our study. This approach is the combination of descriptive and interpretive phenomenology [19].

2.1. Participants. The participants were Iranian infertile women who experienced pregnancy through ARTs. Using purposive sampling, 12 married women were recruited in the study. The inclusion criteria were the first and single pregnancy via ARTs, history of primary and female-related infertility, and the ability to speak Persian fluently. Exclusion criteria were history of miscarriage, assisted pregnancy through donated gametes, severe complication during pregnancy, and fetal abnormalities. Participants with female etiology of infertility including polycystic ovarian syndrome, blocked tubes, fibroids, decreased ovarian reserve, and immunological factors participated in our study.

2.2. Data Collection. The study was conducted in Avicenna Infertility Clinic in Tehran, Iran. The setting was a semipublic and nonacademic referral center affiliated to the Academic Center for Education, Culture and Research (ACECR). The first inclusion criterion was based on the patients' medical records. The convenient time for the interview was suggested by participants. All interviews were conducted by the first author in a private room in the clinic.

Most of the participants were from cities other than Tehran and all interviews were conducted in the infertility center. Data redundancy was recognized after interview with 10 participants, but two other participants were interviewed for assurance. Finally, 12 women were recruited in the study.

Semistructured interviews were performed in 17 sessions and during a six-month process from August 2013 to February 2014. Data were collected by in-depth interviews with approximate duration of 30 to 60 minutes. Participants were asked to talk about their experience with assisted pregnancy after infertility. Interviews began with questions about their initial feelings and perception toward pregnancy. The interviewer summarized participants' speaking at the end of sessions for data confirmation. Participants were encouraged to provide new information. Participants were free to ask questions or leave the rest of interview at any time. We wrote field notes after each interview and all interviews were recorded and transcribed verbatim immediately and then converted to Rich Text Format for MAXQDA 10 software (VERBI GmbH, Marburg, Germany) to facilitate data management.

2.3. Data Analysis. Data were analyzed using van Manen interpretative phenomenological strategies. According to van Manen, the selective and detailed or line-by-line approach was used to isolate thematic statements. van Manen has suggested the following 6 inseparable steps for researchers which are used in our study:

(1) Focusing on the phenomenon that deeply interests us and makes our minds engaged: in this regard, the researcher's mind was constantly engaged with this question: what is the meaning of assisted pregnancy after infertility?

(2) Exploring the phenomenon as something alive rather than what we conceptualize: to make the researcher interact with the main experience, women who actually had experience with this phenomenon were invited to our research.

(3) Reflecting on the themes that reveal inherent characteristics of the phenomenon: researchers must constantly ask themselves what the nature of experience with assisted pregnancy after infertility is. In answering this question, inherent themes will be understood.

(4) Describing the phenomenon with the art of writing and rewriting: phenomenological analysis is primarily an exercise in writing and thereby the researchers can achieve the meaning of experience through the practice. The researcher should try to reflect experience in such a way that the reader feels that he/she has experienced the phenomenon under study and is able to have the same result about its meaning.

(5) Establishing and maintaining a conscious connection with the phenomenon: the researcher should be preoccupied with the lived experience of pregnant women via ARTs. Creating a strong connection between the text and the phenomenon and using rich and in-depth descriptions of the findings reduce the likelihood of deviation from the main path.

(6) Balancing the research context by considering the parts and the whole: in the last step, both the whole and contextual data are considered and the relationship of each part in the formation of phenomenon is examined [20].

2.4. Trustworthiness. Lincoln and Guba explained that credibility, confirmability, dependability, and transferability ensure the rigor in qualitative research. In order to achieve credibility in our research, maximum variation sampling, immersion and long engagement of researcher in the field, persistent observation, data triangulation, peer-checking, and member-checking were done. Experience of the authors in the field of infertility, ARTs, prenatal care, and qualitative research methods enhanced the confirmability. The data analysis process has been approved by all members of the team. All interviews were recorded and transcribed immediately by the first author to ensure dependability. The first author wrote her preunderstanding regarding pregnancy through ARTs prior to study and made efforts to bracket them in data analysis process. So as to meet transferability, the context of information collection is fully described.

TABLE 1: Demographic characteristics of subjects.

Participant	Age	Level of education	Gestational age (week)	Marriage duration	Infertility duration (year)	The cause of infertility	History of treatment failure (N)	Ethnicity
1	33	M.S.	4, 8	5	5	Hypothalamic amenorrhea	—	Kurd
2	24	B.S.	5	3	1	PCO	IO (1)	Fars
3	30	HS	4	3	1	DOR	Io (3)	Fars
4	28	HS	20, 29	13	10	Tubal factor	IUI (1)	Fars
5	36	HS	13, 19, 28	15	14	Tubal factor	Io (3)	Fars
6	28	HS	20	9	5	PCO	ICSI (1)	Fars
7	30	B.S.	20	14	11	PCO, tubal factor	ICSI (3)	Kurd
8	26	B.S. student	16, 20	6	5	Fibroma	IUI (5)	Fars
9	32	HS	9	13	12	Immunological	IUI (5) ICSI (1)	Turk
10	25	HS	4	7	6	Immunological	ICSI (5)	Turk
11	28	9th grade	12	12	11	Fibroma and adhesion in uterus	IUI (1) ICSI (1)	Lor
12	31	M.A. student	28	7	3.5	DOR	IUI (3)	Turk

HS: high school, B.S.: Bachelor of Science, M.A.: Master of Art, and M.S.: Master of Science.
IO: induction ovulation, IUI: intrauterine insemination, and ICSI: intracytoplasmic sperm injection.

2.5. Ethical Consideration. Ethics Committee of the Tehran University of Medical Sciences and the Avicenna Research Institute approved the research proposal. Participants were assured about confidentiality of their responses. The purpose of the study was explained verbally and written consent was obtained from all participants. The participants were ensured that audio files and their transcriptions were stored anonymously and separated from consent forms.

3. Results

The mean age of participants was 29.2 years at the time of interview. Only two participants were employees. The treatment method resulting in pregnancy was ICSI for all participants. Women's characteristics are summarized in Table 1.

3.1. Emergent Themes. After data analysis using MAXQDA software and reviewing over 700 meaning units, three themes were generated: finding peace in life, paradoxical feelings, and struggling to realize a dream (Table 2).

3.2. Finding Peace in Life. Women became relieved by this new experience. They ultimately got pregnant after struggling with infertility and their stress level declined. The fear that they would never become pregnant anymore was alleviated. Subthemes within this theme were feeling of becoming a mother, security and power, self-confidence, and finding meaning in life.

Participants showed more affection to the fetus. They described the feeling of becoming a mother as a new and the best feeling in the world. Some women had the affection even before embryo transfer and had a good feeling after seeing the embryos on the screen. Women had a sense of responsibility toward their fetus especially after the first trimester of pregnancy. They talked, read, and sang to their baby and were very excited when their babies kicked. One of the participants described the sense of being a mother as below: "Something is growing in your body; you are the person giving life, sense and peace to that. It is just a flower to which you are giving water and light. You give everything to that and if you take care and give it everything, you will have a very beautiful, healthy, and fragrant flower."

Sense of power and security was the greatest achievement of pregnancy for these women. This sense was connected with satisfying the husband, improving marital satisfaction, and keeping marriage alive. They did not want infertility to ruin their marriage and they frequently burst into tears when describing the strong feelings of their spouse about children. Some narratives, such as "My husband was jealous of others' babies... I thought that his attention toward children would become more and more... He played with babies and kissed them... He did not say anything to me about infertility, but I knew that he loves children a lot," were common in all the interviews. One of the participants declared her happiness because of satisfying her husband: "My husband was so upset that we would never have a child, and I was sad because of him (bursting into tears). I am glad he achieved his wish." Another participant said: "My husband is more motivated to live with me and my new baby now. I was sure that he was not happy before and maybe he thought we would be separated finally." Marital satisfaction had also increased with the change in husband's behavior and his support during pregnancy. They said that their relation would become better and pregnancy or the presence of a child can bring them closer at times. One participant stated the following: "From the time I got

TABLE 2: Themes arising from women's perceptions of assisted pregnancy.

Theme	Category	Subcategory
Finding peace in life	Power and security	Satisfying husband
		Marital satisfaction
		Keeping the marriage alive
	Finding self-confidence	Feeling lack of something
		Being the center of attention
		Getting rid of the stigma of infertility
	Finding meaning in life	Escape from isolation and loneliness
		Getting rid of monotonous life
		Finding hope
	Feeling of being a mother	Bonding to the fetus
		Sense of responsibility toward the fetus
Paradoxical feelings	Joy and fear	Surprise
		Joy and Fear
	Hope and uncertainty	Uncertainty of being pregnant
		Doubt about the baby's health and safety
		Uncertainty to continue pregnancy to the end of the third trimester
		Uncertainty in bonding with unborn baby
Struggle to realize a dream	Enduring all challenges	Difficult physical, emotional, and financial treatment
		Stigma
		Seeking help out of desperation
	Change in the life style	Low physical activity
		Adaptive behaviors in pregnancy
	Spirituality	Thanks giving to God
		Caring for other people
		Trusting in God

pregnant it seems that there is a sense of happiness in him. He takes care of me more now. He asks me whether the baby moves in my belly. How do you feel now? Does anything bother you?"

The extra attention that the society draws to pregnant women results in a feeling of self-confidence and self-worth. They got rid of the stigma of infertility and nothing was missed in their life anymore. One participant declared her self-confidence with these sentences: "I feel more confident in my life now; it was a nice experience for me. While I was walking in the streets I thought all the people were looking at me." One woman stated how pregnancy was a means of escaping from infertility stigma: "In every party or religious ceremony people came to me and said we bring this for you because of your pregnancy. The feeling and opinion of people toward me has changed now." Another informant said: "Maybe it is not the case, but before pregnancy I thought something has been missed in my life." One woman mentioned: "I think everything is peaceful now. I have the authority to make decisions and to have the last say. All the attentions are on my child and me."

Women remarked finding meaning in life. They found hope in life and it was time to say goodbye to isolation, loneliness, and monotonous life. For example, one of the women discussed: "We are more hopeful. We look at life in another

way. Our life became really monotonous. Now it is more exciting."

3.3. Paradoxical Feelings. Participants have experienced mood swings and irritability during pregnancy. The joy, fear, hope, and uncertainty are some paradoxical feelings. Women were excited and scared after the shock and disbelief. One woman described the paradox of joy and fear as follows: "They said ok madam you are pregnant. At that time I had a feeling that I could neither cry nor laugh. I did not know what to do. You know? I was a little bit surprised...It was positive...I was so happy because of the positive pregnancy test, but suddenly I said to myself what if I have an ectopic pregnancy." Another woman stated the paradoxical feeling as follows: "It is obvious that it is a stressful situation. It is really difficult. Will this pregnancy last? I am really worried whether something happens until the day of childbirth... There are a lot of beautiful fantasies like embracing my child and of course there are some stresses."

Despite the fear and joy, the women's stories revealed that they also experienced hope and uncertainty. There was a great deal of uncertainty, especially about losing the pregnancy. They seemed to be caught between fertile and infertile worlds. Some issues, such as hCG level and its titration, ectopic pregnancy, hearing the baby's heartbeat, miscarriage, birth defects, feeling the baby's kicks, and premature labor, were almost paralyzed at times. One woman stated: "The paradox is that sometimes you say to yourself ok, I have passed all the steps, I did what the doctors recommended and there is no need to be upset and worried, but you think to yourself that the other woman also did all these steps and it was her sixth time. Will this pregnancy last? What if I also become like that woman." Sometimes women were not convinced that they were pregnant even after a positive pregnancy test. They described it was so difficult to believe a positive pregnancy test after experiencing infertility. For instance, one of the participants said: "I did not believe that. I thought to myself if it is possible for me to have an embryo. I said they have made a mistake and I am not pregnant or I said the embryo does not have heartbeat." They had doubts about being pregnant and they did not speak with certainty about their pregnancy. Many times the fear of miscarriage changed their decision to reveal pregnancy to others. One participant said: "I have some friends and during these 2 or 3 weeks they came to our house, but I did not say anything to them since I was not sure about my pregnancy. I intended to wait at least for two months...Nothing is clear right now. The doctor could not see any special thing via ultrasound." Women were concerned about miscarriage and some of them reported that they had checked for bleeding or spotting every time they went to the bathroom. For example, one participant said: "The first three months passed with difficulty and since we expected some bad experiences, we got worried soon. I always checked my underwear in bathroom to see if there is any problem. Two weeks ago it seemed that I had some brownish spots. It was the time when I just sat and started crying loudly."

Sometimes uncertainty did not allow some women to start to feel attachment to their fetus. The majority of women confessed that they had postponed shopping for baby clothes and supplies until the third trimester. One participant remarked: "Now I am in doubt whether I should bond with her. What if something happens to that or a problem occurs? I am a little bit stressed out." Some found it hard to believe that they might actually end up with hugging a baby. One woman said: "I cannot bond with my unborn child, I am afraid I could not carry it into the third trimester. They had to bear the brunt of the impact." Contrary to the sex of the fetus, the well-being of the baby is a usual concern and priority. At times, women were eased only by an ultrasound showing a healthy baby. One participant said: "I repeat this sentence to myself what if the doctor says there is a problem. It was killing. Until the day of ultrasound, my heart will stop beating since I am really stressed out."

3.4. Struggle to Realize a Dream. The lived experience of the women who became pregnant through ARTs is a process of struggling to realize a dream which includes going through all difficulties, change in life style, and spirituality. The participants started a deliberate attempt to become a mother. They endured all the challenges of ARTs including the multiple, long, and difficult cycles of treatment, its high costs, pain and discomfort, and finally the worst kind of waiting to fulfill

their dream. They had to go through the difficult physical, emotional, and financial treatment and did not give up their dream until they put it into reality. They did not complain about the loss of freedom and loss of attractiveness during pregnancy or common physical changes and discomforts in early pregnancy. For example, one participant said: "My situation was very difficult because I was struggling to achieve something; I had to start receiving the everyday shots. It was really difficult at first, but it is pretty ok now. Pain had no meaning to me because of baby."

Financial stress related to incomplete health insurance coverage in Iran was the other concern. Sometimes finding the drugs was difficult for women struggling with fertility problems. One participant remarked: "I do not like being a burden on other people. In the time of infertility sometimes the expenses became so high that we did not afford to pay for them. My husband borrowed some money from someone and when I did not become pregnant, it was a burden on my husband's shoulder."

One woman remarked that despite her discontent, she has accepted help from her mother-in-law: "My husband is in another city for work and it is about six months that I am living in my mother-in-law's house. They are really kind to me, but it is difficult for me. This is not their responsibility to take care of me. Sometimes we have to bear something not for the sake of ourselves but for the sake of our children."

Announcing the pregnancy to others was even a more complex problem. Fear of miscarriage was the most common reason for not sharing pregnancy news early. They were also worried about the negative community reactions to the test tube babies. Sometimes women managed not to reveal the assisted pregnancy. In case of disclosing assisted pregnancy, women were stigmatized by their in-laws, relatives, and friends. In case of prolonged infertility, pregnancy has been repeatedly denied by others in early stages and people asked about the origins of the child or sometimes thought that these women used the donated gametes. One woman said: "in the area that we live, people think that in assisted pregnancy the embryo belongs to someone else. I said to them that I got pregnant naturally, but they thought that I had implanted another one's embryo."

Women experienced a wide variety of adjusting behaviors such as decline in physical activity, sexual intercourse, change in diet, and avoiding high-risk behavior. Now all have gone aside, and the focus is just on the baby. One participant described her adjustment to pregnancy after infertility as follows: "Before that we traveled a lot, but during the past 6 or 7 months we have not travelled at all. I myself stayed at home most of the time and so did my husband. We had to put aside many things that we did before in order to have a child." Another woman mentioned: "I had a headache for about 3 or 4 days, but I did not take any kinds of tablets due to the fear of its side effects on baby. When I made a phone call to my doctor, she told me to take a pill but I did not."

The results illustrated that thanks giving and trust in God, reading holy Quran, and praying for their fetus and other infertile patients are the most cited sources of spiritual experiences. All the participants were Muslim. One participant declared the trust in God as follows: "When I became desperate, there was a feeling that told me to move on and not to be frustrated. There is always the one who can help you from the above. I was hopeful. The day that I went for the transfer I said oh God I just rely on you, do not send me back empty-handed from here." Another woman remarked the sense of her inability to keep the fetus in this way: "Sometimes I feel that I can do nothing more myself. I read holy Quran and say prayers. I rely on the strength from God. When you see you cannot do anything more for yourself, you start asking help from God." Some participants encouraged their friends with fertility problems to pursue the treatment process. Participants felt uncomfortable talking about their pregnancies with infertile friends who are still undergoing treatments. Sometimes participants were upset because of the treatment failure in their friends and also the financial problem that does not permit them to repeat ARTs cycles. One participant mentioned: "Many times I thought about those people who have the same problem as mine and cannot afford the expenses and I told myself what if all of them could come here." Another woman said: "One of my friends did not get pregnant. I was really sad about her. Why should I get pregnant, but she does not. Her husband had told her that this is the last time. I spoke with her a lot, but she said she would not pursue."

4. Discussion

Our study discussed how Iranian pregnant women undergoing ARTs make sense of their conditions. The meaning of assisted pregnancy manifested itself as finding partial peace in life. The findings of our study support previous research on women's lived experiences by assisted pregnancy. Pregnancy had given women a sense of shock and surprise consistent with what was found in the study of Toscano and Montgomery [3]. Also, Redshaw et al. noticed the sense of being complete among women who successfully became pregnant as one of the findings in their study [21]. In the present study, women were very relieved and pregnancy had given women a sense of peace especially because of the power and security in marriage. Most of the women had the risk of this treatment as the unequally shared burden against security in marriage. In patriarchal societies like Iran, women have been identified with their role as mothers, and sometimes they are coerced to be mothers [22]. Children are actually seen as the link between women and their husbands in Iran, and infertility threats marriage [23]. Some participants in the present study said that they had a friendly relationship with their husband before, but they were concerned that infertility may become a problem over time and they may lose their spouses in the future. They wanted to achieve a stable home and family. Consistent with the present study, Hasanpoor-Azghdy et al. found out that pregnancy can stabilize the women status in the family and community [14]. Some participants reported that pregnancy is an end to coldness in marital relationships and the end of the pressures from their relatives and in-laws. Women referred also to the more supportive role of husbands during pregnancy that caused strength and feelings of security in them. Such support was less during infertility

treatment. These findings are similar to other studies in Iran and Taiwan [1, 23, 24].

Results showed that women experienced an increase in self-confidence. Although some studies reported similar self-confidence in assisted pregnancies in comparison with the control group, these studies also considered the increased confidence as pregnancy progresses [7, 25, 26]. Lower level of self-esteem and the feeling of personal deficiency have been reported in infertile women [3, 15]. In the present study, this feeling of lack disappeared in pregnant women.

The emotional pain women experienced when going through assisted pregnancy was hard. Most of the participants in the present study did not inform others of their pregnancy through ARTs. Majority of concerns related to pregnancy announcement were due to social stigma. Women with short infertility period were more successful in hiding assisted pregnancy and tried to keep their secret from others especially their in-laws. As discussed before, the most important duty for an Iranian woman is becoming a mother and infertility or assisted pregnancy can stigmatize her status in the community [23]. In the present study, the main reason for disclosing pregnancy through ARTs was to receive support during pregnancy. Providing counseling with regard to disclosure issues has been emphasized in pregnancy after infertility [5]. As women do not like to share their problem with relatives or people who are close to them, their privacy and confidentiality should be respected more in the prenatal visits. Providing some practical coping tips may be helpful in case of stigma.

The woman's emotions were often unstable. This is also in accordance with other studies stating the experience of joy, fear, uncertainty, ambiguity, and confusion during assisted pregnancies [1, 3, 24]. Uncertainty in bonding to the fetus was also visible in the present study. Mothers tried not to have strong emotional attachment with baby especially in early stage of pregnancy because of the fear of losing the baby. Uncertainty can remain until a healthy baby is delivered. Difficulty in bonding to the fetus has been documented before [27], but there is a controversy and some researchers believe that the attachment to the fetus is similar to other pregnancies [7]. Emotional support of couples who conceive through ARTs has been emphasized because of postnatal mood disturbance and difficulties in early mothering [4, 5, 9, 28, 29]. Participants need support from health care providers in adjustment to pregnancy to reduce the stress. Anyhow, health care providers should reassure the clients in counseling meetings that the bond between mother and fetus sometimes does not happen instantly after the positive pregnancy test and it may be extended until the second or third trimester.

Pregnancy is the beginning of a new and hard struggle for women with fertility problems. Women in the present study have to deal with the ARTs challenges to fulfill the dream of becoming a mother. Although some of the participants described their pregnancy as abnormal, they had no intention of adopting a child and wanted to have their own pregnancy experience. Similarly, in a study conducted in India, women tried to overcome the hardships and challenges despite the high physical, emotional, and financial difficulties and the low success rate of the treatment process. These women never thought about stopping their treatment also [30].

Women had to go through the change in their life style and spirituality which had been also reported in similar studies [1, 24]. Regardless of the fact that women's daily life had been strongly affected by pregnancy, they were not complaining about change in life style, resting at home, isolation during pregnancy, or elimination of all their freedom. These results were inconsistent with findings of other studies in which women were inconvenient about physical changes [1, 24]. Participants noted that spirituality helped them struggle with their challenges. Many of them were willing to help those having similar problems. Some studies have also looked at the role of spirituality as a protective factor during pregnancy [31]. As a result, we can support the client's spirituality to enhance the patient care.

5. Conclusion

The findings of the present study lead to a preliminary understanding of Iranian women's experiences from pregnancy through ARTs. This concept may be of much value to health care providers supporting women during an assisted pregnancy. Pregnancy is one of the hardest parts of realizing the dream of having a child for former infertile women. On the one hand, pregnant women get relieved and find more power and security in marriage. Nevertheless, women's emotions were often unstable and pregnant women with history of assisted reproductive techniques did not have a more positive experience. Pregnancy as a shocking surprise, a feeling of great relief, uncertainty about the outcome of the fetus, difficulty in pregnancy announcement, change in life style, and turning to religious beliefs had been documented in similar studies, but senses of power and security, marital satisfaction, and IVF stigma are some of the new issues in the present study due to the sociocultural differences. It seems that empowering pregnant women, handling stress, noticing attachment to their babies, managing paradoxical feelings, respecting women's confidentiality, reinforcing the coping strategies in case of stigma, and providing spiritual care to mothers should be construed as extra care in assisted pregnancies. As pregnancy may be influenced by the infertility treatment, the special care needed in an assisted pregnancy should be never taken for granted by health care providers. Health care providers should be well aware of the unavoidable effects of infertility on the experience of pregnancy. Developing new midwife roles and continued research in different contexts would enable health workers to provide a good care in assisted pregnancies.

5.1. Limitations of the Study. The two main limitations of the qualitative research methods are related to the issues of generalizability and replicability of the study [32]. In this respect we followed the purposive sampling approach and we also provide information about the context in which we were collecting the data to address some of these concerns. Anyhow all participants were recruited from one infertility center and their experiences might differ from those who became pregnant in other centers. Sadly enough, fewer women followed their pregnancy care inside the infertility center. Therefore, accessing to all of the women who got pregnant in this clinic and organizing the interviews in the last months of pregnancy were not possible.

Conflict of Interests

The authors declare that they have no conflict of interests.

Acknowledgments

The authors are highly grateful to all of the colleagues at Avicenna Fertility Clinic for their inspiration and contribution and to all the women who shared their experiences with them.

References

[1] L.-H. Wang and T. Y. Lee, "Assisted pregnancy after infertility: Taiwanese women's experience," *Journal of Medical Sciences*, vol. 24, no. 5, pp. 249–256, 2004.

[2] J. Bernstein, J. Lewis, and M. Seibel, "Effect of previous infertility on maternal-fetal attachment, coping styles, and self-concept during pregnancy," *Journal of Women's Health*, vol. 3, no. 2, pp. 125–133, 1994.

[3] S. E. Toscano and R. M. Montgomery, "The lived experience of women pregnant (including preconception) post in vitro fertilization through the lens of virtual communities," *Health Care for Women International*, vol. 30, no. 11, pp. 1014–1036, 2009.

[4] A. Hjelmstedt, A.-M. Widström, H. Wramsby, A.-S. Matthiesen, and A. Collins, "Personality factors and emotional responses to pregnancy among IVF couples in early pregnancy: a comparative study," *Acta Obstetricia et Gynecologica Scandinavica*, vol. 82, no. 2, pp. 152–161, 2003.

[5] A. Hjelmstedt, A.-M. Widström, H. Wramsby, and A. Collins, "Emotional adaptation following successful in vitro fertilization," *Fertility and Sterility*, vol. 81, no. 5, pp. 1254–1264, 2004.

[6] M. P. Lukse and N. A. Vacc, "Grief, depression, and coping in women undergoing infertility treatment," *Obstetrics and Gynecology*, vol. 93, no. 2, pp. 245–251, 1999.

[7] K. Hammarberg, J. R. W. Fisher, and K. H. Wynter, "Psychological and social aspects of pregnancy, childbirth and early parenting after assisted conception: a systematic review," *Human Reproduction Update*, vol. 14, no. 5, pp. 395–414, 2008.

[8] S. Tremayne, "The dilemma of assisted reproduction in Iran," in *Facts, Views & Visions in ObGyn*, Monographs, pp. 70–74, 2012.

[9] M. Barnes, A. Roiko, R. Reed, C. Williams, and K. Willcocks, "Outcomes for women and infants following assisted conception: implications for perinatal education, care, and support," *The Journal of Perinatal Education*, vol. 21, no. 1, pp. 18–23, 2012.

[10] T. M. Cousineau and A. D. Domar, "Psychological impact of infertility," *Best Practice and Research: Clinical Obstetrics and Gynaecology*, vol. 21, no. 2, pp. 293–308, 2007.

[11] M. M. Akhondi, K. Kamali, F. Ranjbar et al., "Prevalence of primary infertility in Iran in 2010," *Iranian Journal of Public Health*, vol. 42, no. 12, pp. 1398–1404, 2013.

[12] S. Vahidi, A. Ardalan, and K. Mohammad, "Prevalence of primary infertility in the Islamic Republic of Iran in 2004-2005," *Asia-Pacific Journal of Public Health*, vol. 21, no. 3, pp. 287–293, 2009.

[13] L. Mosalanejad, N. Parandavar, M. Gholami, and S. Abdollahifard, "Increasing and decreasing factors of hope in infertile women with failure in infertility treatment: a phenomenology study," *Iranian Journal of Reproductive Medicine*, vol. 12, no. 2, pp. 117–124, 2014.

[14] S. B. Hasanpoor-Azghdy, M. Simbar, and A. Vedadhir, "The emotional-psychological consequences of infertility among infertile women seeking treatment: results of a qualitative study," *Iranian Journal of Reproductive Medicine*, vol. 12, no. 2, pp. 131–138, 2014.

[15] Z. Behboodi-Moghadam, M. Salsali, H. Eftekhar-Ardabily, M. Vaismoradi, and F. Ramezanzadeh, "Experiences of infertility through the lens of Iranian infertile women: a qualitative study," *Japan Journal of Nursing Science*, vol. 10, no. 1, pp. 41–46, 2013.

[16] B. Morshed-Behbahani, L. Mossalanejad, S. Shahsavari, and M. Dastpak, "The experiences of infertile women on assistant reproductive treatments: a phenomenological study," *Iranian Red Crescent Medical Journal*, vol. 14, no. 6, pp. 382–383, 2012.

[17] N. Khodakarami, S. Hashemi, S. Seddigh, M. Hamdiyeh, and R. Taheripanah, "Life experience with infertility; a phenomenological study," *Journal of Reproduction & Infertility*, vol. 10, no. 4, pp. 287–298, 2010.

[18] E. Van Teijlingen and K. Forrest, "The range of qualitative research methods in family planning and reproductive health care," *Journal of Family Planning and Reproductive Health Care*, vol. 30, no. 3, pp. 171–173, 2004.

[19] M. van Manen, *Researching Lived Experience: Human Science for Action Sensitive Pedagogy*, Althouse, London, UK; State University of New York Press, Albany, NY, USA, 1990.

[20] M. van Manen, *Researching Lived Experience: Human Science for an Action Sensitive Pedagogy*, Suny Press, London, UK, 2001.

[21] M. Redshaw, C. Hockley, and L. L. Davidson, "A qualitative study of the experience of treatment for infertility among women who successfully became pregnant," *Human Reproduction*, vol. 22, no. 1, pp. 295–304, 2007.

[22] "Current practices and controversies in assisted reproduction," in *Proceedings of the WHO Meeting on Medical, Ethical and Social Aspects of Assisted Reproduction*, Geneva, Switzerland, September 2001.

[23] M. J. Abbasi-Shavazi, M. C. Inhorn, H. B. Razeghi-Nasrabad, and G. Toloo, "The 'Iranian ART Revolution': infertility, assisted reproductive technology, and third-party donation in the Islamic Republic of Iran," *Journal of Middle East Women's Studies*, vol. 4, no. 2, pp. 1–28, 2008.

[24] Y.-N. Lin, Y.-C. Tsai, and P.-H. Lai, "The experience of taiwanese women achieving post-infertility pregnancy through assisted reproductive treatment," *Family Journal*, vol. 21, no. 2, pp. 189–197, 2013.

[25] S. J. Cox, C. Glazebrook, C. Sheard, G. Ndukwe, and M. Oates, "Maternal self-esteem after successful treatment for infertility," *Fertility and Sterility*, vol. 85, no. 1, pp. 84–89, 2006.

[26] S. C. Klock and D. A. Greenfeld, "Psychological status of in vitro fertilization patients during pregnancy: a longitudinal study," *Fertility and Sterility*, vol. 73, no. 6, pp. 1159–1164, 2000.

[27] E. F. Olshansky, "Psychosocial implications of pregnancy after infertility," *NAACOG's Clinical Issues in Perinatal and Women's Health Nursing*, vol. 1, no. 3, pp. 342–347, 1990.

[28] I. Kowalcek, "Experience of pregnancy and delivery after ART," *Zeitschrift fur Geburtshilfe und Neonatologie*, vol. 215, no. 5, pp. 183–186, 2011.

[29] J. R. W. Fisher, K. Hammarberg, and H. W. G. Baker, "Assisted conception is a risk factor for postnatal mood disturbance and early parenting difficulties," *Fertility and Sterility*, vol. 84, no. 2, pp. 426–430, 2005.

[30] A. Widge, "Seeking conception: Experiences of urban Indian women with in vitro fertilisation," *Patient Education and Counseling*, vol. 59, no. 3, pp. 226–233, 2005.

[31] D. E. Jesse, J. Walcott-McQuigg, A. Mariella, and M. S. Swanson, "Risks and protective factors associated with symptoms of depression in low-income African American and Caucasian women during pregnancy," *Journal of Midwifery and Women's Health*, vol. 50, no. 5, pp. 405–410, 2005.

[32] K. F. Keenan and E. van Teijlingen, "The quality of qualitative research in family planning and reproductive health care," *Journal of Family Planning and Reproductive Health Care*, vol. 30, no. 4, pp. 257–259, 2004.

4

Implementation of the International Association of Diabetes and Pregnancy Study Groups Criteria: Not Always a Cause for Concern

Pooja Sibartie[1] and Julie Quinlivan[1,2]

[1]Department of Obstetrics and Gynaecology, Joondalup Health Campus, Joondalup, WA 6027, Australia
[2]Institute for Health Research, University of Notre Dame Australia, Fremantle, WA 6160, Australia

Correspondence should be addressed to Julie Quinlivan; julie.quinlivan@nd.edu.au

Academic Editor: Ellinor Olander

Background. Controversy surrounds the decision to adopt the International Association of Diabetes and Pregnancy Study Groups (IADPSG) criteria for the diagnosis of gestational diabetes mellitus (GDM) as fears that disease prevalence rates will soar have been raised. *Aims*. To investigate the prevalence of pregnancy complicated with GDM before and after the introduction of the IADPSG 2010 diagnostic criteria. *Materials and Methods*. A prospective audit of all women who delivered from July 1, 2010, to June 30, 2014, in a predefined geographic region within the North Metropolitan Health Service of Western Australia. Women were diagnosed with GDM according to Australian Diabetes in Pregnancy Society (ADIPS 1991) criteria until December 31, 2011, and by the IADPSG 2010 criteria after this date. Incidence of GDM and predefined pregnancy outcomes were audited. *Results*. Of 10,296 women, antenatal oral glucose tolerance test (OGTT) results and follow-up data were obtained for 10,103 women (98%), of whom 349 (3.5%) were diagnosed with GDM. The rate of GDM utilising ADIPS criteria was 3.4% and the rate of utilising IADPSG criteria was 3.5% ($p = 0.92$). *Conclusion*. IADPSG diagnostic criteria did not significantly increase the incidence of GDM in this low prevalence region.

1. Introduction

Gestational diabetes mellitus (GDM) is a common medical complication of pregnancy defined as "any degree of glucose intolerance with onset or first recognition during pregnancy" [1, 2]. The initial criteria for diagnosis were established more than 40 years ago [3]; however, these criteria did not necessarily identify pregnancies with increased risk of adverse pregnancy outcome [4].

The hyperglycaemia and adverse pregnancy outcome (HAPO) study was conducted to clarify the associations between maternal hyperglycaemia and adverse outcomes. The study showed associations between increasing levels of fasting blood glucose (FBG), 1-hour and 2-hour plasma glucose obtained following an oral glucose tolerance test (OGTT), and birthweight >90th centile and cord-blood serum C-peptide level >90th centile [5]. The secondary

outcomes of premature delivery, shoulder dystocia or birth injury, admission to intensive neonatal care unit, hyperbilirubinemia, and preeclampsia were also increased by maternal hyperglycaemia [5].

The consideration of HAPO data led to a recommendation in 2010 by the International Association of Diabetes and Pregnancy Study Groups (IADPSG) for the FBG and 1 h and 2 h glucose levels to diagnose GDM [4]. The diagnostic threshold values were the average glucose values at which the odds for birthweight >90th centile, cord C-peptide >90th centile, and percent body fat >90th centile reached 1.75 times the estimated odds of the outcomes at mean glucose values [4, 5].

However, concern has been expressed that adoption of the new diagnostic criteria would lead to a dramatic increase in the incidence of GDM. One Australian study reported that the change in diagnostic criteria from the previously utilised Australasian Diabetes in Pregnancy Society (ADIPS) 1999 criteria [6] to the new IADPSG 2010 criteria [4] would increase the prevalence of GDM from 9.6% to 13.0% [7]. A NZ study reported that the incidence might rise from 6% to 10% [8]. National debate continues on the workforce implications of the revised criteria and their clinical impact [9, 10].

The aim of this study was to audit the impact of the change from the ADIPS 1999 criteria [6] to the IADPSG 2010 diagnostic criteria [4] within a geographically defined region.

2. Methods

A prospective audit of all pregnancies diagnosed with GDM commenced from July 1, 2010, following publication of HAPO and the IADPSG recommendations. The Institutional Ethics Committee determined that the project fulfilled the criteria of an audit project as pregnancy outcomes were being audited and no intervention other than routine care according to existing clinical protocols was planned. Therefore, the project was exempted from formal ethics committee approval.

All pregnant women greater than 20-week gestation referred for public maternity care who resided within the postcodes 6001–6007, 6147, 6148, 6151, 6152, and 6155 within the North Metropolitan Health Service of the Western Australian Department of Health between July 1, 2010, to June 30, 2014, were included in the audit. Women with a history of preexisting diabetes mellitus (type 1 or 2) were specifically excluded from the project.

All women had an OGTT between 24 and 28 weeks of gestation in accordance with the existing clinical protocol [11].

The ADIPS 1999 criteria were used to diagnose GDM in the period from July 1, 2010, to December 31, 2011 [6]. Women had a 75-gram OGTT with glucose samples taken after an overnight fast and at 2 hr postprandially. GDM was diagnosed if the fasting glucose was $\geq$5.5 mmol/L (100 mg/dL) and/or the 2 h glucose was $\geq$8.0 mmol/L (~145 mg/dL) [6].

From January 1, 2012, to June 30, 2014, all patients were diagnosed with GDM using the IADPSG 2010 diagnostic criteria [4]. Women had a 75-gram OGTT with glucose samples taken after an overnight fast and at 1 hr and 2 hr postprandially. One or more abnormal values were needed for a diagnosis of GDM to be made: FBG > 5.0 mmol/L and/or 1-hour BSL > 10 mmol/L and/or 2-hour BSL $\geq$ 8.5 mmol/L.

The majority of OGTT in the audit period was performed at the Western Diagnostics Pathology laboratories. A small number (2.8%) was performed at other private accredited pathology providers.

All patients had their weight (kg) and height (m) recorded at their booking visit to calculate their body mass index (BMI). Patients with a BMI greater than 40 had their antenatal care at the local maternity hospital but were referred for delivery to the regional tertiary hospital. These patients remained within the audit study.

All pregnancies diagnosed with GDM across the audit period received identical clinical care according to a written protocol. This involved an initial consultation with a diabetic educator, dietician, and obstetric doctor. Patients commenced self-monitoring of blood sugar levels and adopted a diabetic diet. A review visit a fortnight later determined if medication was required in addition to diet.

Delivery outcomes were entered into a computerized database called Meditec by attending midwifery staff as part of routine practice. Delivery outcomes were subsequently extracted from Meditec, case note audit, and a postnatal clinical service for all women with GDM conducted by one author (Julie Quinlivan).

Predefined maternal outcomes were audited. These were mode of delivery, elective or emergency caesarean section, estimated blood loss, and 3rd or 4th degree perineal tear. Predefined newborn outcomes were audited. These were gestational age at birth, birthweight, birthweight >90th centile adjusted for gestational age, Apgar at 1 and 5 minutes, umbilical artery and vein pH, admission to Special Care Unit, and serious perinatal complications such as stillbirth, neonatal death, or birth trauma including shoulder dystocia.

A power calculation assumed that the change in incidence of GDM would be 30%, a conservative estimate based on the previous Australian and New Zealand studies [7, 8]. The baseline rate of GDM in the audit region was approximately 3.5%. Assuming a power of 80% and alpha error of 0.05, a sample of 10,994 women was required across the audit period to detect a change in incidence from 3.5 to 4.6%.

Data were presented as number and percentage for the incidence of GDM. Descriptive statistics of predefined clinical outcomes were compared using Student's t-test for continuous variables and Chi Square test or Fisher exact test for discrete data. A p value of 0.05 was considered significant.

3. Results

Of 10,296 women delivering in the audit period, antenatal OGTT results could be traced for 10,277 women (99.8%). The remaining 19 (0.2%) women did not have an antenatal OGTT, in violation of national clinical protocol. Of these women, 5 attempted an OGTT and were unable to complete the test due to nausea and/or vomiting. They subsequently declined a repeat test. The other 14 women either presented for care too late for testing or declined testing.

Table 1 summarizes the incidence of GDM under the two diagnostic criteria. The overall incidence was not significantly different with 3.4% diagnosed under the ADIPS 1999 criteria and 3.5% under the IADPSG 2010 criteria. In the subgroup of 342 women with a BMI > 40 (representing 3.3% of the study population) the incidence of GDM was 3.7% using ADIPS 1999 criteria and 8.5% using IADPSG 2010 criteria. This difference was not statistically significant (p = 0.11); however, the audit was not adequately powered to detect a difference in the subgroup of women with high BMI.

TABLE 1: Incidence of GDM under ADIPS 1999 and IADPSG 2010 criteria.

	ADIPS	IADPSG	p value
All women	N = 3,553	N = 6,724	
GDM	121 (3.4%)	236 (3.5%)	0.78
No GDM	3,432 (96.6%)	6488 (96.5%)	
Women with BMI ≤ 40	N = 3446	N = 6489	
GDM	117 (3.4%)	216 (3.3%)	0.86
No GDM	3,329 (96.6%)	6,273 (96.7%)	
Women with BMI > 40	N = 107	N = 235	
GDM	4 (3.7%)	20 (8.5%)	0.11
No GDM	103 (96.3%)	215 (91.5%)	

Across the audit period the proportion of women with GDM who required management with medication (metformin or insulin) in addition to diet was not significantly different (25% in women diagnosed by ADIPS 1999 criteria and 28% in women diagnosed by IADPSG 2010 criteria, resp.).

Delivery data for 10,277 (98%) women were available for audit through Meditec, case note audit, or the postnatal clinical service.

Table 2 summarizes predefined delivery outcomes. Babies born to women diagnosed with GDM according to the IADPSG 2010 criteria had significantly higher umbilical artery pH (7.28 versus 7.21; $p = 0.01$). They had a significant lower birthweight (3360 gms versus 3470 gms; $p = 0.02$) and birthweight above the >90th centile adjusted for gestational age (11% versus 18%; $p = 0.04$). Other predefined maternal and newborn outcomes were not significantly different between groups.

4. Discussion

The audit found no significant difference in the incidence of GDM before and after the introduction of the IADPSG 2010 criteria, with the overall incidence being low at 3.5%. Our results differ from the previous Australian and New Zealand studies [7, 8].

One explanation may be that prevalence of GDM in our region is low compared to many other sites. Our rate of 3.5% contrasts higher background rates in the sites involved in the HAPO trial where incidences ranged from 8 to 25% [12]. However, HAPO study sites were specifically included because of their high rates of GDM. They were tertiary sites where women with high BMI and other pregnancy complications were referred for antenatal and delivery management [5, 12]. Our study was based upon a geographical region rather than a hospital cohort and thus captured women of all risk levels, including a majority who were of "normal" risk, unlike the patient population within a tertiary centre.

A second explanation for the observed difference in outcome between our study and previous ones may be the racial mix of the population. Although our geographic maternity cohort reflected the wider Australian public maternity cohort in terms of maternal age and parity [13], racial background was overwhelmingly English speaking Caucasian.

A third explanation may be due to maternal obesity levels. Our geographic catchment has a low prevalence of overweight and obese patients compared to many sites. Lower obesity levels mean that the underlying risk of metabolic hyperglycaemia is lowered. Of note, in our subgroup of women with a BMI > 40 the incidence of GDM rose from 3.7% to 8.5% under the IADPSG 2010 criteria, more in line with studies elsewhere [7, 8].

As a secondary consideration, the adoption of the IADPSG 2010 criteria did not adversely impact upon our predefined maternal and newborn outcomes. There was a significant improvement in three newborn outcomes, being an increase in umbilical artery pH and a reduction in birthweight and birthweight >90th centile adjusted for gestational age. There were no significant changes in maternal outcomes. This provides reassuring safety data for the change.

The study had several strengths. Firstly, data were extracted from a defined geographic region before and after implementation of the IADPSG 2010 diagnostic criteria. Secondly, all women received treatment using identical clinical protocols throughout the audit period. Thirdly, there was high compliance with screening for GDM (99.8%) and ascertainment of outcome (98% of women). A study limitation is the low background incidence of GDM that limits generalizability to regions where incidence rates are higher. A second limitation is that only 3.3% of women presented with a BMI > 40. In this subgroup of women, the incidence of GDM was higher at 8.5%. Centres where the obstetric population has a higher incidence of obesity may report an increase in the incidence in GDM utilising the new diagnostic criteria. However, it is likely that this reflects a genuine increase in metabolic pathology, as obesity is a major risk factor for GDM and adverse pregnancy outcome [14].

5. Conclusion

The IADPSG used a consensus process to redefine GDM based on its association with adverse pregnancy outcomes. There has been controversy about the adoption of the new guidelines. However, in our audit study of 10,296 women, we observed no significant increase in the incidence of GDM. The adoption of the new criteria was associated with improvements in three newborn outcomes.

Conflict of Interests

The authors declare that there is no conflict of interests regarding the publication of this paper.

TABLE 2: Delivery outcomes.

	GDM ADIPS N = 121	GDM IADPSG N = 236	p value
Maternal outcomes			
Maternal age (years) Mean (sd)	31.0 (5.3)	31.1 (5.6)	0.75
Parity Median (IQR)	1 (1–2.5)	1 (1–2.5)	0.34
Caesarean section N (%)	30 (25%)	64 (27%)	0.64
Blood loss (mL) Median (IQR)	300 (200–380)	300 (200–400)	0.25
Birth trauma (3rd/4th degree tear) N (%)	2 (2%)	5 (2%)	1.00
Newborn outcomes			
Gestational age (days) Mean (sd)	274 (7)	275 (6)	0.82
Birthweight (grams) Mean (sd)	3470 (345)	3360 (321)	0.02
Birthweight >90th centile for gestational age N (%)	22 (18%)	25 (12%)	0.04
Apgar 1 Mean (sd)	9 (8.25–9)	9 (9-9)	0.17
Apgar 5 Mean (sd)	9 (8.40–9)	9 (9-9)	0.21
Arterial cord blood Mean (sd)	7.21 (0.6)	7.28 (0.6)	0.01
Venous cord blood Mean (sd)	7.33 (0.2)	7.34 (0.2)	0.89
Admission to neonatal nursery N (%)	14 (12%)	28 (12%)	0.93

Acknowledgments

The authors acknowledge Research Assistant Ms. Ronni Highet and Research Student Ms. Danielle Lam who contributed towards extraction of audit data. They also acknowledge Joondalup Health Campus for providing the GDM follow-up clinical service during the audit period and for funding the gestational diabetes postnatal audit clinics.

References

[1] American Diabetes Association, "Diagnosis and classification of diabetes mellitus," *Diabetes Care*, vol. 32, supplement 1, pp. S62–S67, 2008.

[2] B. E. Metzger and D. R. Coustan, "Summary and recommendations of the Fourth International Workshop-Conference on Gestational Diabetes Mellitus," *Diabetes Care*, vol. 21, supplement 2, pp. B161–B167, 1998.

[3] J. B. O'Sullivan and C. M. Mahan, "Criteria for oral glucose tolerance test in pregnancy," *Diabetes*, vol. 13, pp. 278–285, 1964.

[4] International Association of Diabetes and Pregnancy Study Groups Consensus Panel, "International Association of Diabetes and Pregnancy study groups recommendations on the diagnosis and classification of hyperglycemia in pregnancy," *Diabetes Care*, vol. 33, no. 3, pp. 676–682, 2010.

[5] B. E. Metzger, L. P. Lowe, A. R. Dyer et al., "Hyperglycemia and adverse pregnancy outcomes," *The New England Journal of Medicine*, vol. 358, no. 19, pp. 1991–2002, 2008.

[6] F. I. R. Martin, A. Vogue, R. Dargaville, and et al, "The diagnosis of gestational diabetes," *Medical Journal of Australia*, vol. 155, no. 2, p. 112, 1991.

[7] R. G. Moses, G. J. Morris, P. Petocz, F. Sangil, and D. Garg, "The impact of potential new diagnostic criteria on the prevalence of gestational diabetes mellitus in Australia," *Medical Journal of Australia*, vol. 194, no. 7, pp. 338–340, 2011.

[8] A. J. Ekeroma, G. S. Chandran, L. McCowan, D. Ansell, C. Eagleton, and T. Kenealy, "Impact of using the International Association of Diabetes and Pregnancy Study Groups criteria in South Auckland: prevalence, interventins and outcomes," *Australian and New Zealand Journal of Obstetrics and Gynaecology*, vol. 55, no. 1, pp. 34–41, 2015.

[9] M. C. D'Emden, "Reassessment of the new diagnostic thresholds for gestational diabetes mellitus: an opportunity for improvement," *The Medical Journal of Australia*, vol. 201, no. 4, pp. 209–211, 2014.

[10] D. A. S. Kevat, A. K. Sinha, and A. G. McLean, "Lower treatment targets for gestational diabetes, is lower really better?" *The Medical Journal of Australia*, vol. 201, no. 4, pp. 204–207, 2014.

[11] Royal Australian College of Obstetricians and Gynaecologists, *Diagnosis of gestational Diabetes Mellitus (GDM) and Diabetes*

Mellitus in Pregnancy, Royal Australian and New Zealand College of Obstetricians and Gynaecologists, Melbourne, Australia, 2014.

[12] D. A. Sacks, D. R. Coustan, D. R. Hadden et al., "Frequency of gestational diabetes mellitus at collaborating centers based on IADPSG consensus panel-recommended criteria: the Hyperglycemia and Adverse Pregnancy Outcome (HAPO) Study," *Diabetes Care*, vol. 35, no. 3, pp. 526–528, 2012.

[13] Z. Li, R. Zeki, L. Hilder, and E. A. Sullivan, "Australia's mothers and babies 2011," Australian Institute of Health and Welfare Canberra, 2013.

[14] J. A. Quinlivan and L. Danielle, "Cholesterol abnormalities are common in women with prior gestational diabetes," *Journal of Diabetes & Metabolism*, vol. 4, no. 4, article 255, 2013.

5

Perinatal Risks Associated with Early Vanishing Twin Syndrome following Transfer of Cleavage- or Blastocyst-Stage Embryos

Nigel Pereira,[1] Katherine P. Pryor,[2] Allison C. Petrini,[2] Jovana P. Lekovich,[1] Jaclyn Stahl,[1] Rony T. Elias,[1] and Steven D. Spandorfer[1]

[1]The Ronald O. Perelman and Claudia Cohen Center for Reproductive Medicine, Weill Cornell Medicine, New York, NY, USA
[2]Department of Obstetrics and Gynecology, Weill Cornell Medical College, New York, NY, USA

Correspondence should be addressed to Nigel Pereira; nip9060@med.cornell.edu

Academic Editor: Keith A. Eddleman

Objective. To investigate whether the perinatal risks associated with early vanishing twin (VT) syndrome differ between cleavage- or blastocyst-stage embryo transfers (ET) in fresh in vitro fertilization (IVF) cycles. *Methods.* Retrospective, single-center, cohort study of IVF cycles with fresh cleavage- or blastocyst-stage ETs resulting in a live singleton birth. The incidence of preterm birth (PTB), low birth weight (LBW), and very low birth weight (VLBW) was compared between cleavage- and blastocyst-stage ET cycles complicated by early VT. *Results.* 7241 patients had live singleton births. Early VT was observed in 709/6134 (11.6%) and 70/1107 (6.32%) patients undergoing cleavage-stage and blastocyst-stage ETs, respectively. Patients in the blastocyst-stage group were younger compared to the cleavage-stage group. The cleavage-stage group had a similar birth weight compared to the blastocyst-stage group. There was no difference in the incidence of PTB (9.87% versus 8.57%), LBW (11.1% versus 11.4%), or VLBW (1.13 versus 1.43%) when comparing the cleavage-stage early VT and blastocyst-stage early VT groups, even after adjustment with logistic regression. *Conclusions.* Our study highlights that the adverse perinatal risks of PTB, LBW, and VLBW associated with early VT syndrome are similar in patients undergoing cleavage-stage or blastocyst-stage ETs during fresh IVF cycles.

1. Introduction

The use of in vitro fertilization (IVF) to overcome infertility continues to increase globally. Over 4,000,000 IVF cycles were initiated worldwide between 2008 and 2010, resulting in the birth of 1,144,858 children [1]. A majority of these IVF cycles involve the transfer of >1 embryo to achieve a pregnancy, often contributing to the pathogenesis of multiple pregnancies, which occurs in up to 23.1% of fresh IVF cycles [1]. With successful advances in culture media, there has been a practice shift in IVF from cleavage-stage to blastocyst-stage embryo transfers (ETs) [2, 3]. Thus, the extended culture of embryos to the blastocyst-stage allows for the selection of fewer embryos for ET compared to cleavage-stage ETs [2, 3]. Yet, the number of single ET cycles remains relatively low (i.e., 21.4% in 2013 (United States) and 30.0% in 2010 (globally) [1, 4]), suggesting that transfer of >1 embryo, either cleavage-stage or blastocyst-stage, remains the norm in IVF cycles.

Approximately one out of every 10 singleton IVF pregnancies are thought to originate from a twin gestation [5] in a phenomenon known as vanishing twin (VT) syndrome [6]. Existing data suggest higher perinatal risks such as low birth weight and preterm birth in the surviving twin of VT syndrome [7–13]. However, it is important to note that these data are primarily generated from studies involving the transfer of >1 cleavage-stage embryo to achieve a pregnancy. Although one study has previously reported a decreased risk of VT syndrome in blastocyst-stage ET when compared to cleavage-stage ET [14], it is currently unknown whether early VT syndrome is associated with different perinatal risks in blastocyst or cleavage-stage ET cycles. Thus, the primary objective of the current study is to investigate whether the perinatal risks associated with early VT syndrome differ between cleavage- and blastocyst-stage ETs in fresh IVF cycles.

2. Materials and Methods

2.1. Cycle Inclusion Criteria. All fresh IVF cycles with transfer of cleavage- or blastocyst-stage embryos between 2004 and 2013 at the Ronald O. Perelman and Claudia Cohen Center for Reproductive Medicine were analyzed for potential inclusion. Only patients with live singleton birth were included. The diagnosis of early VT was made based on criteria described by Petrini et al. [15]. In brief, patients with a positive β-human chorionic gonadotropin (hCG) level on cycle day (CD) 28 underwent a transvaginal sonogram on CD 49 to record the number of fetal poles with cardiac activity in the respective gestational sacs [15]. Patients with spontaneous in utero reduction of one or more embryos before CD 49 were considered to have an early VT. For this study, we only included embryos that spontaneously reduced within the first trimester. All patients utilizing donor oocytes or undergoing frozen-thawed ET were excluded. The retrospective cohort study protocol was approved by the Weill Cornell Medical College Institutional Review Board.

2.2. Clinical and Laboratory Protocols. Previously described protocols for ovarian stimulation, ovulatory trigger, and oocyte retrieval were utilized [16]. Ovarian stimulation began on CD 2 of menses with gonadotropins (Follistim, Merck, Kenilworth, NJ, USA, or Gonal-F, EMD-Serono Inc., Rockland, MA, USA, and Menopur, Ferring Pharmaceuticals Inc., Parsippany, NJ, USA). Dosing of gonadotropins was based on patient age, body mass index (BMI, kg/m^2), antral follicle count, and previous response to stimulation, if any. Ovulation was suppressed with daily injection of 0.25 mg Ganirelix Acetate (Merck, Kenilworth, NJ, USA). The hCG trigger (Pregnyl, Merck, Kenilworth, NJ, USA) was given when the two lead follicles attained a mean diameter >17 mm. Oocyte retrieval was performed under conscious sedation using transvaginal sonogram guidance approximately 34-35 hours after the hCG trigger. The retrieved oocytes were fertilized using intracytoplasmic sperm injection (ICSI) or conventional in vitro insemination depending on the male partner's semen analysis [17]. All embryos were cultured in in-house culture media [18]. Cleavage-stage embryos were graded based on the Veeck criteria, while the blastocyst-stage embryos were graded based on criteria described by Gardner and Schoolcraft [19]. The majority of patients underwent cleavage-stage ET, while those with several good-quality cleavage-stage embryos on day 3 were eligible for blastocyst-stage ET on day 5 [20]. All ETs were performed with Wallace catheters (Smiths Medical Inc., Norwell, MA, USA).

2.3. Study Variables. Baseline demographics recorded for all patients included age, parity, BMI (kg/m^2), and infertility diagnosis. Ovarian stimulation parameters recorded were total days of ovarian stimulation, total dosage of gonadotropins administered (IU), peak estradiol (E$_2$) level (pg/mL), peak endometrial thickness (mm), and total number of oocytes retrieved. The mean number of embryos transferred per patient was recorded, based on which implantation rates were calculated (i.e., the number of embryos with cardiac activity detected via transvaginal sonography on CD49 out of

the total number of embryos transferred). Perinatal outcomes recorded for all live births were mode of delivery, preterm birth (PTB), low birth weight (LBW), very low birth weight (VLBW), and term LBW. Any live birth at <37 weeks of gestational age was defined as PTB [21]. PTB between ≥34 and <37 weeks of gestation was defined as late PTB, while that occurring at <34 weeks of gestation was classified as early PTB [21]. Birth weights <2,500 g and <1,500 g irrespective of gestational age were classified as LBW and VLBW, respectively [22]. Any live singleton born ≥37 weeks of gestational age, but with a birth weight of <2,500 grams, was considered a term LBW singleton [21, 22].

2.4. Statistical Analyses. Continuous variables were checked for normality using Shapiro-Wilk's test and expressed as mean ± standard deviation (SD). Categorical variables were expressed as number of cases (*n*) and percentage (%). Nonparametric variables were expressed as median (interquartile range [IQR]). Independent *t*-tests, Wilcoxon rank-sum tests, and Chi-square tests were used as indicated. Odds ratios (OR) with 95% confidence intervals (CI) were calculated for the incidence of PTB, LBW, VLBW, and term LBW and were adjusted with multiple logistic regression, controlling for the following variables: age (<35 years versus ≥35 years); total days of ovarian stimulation (<9 days versus ≥9 days); total gonadotropins administered (<2000 IU versus ≥2000 IU); peak E$_2$ level (<2000 versus ≥2000 pg/mL); total number of oocytes (<10 versus ≥10); and blastocyst-stage ET (yes versus no). A *P* value < 0.05 was considered statistically significant. All statistical analyses were performed using STATA version 13 (College Station, TX: StataCorp LP).

3. Results

A total of 7241 patients had live singleton births during the study period. Cleavage- and blastocyst-stage ETs contributed to live singleton births in 6134 (84.7%) and 1107 (15.3%) patients, respectively. Early VT was observed in 709 (11.6%) and 70 (6.32%) patients undergoing cleavage-stage and blastocyst-stage ETs, respectively, which represented a 0.51 times lower odds of early VT in the blastocyst-stage group compared to the cleavage-stage group (OR 0.51; 95% CI 0.19–1.41). Of note, these odds are similar to the odds reported by Fernando et al. [14].

Table 1 compares the baseline demographics of all patients undergoing cleavage-stage or blastocyst-stage ETs with early VT. While there were no differences in the mean parity, BMI, and distribution of infertility diagnoses, patients in the blastocyst-stage group (36.2 ± 1.01 years) were younger compared to the cleavage-stage group (38.1 ± 2.98 years; *P* < 0.001).

As highlighted in Table 2, patients undergoing blastocyst-stage ET required a lower dosage of gonadotropins and had higher peak E$_2$ levels compared to the cleavage-stage group. Also, the yield of total and mature oocytes was higher in the latter group compared to the former. These differences suggested a more robust ovarian response in blastocyst-stage ET group. There were no differences in the total days of ovarian stimulation or peak endometrial thickness.

TABLE 1: Baseline demographics of patients undergoing cleavage-stage ETs (n = 709) or blastocyst-stage ETs (n = 70) with early VT.

Parameter	Cleavage-stage (n = 709)	Blastocyst-stage (n = 70)	P
Age (years)	38.1 ($\pm$2.98)	36.2 ($\pm$1.01)	<0.001
Parity	0.71 ($\pm$0.21)	0.59 ($\pm$0.38)	0.11
BMI (kg/m^2)	23.1 ($\pm$2.97)	22.9 ($\pm$1.83)	0.55
Infertility diagnoses			0.28
Ovulatory	198 (27.9%)	15 (21.4%)	
Tubal	38 (5.36%)	8 (11.4%)	
Endometriosis	37 (5.22%)	7 (10%)	
Male factor	262 (37.0%)	22 (31.4%)	
Idiopathic	39 (5.50%)	9 (12.9%)	
Other	135 (19.0%)	9 (12.9%)	

Data are presented as mean ± standard deviation, median (interquartile range), and n (%); BMI: body mass index.

TABLE 2: Comparison of ovarian stimulation parameters of patients undergoing cleavage-stage ETs (n = 709) or blastocyst-stage ETs (n = 70) with early VT.

Parameter	Cleavage-stage (n = 709)	Blastocyst-stage (n = 70)	P
Total days of ovarian stimulation	9.77 ($\pm$1.49)	9.41 ($\pm$1.12)	0.06
Total dosage of gonadotropins (IU)	2992.7 ($\pm$329.1)	2527.2 ($\pm$278.3)	<0.001
Peak E$_2$ level (pg/mL)	1609.2 ($\pm$471.9)	2259.0 ($\pm$512.3)	<0.001
Peak endometrial thickness (mm)	10.8 ($\pm$2.12)	10.7 ($\pm$1.92)	0.71
Total number of oocytes	12 (9–15)	14 (9–17)	<0.001
Total number of mature oocytes	10 (7–13)	12 (7–15)	<0.001

Data are presented as mean ± standard deviation, median (interquartile range), and n (%); E$_2$: estradiol.

Table 3 summarizes the perinatal outcomes of patients undergoing cleavage-stage or blastocyst-stage ETs with early VT. The mean number of embryos transferred was higher in the cleavage-stage group (2.64 ± 0.91) compared to the blastocyst-stage group (1.69 ± 0.42). No difference in the mode of delivery, rate of term birth, rate of late PTB, or rate of early PTB was noted. The cleavage-stage group had a similar birth weight compared to the blastocyst-stage group (3187.1 ± 409.9 grams versus 3198.2 ± 387.2 grams; P = 0.82). Furthermore, the odds of LBW, VLBW, or term LBW were nonsignificant when comparing the groups.

Tables 4, 5, 6, and 7 highlight the adjusted OR for PTB, LBW, VLBW, and term LBW, respectively, after accounting for age, total gonadotropins administered, total days of ovarian stimulation, peak E$_2$ level, total number of oocytes, and blastocyst-stage ET using multiple logistic regression. As evident from the aforementioned tables, no differences in the odds of adverse perinatal outcomes between the cleavage-stage and blastocyst-stage groups were noted.

4. Discussion

Since the recognition of VT syndrome in the 1970s [23], several investigators have reported adverse perinatal outcomes such as LBW, PTB, low APGAR scores, and fetal malformations associated with VT syndrome in a myriad of clinical settings and modes of conception. Several investigators have postulated reasons for the association of perinatal risks and VT syndrome. La Sala et al. [6] proposed that VT syndrome

is a subtype of single fetal demise in twins, resulting in blood shunting from the placenta of the surviving twin, ultimately leading to deleterious effects. Thus, increasing gestational ages of VT would be associated with heightened perinatal risks. For example, the rates of PTB (16.7%) reported by La Sala et al. [6] for VT syndrome occurring after 8 weeks of gestation are higher than the rates of PTB (9.9% for cleavage-stage ET and 8.6% for blastocyst-stage ET) reported in our study after early VT. Another theory suggests that chronic inflammation following VT reduction directly impacts the growth and progression of the surviving twin [10–12]. Finally, Mansour et al. [7] reported that adverse perinatal outcomes associated with VT syndrome may be mediated through early embryonic modification rather than a uterine or placentation etiology.

The impact of ET stage on perinatal outcomes in IVF cycles associated with early VT syndrome is currently unknown. Thus, our study evaluates the perinatal risks associated with early VT in two different implantation models— cleavage-stage ET and blastocyst-stage ET. Historically, cleavage-stage ET was considered standard in IVF-ET cycles, primarily due to limitations in our knowledge of stage-specific culture medium requirements and the low survival of embryos cultured past this stage [2, 3]. Advances in laboratory protocols have enabled extended culture with subsequent increase in blastocyst-stage ET. Yet, the ideal ET stage depends on several factors including consideration of short-term outcomes (including implantation and clinical pregnancy rates, cycle cancellation rates, and likelihood

TABLE 3: Comparison of perinatal outcomes in patients undergoing cleavage-stage ETs ($n = 709$) or blastocyst-stage ETs ($n = 70$) with early VT.

Parameter	Cleavage-stage ($n = 709$)	Blastocyst-stage ($n = 70$)	OR (95% CI)	P
Age (years)	38.1 (±2.98)	36.2 (±1.01)	—	<0.001
Number of embryos transferred	2.64 (±0.91)	1.69 (±0.42)	—	<0.001
Implantation rate	39.7%	43.2%	0.83 (0.47–1.46)	0.52
Mode of delivery				0.87
Vaginal	378 (53.3%)	38 (54.3%)	0.96 (0.59–1.57)	
Cesarean	331 (46.7%)	32 (45.7%)		
Term birth	639 (90.1%)	64 (91.4%)	0.86 (0.33–2.23)	0.75
Preterm birth				0.70
Late preterm	41 (5.78%)	4 (5.71%)	0.71 (0.12–4.12)	
Early preterm	29 (4.09%)	2 (2.86%)		
Overall birth weight (g)	3187.1 (±409.9)	3198.2 (±387.2)	—	0.82
LBW	79 (11.1%)	8 (11.4%)	0.97 (0.40–2.33)	0.95
VLBW	8 (1.13%)	1 (1.43%)	0.79 (0.07–9.43)	0.85
Term LBW	30 (4.69%)	4 (6.25%)	0.74 (0.22–2.53)	0.63

Data are presented as mean ± standard deviation, median (interquartile range), and n (%); LBW: low birth weight; VLBW: very low birth weight; OR: odds ratio; CI: confidence interval.

TABLE 4: Preterm birth and multiple logistic regression to account for confounding variables.

PTB	Standard error	Adjusted OR (95% CI)	P
Age (<35 versus ≥35 years)	0.21	0.87 (0.54–1.41)	0.58
Duration of ovarian stimulation (<9 versus ≥9 days)	0.36	0.83 (0.35–1.97)	0.67
Gonadotropin dose (<2000 versus ≥2000 IU)	0.86	0.93 (0.15–5.71)	0.94
Peak E_2 level (<2000 versus ≥2000 pg/Ml)	0.24	1.12 (0.74–1.71)	0.57
Total number of oocytes (<10 versus ≥10)	0.13	0.70 (0.48–1.11)	0.16
Blastocyst-stage ET (yes versus no)	0.21	0.74 (0.42–1.28)	0.28

PTB: preterm birth; E_2: estradiol; ET: embryo transfer.

TABLE 5: Low birth weight and multiple logistic regression to account for confounding variables.

LBW	Standard error	Adjusted OR (95% CI)	P
Age (<35 versus ≥35 years)	0.59	1.16 (0.43–3.14)	0.77
Duration of ovarian stimulation (<9 versus ≥9 days)	1.25	1.24 (0.17–8.96)	0.83
Gonadotropin dose (<2000 versus ≥2000 IU)	0.76	0.81 (0.13–5.04)	0.82
Peak E_2 level (<2000 versus ≥2000 pg/Ml)	0.30	0.86 (0.44–1.69)	0.66
Total number of oocytes (<10 versus ≥10)	0.20	0.93 (0.18–4.13)	0.77
Blastocyst-stage ET (yes versus no)	0.11	0.85 (0.66–1.99)	0.20

LBW: low birth weight; E_2: estradiol; ET: embryo transfer.

TABLE 6: Very low birth weight and multiple logistic regression to account for confounding variables.

VLBW	Standard error	Adjusted OR (95% CI)	P
Age (<35 versus ≥35 years)	0.47	1.04 (0.17–6.30)	0.97
Duration of ovarian stimulation (<9 versus ≥9 days)	0.54	0.96 (0.19–5.44)	0.75
Gonadotropin dose (<2000 versus ≥2000 IU)	0.41	0.71 (0.44–6.56)	0.44
Peak E_2 level (<2000 versus ≥2000 pg/Ml)	0.19	0.81 (0.55–1.19)	0.29
Total number of oocytes (<10 versus ≥10)	0.26	0.98 (0.59–1.63)	0.94
Blastocyst-stage ET (yes versus no)	0.40	0.88 (0.36–2.17)	0.78

VLBW: very low birth weight; E_2: estradiol; ET: embryo transfer.

TABLE 7: Term low birth weight and multiple logistic regression to account for confounding variables.

Term LBW	Standard error	Adjusted OR (95% CI)	P
Age (<35 versus ≥35 years)	0.46	0.86 (0.59–7.80)	0.76
Duration of ovarian stimulation (<9 versus ≥9 days)	0.73	0.92 (0.35–3.08)	0.33
Gonadotropin dose (<2000 versus ≥2000 IU)	0.42	0.83 (0.44–6.09)	0.38
Peak E_2 level (<2000 versus ≥2000 pg/Ml)	0.32	0.92 (0.16–1.86)	0.48
Total number of oocytes (<10 versus ≥10)	0.39	0.94 (0.09–1.82)	0.25
Blastocyst-stage ET (yes versus no)	0.47	0.91 (0.28–3.83)	0.84

LBW: low birth weight; E_2: estradiol; ET: embryo transfer.

of survival of embryos to blastocyst-stage) and long-term outcomes (including live birth rates, multiple gestations, and perinatal outcomes). Despite improvements in extended culture and growing evidence to support greater use of blastocyst-stage ET, cleavage-stage ET is still utilized in the majority of IVF-ET cycles [2, 3].

Our study demonstrates that the incidence of early VT is lower in blastocyst-stage ET cycles compared to cleavage-stage ET cycles. However, the adverse perinatal risks of PTB, LBW, and VLBW associated with early VT syndrome are similar in patients undergoing cleavage-stage or blastocyst-stage ETs during fresh IVF cycles. Salient strengths of the current study include its large sample size and utilization of multiple logistic regression to account for several confounding variables. Despite these strengths, our study is not without limitations. First, though we attribute the perinatal risks seen in our population to early dizygotic twinning, the chorionicity of the pregnancies included in our study cohort was not evaluated. It is possible that monochorionic gestations, at least in part, may have contributed to the pathogenesis of the aforementioned perinatal risks. Second, given the retrospective nature of this study, we remain uncertain whether our findings would hold true in larger prospective settings.

While previous studies suggest that early VT syndrome confers increased perinatal risks in fresh IVF-ET cycles, out study emphasizes that these outcomes do not differ between cleavage- and blastocyst-stage ETs. It is important to note that the increased odds of LBW noted in our study are still significantly lower than the incidence of LBW associated with VT syndrome reported in previous publications [7–13]. While the stage of ET does not impact the perinatal risks associated with early VT, our study does highlight the need to perform single embryo transfers when possible to minimize adverse outcomes associated with the transfer of >1 embryo in IVF-ET cycles. Finally, patients with early VT syndrome should be counseled about potential perinatal risks. Ultrasonographic surveillance of the surviving twin to confirm adequate growth may be considered as a reasonable clinical strategy in such patients.

Competing Interests

The authors declare that they have no competing interests.

References

[1] S. Dyer, G. M. Chambers, J. de Mouzon et al., "International Committee for Monitoring Assisted Reproductive Technologies world report: assisted reproductive technology 2008, 2009 and 2010," *Human Reproduction*, vol. 31, no. 7, pp. 1588–1609, 2016.

[2] D. Glujovsky, D. Blake, C. Farquhar, and A. Bardach, "Cleavage stage versus blastocyst stage embryo transfer in assisted reproductive technology," *Cochrane Database of Systematic Reviews*, vol. 7, Article ID CD002118, 2012.

[3] D. Glujovsky and C. Farquhar, "Cleavage-stage or blastocyst transfer: what are the benefits and harms?" *Fertility and Sterility*, vol. 106, no. 2, pp. 244–250, 2016.

[4] S. Sunderam, D. M. Kissin, S. B. Crawford et al., "Centers for Disease Control and Prevention (CDC). Assisted reproductive technology surveillance-United States, 2013," *MMWR Surveillance Summaries*, vol. 64, no. 11, pp. 1–25, 2015.

[5] A. Pinborg, Ø. Lidegaard, N. la Cour Freiesleben, and A. N. Andersen, "Consequences of vanishing twins in IVF/ICSI pregnancies," *Human Reproduction*, vol. 20, no. 10, pp. 2821–2829, 2005.

[6] G. B. La Sala, M. T. Villani, A. Nicoli, A. Gallinelli, G. Nucera, and I. Blickstein, "Effect of the mode of assisted reproductive technology conception on obstetric outcomes for survivors of the vanishing twin syndrome," *Fertility and Sterility*, vol. 86, no. 1, pp. 247–249, 2006.

[7] R. Mansour, G. Serour, M. Aboulghar, O. Kamal, and H. Al-Inany, "The impact of vanishing fetuses on the outcome of ICSI pregnancies," *Fertility and Sterility*, vol. 94, no. 6, pp. 2430–2432, 2010.

[8] E. Evron, E. Sheiner, M. Friger, R. Sergienko, and A. Harlev, "Vanishing twin syndrome: is it associated with adverse perinatal outcome?" *Fertility and Sterility*, vol. 103, no. 5, pp. 1209–1214, 2015.

[9] B. Luke, M. B. Brown, D. A. Grainger, J. E. Stern, N. Klein, and M. I. Cedars, "The effect of early fetal losses on twin assisted-conception pregnancy outcomes," *Fertility and Sterility*, vol. 91, no. 6, pp. 2586–2592, 2009.

[10] A. Pinborg, Ø. Lidegaard, and A. N. Andersen, "The vanishing twin: a major determinant of infant outcome in IVF singleton births," *British Journal of Hospital Medicine*, vol. 67, no. 8, pp. 417–420, 2006.

[11] A. Pinborg, Ø. Lidegaard, N. C. Freiesleben, and A. N. Andersen, "Vanishing twins: a predictor of small-for-gestational age in IVF singletons," *Human Reproduction*, vol. 22, no. 10, pp. 2707–2714, 2007.

[12] B. Almog, I. Levin, I. Wagman et al., "Adverse obstetric outcome for the vanishing twin syndrome," *Reproductive BioMedicine Online*, vol. 20, no. 2, pp. 256–260, 2010.

[13] O. Shebl, T. Ebner, M. Sommergruber, A. Sir, and G. Tews, "Birth weight is lower for survivors of the vanishing twin syndrome: a case-control study," *Fertility and Sterility*, vol. 90, no. 2, pp. 310–314, 2008.

[14] D. Fernando, J. L. Halliday, S. Breheny, and D. L. Healy, "Outcomes of singleton births after blastocyst versus nonblastocyst transfer in assisted reproductive technology," *Fertility and Sterility*, vol. 97, no. 3, pp. 579–584, 2012.

[15] A. C. Petrini, N. Pereira, J. P. Lekovich, R. T. Elias, and S. D. Spandorfer, "Early spontaneous multiple fetal pregnancy reduction is associated with adverse perinatal outcomes in in vitro fertilization cycles," *Women's Health*, vol. 12, no. 4, pp. 420–426, 2016.

[16] J. Y. J. Huang and Z. Rosenwaks, "Assisted reproductive techniques," *Methods in Molecular Biology*, vol. 1154, pp. 171–231, 2014.

[17] G. D. Palermo, Q. V. Neri, P. N. Schlegel, and Z. Rosenwaks, "Intracytoplasmic Sperm Injection (ICSI) in extreme cases of male infertility," *PLoS ONE*, vol. 9, no. 12, Article ID e113671, 2014.

[18] L. V. Gosden, "Oocyte retrieval and quality evaluation," *Methods in Molecular Biology*, vol. 1154, pp. 343–360, 2014.

[19] D. K. Gardner and W. B. Schoolcraft, "In vitro culture of human blastocysts," in *Toward Reproductive Certainty: Fertility and Genetics Beyond*, R. Jansen and D. Mortimer, Eds., pp. 378–388, Parthenon, London, UK, 1999.

[20] N. Pereira, D. E. Reichman, D. E. Goldschlag, J. P. Lekovich, and Z. Rosenwaks, "Impact of elevated peak serum estradiol levels during controlled ovarian hyperstimulation on the birth weight of term singletons from fresh IVF-ET cycles," *Journal of Assisted Reproduction and Genetics*, vol. 32, no. 4, pp. 527–532, 2015.

[21] C. Y. Spong, B. M. Mercer, M. D'Alton, S. Kilpatrick, S. Blackwell, and G. Saade, "Timing of indicated late-preterm and early-term birth," *Obstetrics and Gynecology*, vol. 118, no. 2, part 1, pp. 323–333, 2011.

[22] G. R. Alexander, J. H. Himes, R. B. Kaufman, J. Mor, and M. Kogan, "A United States national reference for fetal growth," *Obstetrics and Gynecology*, vol. 87, no. 2 I, pp. 163–168, 1996.

[23] L. M. Hellman, M. Kobayashi, and E. Cromb, "Ultrasonic diagnosis of embryonic malformations," *American Journal of Obstetrics & Gynecology*, vol. 115, no. 5, pp. 615–623, 1973.

6

Mild Anemia and Pregnancy Outcome in a Swiss Collective

Gabriela Bencaiova and Christian Breymann

Division of Obstetrics, Department of Obstetrics and Gynecology, University Hospital of Zurich, Frauenklinikstrasse 10, 8091 Zurich, Switzerland

Correspondence should be addressed to Gabriela Bencaiova; benca@bluewin.ch

Academic Editor: Sinuhe Hahn

Background. Over half of all women in the world experience anemia during their pregnancy. Our aim was to investigate the relation between hemoglobin and iron status examined in second trimester and pregnancy outcome. *Methods.* In a prospective longitudinal study, 382 pregnant women were included. Blood samples were examined for hematological status and serum ferritin between 16 and 20 weeks and for hemoglobin before delivery. The adverse maternal and perinatal outcomes were determined. Regression analysis was performed to establish if anemia and low serum ferritin are risk factors for pregnancy complications. *Results.* There was no increase of complications in women with mild anemia and in women with depleted iron stores. The finding showed that mild iron deficiency anemia and depleted iron stores are not risk factors for adverse outcomes in iron supplemented women. *Conclusions.* Mild anemia and depleted iron stores detected early in pregnancy were not associated with adverse maternal and perinatal outcomes in iron supplemented women.

1. Introduction

Over half of all women in the world experience anemia during their pregnancy [1–4]. The association between the gestational age at which anemia is diagnosed and adverse pregnancy outcomes is an important issue [5, 6]. Some of the increase in anemia and iron deficiency anemia (IDA) with gestation is a consequence of the normal physiological changes of pregnancy [7]. To avoid the difficulties in anemia detection caused by plasma volume increase, the examination should be conducted until 20 weeks of gestation.

Findings from the studies on the relationship between anemia and adverse pregnancy outcome are contradictory. Several studies have shown that preterm delivery, small for gestational age, and low birth weight are increased for women with anemia during the 1st trimester and risk depends on the severity of the hemoglobin deficit [6, 8–11]. Women with hemoglobin between 8.0 and 9.9 g/dL had significantly higher risk for low birth weight, preterm birth, and small for gestational age than women with hemoglobin between 10.0 and 11.9 g/dL [12]. The observation by Scholl et al. showed that only iron deficiency anemia, not any other anemia, was related to preterm birth, which suggests that some iron specific mechanism may be at play [12].

Severe anemia is also associated with adverse maternal outcome and may contribute directly or indirectly to a significant proportion of maternal cardiac failure, hemorrhage, and infection. On the other hand, higher rates of placental problems (abnormal placentation and placental abruption) were found among the anemic women [13].

The aim of this study was to investigate the relationship between hemoglobin concentration and serum ferritin and adverse outcomes. The logistic regression analysis was performed to establish if anemia and low serum ferritin are risk factors for well-known adverse pregnancy outcome.

2. Methods

2.1. Study Population. A prospective longitudinal study was performed at the Department of Obstetrics, University Hospital of Zurich, to determine the relationship between hemoglobin concentration and serum ferritin and adverse outcome. The study was approved by the Human Research Ethics Committee at the Women's Hospital in Zurich.

The women were asked for their consent to participate in our study and the informed consent was obtained before study enrolment.

The hematological status and serum ferritin were examined in 382 pregnant women between 16 and 20 pregnancy weeks and hemoglobin concentration before delivery. All women were presented with singleton pregnancies. Exclusion criteria included chronic renal disease and malignancies and having a blood transfusion at least 3 months before enrolment in the study. Women with hemoglobin (Hb) between 10.0 and 11.0 g/dL received oral iron supplementation. Women with hemoglobin <10.0 g/dL were treated directly with intravenous iron in the anemia clinic if they agreed with intravenous therapy.

2.2. Study Criteria.
According to current guidelines based on recommendations of the CDC, anemia in pregnancy is defined by a hemoglobin value less than 11.0 g/dL in both the first and third trimesters and less than 10.5 g/dL in the second trimester [14]. On the basis of our experiences determining Hb (error of measurement of Hb ±0.5 g/dL) and the related high intraindividual variations, we chose Hb < 11.0 g/dL as the cut-off. Iron deficiency anemia was defined as Hb < 11.0 g/dL and a serum ferritin ≤ 15 μg/L. Depleted iron stores was defined as a serum ferritin < 20 μg/L. Anemia for other reasons was defined as Hb < 11.0 g/dL and ferritin > 15 μg/L. The category anemia for other reasons included the following: thalassemia and hemoglobinopathies, vitamin B12 deficiency anemia, folic acid deficiency anemia, and chronic inflammatory diseases (particularly HIV positive women, active hepatitis B).

The women were divided according to hemoglobin concentration and ferritin levels into women with iron deficiency anemia (Hb < 11.0 g/dL and ferritin ≤ 15 μg/L) (Group 1), women with depleted iron stores without anemia (Hb ≥ 11.0 g/dL and ferritin < 20 μg/L) (Group 2), women with anemia for other reasons (Hb < 11.0 g/dL and ferritin > 15 μg/L) (Group 3), and women with normal status (Group 4: control group).

2.3. Laboratory Assessment.
Blood samples were collected by venipuncture. Hb, red blood cells (RBC), hematocrit (HCT), mean corpuscular volume (MCV), percentage of red cells, microcytic, macrocytic, hypochromic, and hyperchromic erythrocytes, hemoglobin content of reticulocytes (CHr), and red blood cell distribution width (RDW) were measured using an ADVIA hematology analyser system (Bayer Diagnostics, Leverkusen, Germany). Mean corpuscular hemoglobin (MCH) was automatically calculated from Hb and RBC. Ferritin was assessed by chemiluminescence immunoassay (ACS 190; Ciba/Corning Diagnostic Corp., Cleveland, OH).

2.4. Maternal and Perinatal Outcomes.
Postpartum hemorrhage was defined as Hb decrease of more than 3.0 g/dL on the second day after delivery. Abnormal site of placental implantation (placenta praevia) and abnormal placental penetration (placenta accreta/increta/percreta) were described as abnormal placental invasion or abnormal placentation. Gestational age was determined on the basis of early ultrasound examination. Low birth weight (LBW) was defined as birth weight <2500 g. Preterm birth was defined as birth before 37 completed weeks of gestation. Preterm premature rupture of fetal membranes (PPROM) was defined as rupture of fetal membranes before 37 completed weeks of gestation. Intrauterine growth restriction (IUGR) was defined as birth weight below the sex-specific 5th percentile of weights for gestational age, decreased amniotic fluid volume, or abnormal Doppler. Macrosomia was defined as birth weight above the sex-specific 95th percentile of weights for gestational age.

The Statistical Package for the Social Sciences (SPSS) (Version 12.0.1. for Windows, SPSS Inc.) was used for all data analyses. Demographic characteristics were expressed as means (±standard deviation) and range. The outcome variables were expressed as the absolute number (percentage). P value was based on Fisher's exact test for categorical data and the Mann-Whitney U test for quantitative variables. Univariate logistic regression analysis was performed to compute odds ratios with 95% confidence intervals of women in Groups 1, 2, and 3 versus nonanemic women (Group 4) for well-known adverse maternal and perinatal outcomes. No correction for multiple testing was performed when comparing single groups with nonanemic women. Those P values are only descriptive.

3. Results

The demographic and clinical characteristics are shown in Table 1. Iron deficiency anemia was observed in 6.5%, depleted iron stores in 32.2%, and anemia for other reasons in 11.8%. The mean gestational age at study enrolment was 16.3 ± 1.4 weeks. The mean hemoglobin concentration at enrolment was 11.8 ± 0.9 g/dL and serum ferritin was 33.5 ± 27.8 μg/L. Out of 70 anemic women, only mild anemia was observed at enrolment. A higher parity was observed in women with iron deficiency anemia and with depleted iron stores (Table 1). Women in Groups 1, 2, and 3 came more often from former Yugoslavia and developing countries than women in Group 4 ($P = 0.001$).

The maternal outcomes are shown in Table 2. The mean hemoglobin level before delivery was 12.1 ± 1.2 g/dL (7.9–15.4). The prevalence of anemia before delivery was 9.7%, namely, mild anemia in 8.8% and moderate anemia in 0.9% (Hb < 9.0 g/dL). Although iron therapy was given in anemic women, a significantly lower Hb before delivery was observed in these women ($P = 0.001$). There was also a significant difference of hemoglobin concentration before delivery between women with depleted iron stores and normal women ($P = 0.005$). There was no increase of maternal complications in women with anemia and in women with depleted iron stores.

The mean gestational age at delivery was 38.7 ± 2.9 weeks (25–42) and birth weight was 3320 ± 646 g (730–5250) (Table 3). Preterm delivery was observed in 7.6% (29/382), low birth weight in 8.1% (31/382), and perinatal mortality in 0.5% (2/382). There was a significant difference of meconium stained amniotic fluid between women with

TABLE 1: Demographic and clinical characteristics.

(a)

	Group 1	Group 2	Group 3	Group 4	All women
Pregnant women	25/382 (6.5)	123/382 (32.2)	45/382 (11.8)	189/382 (49.5)	382
Maternal age (years)	30.3 ± 5.9 (21.2–38.7)	29.7 ± 5.7 (21.2–44.9)	30.1 ± 6.3 (20.2–41.9)	30.8 ± 5.9 (18.9–44.3)	30.3 ± 5.9 (18.9–44.9)
Gravidity	2.8 ± 1.8 (1–7)	2.4 ± 1.4 (1–7)	2.3 ± 1.5 (1–8)	2.3 ± 1.7 (1–14)	2.4 ± 1.6 (1–14)
=1	7/25 (28.0)	36/123 (29.2)	18/45 (40.0)	74/189 (39.2)	135/382 (35.3)
2–4	14/25 (56.0)	77/123 (62.6)	24/45 (53.3)	100/189 (52.9)	215/382 (56.3)
≥5	4/25 (16.0)	10/123 (8.2)	3/45 (6.7)	15/189 (7.9)	32/382 (8.4)
Parity	2.3 ± 1.3 (1–5)	1.9 ± 0.9 (1–5)	1.7 ± 0.8 (1–4)	1.7 ± 1.0 (1–6)	1.8 ± 0.9 (1–6)
=1	9/25 (36.0)	43/123 (35.0)	22/45 (48.9)	101/189 (53.4)	175/382 (45.8)
2–3	12/25 (48.0)	72/123 (58.5)	22/45 (48.9)	78/189 (41.3)	184/382 (48.2)
≥4	4/25 (16.0)	8/123 (6.5)	1/45 (2.2)	10/189 (5.3)	23/382 (6.1)
Gestational age at delivery (wk)	38.6 ± 2.3 (30–41)	38.9 ± 1.9 (29–42)	38.7 ± 1.8 (33–41)	38.7 ± 2.6 (25–42)	38.7 ± 2.9 (25–42)
<37	2/25 (8)	7/123 (5.7)	2/45 (4.4)	18/189 (9.5)	29/382 (7.6)
37–42	23/25 (92)	116/123 (94.3)	43/45 (95.6)	171/189 (90.5)	353/382 (92.4)
Gestational age at enrolment (wk)	16.3 ± 1.3 (15–19)	16.4 ± 1.3 (15–20)	16.4 ± 1.3 (15–19)	16.2 ± 1.2 (15–19)	16.3 ± 1.4 (15–20)
BMI (kg/m²)	22.9 ± 4.8 (18.2–35.5)	23.5 ± 5.5 (15.4–50.9)	24.1 ± 4.3 (17.6–32.6)	24.2 ± 5.1 (17.8–45.2)	23.9 ± 5.1 (15.4–50.9)
Origin of mother					
Europe + North America	2/25 (8.0)	37/123 (30.1)	7/45 (15.6)	76/189 (40.2)	122/382 (31.9)
Former Yugoslavia	12/28 (48.0)	49/123 (39.8)	16/45 (35.6)	50/189 (26.5)	127/382 (33.2)
Developing countries	11/25 (44.0)	37/123 (30.1)	22/45 (48.9)	63/189 (33.3)	133/382 (34.8)

Data expressed as mean ± s.d. (range) or number (%).

(b)

P value	1 versus 4	2 versus 4	3 versus 4	1, 2, and 3 versus 4
Maternal age	0.827	0.068	0.336	0.082
Gravidity	0.121	0.144	0.913	0.153
Parity	0.029*	0.005**	0.797	0.006*
Gestational age at delivery	0.633	0.687	0.485	0.919
BMI	0.19	0.383	0.941	0.31
Origin of mother	0.05	0.038*	0.008*	0.001**

*P value < 0.05; **P value < 0.005.
Group 1: iron deficiency anemia.
Group 2: depleted iron stores.
Group 3: anemia for other reasons.
Group 4: normal status.

depleted iron stores and nonanemic women (1/123 versus 14/189) (P = 0.006) (Table 3). No difference of low birth weight, IUGR, preterm delivery, or PPROM between anaemic and nonanemic women was ascertained. Macrosomia was more often in women with iron deficiency anemia and with depleted iron stores (16% and 11.4%).

The logistic regression analysis showed that anemia and depleted iron stores are not significant risk factors for adverse pregnancy outcome (Table 4). The upper limits of the 95% confidence intervals of the odds ratios for preterm delivery, LBW, IUGR, and caesarean section showed that mild anemia and depleted iron stores are not associated with those adverse outcomes in iron supplemented women. Placental abruption, abnormal placentation, and puerperal infection were too rare to draw any conclusions.

4. Discussion

The prevalence of anemia and depleted iron stores in the present study was 50.5% (193/382), namely, anemia in 18.3% (70/382) and depleted iron stores in 32.2% (123/382). Our results are in accordance with other studies performed in European countries [15]. A higher parity was observed in women with iron deficiency anemia and depleted iron stores.

TABLE 2: Maternal outcome (%).

(a)

	Group 1	Group 2	Group 3	Group 4	All women
Hb at delivery (g/dL)	10.9 ± 1.1 (8.8–12.7)	12.1 ± 1.2 (7.9–15.4)	11.3 ± 0.9 (9.1–12.9)	12.5 ± 0.9 (9.5–15.1)	12.1 ± 1.2 (7.9–15.4)
Placental abruption	0/25 (0.0)	1/123 (0.8)	0/45 (0.0)	1/189 (0.5)	2/382 (0.5)
Abnormal placentation	2/25 (8.0)	4/123 (3.3)	0/45 (0.0)	2/189 (1.1)	8/382 (2.1)
Preeclampsia, eclampsia	0/25 (0.0)	1/123 (0.8)	3/45 (6.7)	4/189 (2.1)	8/382 (2.1)
Cardiac failure	0/25 (0.0)	0/123 (0.0)	0/45 (0.0)	0/189 (0.0)	0/382 (0.0)
Delivery modus					
Nonoperative vaginal delivery	16/25 (64.0)	69/123 (56.1)	23/45 (51.1)	91/189 (48.1)	199/382 (52.1)
Operative vaginal delivery	1/25 (4.0)	9/123 (7.3)	3/45 (6.7)	31/189 (16.4)	44/382 (11.5)
Caesarean section prim.	6/25 (24.0)	25/123 (20.3)	14/45 (31.3)	37/189 (19.6)	82/382 (21.5)
Caesarean section sec.	2/25 (8.0)	20/123 (16.3)	5/45 (11.1)	30/189 (15.9)	57/382 (14.9)
Postpartum hemorrhage	1/25 (4.0)	7/123 (5.7)	6/45 (13.3)	21/189 (11.1)	35/382 (9.2)
Puerperal sepsis	0/25 (0.0)	0/123 (0.0)	0/45 (0.0)	0/189 (0.0)	0/382 (0.0)
Puerperal infection	0/25 (0.0)	6/123 (4.9)	1/45 (2.2)	6/189 (3.2)	13/382 (3.4)
Urinary tract infection	0/25 (0.0)	1/123 (0.8)	0/45 (0.0)	1/189 (0.5)	2/382 (0.5)
Wound infection	0/25 (0.0)	1/123 (0.8)	0/45 (0.0)	2/189 (1.1)	3/382 (0.8)
Mastitis	0/25 (0.0)	2/123 (1.6)	1/45 (2.2)	2/189 (1.1)	5/382 (1.3)
Endometritis	0/25 (0.0)	1/123 (0.8)	0/45 (0.0)	0/189 (0.0)	1/382 (0.3)
Thrombophlebitis	0/25 (0.0)	1/123 (0.8)	0/45 (0.0)	1/189 (0.5)	1/382 (0.3)
Infection of unclear etiology	0/25 (0.0)	1/123 (0.8)	0/45 (0.0)	0/189 (0.0)	1/382 (0.3)
Subinvolution	1/25 (4.0)	3/123 (2.4)	0/45 (0.0)	2/189 (1.1)	6/382 (1.6)

(b)

P value	1 versus 4	2 versus 4	3 versus 4	1, 2, and 3 versus 4
Hb at delivery	0.001***	0.005**	0.001***	0.001***
Placental abruption	1	1	1	1
Abnormal placentation	0.068	0.217	1	0.284
Preeclampsia, eclampsia	1	0.652	0.132	1
Delivery modus	0.211	0.125	0.157	0.021*
Postpartum hemorrhage	0.482	0.11	0.613	0.217
Puerperal infection	1	0.55	1	1
Subinvolution	0.312	0.386	1	0.685

*P value < 0.05; **P value < 0.005; ***P value < 0.001.

Depleted iron stores were higher in women from former Yugoslavia and anemia for other reasons in women from developing countries.

Mild anemia and depleted iron stores detected early in pregnancy were not associated with adverse outcomes in iron supplemented women. In our study, macrosomia was more often in nondiabetic women with iron deficiency anemia (16.0%). Early nonexcessive placental hyperplasia in women with mild anemia might lead to increased nutrition support in later pregnancy if a stress situation is experienced. To our knowledge, no studies exist observing the increased prevalence of macrosomia in women with iron deficiency anemia.

There is a lot of controversial information about anemia in pregnancy and adverse outcomes. Two points are important for assessment of this relationship: the gestational age at which the determination of hemoglobin is performed and the degree of anemia.

Hemoglobin and hematocrit decline due to physiologic expansion of the plasma volume throughout the 1st and 2nd trimesters [7]. Plasma volume expansion reaches its lowest point late in the second to early in the third trimester and then rises again nearer to term. It is thus becoming clear that the best time to detect any risk associated with maternal anemia may be early in pregnancy. This was also confirmed in the following current studies [10, 16]. Any estimation of hemoglobin concentration taken after 20 weeks' gestation will be reasonably representative of the fall induced by pregnancy [17]. The mean gestational age at enrolment in our study was 16 weeks.

The second important point is the degree of anemia in pregnancy. This is the reason why there is a lot of controversial information about the relationship between anemia and adverse outcomes. The extensive literature review presented strong evidence for an association between maternal hemoglobin and birth weight as well as between maternal

TABLE 3: Perinatal outcome (%).

(a)

	Group 1	Group 2	Group 3	Group 4	All women
Gestational age at delivery (wk)	38.6 ± 2.3	38.9 ± 1.9	38.7 ± 1.8	38.7 ± 2.6	38.7 ± 2.9 (25–42)
Birth weight (g)	3412 ± 605	3369 ± 625	3218 ± 546	3299 ± 687	3320 ± 646 (730–5250)
Meconium in amniotic fluid	3/25 (12.0)	1/123 (0.8)	3/45 (6.7)	14/189 (7.4)	21/382 (5.5)
LBW	2/25 (8.0)	7/123 (5.7)	3/45 (6.7)	19/189 (10.1)	31/382 (8.1)
IUGR	0/25 (0.0)	7/123 (5.7)	3/45 (6.7)	12/189 (6.3)	22/382 (5.8)
Macrosomia	4/25 (16.0)	14/123 (11.4)	0/45 (0.0)	15/189 (7.9)	33/382 (8.6)
Preterm delivery	2/25 (8.0)	7/123 (5.7)	2/45 (4.4)	18/189 (9.5)	29/382 (7.6)
PPROM	1/25 (4.0)	2/123 (1.6)	0/45 (0.0)	7/189 (3.7)	10/382 (2.6)
Still birth	0/25 (0.0)	0/123 (0.0)	1/45 (2.2)	0/189 (0.0)	1/382 (0.3)
Neonatal death	0/25 (0.0)	0/123 (0.0)	0/45 (0.0)	1/189 (0.5)	1/382 (0.3)
NICU admissions	0/25 (0.0)	0/123 (0.0)	0/45 (0.0)	1/189 (0.5)	1/382 (0.3)
Apgar score at 1'	8.1 ± 0.8 (6–9)	7.9 ± 0.9 (3–9)	7.9 ± 1.5 (0–10)	7.7 ± 1.3 (1–9)	7.9 ± 1.2 (0–10)
Apgar score at 5'	8.8 ± 0.7 (7–10)	9.0 ± 0.5 (7–10)	8.8 ± 1.5 (0–10)	8.9 ± 0.9 (3–10)	8.9 ± 0.9 (0–10)
Apgar score <5 at 5'	0/25 (0.0)	0/123 (0.0)	1/45 (2.2)	3/189 (1.6)	4/382 (1.0)

(b)

P value	1 versus 4	2 versus 4	3 versus 4	1, 2, and 3 versus 4
Meconium in amniotic fluid	0.428	0.006*	1	0.12
LBW	1	0.211	0.583	0.192
IUGR	0.368	1	1	0.666
Macrosomia	0.25	0.324	0.82	0.717
Preterm delivery	1	0.287	0.38	0.179
PPROM	1	0.491	0.351	0.216
Still birth	NoS	NoS	0.192	1
Neonatal death	1	1	1	0.495
NICU admissions	1	1	1	0.495
Apgar score <5 at 5'	1	0.281	0.577	0.368

*P value < 0.05.

NoS: no statistics are computed because variable is a constant.

TABLE 4: Logistic regression analysis of adverse outcomes among anemic women and women with depleted iron stores (Groups 1, 2, and 3) versus nonanemic women (Group 4).

Adverse outcome	Groups 1, 2, and 3 (n = 193)	Group 4 (n = 189)	O.R. (95% CI)	P value
Preterm delivery	11/193 (5.7)	18/189 (9.5)	0.58 (0.26–1.25)	0.162
LBW	12/193 (6.2)	19/189 (10.1)	0.59 (0.28–1.26)	0.174
IUGR	10/193 (5.2)	12/189 (6.4)	0.81 (0.34–1.91)	0.625
Caesarean section	72/193 (37.3)	67/189 (35.5)	0.92 (0.60–1.43)	0.75

hemoglobin and preterm delivery [18]. Mild anemia, which was present in our study, was not associated with adverse outcomes in iron supplemented women. Therefore, we assume that iron supplementation had a protective effect on adverse outcome. On the other hand, severe maternal anemia, particularly in the first trimester, is associated with adverse outcomes, namely, preterm birth, low birth weight, intrauterine growth restriction, low Apgar score, and operative deliveries [5, 9, 10, 16, 19, 20]. The association between the degree of anemia and adverse outcome was investigated by many studies, in which this association was confirmed [5, 9, 10, 21]. Extremely high maternal mortality (6.2%) and perinatal mortality (60%) were determined in the study by Patra et al., in which severe maternal anemia was determined in the third trimester [20].

A meta-analysis of studies on the association between hemoglobin concentration and adverse outcome, conducted between 1985 and 1998, showed that maternal anemia during early pregnancy is associated with slightly increased preterm delivery but not with significantly increased low birth weight or with fetal growth restriction [16]. This meta-analysis did not consider the degree of anemia nor did it use different parameters for the definition of anemia. Generally, the hematological parameters and criteria for anemia differ widely. Some authors use hematocrit <33% as criteria for anemia [22], and others use hemoglobin concentration with a different cut-off, namely, less than 11.0 g/dL, 10.5, or 10.0 g/dL [5, 6, 8–10, 17, 19]. We defined anemia as hemoglobin concentration of 11.0 g/dL or less, since we previously saw high intraindividual variations between Hb 10.5 and 11.0 g/dL and there was a large group of women with hemoglobin between 10.5 and 10.9 g/dL (39/382; 10.2%).

The limitation of our study is the absence of CRP determination, since ferritin is a marker of inflammation. Consequently, high serum ferritin could actually be a false positive in patients with inflammation. The second disadvantage is the lack of any comparison of our results with an untreated group of anemic women. However, if we compare our results with other studies, we can say that iron supplementation had a protective effect on adverse pregnancy outcome. Since we wished to simulate normal supplementation, the women did not have to return any residual supplementation. Thus, compliance was not monitored in this study.

Systematic iron prophylaxis and iron-folic acid supplementation during pregnancy has been debated [23–26]. The first choice in the prophylaxis of iron deficiency anemia for almost all women is oral iron replacement because of its effectiveness, safety, and low cost [24]. However, in practice, physicians are frequently faced with poor compliance, which can lead to anemia. The second choice is intravenous iron supplementation with no drug-related serious adverse effects [25]. The commonly cited disadvantages of intravenous iron supplementation are high cost and the invasive nature of the procedure.

We recommend screening for hemoglobin and iron status in early pregnancy. When there is a good compliance with iron supplementation and the pregnancy is uncomplicated, there is no need for hematological tests during further prenatal visits, even in cases of mild iron deficiency anemia and depleted iron stores detected in early pregnancy. One clear set of hematological test results early in pregnancy indicates that there is no increased risk of adverse maternal and perinatal outcomes due to mild iron deficiency anemia and depleted iron stores in iron supplemented women; further testing later in pregnancy is therefore superfluous.

5. Conclusions

Mild anemia and depleted iron stores detected early in pregnancy were not associated with adverse maternal and perinatal outcomes.

Conflict of Interests

The authors declare that there is no conflict of interests regarding the publication of this paper.

References

[1] E. DeMaeyer and M. Adiels-Tegman, "The prevalence of anaemia in the world," *World Health Statistics Quarterly*, vol. 38, no. 3, pp. 302–316, 1985.

[2] T. O. Scholl, "Iron status during pregnancy: setting the stage for mother and infant," *The American Journal of Clinical Nutrition*, vol. 81, no. 5, pp. 1218S–1222S, 2005.

[3] A. C. Looker, P. R. Dallman, M. D. Carroll, E. W. Gunter, and C. L. Johnson, "Prevalence of iron deficiency in the United States," *The Journal of the American Medical Association*, vol. 277, no. 12, pp. 973–976, 1997.

[4] F. E. Viteri, "The consequences of iron deficiency and anaemia in pregnancy on maternal health, the foetus and the infant," *SCN News*, no. 11, pp. 14–18, 1994.

[5] L.-M. Zhou, W.-W. Yang, J.-Z. Hua, C.-Q. Deng, X. Tao, and R. J. Stoltzfus, "Relation of hemoglobin measured at different times in pregnancy to preterm birth and low birth weight in Shanghai, China," *American Journal of Epidemiology*, vol. 148, no. 10, pp. 998–1006, 1998.

[6] H. Hämäläinen, K. Hakkarainen, and S. Heinonen, "Anaemia in the first but not in the second or third trimester is a risk factor for low birth weight," *Clinical Nutrition*, vol. 22, no. 3, pp. 271–275, 2003.

[7] M. F. McMullin, R. White, T. Lappin, J. Reeves, and G. MacKenzie, "Haemoglobin during pregnancy: relationship to erythropoietin and haematinic status," *European Journal of Haematology*, vol. 71, no. 1, pp. 44–50, 2003.

[8] F. W. Lone, R. N. Qureshi, and F. Emmanuel, "Maternal anaemia and its impact on perinatal outcome in a tertiary care hospital in Pakistan," *Eastern Mediterranean Health Journal*, vol. 10, no. 6, pp. 801–807, 2004.

[9] M. Malhotra, J. B. Sharma, S. Batra, S. Sharma, N. S. Murthy, and R. Arora, "Maternal and perinatal outcome in varying degrees of anemia," *International Journal of Gynecology & Obstetrics*, vol. 79, no. 2, pp. 93–100, 2002.

[10] A. Levy, D. Fraser, M. Katz, M. Mazor, and E. Sheiner, "Maternal anemia during pregnancy is an independent risk factor for low birthweight and preterm delivery," *European Journal of Obstetrics & Gynecology and Reproductive Biology*, vol. 122, no. 2, pp. 182–186, 2005.

[11] V. R. Lops, L. P. Hunter, and L. R. Dixon, "Anemia in pregnancy," *American Family Physician*, vol. 51, no. 5, pp. 1189–1197, 1995.

[12] T. O. Scholl, M. L. Hediger, R. L. Fischer, and J. W. Shearer, "Anemia vs iron deficiency: increased risk of preterm delivery in a prospective study," *The American Journal of Clinical Nutrition*, vol. 55, no. 5, pp. 985–988, 1992.

[13] A. F. Fleming, "Maternal anemia and fetal outcome in pregnancies complicated by thalassemia minor and "stomatocytosis"," *American Journal of Obstetrics and Gynecology*, vol. 116, no. 3, pp. 309–319, 1973.

[14] Centers for Disease Control, "CDC criteria for anaemia in children and childbearing-aged women," *Morbidity and Mortality Weekly Report*, vol. 38, pp. 400–404, 1989.

[15] S. Hercberg, P. Preziosi, and P. Galan, "Iron deficiency in Europe," *Public Health Nutrition*, vol. 4, no. 2, pp. 537–545, 2001.

[16] X. Xiong, P. Buekens, S. Alexander, N. Demianczuk, and E. Wollast, "Anemia during pregnancy and birth outcome: a meta-analysis," *American Journal of Perinatology*, vol. 17, no. 3, pp. 137–146, 2000.

[17] P. Steer, M. A. Alam, J. Wadsworth, and A. Welch, "Relation between maternal haemoglobin concentration and birth weight

in different ethnic groups," *British Medical Journal*, vol. 310, no. 6978, pp. 489–491, 1995.

[18] K. M. Rasmussen, "Is there a causal relationship between iron deficiency or iron-deficiency anemia and weight at birth, length of gestation and perinatal mortality?" *Journal of Nutrition*, vol. 131, no. 2, pp. 590S–601S, 2001.

[19] O. I. Fareh, D. E. E. Rizk, L. Thomas, and B. Berg, "Obstetric impact of anaemia in pregnant women in United Arab Emirates," *Journal of Obstetrics & Gynaecology*, vol. 25, no. 5, pp. 440–444, 2005.

[20] S. Patra, S. Pasrija, S. S. Trivedi, and M. Puri, "Maternal and perinatal outcome in patients with severe anemia in pregnancy," *International Journal of Gynecology and Obstetrics*, vol. 91, no. 2, pp. 164–165, 2005.

[21] K. S. Scanlon, R. Yip, L. A. Schieve, and M. E. Cogswell, "High and low hemoglobin levels during pregnancy: differential risks for preterm birth and small for gestational age," *Obstetrics & Gynecology*, vol. 96, no. 5, pp. 741–748, 2000.

[22] G. T. Bondevik, R. T. Lie, M. Ulstein, and G. Kvale, "Maternal hematological status and risk of low birth weight and preterm delivery in Nepal," *Acta Obstetricia et Gynecologica Scandinavica*, vol. 80, no. 5, pp. 402–408, 2001.

[23] A. Kumar, S. Jain, N. P. Singh, and T. Singh, "Oral versus high dose parenteral iron supplementation in pregnancy," *International Journal of Gynecology and Obstetrics*, vol. 89, no. 1, pp. 7–13, 2005.

[24] N. Milman, "Iron prophylaxis in pregnancy—general or individual and in which dose?" *Annals of Hematology*, vol. 85, no. 12, pp. 821–828, 2006.

[25] R. M. Schaefer, R. Huch, A. Krafft et al., "The iron letter—an update on the treatment of iron deficiency anemia," *Praxis*, vol. 95, no. 10, pp. 357–364, 2006.

[26] T. G. Sanghvi, P. W. J. Harvey, and E. Wainwright, "Maternal iron-folic acid supplementation programs: evidence of impact and implementation," *Food and Nutrition Bulletin*, vol. 31, no. 2, pp. S100–S107, 2010.

7

Postpartum Visit Attendance Increases the Use of Modern Contraceptives

Saba W. Masho,[1,2,3] **Susan Cha,**[2] **RaShel Charles,**[1] **Elizabeth McGee,**[4] **Nicole Karjane,**[3] **Linda Hines,**[5] **and Susan G. Kornstein**[1,3,6]

[1]*Virginia Commonwealth University Institute of Women's Health, P.O. Box 980319, Richmond, VA 23298, USA*
[2]*Division of Epidemiology, Department of Family Medicine and Population Health, Virginia Commonwealth University, 830 E. Main Street, P.O. Box 980212, Richmond, VA 23298, USA*
[3]*Department of Obstetrics and Gynecology, Virginia Commonwealth University School of Medicine, P.O. Box 980034, Richmond, VA 23298, USA*
[4]*Division of Reproductive Endocrinology & Infertility, Department of Obstetrics, Gynecology and Reproductive Sciences, The University of Vermont College of Medicine, Smith 410, Main Campus, 111 Colchester Avenue, Burlington, VT 05401, USA*
[5]*Virginia Premier Health Plan, Inc., 600 E. Broad Street, 4th Floor, Suite 400, Richmond, VA 23219, USA*
[6]*Department of Psychiatry, Virginia Commonwealth University School of Medicine, 1200 E. Broad Street, P.O. Box 980710, Richmond, VA 23298, USA*

Correspondence should be addressed to Saba W. Masho; saba.masho@vcuhealth.org

Academic Editor: Fabio Facchinetti

Background. Delays in postpartum contraceptive use may increase risk for unintended or rapid repeat pregnancies. The postpartum care visit (PPCV) is a good opportunity for women to discuss family planning options with their health care providers. This study examined the association between PPCV attendance and modern contraceptive use using data from a managed care organization. *Methods.* Claims and demographic and administrative data came from a nonprofit managed care organization in Virginia (2008–2012). Information on the most recent delivery for mothers with singleton births was analyzed ($N = 24,619$). Routine PPCV (yes, no) and modern contraceptive use were both dichotomized. Descriptive analyses provided percentages, frequencies, and means. Multiple logistic regression was conducted and ORs and 95% CIs were calculated. *Results.* More than half of the women did not attend their PPCV (50.8%) and 86.9% had no modern contraceptive use. After controlling for the effects of confounders, women with PPCV were 50% more likely to use modern contraceptive methods than women with no PPCV (OR = 1.50, 95% CI = 1.31, 1.72). *Conclusions.* These findings highlight the importance of PPCV in improving modern contraceptive use and guide health care policy in the effort of reducing unintended pregnancy rates.

1. Introduction

Unintended pregnancy is a major public health problem in the US. According to a recent study analyzing data from the National Survey of Family Growth, in 2008, over half (51%) of the 6.6 million pregnancies in the US were unintended [1]. Additionally, a report using data from the National Survey of Family Growth that compared the proportion of US unintended pregnancies between 1982 and 2006–2010 found no significant improvements in the rates of unintended pregnancies over this extended time period [2]. Moreover, despite the availability of effective modern contraceptive methods, the rate of unintended pregnancies increased from 48% in 2001 to 51% in 2008 [1].

Unintended pregnancies are major public health concerns with potential detrimental effects on the health and wellbeing of infants, mothers, and society as a whole. Unintended pregnancy is associated with delayed prenatal care, smoking or drinking during pregnancy, preterm birth and low birth weight, poor attitudes towards parenting, poor infant development, and poor mother-infant relationships [3–6]. These levy a heavy burden on both state and federal economies. For instance, in 2010, total government expenditures on unintended pregnancies amounted to $21.0 billion, accounting for more than half of the $40.8 billion spent on all publicly funded pregnancies in 2010 [7].

Most women and couples want to have control over the timing and spacing of their childbearing for both economic and social reasons [8, 9]. The postpartum care visit (PPCV) is a good opportunity for patients and their significant others to have important conversations about family planning with their health care providers. The PPCV also allows providers to give necessary counseling and resources to women. Fundamentally, the best way of preventing unintended pregnancies is to provide women with an effective modern contraceptive method, which can be done through contraceptive counseling at a routine PPCV.

Delays in postpartum contraceptive use create a risky environment for women to have unintended or rapid repeat pregnancies [10, 11]. Although ovulation can occur within six weeks after delivery, it can occur as early as four weeks in nonbreastfeeding women [11]. Therefore, providing women with modern contraceptive methods shortly after they give birth is an effective way of curtailing the risk of an unintended pregnancy.

Some studies have shown the beneficial impact of PPCV attendance on greater contraceptive use [12–14] and reduced likelihood of rapid repeat pregnancy [15, 16] in select subgroups of women. Even women with no insurance or Medicaid were found to increase their use of an effective method after delivery if they attended counseling sessions [14]. However, the results did not account for important factors that could have affected postnatal services such as substance use or mental health problems (e.g., depression). Moreover, receipt of counseling was based on self-report data and did not necessarily indicate PPCV compliance or attendance. The fact remains that the PPCV is part of the standards of care for postpartum women and presents a suitable opportunity for contraceptive counseling. Strategies designed to reduce high rates of unintended pregnancies would benefit from targeting the postpartum period since women's opinions of subsequent pregnancies change over time [10].

The purpose of this study is to examine the association between PPCV attendance and the use of modern contraceptives among women who received care from a nonprofit managed care organization in the state of Virginia. These findings could provide a better understanding of the influence of the PPCV on modern contraceptive use and guide health care policy in the effort of reducing unintended pregnancy rates.

2. Materials and Methods

Data came from Virginia Premier, a managed care organization that coordinates health care services for low-income individuals enrolled in Virginia Medicaid. Claims and demographic and administrative information were available for women with singleton births between the years of 2008 to 2012. Information on the most recent birth was analyzed for mothers who gave birth to more than one infant during the study period. Thus, the total sample size was comprised of 24,619 women. This study was approved by the Virginia Commonwealth University Institutional Review Board.

The demographic dataset included information on maternal characteristics such as age, race, and region of residence. The birth event dataset included birthing information, such as delivery date, delivery type (vaginal, C-section), gestational age, and birth weight of infant, as well as NICU status and length of stay. Medical claims data were also included and provided the International Classification of Diseases, Ninth Revision (ICD-9) codes used to determine postpartum visit attendance, pregnancy complications, and substance abuse. Additionally, interview data was collected by case managers during both prenatal and postpartum period for clinical administrative purposes. These consisted of personal information such as education level, primary language spoken, smoking status, alcohol use, breastfeeding intention during pregnancy and actual feeding method (i.e., breastfeeding, bottle feeding, or both), depression, and birth control use, as well as the instances and types of case management.

The exposure of interest, PPCV attendance, came from medical claims data containing ICD-9-Clinical Modification (ICD-9-CM) for medical diagnoses and procedures on claims for services. Postpartum care and evaluation at the follow-up visit were determined by an ICD-9 code for routine postpartum follow-up (V24.2). This information was categorized as "yes" or "no."

The outcome, modern contraceptive use, came from the interview data which were collected by case managers for clinical administrative purposes. Women who reported using any modern contraceptive methods such as "birth control pill," "Depo-Provera," "Norplant," "patch," "ring," "IUD" (i.e., intrauterine device), "condoms and foam," and "diaphragm" were classified as "users." Those who did not indicate the use of any methods were considered "nonusers."

Sociodemographic factors included maternal age (≤20 years; 21–29 years; ≥30 years), race/ethnicity (White; Black; Hispanic; other), and the highest educational level (less than high school; high school graduate; greater than high school). Maternal region of residence in Virginia was categorized into seven regions: Danville/Lynchburg, Far Southwest, Fredericksburg, Richmond, Roanoke, Tidewater, and Western. Location of the majority of medical services was defined as the type of health care system most utilized by each individual patient (private office; hospital; health department; or federally qualified health centers (FQHC)). This was based on the total number of visits to each health care setting calculated for each woman. Substance use and mental health problems included tobacco use disorder (yes, no), drug abuse/dependence (yes, no), alcohol abuse/dependence (yes, no), and history of depression (yes, no). Pregnancy complications including preeclampsia, eclampsia, hypertension, diabetes, anemia, cervical incompetence, ectopic pregnancy, uterine inertia, premature separation of placenta, and placenta previa (yes; no), type of delivery (normal vaginal, caesarean section), and birth outcomes (normal weight and term; normal weight and preterm; low birth weight and term; low birth weight and preterm), where preterm birth was defined as gestational age of <37 weeks and low birth weight was defined as <2500 grams, were also assessed.

Descriptive analyses were conducted and percentages, frequencies, and means were reported. Bivariate analysis was conducted to examine factors associated with attending a PPCV or modern contraceptive use. To adjust for potential confounders, multivariable logistic regression was conducted and odds ratios (OR) and 95% confidence intervals (CIs) were calculated. Potential confounders were identified and included in the model if the variable resulted in a 10% or greater change in the estimate.

3. Results

The average age of the study population was 24.9 (standard deviation = 5.3) years. The majority of the women were 21–29 years of age (59.8%), had high school education (51.4), used hospitals for the majority of their medical services (87.3%), had normal vaginal deliveries (67.8%), and delivered their babies at normal weight and term (86.7%) (Table 1). Nearly half (49.3%) of the women attended their postpartum visit and 86.9% had no recorded modern contraceptive use.

Factors associated with modern contraceptive use included sociodemographic factors (i.e., age, race, location of majority of services, and region of residence in Virginia; $p < 0.0001$), health behavioral factors (i.e., tobacco use, $p = 0.0010$; drug abuse/dependence, $p = 0.0140$), and pregnancy complications ($p = 0.0202$). Specifically, modern contraceptive users included a greater proportion of women who were aged 20 years or younger and Black or Hispanic. Importantly, a greater proportion of modern contraceptive users attended their PPCV (57.1%) compared to nonusers (48.1%, $p < 0.0001$). Moreover, there was a significant difference in the distribution of region of residence for women who used modern contraceptives and those who did not. Specifically, a greater proportion of women who used contraception resided in highly populated urban regions than women who did not use contraception (Richmond, 17.4% versus 14.3%; Roanoke, 31.1% versus 28.8%). A greater proportion of nonusers resided in regions with smaller populations than women who used contraception (Danville/Lynchburg, 10.3% versus 8.8%; Fredericksburg, 6.8% versus 6.1%).

More than half of the women who were ≤20 years of age (50.0%), Black (50.9%), and highly educated (54.9%) attended their postpartum visits (Table 2). Women who received most of their medical services from a hospital or health department/FQHC had significantly increased odds of attending their postpartum visits than women who utilized mostly health services from private offices (COR [crude odds ratio] = 1.36, 95% CI = 1.24–1.50; COR = 1.99, 95% CI = 1.72–2.30, resp.). Likewise, compared to women from Fredericksburg, those who lived in areas with greater poverty were more likely to attend their postpartum visit, for example, Danville/Lynchburg, Western, and Richmond. In fact, women from Danville/Lynchburg were nearly three times as likely to attend postpartum visits (COR = 3.32, 95% CI = 2.92–3.79). Additionally, women with a history of depression were more likely to attend their postpartum visits when compared with women with no history of depression (COR = 1.13, 95% CI = 1.02–1.24). In terms of health behavioral factors, tobacco users and those diagnosed with drug abuse/dependence were less likely to attend their postpartum visits than nonusers and women not diagnosed with drug abuse/dependence (OR = 0.83, 95% CI = 0.78–0.88; OR = 0.67, 95% CI = 0.60–0.74, resp.). Women who experienced pregnancy complications had 1.23 times the odds of attending their postpartum visit compared with women with no complications during pregnancy (COR = 1.23, 95% CI = 1.17–1.30). There were no significant differences in postpartum visit attendance between women with normal vaginal delivery and women with C-sections. Moreover, when considering birth outcomes, women who delivered infants that were both of low birth weight and preterm were significantly less likely to attend their postpartum visit than women who delivered infants that were of normal weight and term (Table 2).

A significant association between postpartum visit attendance and modern contraceptive use was observed (Table 3). Women who attended their postpartum visit were 44% more likely to use postpartum contraception compared to women with no postpartum visit (OR = 1.44, 95% CI = 1.33–1.55). No covariate changed the estimate by 10% or greater; therefore, the unadjusted model was retained. Nonetheless, estimates remained robust and statistically significant even after controlling for age, race, education, location of majority of services, region of residence, tobacco use, drug abuse/dependence, alcohol abuse/dependence, history of depression, pregnancy complications, method of delivery, and birth outcomes (AOR [adjusted odds ratio] = 1.50, 95% CI = 1.31–1.72). In other words, women attending postpartum visits were 50% more likely to use modern contraceptive methods than women who did not attend their postpartum visit (Table 3).

4. Discussion

Despite the majority of the study population having no postpartum modern contraceptive use, women were 50% more likely to use contraception after delivery if they attended a postpartum appointment compared to those who did not attend their PPCV. This was independent of sociodemographic factors, substance use, depression, and pregnancy or birth complications.

Findings from the current study suggest that the period following childbirth is a crucial and opportune time for new mothers receiving publicly funded health care services to get insurance coverage for contraception and counseling and guidance on effective methods to avoid unintended and rapid repeat pregnancy [17, 18]. For example, Thiel de Bocanegra et al. examined health records for Medicaid recipients in California ($n = 117,644$) and reported that although only 41% had a modern contraceptive claim within 90 days of giving birth, receipt of contraception at the first postpartum clinic visit was significantly associated with avoiding another pregnancy within 6 and 18 months of a previous live birth (AOR = 1.63, 95% CI = 1.49, 1.80; AOR = 1.57, 95% CI = 1.50, 1.65, resp.) [17]. Recognizing the importance of postpartum care, the American Academy of Pediatrics and the American College of Obstetricians and Gynecologists recommend that new mothers have a checkup four to six weeks after delivery [19].

TABLE 1: Distribution of population characteristics by postpartum contraceptive use.

	Contraceptive use		Total population $N = 24{,}619$	χ^2	p value
	Yes $N = 3{,}232$	No $N = 21{,}387$			
	Column %				
Age				84.43	<0.0001
≤20 years	26.1	21.6	22.2		
21–29 years	61.2	59.6	59.8		
≥30 years	12.7	18.8	18.0		
Race				52.49	<0.0001
White	51.6	56.2	55.7		
Black	28.3	25.1	25.5		
Hispanic	5.6	3.0	3.3		
Other	14.5	15.7	15.5		
Education				0.90	0.6388
<High school	19.2	19.4	19.3		
High school	50.9	51.8	51.4		
>High school	29.9	28.8	29.3		
Location of majority of services				23.32	<0.0001
Private	5.9	7.9	7.7		
Hospital	89.9	86.9	87.3		
Health department/FQHC	4.3	5.2	5.1		
Region of residence in Virginia				107.36	<0.0001
Danville/Lynchburg	8.8	10.3	10.1		
Far Southwest	0.9	3.9	3.5		
Fredericksburg	6.1	6.8	6.7		
Richmond	17.4	14.3	14.7		
Roanoke	31.1	28.8	29.1		
Tidewater	17.4	18.6	18.4		
Western	18.3	17.4	17.5		
Tobacco use	24.7	27.5	27.1	10.88	0.0010
Drug abuse/dependence	5.0	6.1	6.0	6.04	0.0140
Alcohol abuse/dependence	1.0	1.0	1.0	0.08	0.7831
History of depression	7.3	6.6	6.7	2.12	0.1454
Pregnancy complications	42.4	40.3	40.6	5.39	0.0202
Delivery				2.11	0.1463
Normal vaginal	68.9	67.6	67.8		
C-section	31.1	32.4	32.2		
Birth outcomes				6.79	0.0787
Normal weight & term	88.1	86.5	86.7		
Normal weight & preterm	3.3	3.9	3.9		
Low birth weight & term	3.2	3.6	3.6		
Low birth weight & preterm	5.5	6.0	5.9		
Postpartum visit attendance				91.28	<0.0001
Yes	57.1	48.1	49.3		
No	42.9	51.9	50.8		

FQHC: federally qualified health centers; g: grams; wks: weeks. Normal weight: ≥2500 grams; low birth weight: <2500 grams; term: ≥37 weeks; preterm: <37 weeks.

TABLE 2: Factors associated with postpartum visit attendance.

	Postpartum visit (row %)	Crude OR (95% CI)
Age		
≤20 years	50.0	1.00
21–29 years	49.4	0.97 (0.92–1.04)
≥30 years	48.0	0.92 (0.85–1.00)
Race		
White	49.6	1.00
Black	50.9	1.05 (0.98–1.13)
Hispanic	48.7	0.97 (0.82–1.16)
Other	48.9	0.97 (0.88–1.05)
Education		
<High school	51.8	0.88 (0.76–1.03)
High school	54.3	0.98 (0.87–1.10)
>High school	54.9	1.00
Location of majority of services		
Private	41.9	1.00
Hospital	49.5	1.36 (1.24–1.50)*
Health department/FQHC	58.9	1.99 (1.72–2.30)*
Region of residence in Virginia		
Danville/Lynchburg	70.2	3.32 (2.92–3.79)*
Far Southwest	48.6	1.33 (1.13–1.57)*
Fredericksburg	41.5	1.00
Richmond	49.4	1.38 (1.23–1.55)*
Roanoke	45.0	1.16 (1.04–1.29)
Tidewater	42.8	1.05 (0.94–1.18)
Western	54.1	1.66 (1.48–1.86)
Tobacco use		
No	50.5	1.00
Yes	45.8	0.83 (0.78–0.88)
Drug abuse/dependence		
No	49.9	1.00
Yes	39.9	0.67 (0.60–0.74)
Alcohol abuse/dependence		
No	49.3	1.00
Yes	44.7	0.83 (0.65–1.07)
History of depression		
No	49.1	1.00
Yes	52.0	1.13 (1.02–1.24)
Pregnancy complications		
No	47.2	1.00
Yes	52.3	1.23 (1.17–1.30)
Delivery		
Normal vaginal	49.3	1.00
C-section	49.4	1.00 (0.95–1.06)
Birth outcomes		
Normal weight & term	49.6	1.00
Normal weight & preterm	49.8	1.01 (0.89–1.15)
Low birth weight & term	46.8	0.89 (0.78–1.02)
Low birth weight & preterm	45.7	0.86 (0.77–0.95)

OR: odds ratio; CI: confidence interval; FQHC: federally qualified health centers; g: grams; wks: weeks. Normal weight: ≥2500 grams; low birth weight: <2500 grams; term: ≥37 weeks; preterm: <37 weeks. *$p < 0.05$.

TABLE 3: Association between postpartum visit attendance and contraceptive use.

	[a]OR (95% CI)	[b]OR (95% CI)
Postpartum visit	[*]1.44 (1.33–1.55)	[*]1.50 (1.31–1.72)
No postpartum visit	1.00	1.00

OR: odds ratio; CI: confidence interval.
[a]No factor changed the estimate by 10% or greater.
[b]Fully adjusted model controlling for age, race, education, location of majority of services, region of residence, tobacco use, drug abuse/dependence, alcohol abuse/dependence, history of depression, pregnancy complications, delivery, and birth outcomes.
[*]Statistically significant.

Extant literature supports the results from our study in that patients who do not attend their PPCV are less likely to use contraception or effective methods (e.g., long-acting reversible contraception or LARC) [12–17, 20, 21]. For instance, DePiñeres et al. examined factors associated with postpartum contraception using self-report data from New Mexico PRAMS (1998-1999). Women aged 35 years or more, unmarried and lacking a postpartum visit, had increased risk of no postpartum contraception [21]. Specifically, the odds of postpartum modern contraceptive use were nearly threefold greater in women who reported attending their PPCV than in those who did not attend (AOR = 3.06, 95% CI = 2.17, 4.31) [21]. Likewise, a recent study that assessed women's barriers to receiving LARC in the postpartum period reported common reasons for nonuse being having to come back for another insertion visit (45%) and being unable to afford LARC methods (11%) [20]. Moreover, women who were interested in but not using LARC were more likely to have missed their postpartum visit compared to women using effective methods ($p = 0.001$) [20]. This can be especially problematic when nearly half of the women resume sexual intercourse within six weeks of giving birth, regardless of lactation or delivery method [18]. As such, a delay in effective modern contraceptive method initiation can be detrimental for women of low income or with high-risk pregnancies.

Focused contraceptive counseling and education by health providers is essential to improve women's reproductive health and postnatal care. In a qualitative study comprised of postpartum, urban, and minority women, participants showed preference for frequent contraceptive counseling sessions throughout pregnancy, with reinforcement and reevaluation of decisions after delivery [22]. Thus, public health strategies seeking to reduce high rates of unintended pregnancies should include the postpartum period since women's opinions of subsequent pregnancies change over time [10] and the PPCV is already an important standard of care for postpartum women.

This study was strengthened by the use of claims data rather than self-report data to ensure more objective measures of key variables of interest such as contraception and PPCV. We also considered a myriad of factors that could affect women's use of contraception or attendance such as sociodemographic characteristics, health behaviors, history of depression, and pregnancy/birth outcomes. The focus on a high-risk population receiving publicly funded health care services can provide more useful information on areas to improve in health care delivery and intervention efforts. Nonetheless, there were some study limitations. The dataset did not contain information on the quality of patient-provider interaction during PPCVs (e.g., topics covered, duration of visit, and communication style) that would be better assessed in qualitative studies [23]. Additionally, confounding factors such as breastfeeding were not assessed due to lack of complete data. We were also unable to ascertain whether certain modern contraceptive methods that were claimed under the insurance (e.g., birth control pills, barrier methods) were actually used.

5. Conclusions

In conclusion, among women with Medicaid, those who attended a postpartum visit were 50% more likely to use a modern contraceptive method after delivery. The postpartum visit is an apt setting for health providers to educate women on family planning options to ensure proper birth spacing and prevent unintended or rapid repeat pregnancies. Reducing barriers for access to and use of PPCV is greatly needed in low-income women or other vulnerable populations who face additional challenges with unstable housing, transportation barriers, and language barriers [24]. Future studies are needed to evaluate effective components of care (e.g., multiple counseling sessions) and patient-provider communication.

Competing Interests

The authors declare that there are no competing interests regarding the publication of this paper.

Acknowledgments

This study was funded by Virginia Premier Health Plan, Inc.

References

[1] L. B. Finer and M. R. Zolna, "Shifts in intended and unintended pregnancies in the United States, 2001–2008," *American Journal of Public Health*, vol. 104, supplement 1, pp. S43–S48, 2014.

[2] W. D. Mosher, J. Jones, and J. C. Abma, "Intended and unintended births in the United States: 1982–2010," *National Health Statistics Reports*, no. 55, pp. 1–28, 2012.

[3] J. P. Mayer, "Unintended childbearing, maternal beliefs, and delay of prenatal care," *Birth*, vol. 24, no. 4, pp. 247–252, 1997.

[4] J. S. Barber, W. G. Axinn, and A. Thornton, "Unwanted childbearing, health, and mother-child relationships," *Journal of Health and Social Behavior*, vol. 40, no. 3, pp. 231–257, 1999.

[5] S. T. Orr, C. A. Miller, S. A. James, and S. Babones, "Unintended pregnancy and preterm birth," *Paediatric and Perinatal Epidemiology*, vol. 14, no. 4, pp. 309–313, 2000.

[6] C. Logan, E. Holcombe, J. Manlove, and S. Ryan, "The consequences of unintended childbearing: a white paper," Child Trends Web site, http://eric.ed.gov/?id=ED510648.

[7] A. Sonfield and K. Kost, *Public Costs from Unintended Pregnancies and the Role of Public Insurance Programs in Paying for Pregnancy-Related Care: National and State Estimates for 2010*, Guttmacher Institute, 2015, http://www.guttmacher.org/pubs/public-costs-of-UP-2010.pdf.

[8] L. B. Finer, L. F. Frohwirth, L. A. Dauphinee, S. Singh, and A. M. Moore, "Reasons U.S. women have abortions: quantitative and qualitative perspectives," *Perspectives on Sexual and Reproductive Health*, vol. 37, no. 3, pp. 110–118, 2005.

[9] A. N. Broen, T. Moum, A. S. Bödtker, and Ö. Ekeberg, "Reasons for induced abortion and their relation to women's emotional distress: A Prospective, Two-year Follow-up Study," *General Hospital Psychiatry*, vol. 27, no. 1, pp. 36–43, 2005.

[10] S. Sober and C. A. Schreiber, "Postpartum contraception," *Clinical Obstetrics and Gynecology*, vol. 57, no. 4, pp. 763–776, 2014.

[11] L. Speroff and D. R. Mishell Jr., "The postpartum visit: it's time for a change in order to optimally initiate contraception," *Contraception*, vol. 78, no. 2, pp. 90–98, 2008.

[12] A. B. Parlier, B. Fagan, M. Ramage, and S. Galvin, "Prenatal care, pregnancy outcomes, and postpartum birth control plans among pregnant women with opiate addictions," *Southern Medical Journal*, vol. 107, no. 11, pp. 676–683, 2014.

[13] A. B. Berenson and C. M. Wiemann, "Contraceptive use among adolescent mothers at 6 months postpartum," *Obstetrics and Gynecology*, vol. 89, no. 6, pp. 999–1005, 1997.

[14] L. B. Zapata, S. Murtaza, M. K. Whiteman et al., "Contraceptive counseling and postpartum contraceptive use," *American Journal of Obstetrics and Gynecology*, vol. 212, no. 2, pp. 171.e1–171.e8, 2015.

[15] L. F. Damle, A. C. Gohari, A. K. McEvoy, S. Y. Desale, and V. Gomez-Lobo, "Early initiation of postpartum contraception: does it decrease rapid repeat pregnancy in adolescents?" *Journal of Pediatric and Adolescent Gynecology*, vol. 28, no. 1, pp. 57–62, 2015.

[16] P. Zutshi, I. Paredes, H. Winn, J. Stoltzfus, and J. Anasti, "Short interval between pregnancies: a search for modifiable risk factors," *Obstetrics & Gynecology*, vol. 123, no. 1, p. 112S, 2014.

[17] H. Thiel de Bocanegra, R. Chang, M. Menz, M. Howell, and P. Darney, "Postpartum contraception in publicly-funded programs and interpregnancy intervals," *Obstetrics and gynecology*, vol. 122, no. 2, pp. 296–303, 2013.

[18] S. B. Teal, "Postpartum contraception: optimizing interpregnancy intervals," *Contraception*, vol. 89, no. 6, pp. 487–488, 2014.

[19] American Academy of Pediatrics and American College of Obstetricians and Gynecologists, *Guidelines for Perinatal Care*, American Academy of Pediatrics and the American College of Obstetricians and Gynecologists, Evanston, III, USA, 7th edition, 2012.

[20] M. L. Zerden, J. H. Tang, G. S. Stuart, D. R. Norton, S. B. Verbiest, and S. Brody, "Barriers to receiving long-acting reversible contraception in the postpartum period," *Women's Health Issues*, vol. 25, no. 6, pp. 616–621, 2015.

[21] T. DePiñeres, P. D. Blumenthal, and M. Diener-West, "Postpartum contraception: the New Mexico Pregnancy Risk Assessment Monitoring System," *Contraception*, vol. 72, no. 6, pp. 422–425, 2005.

[22] L. Yee and M. Simon, "Urban minority women's perceptions of and preferences for postpartum contraceptive counseling," *Journal of Midwifery and Women's Health*, vol. 56, no. 1, pp. 54–60, 2011.

[23] C. Dehlendorf, J. T. Henderson, E. Vittinghoff et al., "Association of the quality of interpersonal care during family planning counseling with contraceptive use," *American Journal of Obstetrics & Gynecology*, vol. 215, no. 1, pp. 78.e1–78.e9, 2016.

[24] A. S. Bryant, J. S. Haas, T. F. McElrath, and M. C. McCormick, "Predictors of compliance with the postpartum visit among women living in healthy start project areas," *Maternal and Child Health Journal*, vol. 10, no. 6, pp. 511–516, 2006.

8

A New Model for Providing Cell-Free DNA and Risk Assessment for Chromosome Abnormalities in a Public Hospital Setting

Robert Wallerstein,[1] Andrea Jelks,[2] and Matthew J. Garabedian[2]

[1] *Department of Pediatrics, Santa Clara Valley Medical Center, San Jose, CA 95128, USA*
[2] *Maternal Fetal Medicine, Department of Obstetrics and Gynecology, Santa Clara Valley Medical Center, San Jose, CA 95128, USA*

Correspondence should be addressed to Matthew J. Garabedian; matthew.garabedian@hhs.sccgov.org

Academic Editor: Sinuhe Hahn

Objective. Cell-free DNA (cfDNA) offers highly accurate noninvasive screening for Down syndrome. Incorporating it into routine care is complicated. We present our experience implementing a novel program for cfDNA screening, emphasizing patient education, genetic counseling, and resource management. *Study Design.* Beginning in January 2013, we initiated a new patient care model in which high-risk patients for aneuploidy received genetic counseling at 12 weeks of gestation. Patients were presented with four pathways for aneuploidy risk assessment and diagnosis: (1) cfDNA; (2) integrated screening; (3) direct-to-invasive testing (chorionic villus sampling or amniocentesis); or (4) no first trimester diagnostic testing/screening. Patients underwent follow-up genetic counseling and detailed ultrasound at 18–20 weeks to review first trimester testing and finalize decision for amniocentesis. *Results.* Counseling and second trimester detailed ultrasound were provided to 163 women. Most selected cfDNA screening (69%) over integrated screening (0.6%), direct-to-invasive testing (14.1%), or no screening (16.6%). Amniocentesis rates decreased following implementation of cfDNA screening (19.0% versus 13.0%, $P < 0.05$). *Conclusion.* When counseled about screening options, women often chose cfDNA over integrated screening. This program is a model for patient-directed, efficient delivery of a newly available high-level technology in a public health setting. Genetic counseling is an integral part of patient education and determination of plan of care.

1. Introduction

Cell-free DNA (cfDNA) is a newly available technology that allows highly accurate screening for the most common chromosome abnormalities without invasive testing. This testing identifies fetal DNA in the maternal circulation and is considered to have a detection rate for trisomy 21 and trisomy 18 of greater than 97% and greater than 80% for trisomy 13 [1–8]. Currently, consideration of cfDNA testing is recommended for women at increased risk for chromosome abnormalities including women of advanced maternal age (AMA), with abnormal serum screening results, ultrasonographic findings suggestive of aneuploidy, or history of a prior pregnancy affected by trisomy [9]. However, the utilization of this new technology and the specifics of incorporating it into routine care are complex, as the information obtained from cfDNA screening may overlap or contradict that from maternal serum screening, nuchal translucency ultrasound, or the genetic sonogram.

We present our experience with implementing a new program for cfDNA screening in a public hospital setting with attention to patient education and early genetic counseling to individualize care and eliminate redundant screening. The aim of this report is to assess implementation of this program in terms of diagnostic testing elected by participating patients in comparison to a cohort of AMA patients seen prior to availability of cfDNA in our practice. In addition, we sought to analyze concurrent trends in prenatal ultrasound practice, specifically whether nuchal translucency utilization and/or the relative importance of ultrasound soft markers at the detailed ultrasound changed after integration of cfDNA.

2. Methods

In response to the availability of cfDNA, beginning in January 2013, we implemented a new patient care program entitled advanced maternal age options (AMA Options) to incorporate cfDNA testing into the existing prenatal diagnosis services at Santa Clara Valley Medical Center (SCVMC) Health and Hospital System. SCVMC is a tertiary care public health hospital with 6 free standing ambulatory health centers providing a full scope of maternal child health services. In addition, there are multiple community partner clinics that refer high-risk women for specialized pregnancy, delivery, and neonatal care. Genetics and maternal fetal medicine ultrasound and consultation services are provided together at a single centralized ambulatory clinic location, which is also designated as a regional prenatal diagnosis center certified by the State of California Department of Health Genetic Disease Screening Program. Genetic counseling is provided by licensed genetic counselors in the patient's preferred language, either with the aid of native speaking counselors or professional translators. Our system provides care to a predominantly Hispanic population (74.0% in 2012; California Maternal Quality Care Collaborative Maternal Data Center; accessed 5 November 2013), as well as a significant number of women of Asian/Pacific Islander decent (13.4% in 2012).

The goal of the AMA Options program was to create a patient-directed plan of care for high-risk women that would allow the greatest access to a variety of testing options and avoid performing redundant screening. Women who were identified as high risk (aged 35 or older at delivery or those with a prior family history of trisomy 13, 18, or 21) were referred for genetic counseling by their primary obstetricians during the late first trimester, ideally between 11 and 12 weeks of gestation. Genetic counselors reviewed the available testing options including cfDNA, first and second trimester serum screening, nuchal translucency (NT) ultrasound, detailed ultrasound, and amniocentesis. During that appointment, a patient-directed plan of care was created according to one of four care pathways: (1) cfDNA; (2) integrated screening (first trimester serum screening with NT ultrasound and second trimester quad screening); (3) direct-to-invasive testing (chorionic villus sampling (CVS) or amniocentesis); or (4) no screening. cfDNA or first trimester serum screening was performed during that visit, if desired. We assumed that this schema of stratifying choices would allow women to choose which testing they preferred while avoiding performance of multiple testing modalities on the same woman (i.e., women would not get first trimester serum screening and NT ultrasound if they were electing cfDNA).

Women were by and large covered through the California medical program which recognized cfDNA as a covered service for high-risk pregnancies. The Harmony Prenatal Test (Ariosa Diagnostics, San Jose, California) was available and, in most cases, was a covered benefit. Results of the cfDNA took approximately 10 days. Women did not have direct access to cfDNA screening without counseling through this program.

All participating women were scheduled for detailed ultrasound between 16 and 22 weeks (ideally between 18 and 20 weeks). Women were seen briefly for a second genetic counseling appointment in coordination with their detailed ultrasound to review the results of first trimester risk assessment and finalize their decision for amniocentesis. If desired, amniocentesis was performed in conjunction with the detailed ultrasound. Second trimester AFP screening for neural tube defects was offered to all patients not having amniocentesis performed. All first and second trimester serum specimens were processed through the California Genetics Disease Screening Program.

We compared high-risk women seen in the AMA Options program between January and September 2013 to advanced maternal age women seen in our clinic during the same period in 2012, prior to the initiation of the AMA Options program and prior to availability of cfDNA in our practice. During 2012, high-risk women were generally offered standard first and second trimester screening by their primary obstetricians and referred and seen for genetic counseling in the second trimester (ideally at 18 weeks) on the same day and immediately prior to a detailed ultrasound, with amniocentesis, if desired. NT ultrasound was offered and scheduled between 11 and 14 weeks as available. Women who had abnormal screening were seen for genetic counseling within 5 days. They were offered CVS (prior to 14 1/7 weeks) or amniocentesis (after 16 0/7 weeks) and detailed ultrasound. For nuchal translucency ≥3.5 mm, patients were also offered fetal echocardiography between 20 and 22 weeks. As all women with screen positive results were covered through California public insurance, their out-of-pocket expense was not a determining factor in test choices.

Choices in prenatal diagnostic testing and indications for invasive testing among all patients seen for genetic counseling prior to and following initiation of the AMA Options program were recorded by the genetic counselors in a prospective interdepartmental database. Indication for invasive testing was classified as fetal anomaly (if any fetal anomalies other than soft markers were found at the time of the detailed ultrasound); ultrasound soft marker (see below); abnormal serum screening (screen positive on first and/or second trimester screening); family history (patient or 1st degree relative with congenital anomaly, mental retardation, genetic syndrome, or aneuploidy); or advanced maternal age only (if absence of any of the above indications).

The presence of fetal anomalies or ultrasound soft markers was recorded by the perinatologist performing the detailed ultrasound. Ultrasound protocols in use by our department during both 2012 and 2013 specified reporting of 6 soft markers in patients undergoing either standard or detailed sonograms between 16 and 22 weeks: echogenic intracardiac focus (unilateral or bilateral, isoechoic to bone) [10]; choroid plexus cyst (unilateral or bilateral, >5 mm diameter) [10]; echogenic bowel (isoechoic to bone) [11]; pyelectasis (renal pelvis ≥4 mm) [12]; shortened humerus (less than 2.5% percentile for BPD) [13]; and nuchal thickness ≥6 mm (on angled axial view of upper cerebellum) [11]. Management and patient counseling upon finding of one or more soft markers was individualized by the perinatologist performing the ultrasound.

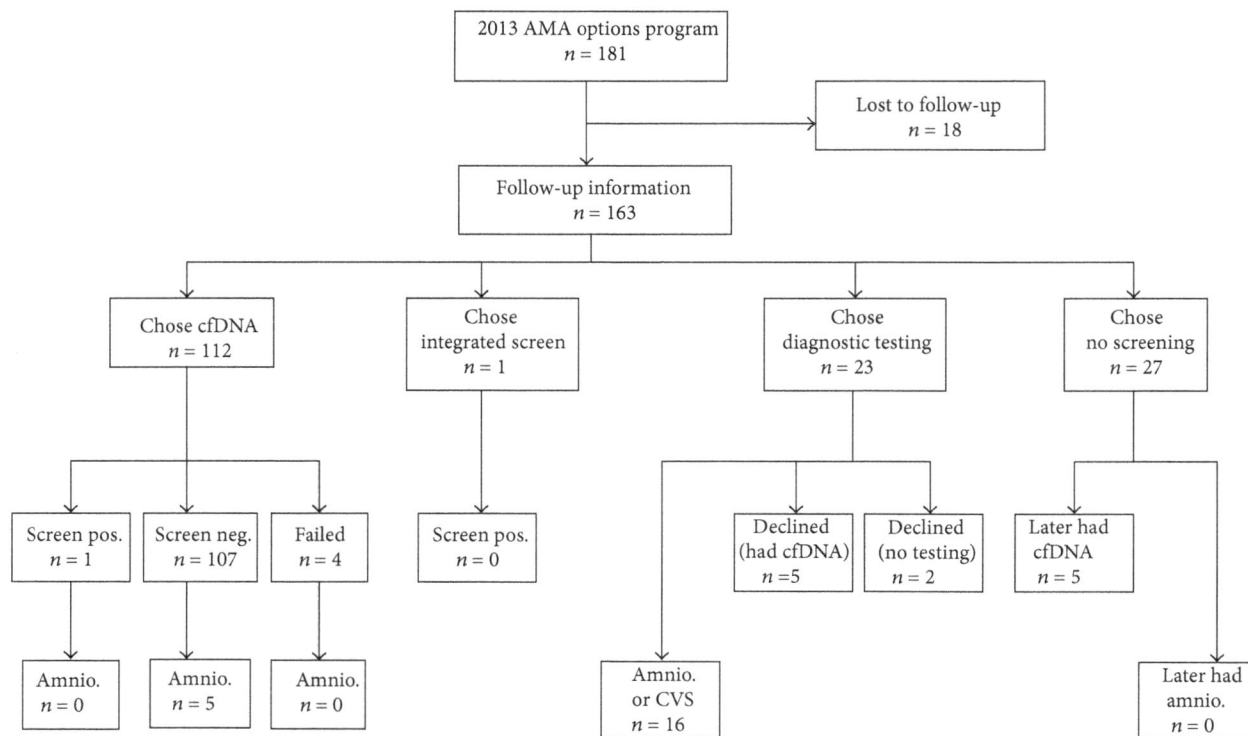

FIGURE 1: Patient eligibility for AMA Options genetic counseling and choice of testing strategy.

The Santa Clara Valley Medical Center Institutional Review Board granted exemption from review for this project. Statistical analysis was performed using STATA/IC 12 (StataCorp, College Station, TX) to test for differences in proportions.

3. Results

In the first 9 months of 2013, 181 women were seen in our unit for AMA Options counseling. For 163 (90%) of these, complete information about ultrasound findings and diagnostic testing choices at the 16–22-week detailed ultrasound were available, and these women are the subject of the current report. Of those who did not follow up for second trimester detailed ultrasound in our unit, there was no difference in patient demographics (age 38.0 versus 38.6 years; gestational age 11.5 versus 12.1 weeks), proportion choosing early cfDNA screening (66.7%) or invasive testing (16.7%), or proportion with abnormal screening (0.0%).

Figure 1 shows the number of women electing the various options presented at the AMA Options counseling session: cell-free fetal DNA screening (112/163, 68.7%), integrated screening (1/163, 0.6%), direct-to-invasive testing (23/163, 14.1%), and no screening (27/163, 16.6%). Of those who initially chose no screening, 5/27 (18.5%) women ultimately did desire and underwent cfDNA; and, of those who initially elected direct-to-invasive testing, 5/23 (21.7%) ultimately chose to undergo cfDNA screening in lieu of amniocentesis in

the second trimester. Overall, a total of 122 women (122/163, 74.8%) underwent cfDNA.

One woman (1/122, 0.8%) was screened positive for trisomy 21 on cfDNA but did not elect invasive testing. She experienced a spontaneous abortion of dichorionic twins at 17 weeks; genetic testing was not performed on the conceptus. Four women (4/122, 4.1%) failed to obtain a result from cfDNA, none of whom underwent invasive testing. Three of these women had normal detailed ultrasounds. The fourth experienced a fetal demise at 15 weeks; karyotype and microarray were normal on the products of conception.

Table 1 shows the 16–22-week ultrasound findings and diagnostic testing elected for women who had undergone AMA Options counseling and the reasons cited for invasive testing. A total of 21/161 (13.0%) women ultimately underwent invasive testing; 16/23 had initially selected this as their preferred testing method. Five additional women elected amniocentesis after normal cfDNA testing and normal detailed ultrasound. Two women chose CVS, one of whom had an unsuccessful procedure and ultimately underwent amniocentesis; a total of 20 amniocenteses were performed. No abnormal karyotypes were found.

Two noteworthy trends in practice were observed in 2013 after initiation of the AMA Options program. We found a significant decrease in the proportion of women who had ultrasound soft markers reported during the detailed ultrasound (37/457, 8.1% versus 5/161, 3.1%, $P = 0.03$). We also noted that, when comparing our overall AMA population between 2012 and 2013, a much lower proportion of AMA

TABLE 1: Amniocentesis utilization and reason: 2013 AMA Options verses 2012 all AMA.

	2013 AMA Options			2012 all AMA			P value
	N	Amnio./CVS, n	% (n/N)	N	Amnio./CVS, n	% (n/N)	
Total	**161**	21	13.0%	**457**	87	19.0%	0.08
Anomaly	0	0	0.0%	9	7	77.8%	
SM + Abnormal screen	0	0	0.0%	9	6	66.7%	
Soft marker only	5	1	20.0%	37	9	24.3%	0.83
Abnormal serum screen only	7	2	28.6%	58	18	31.0%	0.91
Family history	4	0	0.0%	16	3	18.8%	0.35
AMA only	145	18	12.4%	328	44	13.4%	0.77

TABLE 2: Nuchal translucency screen positive results and outcomes: 2012 verses 2013.

	Epoch 1: January–September 2012 N = 683	Epoch 2: January–September 2013 N = 521	P value
Screen positive	14 (2.0%)	13 (2.5%)	**0.56**
Nuchal translucency ≥3.5 mm	1 (0.1%)	2 (0.4%)	**0.28**
Congenital heart disease	0 (0%)	1 (0.2%)	**0.24**
Aneuploidy (Turner's = 1)	0 (0%)	1 (0.2%)	**0.24**

Data reported as n (%).

women overall underwent nuchal translucency ultrasounds in 2013 after initiation of AMA Options (Table 2). Consequently, a higher proportion of available NT ultrasound appointments were allocated to patients aged less than 35.

In 2012 and 2013, a similar small proportion of patients undergoing nuchal translucency ultrasound were screened positive for trisomy 21 or 18 (Table 2), and a similar proportion was found to have nuchal measurement exceeding 3.5 mm. Only one case of congenital heart disease occurred in the group with large nuchal translucency; this case was associated with findings of multiple anomalies and confirmed 45X monosomy at 17 weeks; the patient elected pregnancy termination. Across both epochs, there was only 1 woman who had an infant with trisomy 21 without being prenatally detected. This patient was 32 years of age and had integrated serum screening with normal results.

4. Discussion

In the current report, we describe our experience with implementation of a novel program to incorporate cfDNA screening with patient-specific genetic counseling in a public hospital setting. We believe our AMA Options program can serve as a model for use of a newly available high-level technology in a public health setting. We believe our AMA Options program serves as a model for implementation of cfDNA in a public health setting hospital system. With implementation of this program of patient-directed aneuploidy assessment, we were able to provide first trimester genetic counseling to nearly 40% of our AMA population while minimizing redundant testing strategies. When presented with options for aneuploidy screening, nearly 70% of these patients opted for cfDNA screening and chose to forgo integrated first and second trimester screening. This is consistent with

the anticipated 71.9%–79% of women expressing a desire for cfDNA testing [14, 15]. Our experience has been very different from that of Taylor et al., who offered cfDNA to all women considering genetic testing with a 28% of women opting for cfDNA over integrated screening [16]. Interestingly, 1 in 6 patients initially opted to have no screening or diagnostic testing, suggesting that a significant portion of our patients do not desire antenatal information about aneuploidy risk when provided with genetic counseling.

Integrated algorithms incorporating first and second trimester serum analytes, with and without first trimester nuchal translucency, have been developed [17]. However, these algorithms do not currently incorporate cfDNA, leaving providers and patients to face the question of whether to use cfDNA in addition to or in place of integrated screening. When combining different independent screening tests, one must be cognizant of the additive effect on false positive rates. With our AMA Options program, we have minimized the problem of a compounded false positive rate by offering patients who present for care early in pregnancy the choice of one of several discrete screening pathways. This strategy avoids simply adding a new test on top of existing options in a haphazard manner. Additionally, by providing pre- and posttest genetic counseling, in a manner consistent with ACOG guidelines [17], patients are provided with a clear understanding of rates of detection and false positive results, advantages and disadvantages of the different strategies, and the role of diagnostic procedures.

We also examined how the AMA Options program affected health care delivery within our system. A decrease in utilization of amniocentesis was observed, consistent with published experience [18]. Interestingly, we found an apparent change in practice pattern with respect to the reporting of soft markers for chromosome abnormalities during second trimester ultrasonography. Among women offered cfDNA in the first trimester, soft markers were reported less frequently. Likelihood ratios of soft markers noted on second trimester ultrasound and after first trimester, second trimester, and integrated screening have been calculated [19, 20]. The utility of these findings following cfDNA screening is currently unknown; however, given that the reported risk of selected chromosome abnormalities is 1:10,000 with a negative cfDNA screen, it seems unlikely that the presence of isolated soft markers on genetic ultrasound would increase the risk to a significant level. We speculate that MFM providers performing the second trimester ultrasound on women who had already had negative cfDNA testing were more reluctant to report soft markers to avoid patient confusion.

Current guidelines call for the use of cfDNA in populations considered high risk for chromosome abnormalities [9]. While cfDNA does have appealing characteristics, such as its noninvasive nature, high detection rate for the most common aneuploidies, and low false positive rate, it should be integrated into clinical practice in conjunction with appropriate counseling, to ensure that patients understand the test and its limitations [21]. Currently, ACOG recommends pretest genetic counseling to inform patients of the abilities and limitations of cfDNA [9]. Such counseling is important to guide patients through a very complex decision involving multiple tests that provide similar information. After initiation of our AMA Options program (during which most women declined first trimester screening in favor of cfDNA), we noted increased access to nuchal translucency ultrasound appointments for non-AMA (or low-risk) women. In our public health hospital system, NT appointments are a limited resource, and reallocation of these appointments has helped to further our goal to offer first trimester aneuploidy screening to all women in our system.

Presently, cfDNA screening is not recommended for use in a low-risk population, as the performance of cfDNA in these women has not been adequately evaluated. In contrast, integrated screening has been evaluated and is appropriate for use in women younger than 35 years old [22]. Existing data on the use of cfDNA in non-high-risk women is promising, but further studies are needed to better understand testing performance in low-risk or unselected populations [23]. The false positive rate of cfDNA screening is an important consideration, as acting on a positive result without confirmatory testing may lead to undesired termination of nonaneuploid fetuses [23]. As such, cfDNA must be used as a screening test and confirmatory testing is recommended to inform decisions about pregnancy termination [9, 21].

One potential criticism of our approach is that patients electing cfDNA no longer undergo formal first trimester assessment of nuchal translucency (NT). The NT ultrasound's purpose is primarily for first trimester aneuploidy risk assessment as most women have a dating ultrasound with their primary obstetric provider to assure correct scheduling. It is uncommon to detect congenital heart disease by enlarged NT alone. While a large NT has been associated with congenital heart disease [24–28], this sonographic finding is a poor screening tool for congenital heart disease. While there are multiple definitions for enlarged NT in the literature (e.g., $\geq 3.5\,mm$, >95th percentile, $\geq 2.0\,MoM$, $\geq 2.5\,MoM$, $\geq 3.0\,MoM$), all have a poor specificity ($\leq 20\%$) for isolated congenital heart disease [26–28]. While the first trimester NT may be useful for identifying those fetuses at high risk for congenital heart disease, the patients enrolled in the AMA Options program are all considered sufficiently high risk for congenital anomalies that they receive a detailed second trimester ultrasound, with thorough evaluation of fetal cardiac anatomy. While there may be value in earlier detection of congenital heart disease, given its overall low prevalence in this population, we do not see the NT as a test with sufficient performance as a screening test to be an obligatory part of prenatal care for the purposes of screening for congenital heart disease.

Noninvasive prenatal testing is an evolving technology. Starting with assays of maternal serum AFP to the current era of cfDNA, integration of new technologies has presented challenges. Integrating cfDNA into current practice must be done in a rational manner and in conjunction with appropriate counseling. Patients need this counseling to help inform very difficult decision benefits, risks, and limitations of multiple alternatives for aneuploidy screening [23].

In the context of a public health hospital system, resource allocation is an important consideration. While the actual impact of cfDNA implementation on health care cost is still undetermined, recent cost-benefit analysis supports implementation in high-risk populations over other screening algorithms [23, 29–32]. Based upon a theoretical cohort of 4 million pregnancies, Song et al. demonstrate a higher detection rate and net cost savings when screening for trisomy 21 is done with cfDNA in comparison to traditional approaches. With the AMA Options program, in addition to a high acceptance and utilization of cfDNA screening, we have further been able to provide efficient care through the minimization of redundancy in prenatal diagnosis. Additionally, we have been able to improve availability of aneuploidy screening, in the form of first trimester nuchal translucency screening, to new segments of our patient population. In the era of accountable care organizations, this program furthers the goal of providing high quality care while eliminating redundancy in care provided.

The initial experience with our AMA Options program demonstrates that a rational approach to integration of cfDNA into obstetric practice is feasible and efficient. Master's level genetic counselors can provide patient education and assistance with decision making to create an individualized plan of care. Utilizing this model, our patients have embraced this new screening option. We have found that there may be unanticipated practice changes with adoption of cfDNA, specifically with a decreased frequency of reporting isolated soft markers for aneuploidy; however, the clinical impact of such change is unclear. Moving forward, other systems are encouraged to be cognizant as to how cfDNA is implemented in their systems. With AMA Options, we provide one model for how this can be done in a rational manner.

Conflict of Interests

None of the authors has a conflict of interests to disclose.

References

[1] R. W. K. Chiu, R. Akolekar, Y. W. L. Zheng et al., "Non-invasive prenatal assessment of trisomy 21 by multiplexed maternal plasma DNA sequencing: large scale validity study," *British Medical Journal*, vol. 342, no. 7790, Article ID c7401, 2011.

[2] M. Ehrich, C. Deciu, T. Zwiefelhofer et al., "Noninvasive detection of fetal trisomy 21 by sequencing of DNA in maternal blood: a study in a clinical setting," *American Journal of Obstetrics and Gynecology*, vol. 204, no. 3, pp. 205–e11, 2011.

[3] A. B. Sparks, E. T. Wang, C. A. Struble et al., "Selective analysis of cell-free DNA in maternal blood for evaluation of fetal trisomy," *Prenatal Diagnosis*, vol. 32, no. 1, pp. 3–9, 2012.

[4] G. E. Palomaki, C. Deciu, E. M. Kloza et al., "DNA sequencing of maternal plasma reliably identifies trisomy 18 and trisomy 13 as well as down syndrome: an international collaborative study," *Genetics in Medicine*, vol. 14, no. 3, pp. 296–305, 2012.

[5] G. E. Palomaki, E. M. Kloza, G. M. Lambert-Messerlian et al., "DNA sequencing of maternal plasma to detect Down syndrome: an international clinical validation study," *Genetics in Medicine*, vol. 13, no. 11, pp. 913–920, 2011.

[6] E. Z. Chen, R. W. K. Chiu, H. Sun et al., "Noninvasive prenatal diagnosis of fetal trisomy 18 and trisomy 13 by maternal plasma dna sequencing," *PLoS ONE*, vol. 6, no. 7, Article ID e21791, 2011.

[7] D. W. Bianchi, L. D. Platt, J. D. Goldberg, A. Z. Abuhamad, A. J. Sehnert, and R. P. Rava, "Genome-wide fetal aneuploidy detection by maternal plasma DNA sequencing," *Obstetrics and Gynecology*, vol. 119, pp. 890–901, 2012.

[8] M. E. Norton, H. Brar, J. Weiss et al., "Non-invasive chromosomal evaluation (NICE) study: results of a multicenter prospective cohort study for detection of fetal trisomy 21 and trisomy 18," *The American Journal of Obstetrics and Gynecology*, vol. 207, no. 2, pp. 137-e1–137-e8, 2012.

[9] American College of Obstetricians and Gynecologists Committee on Genetics, "Committee opinion no. 545: noninvasive prenatal testing for fetal aneuploidy," *Obstetrics and Gynecology*, vol. 120, no. 6, pp. 1532–1534, 2012.

[10] M. Bethune, "Literature review and suggested protocol for managing ultrasound soft markers for Down syndrome: thickened nuchal fold, echogenic bowel, shortened femur, shortened humerus, pyelectasis and absent or hypoplastic nasal bone," *Australasian Radiology*, vol. 51, no. 3, pp. 218–225, 2007.

[11] M. Bethune, "Management options for echogenic intracardiac focus and choroid plexus cysts: a review including Australian Association of Obstetrical and Gynaecological Ultrasonologists consensus statement," *Australasian Radiology*, vol. 51, no. 4, pp. 324–329, 2007.

[12] A. M. Vintzileos, J. F. X. Egan, J. C. Smulian, W. A. Campbell, E. R. Guzman, and J. F. Rodis, "Adjusting the risk for trisomy 21 by a simple ultrasound method using fetal long-bone biometry," *Obstetrics and Gynecology*, vol. 87, no. 6, pp. 953–958, 1996.

[13] B. R. Benacerraf, J. Mandell, J. A. Estroff, B. L. Harlow, and F. D. Frigoletto Jr., "Fetal pyelectasis: a possible association with Down syndrome," *Obstetrics and Gynecology*, vol. 76, no. 1, pp. 58–60, 1990.

[14] R. Tischler, L. Hudgins, Y. J. Blumenfeld, H. T. Greely, and K. E. Ormond, "Noninvasive prenatal diagnosis: pregnant women's interest and expected uptake," *Prenatal Diagnosis*, vol. 31, no. 13, pp. 1292–1299, 2011.

[15] L. Kooij, T. Tymstra, and P. D. van Berg, "The attitude of women toward current and future possibilities of diagnostic testing in maternal blood using fetal DNA," *Prenatal Diagnosis*, vol. 29, no. 2, pp. 164–168, 2009.

[16] J. B. Taylor, V. Y. Chock, and L. Hudgins, "NIPT in a clinical setting: an analysis of uptake in the first months of clinical availability," *Journal of Genetic Counseling*, vol. 23, no. 1, pp. 72–78, 2013.

[17] "ACOG Practice Bulletin No. 77: screening for fetal chromosomal abnormalities," *Obstetrics and Gynecology*, vol. 109, no. 1, pp. 217–227, 2007.

[18] S. Chetty, M. J. Garabedian, and M. E. Norton, "Uptake of non-invasive prenatal testing (NIPT) in women following positive aneuploidy screening," *Prenatal Diagnosis*, vol. 33, no. 6, pp. 542–546, 2013.

[19] K. M. Aagaard-Tillery, F. D. Malone, D. A. Nyberg et al., "Role of second-trimester genetic sonography after down syndrome screening," *Obstetrics and Gynecology*, vol. 114, no. 6, pp. 1189–1196, 2009.

[20] D. A. Nyberg and V. L. Souter, "Use of genetic sonography for adjusting the risk for fetal Down syndrome," *Seminars in Perinatology*, vol. 27, no. 2, pp. 130–144, 2003.

[21] M. E. Norton, N. C. Rose, and P. Benn, "Noninvasive prenatal testing for fetal aneuploidy: clinical assessment and a plea for restraint," *Obstetrics and Gynecology*, vol. 121, no. 4, pp. 847–850, 2013.

[22] F. D. Malone, J. A. Canick, R. H. Ball et al., "First-trimester or second-trimester screening, or both, for down's syndrome," *The New England Journal of Medicine*, vol. 353, no. 19, pp. 2001–2011, 2005.

[23] P. Benn, H. Cuckle, and E. Pergament, "Non-invasive prenatal testing for aneuploidy: current status and future prospects," *Ultrasound in Obstetrics and Gynecology*, vol. 42, no. 1, pp. 15–33, 2013.

[24] R. Mogra, N. Alabbad, and J. Hyett, "Increased nuchal translucency and congenital heart disease," *Early Human Development*, vol. 88, no. 5, pp. 261–267, 2012.

[25] G. Makrydimas, A. Sotiriadis, I. C. Huggon et al., "Nuchal translucency and fetal cardiac defects: a pooled analysis of major fetal echocardiography centers," *American Journal of Obstetrics and Gynecology*, vol. 192, no. 1, pp. 89–95, 2005.

[26] M. Westin, S. Saltvedt, G. Bergman, H. Almström, C. Grunewald, and L. Valentin, "Is measurement of nuchal translucency thickness a useful screening tool for heart defects? A study of 16 383 fetuses," *Ultrasound in Obstetrics & Gynecology*, vol. 27, no. 6, pp. 632–639, 2006.

[27] J. Jouannic, A. Thieulin, D. Bonnet et al., "Measurement of nuchal translucency for prenatal screening of congenital heart defects: a population-based evaluation," *Prenatal Diagnosis*, vol. 31, no. 13, pp. 1264–1269, 2011.

[28] L. L. Simpson, F. D. Malone, G. R. Saade, and M. E. D'Alton, "Nuchal translucency and the risk of congenital heart disease," *Obstetrics and Gynecology*, vol. 109, no. 6, pp. 1456–1457, 2007.

[29] K. Song, T. J. Musci, and A. B. Caughey, "Clinical utility and cost of non-invasive prenatal testing with cfDNA analysis in high-risk women based on a US population," *Journal of Maternal-Fetal and Neonatal Medicine*, vol. 26, no. 12, pp. 1180–1185, 2013.

9

Can Obstetric Risk Factors Predict Fetal Acidaemia at Birth?A Retrospective Case-Control Study

Habiba Kapaya ⓘD, Roslyn Williams, Grace Elton, and Dilly Anumba ⓘD

Department of Oncology and Metabolism, Academic Unit of Reproductive & Developmental Medicine, 4th Floor Jessop Wing, Tree Root Walk, Sheffield S102SF, UK

Correspondence should be addressed to Habiba Kapaya; h.kapaya@sheffield.ac.uk

Academic Editor: Luca Marozio

Background. Despite major advances in perinatal medicine, intrapartum asphyxia remains a leading and potentially preventable cause of perinatal mortality and long-term morbidity. The umbilical cord pH is considered an essential criteria for the diagnosis of acute intrapartum hypoxic events. The purpose of this study was to evaluate whether obstetric risk factors are associated with fetal acidaemia at delivery. *Methodology*. In a case-control study, 294 women with term singleton pregnancies complicated by an umbilical artery cord pH < 7.20 at birth were individually matched by controls with umbilical artery cord pH > 7.20. Groups were compared for differences in maternal, obstetric, and fetal characteristics using logistic regression models presented as odds ratio (OR) with 95% confidence intervals (CI). *Results*. The study showed pregestational diabetes (PGDM) [OR: 5.31, 95% CI: 1.15- 24.58, P = 0.018], urinary tract infection (UTI) [OR: 3.21, 95% CI: 1.61- 6.43, P < 0.001], and low Apgar scores to be significantly associated with acidaemia, whereas low maternal BMI [OR: 0.19, 95% CI: 0.04-0.87, P = 0.032], pyrexia in labour [OR 0.23; 95% CI 0.12-0.53; P < 0.001], electronic fetal monitoring (EFM) [OR 0.65; 95% CI 0.43-0.99; P = 0.042], and emergency caesarean section [OR 0.42; 95% CI 0.26-0.66; P < 0.001] were found to be protective of acidaemia. *Conclusion*. Certain obstetric risk factors before and during labour can identify newborns at risk of developing acidaemia. Further research is needed to gain quantitative insight into the predictive capacity of these risks that can inform obstetric clinical management for improved outcomes.

1. Introduction

Intrapartum fetal hypoxia, resulting in permanent neurological impairment, remains a significant source of concern for parents and healthcare professionals [1]. Today, electronic fetal monitoring (EFM) is the most common method used to assess for fetal well-being during labour without substantial evidence to suggest a benefit [2]. Despite its widespread use over the last four decades, the incidence of intrapartum fetal hypoxia culminating in long-term neurological sequelae (cerebral palsy) or perinatal death has remained largely unchanged [3, 4]. Numerous clinical studies have investigated the relationship between neonatal complications and umbilical artery pH [5–7]. However, few studies have analysed the risk factors for fetal acidosis [6, 8]. Our purpose was to employ a case-control design to identify possible risk factors during pregnancy and delivery for fetal acidaemia at birth that could help obstetricians recognise patients who have a higher risk of developing fetal and subsequent neonatal acidaemia. The recognition of an epidemiological profile could help identify women requiring intensive surveillance during labour, thereby enabling expedited delivery before permanent neurological damage ensues [8].

2. Materials and Methods

This was a retrospective case-control study from June 1, 2016, to January 31, 2017. The study was performed at the Jessop Wing of the Sheffield Teaching Hospitals Trust, a tertiary-referral University hospital where approximately 8000 deliveries take place annually. Data was collected from a cohort of consecutive delivering women with a singleton nonanomalous cephalic fetus at more than 37 gestational weeks. Acidaemia was defined as pH < 7.20 on the arterial blood samples obtained from the umbilical cord at birth. This level was used as pH of <7.20 on fetal blood sampling is defined as abnormal in current intrapartum guidelines of the UK and is used to prompt immediate delivery [9]

Cord blood gas samples were analysed using an ABL 800 Series blood gas analysers situated on the labour ward and maternity theatres of the hospital. Cord blood gas results obtained utilising the blood gas analyser were downloaded into a database for this study. For the case group, newborns with umbilical arterial cord blood pH < 7.20 were included. The control group included newborns with a normal umbilical artery cord blood pH > 7.20 born consecutively following each newborn included in the case group. For all cases and controls, data from the standardized antenatal, intrapartum, and birth outcome records were collected from the hospital electronic maternity database and medical notes. Antenatal data were split into several factors: maternal demographic, chronic maternal disease, previous obstetric history, and current pregnancy problems. Maternal demographic included age, BMI, ethnicity, and parity. Maternal age was defined by criteria suggested by the RCOG [10]: normal 20-34 years, teenage <20 years, advanced maternal age I >35 years, and advanced maternal age II >40 years. As recommended by NICE [11], BMI <18.5 was defined as underweight (18.5-24.9), healthy (25-29.9), Class I obesity (30-34.9), Class II obesity (35-39.9), and Class III obesity (40 or more). Parity was grouped according to Bai et al. [12]: nulliparity as 0, low multiparity as 1-3, and grand multiparity as 4-8. Chronic maternal disease included pregestational diabetes mellitus (PGDM), preexisting cardiac, respiratory, autoimmune, haematological, and thyroid disorder whereas past obstetric history included miscarriage, preterm delivery, stillbirth, and caesarean section. Current pregnancy problems included hypertensive disorder, obstetric cholestasis, gestational diabetes mellitus (GDM), intrauterine growth restriction (IUGR), reduced fetal movement, and proven urinary tract infection (UTI). Intrapartum risk factors included induced labour, oxytocin-augmented labour, meconium-stained amniotic fluid, pyrexia in labour, epidural analgesia, and operative deliveries. Several neonatal outcomes were compared between acidaemic and nonacidaemic neonates. Neonatal outcomes that were examined included birth weight, Apgar score at 1 and 5 min, and neonatal intensive care unit (NICU) admission. The relationship between antenatal and intrapartum risk factors for fetal acidaemia was analysed using logistic regression model presented as odds ratio (OR) with 95% confidence intervals (CI). This study was conducted as a service evaluation project so formal ethical approval was not required.

2.1. Statistical Analysis. SPSS version 24 statistical package was used for all analyses. Baseline characteristics were determined using descriptive statistics and presented as mean ± a standard deviation for continuous variables and as numbers and percentages for categorical and dichotomous variables. A comparison between cases and controls was performed with chi-square or Fisher exact tests, when appropriate for categorical variables. Fisher's exact test was used when assumptions of the chi-square test were violated. A probability value of <0.05 was considered statistically significant. Binary logistic regression was used to investigate the independent

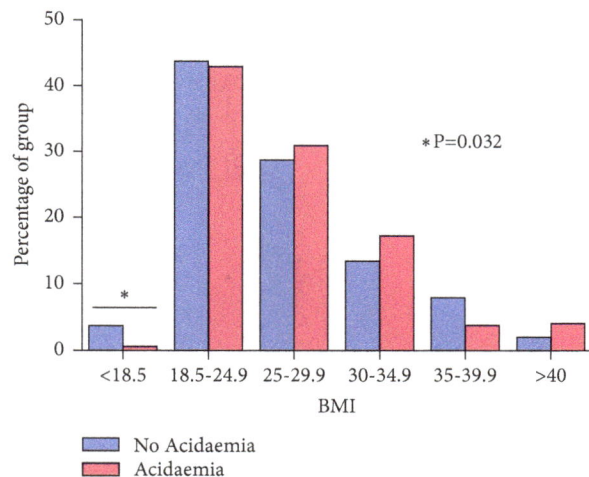

Figure 1: Distribution of maternal BMI between the two groups.

contribution of obstetric factors to the occurrence of fetal acidaemia. Odds ratios and their 95% CIs were calculated from the regression coefficient to estimate the strength of association with each parameter.

3. Results

Between June 1, 2016, and January 31, 2017, there were 3184 singleton term live births at the Jessop Wing. Of 3184, 2115 sets of data were recorded by the blood gas analysing machine. After excluding insufficient, poor quality, and incorrectly labelled umbilical cord blood samples, there were 1112 umbilical cord results. Of 1112 umbilical cord results, 328 cord blood values had a pH less than 7.20; 294 of these were arterial cord gases. Thus 294 cord blood values made up the acidaemia group of this study.

Maternal demographics, obstetric characteristics, delivery and neonatal outcomes according to the study groups are shown in Tables 1, 2, and 3, respectively. There were no differences between the case and controls in terms of age, parity, ethnicity, rates of gestational diabetes, obstetric cholestasis, thyroid, cardiac, respiratory, rheumatology, haematology, and hypertensive disorders but a difference in maternal BMI, UTI, and PGDM was observed between the two groups. With regard to maternal BMI, although we had only 13 women in the study with a BMI of <18.5, underweight women seemed to be protective against neonatal acidaemia (OR 0.19; 95% CI 0.04-0.87; P=0.032). On the other hand, a stepwise trend towards acidaemia with increasing BMI was observed; odds ratios increased from 1.10 in the group with a BMI between 25 and 30 to 1.30 between 30 and 35 to 2.07 with BMI > 40 (see Figure 1).

Although number of women with chronic health conditions such as thyroid, rheumatology, respiratory, and haematology problems were slightly higher in the acidaemia group, this difference was not statistically significant. However, a significantly increased proportion of women with PGDM were observed in the acidaemia group (5.3%) compared to the controls (1.1%); P = 0.018. From logistic regression analysis,

TABLE 1: Maternal demographic risk factors.

	Non-acidaemia pH > 7.20 (N = 294)	Acidaemia pH < 7.20 (N = 294)	Missing %	p-value	Odds ratios (95% CI)
		Maternal demographic risk factors			
Maternal age (years) mean ± SD	29 [5.19]	29 [5.82]		0.664	
Maternal Age					
Reference age					REFERENCE
Teenage pregnancy	6 (2.0%)	6 (2.0%)	0.3%	0.988	1.01 (0.32 - 3.17)
Advanced age I	44 (15.0%)	42 (14.3%)		0.872	0.96 (0.61 - 1.53)
Advanced age II	12 (4.1%)	16 (5.5%)		0.451	1.35 (0.62 - 2.91)
Ethnicity					
White	156 (65.3%)	161 (68.5%)			REFERENCE
Black	20 (8.4%)	17 (7.2%)	19.4%	0.58	0.82 (0.42 - 1.63)
Asian	43 (18.0%)	35 (14.9%)		0.350	0.79 (0.48 - 1.30)
Mixed	8 (3.3%)	6 (2.6%)		0.563	0.73 (0.25 - 2.14)
Other	12 (5.0%)	16 (6.8%)		0.520	1.29 (0.59 - 2.82)
BMI (kg/m²) mean ±SD	25.3 [4.95]	25.7 [5.7]		0.496	
BMI (kg/m²)					
Healthy weight	126 (43.8%)	122 (43.0%)			REFERENCE
Underweight	11 (3.8%)	2 (0.7%)		**0.032**	0.19 (0.04 - 0.87)
Overweight	83 (28.8%)	88 (31.0%)	2.7%	0.648	1.10 (0.74 - 1.62)
Obesity I	39 (13.5%)	49 (17.3%)		0.296	1.30 (0.80 - 2.12)
Obesity II	23 (8.0%)	11 (3.9%)		0.069	0.49 (0.23 - 1.06)
Obesity III	6 (2.1%)	12 (4.2%)		0.160	2.06 (0.75 - 5.68)
Parity					
Nulliparity	182 (63.2%)	169 (59.5%)	2.7%	0.365	0.86 (0.61 - 1.20)
Low multiparity	100 (34.7%)	111 (39.1%)	2.7%	0.280	1.21 (0.86 - 1.70)
High multiparity	6 (2.1%)	4 (1.4%)	2.7%	0.752	0.67 (0.19 - 2.41)

Demographic variables for acidaemia where the cutoff for acidaemia is pH = 7.20. Independent t-test was performed for maternal age and BMI and binary logistic regression was performed for all variables.

TABLE 2: Obstetric risk factors.

		Obstetric risk factors				
		Non-acidaemia pH > 7.20 (N = 294)	Acidaemia pH < 7.20 (N = 294)	Missing %	p-value	Odds ratios (95% CI)
Past medical history	Pre-gestational diabetes (PGDM)	2 (1.1%)	10 (5.3%)	39.3%	0.018	5.31 (1.15 - 24.58)
	Thyroid disease	10 (5.5%)	15 (8.4%)	38.4%	0.274	1.58 (0.69 - 3.62)
	Rheumatological disease	0 (0.0%)	5 (2.8%)	39.1%	0.061	0.99 (0.97 - 0.99)
	Cardiac disease	17 (9.2%)	11 (6.1%)	38.3%	0.269	0.64 (0.29 - 1.76)
	Asthma	40 (21.4%)	41 (22.4%)	37.1%	0.814	1.06 (0.65 - 1.74)
Past obstetric history	Caesarean section	38 (20.1%)	37 (19.8%)	36.1%	0.938	0.98 (0.59 - 1.63)
	Preterm	8 (4.4%)	8 (4.5%)	38.9%	0.936	1.04 (0.38 - 2.84)
	Stillbirth	5 (2.8%)	3 (1.7%)	39.1%	0.724	0.61 (0.14 - 2.58)
	Miscarriage	57 (29.8%)	50 (27.2%)	36.2%	0.567	0.88 (0.56 - 1.37)
	Smoking	35 (13.9%)	33 (11.6%)	8.8%	0.412	0.81 (0.49 - 1.35)
	Other recreational drugs	12 (6.2%)	19 (9.5%)	33.0%	0.233	1.58 (0.74 - 3.34)
	Anaemia	50 (27.2%)	52 (28.1%)	37.2%	0.841	1.05 (0.66 - 1.65)
	Urinary tract infection (UTI)	12 (6.6%)	34 (18.5%)	37.76%	0.001	3.21 (1.61 - 6.43)
	Pre-eclampsia	35 (18.9%)	50 (27.3%)	37.80%	0.056	1.61 (0.99 - 2.63)
Prenatal risks	Antepartum haemorrhage (APH)	16 (8.6%)	11 (6.1%)	37.93%	0.370	0.70 (0.31 - 1.54)
	GDM (Gestational diabetes mellitus)	14 (7.7%)	11 (6.1%)	38.27%	0.563	0.79 (0.35 - 1.78)
	Obstetric cholestasis	5 (2.8%)	8 (4.5%)	38.95%	0.380	1.66 (0.53 - 5.16)
	IUGR (Intrauterine growth restriction)	19 (10.3%)	7 (4.0%)	38.6%	0.629	0.36 (0.15 - 0.87)
	RFM (Reduced Foetal Movement)	42 (22.6%)	56 (29.8%)	36.4%	0.113	1.46 (0.91 - 2.32)

Obstetric risk factors for acidaemia where the cutoff for acidaemia is pH = 7.20. Binary logistic regression was performed for all variables.

TABLE 3: Delivery and neonatal outcome.

Intrapartum factors		Non-acidaemia pH > 7.20 (N = 294)	Acidaemia pH < 7.20 (N = 294)	Missing %	p-value	Odds ratios (95% CI intervals)
Induction		93 (32.3%)	90 (30.8%)	1.36%	0.703	0.93 (0.69 - 1.37)
Epidural		129 (44.5%)	135 (46.4%)	1.19%	0.644	1.08 (0.78 - 1.50)
Meconium staining		64 (30.3%)	71 (34.0%)	28.57%	0.425	1.18 (0.78 - 1.78)
FBS (Foetal blood sample)		47 (16.3%)	46 (15.9%)	1.70%	0.910	0.98 (0.63 - 1.52)
Pyrexia		30 (61.2%)	21 (28.0%)	80.10%	<0.001	0.23 (0.12 - 0.53)
Continuous intrapartum CTG		239 (83.6%)	218 (76.8%)	3.1%	0.042	0.65 (0.43 - 0.99)
Median duration of labour in minutes (interquartile range)		811 (279-722)	705 (233-636)	19.00%	0.021	
Syntocinon		183 (64.7%)	170 (60.9%)	0.00%	0.360	0.85 0.61 - 1.20
Method of delivery	Unassisted	45 (15.5%)	64 (22.0%)	0.00%		REFERENCE
	Instrumental	83 (28.5%)	131 (45.0%)		0.664	1.11 (0.69 - 1.78)
	Emergency caesarean	160 (55.0%)	95 (32.6%)		<0.001	0.42 (0.26 - 0.66)
	Elective caesarean	3 (1.0%)	1 (0.3%)		0.215	0.23 (0.02 - 2.33)
Median APGAR at 1 minute (interquartile range)		8 (7-9)	7 (6-9)	1.28%	<0.001	
Median APGAR at 5 minutes (interquartile range)		9 (9-9)	9 (9-9)	1.28%	0.025	
NICU admission		26 (9.1%)	25 (8.7%)	2.7%	0.863	0.95 (0.54 - 1.69)
Mean birthweight in grams ± (SD)		3201 (512)	3042 (481)	0.0%	0.138	

Intrapartum and postpartum analysis. Binary logistic regression was performed for categorical variables. Independent *t*-test was performed for birth weight and Mann-Whitney *U* test was performed for duration of labour and APGAR scores.

we estimated that infants of women with PGDM were five times more likely to be acidotic (OR 5.31; 95% CI 1.15-24.58) compared to the controls.

Interestingly, women with UTI during pregnancy showed a significantly increased occurrence of neonatal acidaemia compared to the control group (18.5% versus 6.6%; P < 0.001). However the presence of other obstetric risk factors in the previous or current pregnancy was broadly comparable between the two groups.

Antenatal risk factors were included in a logistic regression model to find independence of results. The results of multivariable analysis demonstrated antenatal UTI to be a significant predictor for neonatal acidaemia (OR 3.62; 95% CI 1.57-8.34; P = 0.003).

Surprisingly, most of the intrapartum risk factors showed a significant trend towards nonacidaemia. Among all intrapartum variables, pyrexia in labour had the largest amount of missing data. However, this variable was significantly associated with nonacidaemia (OR 0.23; 95% CI 0.12-0.53; P < 0.001). In addition, the number of women who had continuous CTG monitoring during labour was significantly higher in the control group compared to the cases (83.6% versus 76.8%; P = 0.042). Women in the acidaemia group had significantly shorter labours than women in the nonacidaemia group (705 minutes compared to 811 minutes; P = 0.011). The majority of deliveries in the nonacidaemia group were emergency caesarean sections (55%). However, in the acidaemia group, instrumental delivery made up the largest group (45.0%). A binary logistic regression was carried out to compare instrumental, emergency caesarean, and elective caesarean section delivery with unassisted delivery. The logistic regression showed that emergency caesarean section compared to unassisted deliveries was significantly associated with nonacidaemia (OR 0.42; 95% CI 0.26-0.66; P < 0.001).

With regard to neonatal outcomes low Apgar scores at 1 and 5 minutes were significantly associated with neonatal acidaemia (P < 0.001 and P = 0.025). However, there were no significant differences in the neonatal birthweight and NICU admissions between the two groups.

4. Discussion

The data from this study demonstrates that several obstetric risk factors such as urinary tract infection during pregnancy, pregestational diabetes mellitus, and instrumental delivery increase a higher risk of acidaemia at birth.

Fetal oxygenation and umbilical cord pH usually decline during the course of normal labour [13]. The exact pH value which defines significant acidosis remains unclear. Most studies quote arterial cord pH < 7.20 as a cut-off for significant acidosis [13, 14], whereas Goldaber et al. [15] suggest that most fetuses would tolerate intrapartum acidaemia with a pH as low as 7.00. From an important systematic review and meta-analysis [16], it is known that low umbilical artery cord pH is strongly associated with clinically important neonatal and long-term adverse outcomes. Hence prevention of low cord pH at birth by recognising woman's individual risk of developing such adverse outcome, preferably at an early

stage, optimises the intrapartum monitoring, decision and management process.

During pregnancy, obesity has been related to several obstetric and fetal complications, and the effect is dose-dependent [17]. On the other hand, there is only a small amount of data available about the relationship between being underweight during pregnancy and perinatal complications [18]; in fact the risk of several pregnancy, intrapartum, postnatal, and neonatal complications are less common in underweight women [19]. Results from our study support this notion and demonstrate that low maternal BMI was protective of acidaemia at birth.

Pregnancies affected by diabetes mellitus are at increased risk of perinatal morbidity and mortality as a consequence of poor maternal blood sugar control [20]. Fetuses of PGDM appear to be exposed to chronic intrauterine hypoxia and have been found to be acidaemic at cordocentesis even in the presence of normal biophysical score [21]. A recent study found significant association between fetal acidaemia at delivery and decreased neonatal heart rate variability in infants of PGDM [22]. Landon et al. [23] demonstrated a linear relationship between maternal glucose levels and adverse pregnancy outcome. In addition, a large population based study demonstrated significantly increased maternal and perinatal morbidity in women with PGDM compared to GDM [24]. Thus, it would be logical that PGDM, which is more likely to have elevated glucose levels in early pregnancy, would have increased adverse perinatal outcome compared to GDM. Our results confirm this expectation.

The incidence of UTI in pregnancy can be as high as eight percent and maternal and neonatal complications associated with UTI can be devastating [25]. Our study confirm that UTI at any stage in pregnancy increases the odds of acidaemia at birth threefold compared to women who never had a UTI. The significant association between UTI and acidaemia at birth persisted when multivariable analyses were performed to control for potential confounding factors such as age and parity. This finding is unique and there is no literature to confirm or refute this observation.

When instrumental and caesarean deliveries were compared, whether the indication for operative delivery was fetal compromise or failure to progress in labour, arterial cord pH was worse in the instrumental group. These results are in agreement with existing evidence in literature [1, 14] and are explained by longer period of in utero resuscitation following a decision to deliver by caesarean section in contrast to shorter decision to delivery interval for babies delivered by instrumental delivery. This further explains why we observed shortened labour duration in the acidaemia group compared to the nonacidaemia group.

The presence of maternal fever in labour (chorioamnionitis) is a strong risk factor for adverse neonatal outcome including cerebral palsy and neonatal death [26]. However, studies evaluating its association with umbilical cord gases at birth have found no significant effect on cord pH [27]. Strikingly, our study found pyrexia in labour to have protective effect on acidaemia. It is plausible that women with pyrexia in labour were closely monitored and a threshold of intervention (delivery by caesarean section) was probably lower in this group resulting in better neonatal outcome. Furthermore, this variable had a lot of missing data, meaning that the accuracy of this association cannot be conclusively established.

In our study, EFM was performed in 76.8% of the cases and in 88.6% of the control group. The impact of EFM on neonatal outcome continues to be controversial [28]. A recent Cochrane review have failed to show any improvement in perinatal outcome with their use [4]. Intrapartum CTG has low specificity with many nonacidaemic fetuses having CTG changes [29].

With regard to delivery variables, we observed a clear reduction of Apgar scores with lower values of umbilical artery cord pH. This finding is consistent with previous studies [5, 14].

We acknowledge several limitations of this study. First, cord gas sampling was poor, incomplete, and incorrectly labelled in 47.4% of the cases. This data was excluded from the analysis, which raises a possibility of missing some subtle but potentially clinically interesting information that may have given us a better insight and helped obstetricians in recognising patients at higher risk of developing fetal and subsequent neonatal acidaemia.

Second, because of the retrospective nature of this study, we were unable to control for all possible confounding variables and were limited to information previously obtained. Third, we analysed only arterial pH as this is the most commonly used measure instead of taking into consideration other criteria of intrapartum asphyxia [30]. In addition, we defined acidaemia as an umbilical artery pH < 7.20 which is slightly higher than the definition used by the majority of publications on this subject. Nonetheless, there is no consensus on a single umbilical cord artery pH that clearly distinguishes acidotic babies from those that are nonacidotic [31]. Furthermore, if we had chosen pH < 7.0 instead of pH < 7.20 as an outcome measure, although we may have observed significant risk factors for acidaemia, the reliability and significance of these results would have been questioned due to limited sample size as there were only 17 cases with an umbilical artery pH < 7.0 between June 1, 2016, January 31, 2017.

Fourth, the study was not population based, with limited sample size and missing data for most of the variables ranged from 0 to 82.1%; therefore the possibility that bias affected the results of this study must be considered. Fifth, we were unable to assess long-term neonatal outcomes that include developmental delay, neurological morbidity, and cerebral palsy. Finally, cord gas data were not available for many women, because, in our institution, it is not common practice to obtain cord blood gas, as a means of additional assessment in deliveries with an Apgar score of ≥7. Although most neonates who are born with acidaemia will not require additional intervention or develop subsequent morbidity, conclusion from a systematic review and meta-analysis [16] indicates that "initial surveillance of neonates born with a low arterial cord pH, regardless of their clinical condition, is warranted as the odds of complications have been shown to be higher in this group". Based on this conclusion, we find merit in universal umbilical cord blood sampling as a method of identifying neonates who are at risk.

In conclusion, our study has shown that, in women with singleton term pregnancy, factors both before and during labour influence the possibility of developing acidosis of the newborn at birth. While association does not necessarily imply causation, there are good physiological grounds for expecting some causal relationship to be operating. Further studies are needed to validate our results, establish that causality of this association and to assess long-term outcome of these babies.

Conflicts of Interest

The authors declare that they have no conflicts of interest.

References

[1] T. Prior and S. Kumar, "Mode of delivery has an independent impact on neonatal condition at birth," *European Journal of Obstetrics & Gynecology and Reproductive Biology*, vol. 181, pp. 135–139, 2014.

[2] A. G. Cahill and J. Spain, "Intrapartum Fetal Monitoring," *Clinical Obstetrics and Gynecology*, vol. 58, no. 2, pp. 263–268, 2015.

[3] A. Pinas and E. Chandraharan, "Continuous cardiotocography during labour: Analysis, classification and management," *Best Practice & Research Clinical Obstetrics & Gynaecology*, vol. 30, pp. 33–47, 2016.

[4] Z. Alfirevic, D. Devane, and G. M. Gyte, "Continuous cardiotocography (CTG) as a form of electronic fetal monitoring (EFM) for fetal assessment during labour," *Cochrane Database of Systematic Reviews*, vol. 2, Article ID CD006066, 2006.

[5] J. W. Dudenhausen and T. Milz, "Consequences of intrauterine acidosis for early morbidity of term newborn infants," *Zeitschrift für Geburtshilfe und Neonatologie*, vol. 211, no. 4, pp. 153–156, 2007.

[6] E. Maisonneuve, F. Audibert, L. Guilbaud et al., "Risk factors for severe neonatal acidosis," *Obstetrics & Gynecology*, vol. 118, no. 4, pp. 818–823, 2011.

[7] B. A. Sabol and A. B. Caughey, "Acidemia in neonates with a 5-minute Apgar score of 7 or greater – What are the outcomes?" *American Journal of Obstetrics & Gynecology*, vol. 215, no. 4, pp. 486–486.e6, 2016.

[8] F. Crovetto, M. Fumagalli, A. De Carli et al., "Obstetric risk factors for poor neonatal adaptation at birth," *The Journal of Maternal-Fetal and Neonatal Medicine*, pp. 1–7, 2017.

[9] NICE, *Clinical guideline 190: intrapartum care for healthy women and babies*, NICE, 2014.

[10] RCOG statement on increased maternal age, 2017.

[11] National Institute for Health and Care Excellence, *Health and Care Excellence., Obesity, Identification, assessment and management pf overweight and obesity in children, young people and adults*, 2017.

[12] J. Bai, F. W. S. Wong, A. Bauman, and M. Mohsin, "Parity and pregnancy outcomes," *American Journal of Obstetrics & Gynecology*, vol. 186, no. 2, pp. 274–278, 2002.

[13] C.-F. Su, H.-J. Tsai, C.-C. Huang, K.-H. Luo, and L.-Y. Lin, "Fetal acidosis from obstetric interventions during the first vaginal

delivery," *Taiwanese Journal of Obstetrics and Gynecology*, vol. 47, no. 4, pp. 397–401, 2008.

[14] S. N. Khan, G. S. Ahmed, A. M. Abutaleb, and M. A. Hathal, "Is the determination of umbilical cord arterial blood gases necessary in all deliveries? Analysis in a high-risk population," *J Perinatol*, vol. 15, no. 1, pp. 39–42, 1995.

[15] K. G. Goldaber, L. C. Gilstrap, K. J. Leveno, J. S. Dax, and D. D. McIntire, "Pathologic fetal acidemia," *Obstetrics & Gynecology*, vol. 78, no. 6, pp. 1103–1107, 1991.

[16] G. L. Malin, R. K. Morris, and K. S. Khan, "Strength of association between umbilical cord pH and perinatal and long term outcomes: Systematic review and meta-analysis," *BMJ*, vol. 340, no. 7756, Article ID c1471, p. 1121, 2010.

[17] R. K. Edwards, J. Cantu, S. Cliver, J. R. Biggio Jr., J. Owen, and A. T. N. Tita, "The association of maternal obesity with fetal pH and base deficit at cesarean delivery.," *Obstetrics & Gynecology*, vol. 122, no. 2, pp. 262–267, 2013.

[18] S. M. Galán, Á. S. Hernández, I. V. Zúñiga, M. S. Löpez Criado, A. P. Lloréns, and V. José Luis Gallo, "Abnormal maternal body mass index and obstetric and neonatal outcome," *The Journal of Maternal-Fetal and Neonatal Medicine*, vol. 25, no. 3, pp. 308–312, 2012.

[19] N. J. Sebire, M. Jolly, J. Harris, L. Regan, and S. Robinson, "Is maternal underweight really a risk factor for adverse pregnancy outcome? A population-based study in London," *British Journal of Obstetrics and Gynaecology*, vol. 108, no. 1, pp. 61–66, 2001.

[20] A. Ruozi-Berretta, J. J. Piazze, E. Cosmi, A. Cerekja, A. Kashami, and M. M. Anceschi, "Computerized cardiotocography parameters in pregnant women affected by pregestational diabetes mellitus," *Journal of Perinatal Medicine*, vol. 32, no. 5, pp. 426–429, 2004.

[21] K. H. Nicolaides, J. Freeman, and J. M. Brudenell, "Prediction of fetal acidaemia in pregnancies complicated by maternal diabetes mellitus by biophysical profile scoring and fetal heart rate monitoring," *BJOG: An International Journal of Obstetrics & Gynaecology*, vol. 100, no. 3, pp. 227–233, 1993.

[22] N. E. Russell, M. F. Higgins, B. F. Kinsley, M. E. Foley, and F. M. McAuliffe, "Heart rate variability in neonates of type 1 diabetic pregnancy," *Early Human Development*, vol. 92, pp. 51–55, 2016.

[23] M. B. Landon, L. Mele, and C. Y. Spong, "The Relationship Between Maternal Glycemia and Perinatal Outcome," *Obstetrics & Gynecology*, vol. 117, no. 5, pp. 1230-1231, 2011.

[24] A. Fong, A. Serra, T. Herrero, D. Pan, and D. Ogunyemi, "Pregestational versus gestational diabetes: a population based study on clinical and demographic differences," *Journal of Diabetes and its Complications*, vol. 28, no. 1, pp. 29–34, 2014.

[25] J. E. Delzell Jr. and M. L. Lefevre, "Urinary tract infections during pregnancy," *American Family Physician*, vol. 61, no. 3, pp. 713–721, 2000.

[26] L. W. M. Impey, C. E. L. Greenwood, R. S. Black, P. S.-Y. Yeh, O. Sheil, and P. Doyle, "The relationship between intrapartum maternal fever and neonatal acidosis as risk factors for neonatal encephalopathy," *American Journal of Obstetrics & Gynecology*, vol. 198, no. 1, pp. 49–e6, 2008.

[27] C. T. Johnson, I. Burd, R. Raghunathan, F. J. Northington, and E. M. Graham, "Perinatal inflammation/infection and its association with correction of metabolic acidosis in hypoxic-ischemic encephalopathy," *Journal of Perinatology*, vol. 36, no. 6, pp. 448–452, 2016.

[28] S. L. Clark, E. F. Hamilton, T. J. Garite, A. Timmins, P. A. Warrick, and S. Smith, "The limits of electronic fetal heart rate monitoring in the prevention of neonatal metabolic acidemia," *American Journal of Obstetrics & Gynecology*, vol. 216, no. 2, pp. 163–163.e6, 2017.

[29] M. Holzmann, S. Wretler, S. Cnattingius, and L. Nordström, "Neonatal outcome and delivery mode in labors with repetitive fetal scalp blood sampling," *European Journal of Obstetrics & Gynecology and Reproductive Biology*, vol. 184, pp. 97–102, 2015.

[30] A. MacLennan, "A template for defining a causal relation between acute intrapartum events and cerebral palsy: International consensus statement," *British Medical Journal*, vol. 319, no. 7216, pp. 1054–1059, 1999.

[31] S. Kumar and S. Paterson-Brown, "Obstetric aspects of hypoxic ischemic encephalopathy," *Early Human Development*, vol. 86, no. 6, pp. 339–344, 2010.

10

Determinants and Outcomes of Emergency Caesarean Section following Failed Instrumental Delivery: 5-Year Observational Review at a Tertiary Referral Centre in London

Sian McDonnell and Edwin Chandraharan

St. George's University Hospitals NHS Foundation Trust, Blackshaw Road, London SW 17 0RE, UK

Correspondence should be addressed to Edwin Chandraharan; edwin.c@sky.com

Academic Editor: Deborah A. Wing

Objectives. To review the determinants for a failed operative vaginal delivery and to examine associated fetal and maternal morbidity. *Design.* Retrospective observational study. *Setting.* Large London Teaching Hospital. *Method.* A retrospective review of case notes during a 5-year period was carried out. *Results.* Overall 119 women (0.44%) out of 26,856 births had a caesarean section following a failed instrumental delivery, which comprised 5.1% of all operative vaginal births. 73% had a spontaneous onset of labour and 63% required syntocinon at some time prior to delivery. 71.5% of deliveries were complicated by malposition. Only 20% of deliveries were attended by a consultant obstetrician. Almost 50% of women and 8.4% of neonates sustained trauma at the time of either their failed instrumental delivery or the caesarean section. *Conclusions.* Emergency caesarean section during the second stage of labour is associated with maternal and fetal complications. A 'failed instrumental delivery score' (FIDS) may aid practitioners in predicting an increased likelihood of a failed operative vaginal birth and therefore to consider a trial of operative vaginal delivery in the theatre. Senior input should also be sought because a failed operative vaginal birth is associated with increased maternal and fetal morbidity.

1. Introduction

Caesarean section in the second stage of labour is a technically difficult procedure, especially when performed after an operative vaginal delivery has been attempted and when the fetal head is deeply impacted within the pelvis. Therefore, a "second stage" caesarean section may be associated with increased maternal and fetal morbidity [1–4]. Although operative vaginal births are also associated with fetal trauma [5, 6], significant maternal and fetal trauma can also occur during a caesarean section that is performed during late second stage of labour. The rising rates of caesarean section at full dilatation not only are a concern for the delivery in question but also may have a negative impact on woman's future pregnancies and deliveries [7].

A recent 10-year study of operative delivery in a large London teaching hospital has shown a trend to choose a ventouse (vacuum extractor) over forceps and opting for delivery in the operating theatre as well as a small increase in the rate of caesarean section at full dilatation [8]. This study also showed an increase in failed instrumental delivery (correlation coefficient 0.93, $p < 0.05$) which was thought to be due to both instrument failure and a reluctance to attempt instrumentation during second stage of labour.

Other studies have also noted the rise in numbers of caesarean sections at full dilatation [9, 10] and both the Royal College of Obstetricians and Gynaecologists [11] and the American College of Obstetricians and Gynaecologists [12] have advocated the need for further training on instrumental vaginal deliveries.

The aim of this study is to review the determinants for a failed operative vaginal delivery and thereby emergency caesarean sections at full dilatation as well as to determine associated fetal and maternal morbidity.

2. Methods

All women who delivered by caesarean section after a failed instrumental delivery at St. Georges Hospital, London, between July 2007 and June 2012, were identified. This London teaching hospital has over 5000 deliveries a year, with three tiers of obstetricians (registrar ST3-5, senior registrar ST6-7, and consultant) working on labour ward. There was always at least the registrar plus senior registrar or consultant on site 24 hours a day, seven days a week. All of the women whose case notes were obtained were over 37 weeks of gestation and had a cephalic presentation.

A proforma was created and completed from the case notes of each woman, detailing background characteristics as well as details surrounding the labour and delivery. Maternal complications that were considered were haemorrhage, intra-operative complications, and genital tract trauma. Neonatal morbidity included Apgar scores, cord arterial pH, and evidence of scalp or fetal lacerations and cephalhematoma.

Information regarding the use of instruments, the total number of instruments (with different types of forceps being classed as two separate instruments), the number of pulls with each instrument during the delivery, and the number of times the cup detached from the fetal head was also recorded. All ventouse deliveries at St. Georges Hospital are performed using the Kiwi Omnicup and metal and silastic cups are not used.

This study was deemed exempt from the need for ethical approval as it is a retrospective observational analysis performed by review of case notes with no clinical interventions and with results showing no identifiable patient data.

3. Results

A total of 119 women from a cohort of 26,856 deliveries required a caesarean section (0.44%) after failed operative delivery. This is compared to 3881 successful operative vaginal deliveries over this time. Our overall failed instrumental delivery rate (total number of failed instrumental deliveries/total number of instrumental deliveries) was 5.1%.

Case notes were obtained for a total of 119 women. Of these 119 women, 22 were delivered for CTG (cardiotocograph) abnormalities and the other 97 because of failure to progress in the second stage of labour.

3.1. Determinants of Failed Instrumental Delivery. 105 women were primiparous and 14 were multiparous. Of these 14 multiparous women, only one woman had had two previous deliveries. The other 13 women had only one previous delivery; therefore in total there had been 15 previous deliveries.

With respect to their previous deliveries, 5 women had had a previous caesarean section at ≥8 cm, 2 had an elective caesarean section for breech, 4 had a spontaneous vaginal delivery, and 4 had required an operative vaginal delivery during their previous labour. Characteristics of women who had a failed instrumental vaginal delivery (FID) are given in Table 1.

3.2. Adverse Outcomes. 25% of women in our study had a postpartum haemorrhage (Table 2) and almost half of all women sustained maternal trauma at the time of the attempted operative vaginal delivery or caesarean section (Table 3).

Overall, 8.4% of neonates sustained trauma (Table 4) following FID. 40 out of 106 neonates had a low Apgar score or an umbilical cord arterial pH of < 7.1 (Table 5). In 13 cases (10.9%), cord blood gases were not available.

4. Discussion

To the best of our knowledge, our study is the largest study that analyzed the determinants as well as maternal and fetal outcomes for emergency caesarean sections performed for FID over a 5-year period. A number of studies have previously looked at predictors of failed operative vaginal delivery [1, 3, 13] and have concluded that risk factors for FID included

(i) persistent OP presentation;

(ii) birthweight > 4 kg;

(iii) maternal body mass index >30;

(iv) mid-cavity delivery or when 1/5th of the fetal head is palpable per abdomen.

Murphy et al. [1] also concluded that instrumental delivery, whether successful or not, was associated with increased risk of maternal trauma and increased neonatal trauma (if there were >3 pulls). Multiple instrument usage was associated with increased neonatal trauma as well as initial attempt at vaginal delivery by an inexperienced operator.

Considering previous deliveries in multiparous women, Hoskins and Gomez [14] in 1997 found that having a previous caesarean section at full dilatation reduced the chance of a successful subsequent vaginal delivery to 13%. This is compared to a success rate of 73% and 67%, respectively, if their previous caesarean section was at 6–9 cm or 5 cm or less.

Malposition was a key factor in our cohort of women who had a failed instrumental delivery. In only 29% of women was the fetal head in a direct, right, or left occipitoanterior position. There are no randomized control trials looking at the optimal method of delivery when there is malposition. Options include manual rotation and direct traction forceps, rotational vacuum extractor, or Keilland forceps and each of these options has its own relative merits and demerits. However, Keilland forceps require additional expertise because of the additional risks they confer. Therefore, in our unit, only those who can demonstrate competency and regularly perform Keilland forceps delivery are permitted to do so. Tempest et al. [15] suggest that women are more likely to need a caesarean section if rotational ventouse rather than Keilland forceps is used to assist the birth (OR 8.2; 95%CI 4.54–14.79) and the adverse maternal and neonatal outcomes are comparable when delivery is by Keilland forceps compared to failed rotational ventouse and subsequent caesarean section.

In our unit, the Kiwi Omnicup is the recommended instrument for rotational deliveries. It was chosen as the first instrument in 91 of the 119 cases (76%) with 36 (40%) of them

TABLE 1: Characteristics of women who had a failed instrumental vaginal delivery.

Characteristics		
Body mass index	>30 Kg/m^2	10 (8.4%)
Onset of labour	Spontaneous	87 (73.1%)
	Induced	21 (17.6%)
	Augmented	11 (9.2%)
Use of oxytocin	None	44 (37.0%)
	Yes	75 (63.0%)
	<4 cm = 19, 4–7 cm = 30, 8–10 cm = 26	
Position of fetal head	Right/left/direct occipitoanterior	34 (28.5%)
	Right//left/direct occipitoposterior	40 (33.6%)
	Occipitotransverse	43 (36.1%)
	Others	2 (1.8%)
Station of the fetal head (distance of the leading bony point of fetal skull below the ischial spines, measured in centimeters)	Above −1	1
	−1	2
	0	68
	+1	48
	+2	2
Fetal size	Mean 3588 g (2365 g–4840 g)	
Operator experience	Trainee <5 years	13 (10.9%)
	Trainee 6-7 years	82 (68.9%)
	Consultant (>8 years)	24 (20.2%)
Time of decision to perform operative vaginal birth	0800–1700	36 (30.3%)
	1701–2000	11 (9.2%)
	2001–0759	72 (60.5%)
Length of second stage of labour (in cases where the indication was "failure to progress")	<3 hr	5.2%
	3.01–≤4 hr	14.4%
	≥4.01 hr	80.4%

TABLE 2: Maternal outcomes: postpartum haemorrhage (%).

Estimated blood loss	Total	Trainee (<5 years)	Trainee (6 or 7 years)	Consultant (<8 years)
<500	19 (16.0%)	2 (18.2)	13 (15.4)	4 (16.7)
500–999 ml	69 (58.0%)	7 (63.6)	48 (57.1)	14 (58.3)
1000–1999 ml	30 (25.2%)	2 (18.2)	22 (26.2)	6 (25.0)
≥2000 ml	1 (0.8%)	0	1 (1.2)	0

having a second instrument (nonrotational or rotational forceps) applied. In 2001 Vacca reported a 98% success rate [16] for the Kiwi Omnicup in his cohort which included 18 nonrotational and 32 rotational deliveries. However, more recent randomized control trials in the United Kingdom concluded that the Kiwi Omnicup was less successful at achieving a successful vaginal delivery when compared to a "standard" cup (34% versus 21%) and thereby increases the rates of sequential instrument use [17]. However, operator experience and skill need to be considered whilst interpreting the data. Whether the use of the Kiwi cup rather than other rotational instruments is a factor for the failed instrumental rate cannot be determined from our data as this comparison could not be made.

From our data, it can also be seen that failed instrumental deliveries are more common out-of-hours with 60% occurring between 2001 and 0759. Whilst it is not possible to conclude that lack of competency and experience contributed to failed instrumental births, instrumental deliveries are predominantly undertaken by trainees during out-of-hours. Lack of consultant presence on labour ward during out-of-hours has been an issue which the Royal College of Obstetrics and Gynaecology has been attempting to address over recent years [18].

In our study, a large proportion of trials of instrumental delivery were by trainees, although most of these were by obstetricians with over 5-year experience. The impact of the shortening of obstetric training within the UK as a result

TABLE 3: Maternal outcomes: birth trauma.

Complication	Indication: abnormal CTG (%)	Indication: failure to progress (%)
Nil	11 (50)	50 (48.5)
Episiotomy	2 (9.1)	2 (2.1)
Perineal tear/graze	1 (4.5)	12 (12.8)
Uterine extension	8 (36.4)	30 (30.9)
Delivered as breech	2 (9.1)	2 (2.1)
Broad ligament haematoma	0	3 (3.1)
Wound dehiscence	0	1 (1.0)
Inverted T	0	1 (1.0)
Bladder injury	0	1 (1.0)
Urethral tear	0	1 (1.0)

TABLE 4: Neonatal outcomes: trauma.

Trauma	Number (out of a total of 119 babies)
Scalp loss	5
Laceration over eye	3
NNU admission	1
Neonatal death (sepsis)	1
Total	10 (8.4%)

TABLE 5: Neonatal condition at birth: Apgar scores and umbilical cord arterial pH.

	Number (1 unable to obtain; umbilical cord gases were not documented in 12 cases)
Arterial pH <7.1	14/106
Apgar <7 at 1 min	20/106
Apgar <7 at 5 min	6/106

of the European Working Time Directive may have resulted in trainees being less skilled and consequently having a higher failure rate of instrumental deliveries compared to their consultant colleagues.

Of the women that required syntocinon, 35% commenced syntocinon in the later stages of labour (at or more than 8 cm). This illustrates the importance of carefully assessing the causes of "secondary arrest" of labour and having senior input if instrumental vaginal delivery is subsequently required in these cases.

More than 80% of women also had a second stage lasting for more than four hours. The National Institute for Clinical Excellence Intrapartum Guidelines [19] stated that after 2 hours of active pushing, primiparous women should have a diagnosis of "delay" made (i.e., failure to progress) and plans should be put in place for an operative delivery to occur enabling primiparous women to be delivered within 3 hours of the active second stage starting. This illustrates the importance of having definite endpoints in the second stage of labour and to strike the right balance between promoting normality and reducing the risks of a prolonged second stage of labour.

The station of the fetal head may also be a determinant of failed instrumental delivery. According to the Royal College of Obstetrics and Gynaecology [11], mid-cavity delivery is defined as when the leading point of the fetal skull is above station plus 2 cm but not above the ischial spine. Just over 95% of our cases are therefore defined as mid-cavity and therefore, should be performed by an experienced operator because of the need for a high level of clinical and technical skill.

Body mass index of over 30 is generally thought to be a risk factor for failed instrumental delivery although this was not borne out in our analysis.

Fetal factors that contribute to a failed instrumental delivery are difficult to be predicted, both antenatally and during the intrapartum period. For example, a fetal weight of more than 4 kg is associated with increased likelihood of failed instrumental delivery but there is no good evidence to support the use of ultrasound for estimation of fetal weight due to its inaccuracy [20]. Clinical skills therefore remain important in the diagnosis and management of failure to progress in second stage. It has been reported [20] that clinical examination was found to be significantly more likely within 10% of the actual weight than an ultrasound derived estimation of fetal weight (58% versus 32%; RR 1.65; 95% CI 1.42–1.69). It is therefore unlikely that fetal factors such as weight could be used to predict the likelihood of either successful or failed instrumental delivery.

When considering maternal outcomes associated with FID, approximately 25% of women in our study lost more than 1000 mL at the time of their caesarean section. In the study by Murphy et al. [3], only 10% of women lost more than 1000 mL at the time of their caesarean section but this was significantly more than those women who achieved a vaginal delivery (adjusted OR 2.8, 95% CI 1.1–7.6). Their group also showed that increased blood loss was less likely with an experienced obstetrician but in our cohort that did not appear to be the case. This increase in blood loss with a fully dilated caesarean section as compared to vaginal delivery was also noted by Ebulue et al. in 2008 [21] (802.7 ± 100.0 versus 425.4 ± 120.0 mL). We run regular "fire drills" on estimation of blood loss in our unit for all staff and therefore it is very likely that the higher EBL noted in our study reflects a more accurate estimation of blood loss at delivery. In addition, obstetric trainees were involved in delivery of 80% of cases who sustained a postpartum haemorrhage of > 1000 mL (Table 2).

Maternal trauma sustained at the time of delivery can occur either at the time of attempted vaginal delivery or during the emergency caesarean section following FID. In our study, a total of 66 "episodes" of maternal trauma were documented. Eight women sustained trauma via two separate mechanisms whereas 61 women did not sustain any trauma at the time of delivery. Therefore, 48% of women sustained trauma at the time of their failed instrumental vaginal delivery or caesarean section. Over 25% of the women who sustained trauma had vaginal/perineal injuries. There is no evidence to support the routine use of episiotomy at the time of operative vaginal delivery [11]. Macleod and Murphy [22] surveyed practicing obstetricians with regard to operative delivery and the use of episiotomy. They found

TABLE 6: Failed Instrumental Delivery Score.

	0	1	2
Position of presenting part	ROA/LOA/DOA	ROP/LOP/DOP	Others
Commencement of oxytocin at dilatation	≤4 cm	5–7 cm	≥8 cm
Duration of second stage (hrs)	<3	3-4	>4
Experience of the operator (years)	>8	6-7	≤5
Parity	≥3	1-2	<1

that a restrictive approach was preferred for deliveries using a ventouse (72%) but a routine approach for forceps (73%). Even with such an approach, episiotomies should not be performed until the stage where delivery is deemed to be imminent. Therefore, it is essential to avoid an episiotomy when the fetal head is at station 0 or plus 1 cm when there is minimal or no descent with traction, to avoid an inappropriate episiotomy.

Our study highlights the fact that both the incidence and severity of maternal trauma are greater when an emergency caesarean was performed for FID, where the primary indication was failure to progress in labour. Therefore, optimization of management of second stage of labour and providing experienced obstetric input is paramount to avoid these complications.

Neonatal outcomes at the time of failed operative delivery and subsequent caesarean have been considered by a number of studies in the past. Unfortunately, it is difficult to compare our data with these studies due to a wide variation in neonatal complications (neonatal unit admissions, jaundice, sepsis, and seizures) that have been considered by individual studies. Much of the available evidence suggests that sequential instrumentation should be avoided if possible because of the increased neonatal morbidity [1]. Murphy et al. found that the use of sequential instruments was associated with increased neonatal trauma (adjusted OR 3.1, 95% CI 1.5–6.8 and adjusted OR 4.4, 95% CI 1.3–14.4, for completed and failed deliveries, resp.). In our study, 34 women (29%) had sequential instruments with either ventouse and forceps or nonrotational and rotational forceps. In half of these cases, there was malposition of the fetal head. Loss of scalp tissue and laceration of the eye (Table 4) highlight operator factors and the need to determine the fetal position accurately, if necessary, using an ultrasound scan to identify fetal orbits, to avoid these complications.

5. Conclusion

Emergency caesarean section during second stage of labour is associated with maternal and fetal complications and also has the potential to negatively influence a woman's birth experience. Our study has shown that failed instrumental delivery is more likely with fetal malposition, prolonged second stage of labour, use of oxytocin for secondary arrest, and lack of operator experience. It is also associated with maternal and neonatal morbidity. Although current guidelines on operative vaginal delivery do identify "risk factors" that may increase the incidence of failed instrumental delivery, there

are no scoring systems to aid obstetricians in determining the likelihood of failure. Based on the findings of our study that analyzed emergency caesarean sections for FID in 119 women, we have formulated a Failed Instrumental Delivery Score to aid clinicians on the "shop floor" in determining the likelihood of failure (Table 6). We have suggested that if the Failed Instrumental Delivery Score is ≥ 8, there is an increased likelihood of a failed instrumental vaginal birth and hence a trial of instrumental vaginal delivery in the theatre should be considered and the consultant on call should be alerted in view of associated increased maternal and fetal morbidity due to FID. We sincerely hope that use of such clinical scoring system based on key parameters that could be easily determined prior to attempting an instrumental vaginal delivery would help clinicians to ensure availability of an experienced clinician and also to conduct delivery in an appropriate environment with a ready recourse to caesarean section. A larger prospective trial may help in confirming the usefulness of the FID Score.

Abbreviation

FID: Failed instrumental delivery.

Key Message

A proportion of emergency caesarean sections following failed instrumental deliveries may be potentially avoidable. An intrapartum clinical scoring system to determine the adverse factors that are associated with FID may help clinicians to optimize management of second stage of labour.

Conflict of Interests

Sian McDonnell has no conflict of interests. Edwin Chandraharan conducts Ventouse Hands-On Masterclasses at several centres in the United Kingdom.

References

[1] D. J. Murphy, R. E. Liebling, R. Patel, L. Verity, and R. Swingler, "Cohort study of operative delivery in the second stage of labour and standard of obstetric care," BJOG: An International Journal of Obstetrics & Gynaecology, vol. 110, no. 6, pp. 610–615, 2003.

[2] R. E. Liebling, R. Swingler, R. R. Patel, L. Verity, P. W. Soothill, and D. J. Murphy, "Pelvic floor morbidity up to one year after difficult instrumental delivery and cesarean section in the second stage of labor: a cohort study," The American Journal of Obstetrics and Gynecology, vol. 191, no. 1, pp. 4–10, 2004.

[3] D. J. Murphy, R. E. Liebling, L. Verity, R. Swingler, and R. Patel, "Early maternal and neonatal morbidity associated with operative delivery in second stage of labour: a cohort study," *The Lancet*, vol. 358, no. 9289, pp. 1203–1207, 2001.

[4] A. McKelvey, R. Ashe, D. McKenna, and R. Roberts, "Caesarean section in the second stage of labour: a retrospective review of obstetric setting and morbidity," *Journal of Obstetrics and Gynaecology*, vol. 30, no. 3, pp. 263–267, 2010.

[5] M. L. Chiswick and D. K. James, "Kielland's forceps: association with neonatal morbidity and mortality," *British Medical Journal*, vol. 1, no. 6155, pp. 7–9, 1979.

[6] F. O'Mahony, G. J. Hofmeyer, and V. Menon, "Choice of instruments for assisted vaginal delivery," *Cochrane Database of Systematic Reviews*, no. 10, Article ID CD005455, 2010.

[7] J. Unterscheider, M. McMenamin, and F. Cullinane, "Rising rates of caesarean deliveries at full cervical dilatation: a concerning trend," *European Journal of Obstetrics & Gynecology and Reproductive Biology*, vol. 157, no. 2, pp. 141–144, 2011.

[8] J. A. Z. Loudon, K. M. Groom, L. Hinkson, D. Harrington, and S. Paterson-Brown, "Changing trends in operative delivery performed at full dilatation over a 10-year period," *Journal of Obstetrics and Gynaecology*, vol. 30, no. 4, pp. 370–375, 2010.

[9] C. Spencer, D. Murphy, and S. Bewley, "Caesarean delivery in the second stage of labour; better training in instrumental delivery may reduce rates," *British Medical Journal*, vol. 333, no. 7569, pp. 613–614, 2006.

[10] L. Gurney, N. Shivananth, and B. O. Ononeze, "Rising rate of second stage C-section: who is to blame? A questionnaire based study of trainees in the North East of England," *Archives of Disease in Childhood: Fetal and Neonatal Edition*, vol. 95, pp. Fa84–Fa85, 2010.

[11] *Royal College Obstetricians and Gynaecologists Greentop Guideline no. 26: Operative Vaginal Delivery*, RCOG Press, 2011.

[12] The American College of Obstetricians and Gynecologists (ACOG), *Operative Vaginal Delivery*, Practice Bulletin no. 17, ACOG, Washington, DC, USA, 2000.

[13] A. Ben-Haroush, N. Melamed, B. Kaplan, and Y. Yogev, "Predictors of failed operative vaginal delivery: a single-center experience," *The American Journal of Obstetrics and Gynecology*, vol. 197, no. 3, pp. 308.e1–308.e5, 2007.

[14] I. A. Hoskins and J. L. Gomez, "Correlation between maximum cervical dilatation at cesarean delivery and subsequent vaginal birth after cesarean delivery," *Obstetrics and Gynecology*, vol. 89, no. 4, pp. 591–593, 1997.

[15] N. Tempest, A. Hart, S. Walkinshaw, and D. K. Hapangama, "A re-evaluation of the role of rotational forceps: retrospective comparison of maternal and perinatal outcomes following different methods of birth for malposition in the second stage of labour," *BJOG*, vol. 120, no. 10, pp. 1277–1284, 2013.

[16] A. Vacca, "Operative vaginal delivery: clinical appraisal of a new vacuum extraction device," *Australian and New Zealand Journal of Obstetrics and Gynaecology*, vol. 41, no. 2, pp. 156–160, 2001.

[17] G. Attilakos, T. Sibanda, C. Winter, N. Johnson, and T. Draycott, "A randomised controlled trial of a new handheld vacuum extraction device," *BJOG: An International Journal of Obstetrics and Gynaecology*, vol. 112, no. 11, pp. 1510–1515, 2005.

[18] N. Timmins, *Tomorrows Specialist: The Future of Obstetrics, Gynaecology and Womens Health Care*, RCOG Press, 2012.

[19] National Institute of Clinical Excellence (NICE), "Intrapartum care: care of healthy women and their babies during childbirth," Clinical 15 Guideline 55, NICE, 2007.

[20] N. W. Hendrix, C. S. Grady, and S. P. Chauhan, "Clinical vs. sonographic estimate of birth weight in term parturients: a randomized clinical trial," *The Journal of Reproductive Medicine*, vol. 45, no. 4, pp. 317–322, 2000.

[21] V. Ebulue, J. Vadalkar, S. Cely, F. Dopwell, and W. Yoong, "Fear of failure: are we doing too many trials of instrumental delivery in theatre?" *Acta Obstetricia et Gynecologica Scandinavica*, vol. 87, no. 11, pp. 1234–1238, 2008.

[22] M. Macleod and D. J. Murphy, "Operative vaginal delivery and the use of episiotomy—a survey of practice in the United Kingdom and Ireland," *European Journal of Obstetrics Gynecology and Reproductive Biology*, vol. 136, no. 2, pp. 178–183, 2008.

11

Predictors of Perinatal Mortality Associated with Placenta Previa and Placental Abruption: An Experience from a Low Income Country

Yifru Berhan

College of Medicine and Health Sciences, Hawassa University, P.O. Box 1560, Hawassa, Ethiopia

Correspondence should be addressed to Yifru Berhan; yifrub@yahoo.com

Academic Editor: Lee P. Shulman

A retrospective cohort study design was used to assess predictors of perinatal mortality in women with placenta previa and abruption between January 2006 and December 2011. Four hundred thirty-two women (253 with placenta previa and 179 with placental abruption) were eligible for analysis. Binary logistic regression, Kaplan-Meier survival curve, and receiver operating characteristic (ROC) curve were used. On admission, 77% of the women were anaemic (<12 gm/dL) with mean haemoglobin level of 9.0 ± 3.0 gm/dL. The proportion of overall severe anaemia increased from about 28% on admission to 41% at discharge. There were 50% perinatal deaths (neonatal deaths of less than seven days of age and fetal deaths after 28 weeks of gestation). In the adjusted odds ratios, lengthy delay in accessing hospital care, prematurity, anaemia in the mothers, and male foetuses were independent predictors of perinatal mortality. The haemoglobin level at admission was more sensitive and more specific than prematurity in the prediction of perinatal mortality. The proportion of severe anaemia and perinatal mortality was probably one of the highest in the world.

1. Introduction

Placenta previa (placenta implanted over the internal cervical os) and placental abruption (premature separation of normally implanted placenta) are the major causes of antepartum haemorrhage in the third trimester of pregnancies and major contributors of obstetric haemorrhage in general [1]. Each of these conditions has a prevalence rate of 0.5% to 2% in most parts of the world [2–4]. Because of the changes in the lower uterine segment length and placental migration as the pregnancy advances, the prevalence of placenta previa has an inverse relation to the gestational age [5]. In other words, it is suggested that reporting of placenta previa in early gestation is likely to overestimate its actual prevalence at term.

Placenta previa and placental abruption have long been recognized as major obstetric complications that result in maternal and fetal mortality as well as morbidity. The effect of these two bloody obstetric complications on perinatal health is multifactorial: blood loss, premature delivery, intrauterine growth restriction, the risk of perinatal asphyxia, the risk of

sepsis, and hyperbilirubinemia [2, 6–8]. A Danish national cohort study was associated with an increased risk of neonatal mortality, prematurity, low Apgar scores, low birthweight, and transfer to a neonatal intensive care unit [9]. Several other studies from developing countries have also shown that pregnant women complicated by placenta previa are likely to have babies delivered preterm, low birth weight, asphyxiated, and requiring intensive neonatal care, while stillbirth or neonatal mortality may also occur [7, 10, 11]. To be specific, the risk of perinatal mortality in women with placental previa is estimated to be 4% to 8% but, when accompanied by prematurity, the death rate may increase to 50% [12].

On the other hand, the perinatal mortality in placental abruption cases may be as high as 20% to 47% [3, 13]. Specific to developed countries, a recent review has shown that 10–20% of all perinatal deaths are caused by placental abruption [14]. More than a decade back, studies in developed countries concluded that placental abruption had a profound impact on stillbirth [15, 16]. However, a large scale review in the United States in 2001 reported that the high perinatal mortality with abruption was mainly due to its strong association with preterm delivery [17]. But with the advancement of obstetric service, the perinatal mortality has been reported as decreasing [18, 19].

To the best of the author's knowledge, there is no published study that assessed placenta previa and placental abruption associated perinatal mortality and morbidity in Sub-Saharan Africa and in Ethiopia in particular. Thus, this study shades light on the most common complications of placenta previa and placental abruption with emphasis on the primary outcome predictors, the magnitude of perinatal mortality, and associated factors. Secondly, it gives a ground evidence on how soon or late women with placenta previa and placental abruption were coming to the hospital; what interventions were undertaken; and what was the condition of the neonates and mothers at discharge. In short, the findings of this study are instrumental to identify barriers and delays at the community and hospital level. The objective of this study was to determine the predictors of perinatal mortality associated with placenta previa and placental abruption.

2. Methods

This retrospective cohort study included all women with placenta previa and placental abruption who were admitted and managed in Hawassa University Hospital between January 2006 and December 2012. Hawassa University Hospital, located in the capital city of Southern Nation Nationalities and People Regional State of Ethiopia, has a catchment population of more than 16 million. During this study period, 9619 women gave birth in this hospital. Out of these, 511 women with singleton pregnancies were diagnosed to have antepartum haemorrhage (APH) at admission. Multiple births were excluded taking into account that they can have many other complications that might add to the complications attributed to the placenta previa or placental abruption independently.

Further scrutiny of each of the 511 APH labelled patients' charts revealed that there was change of the admission diagnoses through progressive evaluation of the pregnant women and examination of the placenta after delivery. As a result, 21 cases were later on identified as abortion (gestational age < 28 weeks) [20]; 29 cases were due to heavy show; 6 cases were diagnosed to have local causes (cervical infection, polyps, leech infestation, and cervical carcinoma); and 23 cases were excluded because of incomplete documentation. A total of 432 cases were identified as eligible for analysis.

The data sources for this study were individual patient's chart, admission, and discharge record books. Data related to the patients' age, residence, distance travelled for hospital admission, duration of hospital stay, obstetric history, clinical condition, and laboratory results at admission and discharge were collected. When a pregnant woman presented with dark and nonclotting vaginal bleeding after 28 weeks of gestation, placental abruption was diagnosed. The finding of retroplacental clot/bloody jell or depression in the maternal placental surface after delivery was taken as confirmation for atypically presented placenta previa. Whereas ultrasound report of placenta praevia was taken as a final diagnosis. For

the purpose of this study, the degree of maternal anaemia and the survival of babies in the perinatal period were taken as primary outcome indicators.

In this study, APH was defined as any vaginal bleeding due to either placenta previa or placental abruption after 28 weeks of gestation before the delivery of the baby. The total time taken to reach the study hospital after the onset of APH symptoms (painless, bright red, and clotting vaginal bleeding in placenta previa; unexplained lower abdominal pain with or without dark nonclotting vaginal bleeding in placental abruption; and decreased or absent fetal kick in both) was taken as the duration before arrival. In this study, lengthy delay is to mean a period that lasted more than 12 hours since the onset of APH symptoms and long distance travelled implies 50 km or more to reach to the hospital. Gestational ages were categorized as very preterm (28–33 completed weeks), preterm (34–36 completed weeks), and term (37+ weeks). Perinatal status defined the fetal or early neonatal survival (from 28 weeks of pregnancy age up to the first 7 days of newborn age) [21] or otherwise after the onset of vaginal bleeding due to placenta previa or placental abruption.

The mean minimum normal haemoglobin level during pregnancy at sea level is 11-12 gm/dL [22]. In this study, the degree of anaemia was categorized as severe, moderate, mild, and no anaemia when the haemoglobin level was <7 gm/dL, 7–9.9 gm/dL, 10–11.9 gm/dL, and 12+ gm/dL, respectively. In this study, perinatal mortality and perinatal death are used interchangeably.

Ethical approval of this study was obtained from Hawassa University College of Medicine and Health Sciences Institutional Review Board. Written informed consent from the women included in this study was not required as only already registered data were used. Moreover, confidentiality and anonymity are assured by analyzing and disseminating the data in aggregate.

Data analysis was done using SPSS version 16.0 and Microsoft Office Excel 2010 computer software. Whisker and box plot was used to show the relation of perinatal mortality due to placenta previa and placental abruption with delay in arrival, gestational age, haemoglobin level, and fetal birth weight. The binary logistic regression model was applied to assess the association of perinatal mortality as a dependent variable with some selected variables as predictors. Kaplan-Meier survival curve with log rank test and receiver operating characteristic (ROC) curve (nonparametric method) were used to determine the strength of perinatal mortality predictors. P value < 0.05 was taken as indicator of statistically significant association.

3. Results

3.1. General Characteristics. Out of 432 antepartum haemorrhage cases included in this study, placenta previa and placental abruption constituted 253 (58.6%) and 179 (41.4%), respectively. The incidence of placenta previa and placental abruption in the study hospital during the study period was 2.6 and 1.9 per 1000 pregnant women. Placenta previa by type was totalis, partialis, and marginalis/low-lying which accounted for 151 (59.4%), 54 (21.5%), and 48 (19.1%), respectively. The degree of abruption (separation) for 107 (59.8%) was up to 50% or less and for the other 72 (40.2%) cases was over 50%. Twelve cases were diagnosed before the onset of vaginal bleeding. Otherwise, 420 (97.2%) women presented to the hospital after the onset of vaginal bleeding. Of which, 93 (21.5%) were admitted in a state of hemorrhagic shock (with unrecordable blood pressure and severe blood loss anaemia).

Nearly three-fourths of the women were in the age range of 20–34 years and more than three-fifths came from rural areas (Table 1). One hundred forty-five (33.6%) women traveled more than 100 km to reach the study hospital; the mean distance was 96 ± 93 km. When the proportions of mothers' age, residence, and distance travelled were stratified by placenta previa and placental abruption, there was no much difference. Women with placental abruption came relatively earlier than women with placenta previa: >12 hours delay before arrival in placenta previa and placental abruption group was 157 (62.1%) and 81 (45.%), respectively.

Overall, 238 (55.1%) women accessed the study hospital more than 12 hours after onset of their bleeding. The median delay in accessing the study hospital was 16 (interquartile range: 7–48) hours. In more than half of the cases (51.2%), with almost equivalent proportion in both placenta previa and placental abruption, the gestational ages had reached term (37+ weeks). On arrival at the hospital, 142 (32.9%) were fetal demise, and 53 (12.3%) foetuses had abnormal fetal heart rate (persistent bradycardia, persistent tachycardia, or irregularly fluctuating from normal range to bradycardia or tachycardia).

3.2. Degree of Anaemia. On admission, 334 (77.3%) of the women were found to have anaemia and the mean haemoglobin level was 9.0 ± 3.0 gm/dL (Table 2). The distribution of severe, moderate, and mild anaemia was almost proportional. Severe and mild anaemia was detected in the majority of women with placenta previa and placental abruption, respectively. When these women were discharged from the hospital, the severity of anaemia was found even worsening. The proportion of overall severe anaemia increased from 27.8% on admission to 41.2% at discharge and moderate anaemia from 27.1% to 30.6%.

In patients with placenta previa, severe anaemia increased from 33.2% on admission to 51.4% at discharge. In short, the proportion of anaemia increased from 201 (79.4%) to 234 (92.5%) in placenta previa cases and from 133 (74.3%) to 153 (85.5%) in placental abruption cases. Figure 1 summarizes the change in haemoglobin level after delivery. In the majority of women, the haemoglobin levels at discharge were below the level on admission. Specifically, the drops in haemoglobin level were marked in those women who were better with the haemoglobin level >7 gm/dL on admission.

3.3. Interventions in the Hospital. Table 3 shows the specific intervention carried out and fetal outcomes. It was possible to transfuse whole blood for 144 (33.3%) women. Of which,

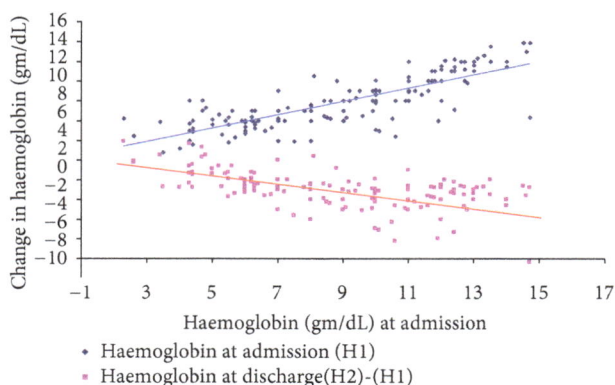

FIGURE 1: The change in haemoglobin level at the time of discharge from the level at the time of admission, 2006–2011, Hawassa University Hospital, Ethiopia.

106 (24.5%) were transfused with 1-2 units of blood (the transfusion criterion of the hospital is haemoglobin <7 gm/dL for blood loss anaemia with or without hemodynamic instability; one unit blood is equivalent to 450 mL). As presented in Figure 2, all women with placenta previa and the majority of women with placental abruption whose haemoglobin level <7 gm/dL at discharge were transfused 1-2 units of blood before having this amount of haemoglobin. Three women with placental abruption were not at all transfused despite having a haemoglobin level of <7 gm/dL.

Eighty-nine (20.6%) women were kept in the maternity ward before delivery for more than two days (median: 2.5 and IQR: 1–24 days). After delivery, 360 (83.3%) women were kept in the hospital for less than a week, with similar proportion in both placenta previa and placental abruption. Three-fourths of women gave birth by caesarean section. Active vaginal bleeding was the highest indication, 79.4% (258/325). One hundred forty-three (66.8%) of the perinatal deaths were delivered by caesarean section. Specifically, 92 (43%) caesarean sections were done for fetal demise and some other indications.

3.4. Perinatal Mortality. As shown in Table 3, there were 214 perinatal deaths, making the total perinatal mortality rate due to placenta previa and abruption about 495/1000 births or nearly 50%. The perinatal mortality rates associated with placenta previa and placental abruption were about 447/1000 births and 564/1000 births, respectively. Of the total perinatal deaths, 164 (38.0%) foetuses were found to be stillbirths (22 foetuses were admitted to the hospital with a positive fetal heart beat and died in utero) and 50 (11.6%) were early neonatal deaths. Out of the total perinatal deaths, placenta previa and placental abruption related deaths were 44.7% (113/253) and 56.4% (101/179), respectively. The proportion of stillbirths and early neonatal deaths in placenta previa and placental abruption were 34.4% versus 43.0% and 10.3% versus 13.4%, respectively.

In Table 4, the univariate analysis revealed that perinatal mortality due to placenta previa and placental abruption

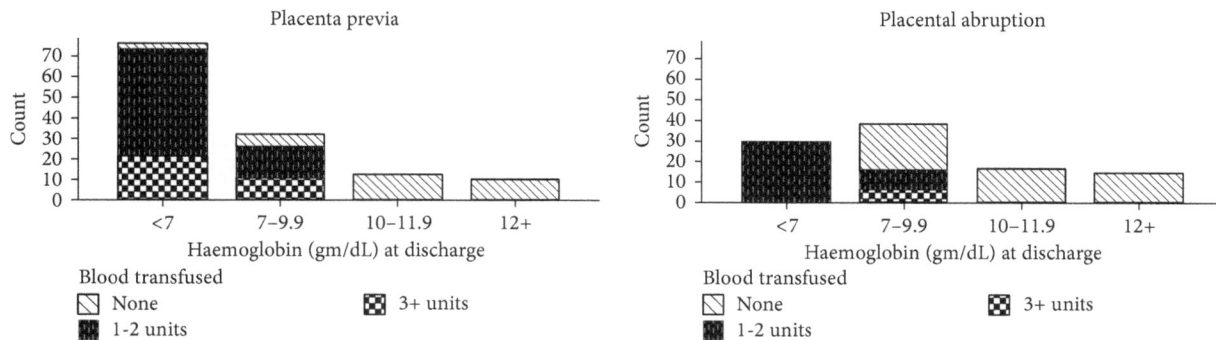

FIGURE 2: The distribution of anaemia* during the time of discharge from the hospital and the amount of blood transfused before achieving this amount of haemoglobin as paneled by type of antepartum haemorrhage (placenta previa and placental abruption). *Severe anaemia (haemoglobin < 7 gm/dL); moderate anaemia (Hb < 7–9.9 gm/dL); mild anaemia (Hb 10–11.9 gm/dL).

was strongly associated with long distance travel, lack of antenatal care, very low birth weight, and maternal severe anaemia. Other variables weakly associated with perinatal mortality due to placenta previa and placental abruption were maternal age above 20 years, rural residence, multiparity, and gestational age of 28–33 weeks during the time of delivery.

For more than three-fifths of the total foetuses (62.5%), their birth weight was above 2500 gm and 259 (60.0%) of the foetuses were male, with comparable proportion in both placental abruption and placenta previa. The gestational age distribution of the perinatal deaths in weeks was 28–33 for 60 (28.0%), 34–36 for 52 (24.3%), and 37+ for 102 (47.7%). The Kaplan-Meier curve demonstrated that the perinatal mortality was the highest among placental abruption cases (log rank: $P < 0.0001$), and in both placenta previa and placental abruption cases, the survival curve dropped sharply in the early period, which may indicate that the majority of the babies died in the first 24 hours of onset of the bleeding (Figure 3).

Figure 4 shows the relation of perinatal mortality with delay in arrival (a), gestational age (b), haemoglobin level (c), and fetal birth weight (d) as stratified by placenta previa and placental abruption. Both the median and IQR hours of delay among perinatal deaths were shorter than the survivors, which is another evidence to strengthen the findings in Figure 3. In women with placental abruption, the median gestational age and fetal birth weight were found to be lower in perinatal deaths than the survivors, whereas in women with placenta praevia, the median gestational ages of perinatal deaths and survivors were comparable. In both placental abruption and placenta previa, however, the median admission haemoglobin level of the cases resulting in perinatal deaths group was much lower than the survivors.

In Table 5, the crude odds ratios in the binary logistic regression have shown that long distance travel, lengthy delay in accessing the hospital, preterm gestational age, low blood pressure, anaemia on admission, and others were strongly associated with perinatal mortality. In the adjusted odds ratios, however, lengthy delay, preterm gestational age, anaemia level, being male, and delivered vaginally were independent predictors of perinatal mortality.

Since the adjusted binary logistic regression model showed highly statistically significant association of perinatal mortality with low gestational age and haemoglobin level (OR 1.4 and 1.9, resp.), receiver operating characteristic curve (ROC) was depicted to test the two variables predictive validity in perinatal mortality (Figure 5). As the area under the curve shows, haemoglobin level on admission was more sensitive and more specific to determine perinatal mortality than the gestational age.

In this series of cases, there was no maternal death reported; couvelaire uterus was detected in 18 women with placental abruption who gave birth by caesarean section; and caesarean hysterectomy was done in 13 cases of placenta previa (12 for placental adherence and one for intractable postpartum haemorrhage).

4. Discussion

This study has shown that the perinatal mortality in women with placenta previa and placental abruption was about 50%, which is probably one of the highest in the world [3, 7, 10–13, 23]. Placenta previa associated perinatal mortality (about 45%) in particular was more than two- to threefold of some less developed countries [6, 23] and more than fifteenfold of a report from developed countries [9, 15, 24]. The perinatal deaths associated with placental abruption alone were also too high but were not as high as those in the recent report from Pakistan [25]. Similarly, the proportion of severely anaemic women both on admission and at discharge was surprisingly high, probably because of the big delay in reporting to the hospital, further blood loss after admission, and inadequate blood transfusion.

Unlike placental abruption, in which bleeding can be concealed and may be complicated with coagulopathy and further blood loss [26], bleeding due to placenta previa is immediately revealed and likely to make many of the pregnant women and their family seek prompt medical care. Relative ease of diagnosis in placenta previa is also an advantage for health professionals to undertake timely appropriate interventions and prevent further blood loss and associated maternal and perinatal complications. In this

TABLE 1: General characteristics of cases stratified by placenta previa and placental abruption, 2006–2011, Hawassa University Hospital, Ethiopia.

Variable	Placenta previa (N = 253)	Abruptio placenta (N = 179)	Total (N = 432)
Mothers' age in years			
<20	12 (4.7)	12 (6.7)	24 (5.6)
20–34	181 (71.6)	140 (78.2)	321 (74.3)
35+	60 (23.7)	27 (15.1)	87 (20.1)
Mothers' residence			
Urban	86 (34.0)	77 (43.0)	163 (37.7)
Rural	167 (66.0)	102 (57.0)	269 (62.3)
Distance traveled in km			
<50	98 (38.7)	80 (44.7)	178 (41.2)
50–100	70 (27.7)	39 (21.8)	109 (25.2)
101–200	37 (14.6)	42 (23.5)	79 (18.3)
>200	48 (19.0)	18 (10.0)	66 (15.3)
Duration before arrival in hours			
≤12	96 (37.9)	98 (54.7)	194 (44.9)
>12	157 (62.1)	81 (45.3)	238 (55.1)
Parity			
0	39 (15.4)	48 (26.8)	87 (20.1)
I–IV	111 (43.9)	93 (52.0)	204 (47.2)
V+	103 (40.7)	38 (21.2)	141 (32.6)
Gestational age in weeks			
28–33	54 (21.3)	30 (16.8)	84 (19.4)
34–36	74 (29.3)	53 (29.6)	127 (29.4)
37+	125 (49.4)	96 (53.6)	221 (51.2)
Antenatal care			
Yes	153 (60.5)	128 (71.5)	281 (65.0)
No	100 (39.5)	51 (28.5)	151 (35.0)
Diastolic BP in mmHg			
Unrecordable	13 (5.1)	3 (1.7)	16 (3.7)
<60	65 (25.7)	12 (6.7)	77 (17.8)
60+	175 (69.2)	164 (91.6)	339 (78.5)
Fetal heart beat			
Negative	71 (28.1)	71 (39.7)	142 (32.9)
Abnormal	32 (12.6)	21 (11.7)	53 (12.3)
Normal	150 (59.3)	87 (48.6)	237 (54.8)

BP: blood pressure.

TABLE 2: The proportion and degree of anaemia at the time of admission and discharge as stratified by placenta previa and placental abruption, 2006–2011, Hawassa University Hospital, Ethiopia.

Haemoglobin in gm/dL	Mean	Severe anaemia (<7)	Moderate anaemia (7–9.9)	Mild anaemia (10–11.9)	No anaemia (12+)
At admission					
Total	9.0 ± 3.0	120 (27.8)	117 (27.1)	97 (22.4)	98 (22.7)
PP	8.7 ± 3.0	84 (33.2)	75 (29.6)	42 (16.6)	52 (20.6)
PA	9.5 ± 3.0	36 (20.1)	42 (23.5)	55 (30.7)	46 (25.7)
At discharge					
Total	7.9 ± 2.6	178 (41.2)	132 (30.6)	77 (17.8)	44 (10.2)
PP	7.6 ± 2.6	130 (51.4)	62 (24.5)	42 (16.6)	19 (7.5)
PA	8.4 ± 2.5	48 (26.8)	70 (39.1)	35 (19.6)	26 (14.5)

PP: placenta previa (N = 253).
PA: placental abruption (N = 179).

TABLE 3: Specific interventions and fetal outcome stratified by placenta previa and placental abruption, 2006–2011, Hawassa University Hospital, Ethiopia.

Variable	Placenta previa ($N = 253$)	Abruptio placenta ($N = 179$)	Total ($N = 432$)
Whole blood transfused			
1-2 units	67 (26.5)	39 (21.8)	106 (24.5)
3+ units	32 (12.6)	6 (3.4)	38 (8.8)
Hospital arrival to delivery time (days)			
≤1	188 (74.3)	155 (86.6)	343 (79.4)
2–7	34 (13.4)	15 (8.4)	49 (11.3)
≥8	31 (13.3)	9 (5.0)	40 (9.3)
Hospital stay after delivery (days)			
≤6	211 (83.4)	149 (83.2)	360 (83.3)
≥7	42 (16.6)	30 (16.8)	72 (16.7)
Mode of delivery			
Vaginal**	18 (7.1)	89 (49.7)	107 (24.8)
Caesarean section	235 (92.9)	90 (50.3)	325 (75.2)
Fetal outcome			
Alive	140 (55.3)	78 (43.6)	218 (50.4)
Still birth	87 (34.4)	77 (43.0)	164 (38.0)
Early neonatal death*	26 (10.3)	24 (13.4)	50 (11.6)
Fetal sex			
Male	145 (57.3)	114 (63.7)	259 (60.0)
Female	108 (42.7)	65 (36.3)	173 (40.0)
Fetal weight (gm)			
1000–1499	21 (8.3)	24 (13.4)	45 (10.4)
1500–2499	72 (28.4)	45 (25.1)	117 (27.1)
2500–3999	154 (60.9)	104 (58.1)	258 (59.7)
4000+	6 (2.4)	6 (3.4)	12 (2.8)

*Within seven days of birth. **Including two vacuum and one forceps assisted delivery.

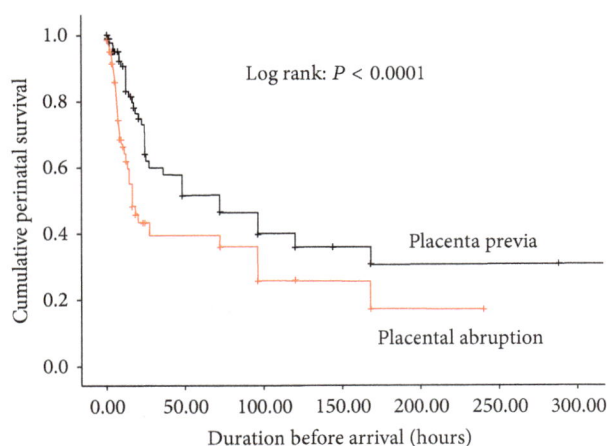

FIGURE 3: Kaplan-Meier estimates of the cumulative perinatal survival stratified by placenta previa and placental abruption, 2006–2011, Ethiopia.

why perinatal deaths were nearly proportional or higher than previously reported [3, 12, 13, 17–19, 23].

In general, the number of women with severe anaemia was quite large in both placenta previa and placental abruption group, which both contributed to about 50% of perinatal mortality. Among others, the adjusted binary logistic regression model also demonstrated that severe anaemia and delay in arrival were strong predictors for high perinatal mortality. Due to the excessive blood loss characteristic of these two obstetric problems, some degree of anaemia is inevitable regardless of the quality of care available in the country where the pregnant women reside.

Maternal anaemia resulting from bleeding was not reported to be contributors to perinatal mortality in some of the previous studies of placental previa and placental abruption [3, 12, 13, 23, 25]. This is probably because of the settings of advanced obstetric care and easy access of health facilities for the majority of pregnant women reported [9]; it might have resulted in a reduction of placenta previa and placental abruption related complications.

In the author's opinion, delay in arrival was probably at the epicenter of the whole problem of the patients included in this study. This is because, the longer pregnant women stay bleeding at home, the more they are likely to be severely

study, however, among women with placenta previa, more than one-third on admission and more than half at discharge were severely anaemic, which is probably the major reason

TABLE 4: Univariate analysis on perinatal mortality in relation to selected demographic and obstetric factors among women with antepartum haemorrhage (APH), 2006–2011, Hawassa University Hospital, Ethiopia.

Variable	Total APH* (N = 432)	Perinatal deaths (N = 214)	P value
Mothers' age in years			
<20	24	6 (25.0)	
20–34	321	166 (51.7)	0.04
35+	87	42 (48.3)	
Mothers' residence			
Urban	163	69 (42.3)	
Rural	269	145 (53.9)	0.02
Distance traveled in km			
<50	178	66 (37.1)	
≥50	254	148 (58.3)	<0.0001
Antenatal care			
Yes	283	124 (43.8)	
No	149	90 (60.4)	0.001
Parity			
0	87	31 (35.6)	
I–IV	204	104 (51.0)	0.04
V+	141	79 (56.0)	
Gestational age in weeks			
28–33	84	60 (71.4)	
34–36	127	52 (40.9)	<0.0001
37+	221	102 (46.2)	
Maternal anaemia on admission			
Severe	113	104 (92.0)	
Moderate	121	52 (43.0)	<0.0001
Mild	91	27 (30.0)	
No anaemia	107	31 (29.0)	
Fetal weight (gm)			
1000–1499	45	36 (80.0)	
1500–2499	117	66 (56.4)	<0.0001
2500–3999	258	112 (43.4)	
4000+	12	0	

*Placenta previa + placental abruption; APH: antepartum haemorrhage.

TABLE 5: Binary logistic regression on predictors of perinatal mortality in women with placenta previa and placental abruption, 2006–2011, Hawassa University Hospital, Ethiopia.

Variable	Crude		Adjusted**	
	P value	OR (95% CI)	P value	OR (95% CI)
Long distance traveled*	0.002	0.8 (0.63, 0.90)	0.31	1.0 (0.99, 1.01)
Lengthy delay before arrival*	0.005	1.01 (1.00, 1.02)	0.003	1.01 (1.005, 1.02)
Low gestational age*	<0.0001	1.1 (1.08, 1.22)	<0.0001	1.4 (1.16, 1.65)
No antenatal care	0.008	0.6 (0.39, 0.87)	0.07	0.34 (0.11, 1.09)
Low blood pressure*	<0.0001	1.02 (1.01, 1.03)	0.94	1.0 (0.98, 1.02)
Anaemia*	<0.0001	1.5 (1.41, 1.68)	<0.0001	1.9 (1.42, 2.59)
Male fetal sex	0.009	1.7 (1.14, 2.51)	<0.0001	11.8 (3.13, 44.25)
Vaginal delivery	<0.0001	1.4 (1.16, 1.58)	<0.0001	2.5 (1.55, 3.97)

*Continuous; all others are dichotomous.
**Adjusted for all variables in this table; other variables like maternal age, parity, and residence did not show significant association in the crude odds ratio.

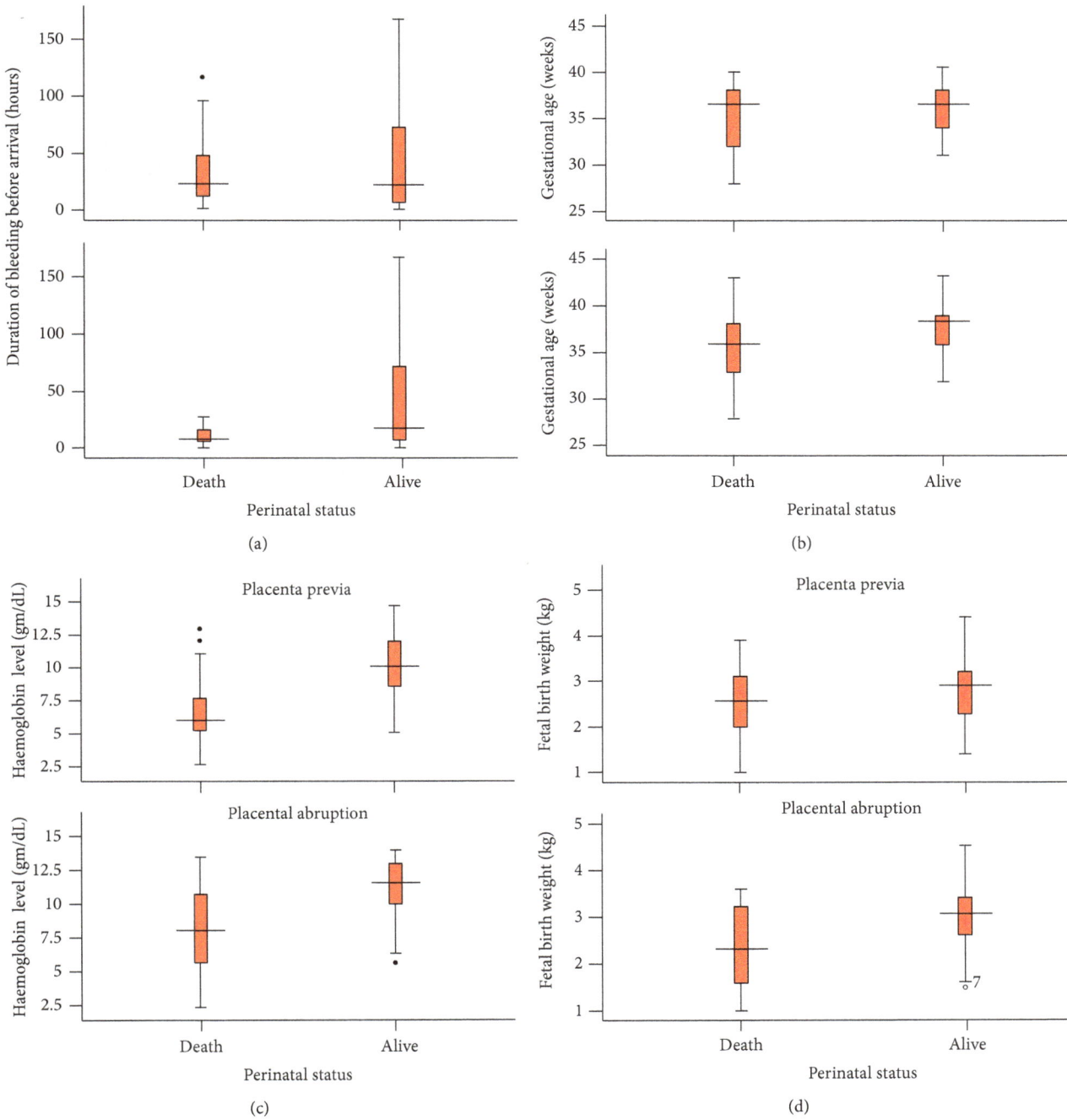

FIGURE 4: The relation of perinatal mortality with delay in arrival (a), gestational age (b), haemoglobin level (c), and fetal birth weight (d) as stratified by women with placenta previa and placental abruption, 2006–2011, Hawassa University Hospital, Ethiopia.

anaemic. As a result, there is a high chance the foetuses will get asphyxiated or dead. Furthermore, since the hospital has been functioning as a referral with blood transfusion and operation facility, it is likely that it has more complicated placenta previa and placental abruption cases that had travelled long distance. Lengthier delay in arriving to the hospital was also observed among women with placenta previa than women with placental abruption, which was probably why many women with placenta previa were found in a severely

anaemic state that has contributed to their significant overall perinatal deaths.

One may pose a question, why was there such significant delay in arrival and long distance travel? Since this study was based on registered data, it was not possible to get an exact answer for this question. However, from day to day observation in the hospital, it is possible to speculate that lack of health care seeking behavior (probably because of unawareness of available health services for this kind of

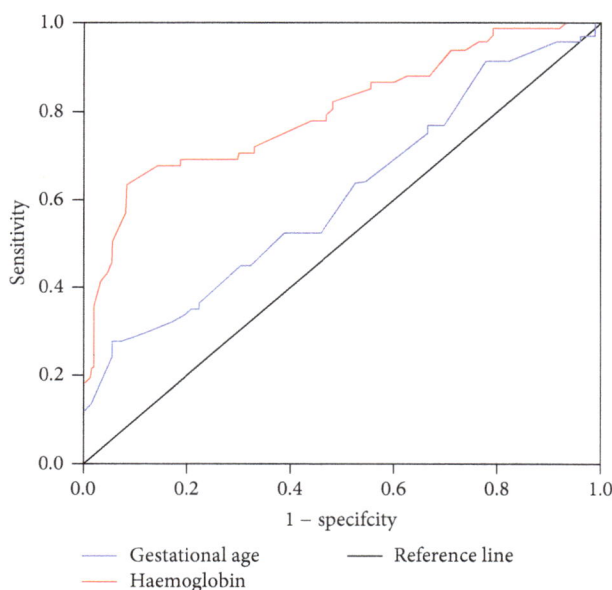

FIGURE 5: Receiver operating characteristics (ROC) curve comparing the sensitivity and specificity of haemoglobin level and gestational age on predicting perinatal mortality in women with placenta previa and placental abruption, 2006–2011, Hawassa University Hospital, Ethiopia.

problem), lack of local midwives for early referral, inability to get access to health facilities (usually due to financial problem and lack of ambulance service in the rural area), and delay in getting proper and satisfying treatment in health facilities including the hospital where these cases were managed might have contributed to high perinatal mortality and high blood loss anaemia. Whatever the barrier for early arrival was, the lengthy delay was the most likely factor for severe blood loss and high perinatal death.

Regardless of the delay in time, however, several studies have shown that placenta previa and placental abruption are known to triple the rate of perinatal mortality primarily due to prematurity [7, 8, 10, 12, 13, 17, 25]. In this study, however, as ROC curve showed, prematurity was not as sensitive and specific as haemoglobin level was in predicting perinatal mortality. The gestational age for more than two-thirds of the perinatal deaths was 34 weeks and above. But this finding has to be interpreted very cautiously. The relatively low perinatal deaths among very premature foetuses (28–33 weeks) may not be a true reflection as there were only a very small number of babies delivered prematurely. Taking into consideration the available intensive neonatal care and the reported neonatal survival rate, by definition, the viable gestational age for foetuses delivered in developed and developing countries including this study starts from 20–24 weeks [9, 15, 24] and 28 weeks [21], respectively. This could mean that if this study had included babies born before 28-week gestation with similar problems, prematurity might have been as well the leading associated problem for high perinatal mortality.

Otherwise, since the area under the curve is said to be an effective and combined measure of sensitivity and specificity for assessing the inherent validity of a predictor [27], above all, haemoglobin level on admission was the strongest predictor of perinatal mortality. The finding of about one-third of the women with severe anaemia and more than one-fifth presenting in shock on admission may also explain how critically ill the women themselves were. Probably it was because of such life threatening anaemia due to blood loss why nearly 80% of the women were subjected to give birth within 24 hours of their arrival to the hospital. Additionally, the finding of the majority of the women with further worsening anaemia indicate the continuous blood loss even after arrival to the hospital (probably due to the high caesarean delivery rate) and lack of adequate blood transfusion.

The explanation for the worsening haemoglobin level at discharge probably goes beyond the continuous blood loss even after arrival. The finding of more than half of women with placenta previa and more than one-fourth of women with placental abruption having severe anaemia at the time of discharge is an objective evidence to show the inadequate blood transfusion in the study hospital. Had it been possible, all women with severe anaemia should have been transfused with blood or had iron infusion and been discharged with haemoglobin level of 7 gm/dL and above. In a clinical setting such as the one in this hospital, like many others in low income countries, getting blood donor is a daily challenge and iron infusion is not yet in routine practice. As a result, many of severely anaemic patients are discharged after assessing only the overall clinical condition.

Limitations of this study are as follows: firstly the findings of this study could not be taken as incidence representing the general population in the hospital's catchment area. This is because the included mothers came mainly from a rural population where about 94% of pregnant women give birth at home [16]. Therefore, the reported cases in this study, if not representative, may reflect the magnitude of similar problems probably with worse outcomes back in the villages. Secondly, some asymptomatic or mild form of abruption may be under reported. Thirdly, some of the women might have variable degrees of anaemia in their pregnancy even before the onset of bleeding due to either placenta previa or placental abruption, which this study was not able to address. In Africa, severely anaemic pregnant women were reported to be between 1% and 5% [28] and 3% in Ethiopia [20]. Fourthly, some of the women discharged with severe anaemia might have had further complications which this study was not able to determine. Fifthly, although perinatal mortality is extended up to 28 weeks of postnatal period; this study was limited to the time the neonates were discharged from the hospital.

5. Conclusions

Low maternal haemoglobin level and delay in arrival were strong predictors of perinatal mortality due to placenta previa and placental abruption. The perinatal mortality was nearly 50% and 76.6% of these were stillbirths. The proportion of severe anaemia and perinatal mortality was probably one of the highest in the world. To reduce the burden of placenta previa and placental abruption related perinatal mortality, (1) comprehensive obstetric care including blood transfusion and iron infusion set up should be availed as close as possible to the villages where the study participants came from, and (2) there should be a strategy to let the community know the importance of antenatal care, maternal, and fetal risks of vaginal bleeding during pregnancy. Future studies should give emphasis on assessing the reasons for the delay in accessing and availing comprehensive obstetric care.

Conflict of Interests

The author would like to declare that there are no competing interests.

References

[1] Q. Yang, S. W. Wen, K. Phillips, L. Oppenheimer, D. Black, and M. C. Walker, "Comparison of maternal risk factors between placental abruption and placenta previa," *The American Journal of Perinatology*, vol. 26, no. 4, pp. 279–286, 2009.

[2] Y. Oyelese and C. V. Ananth, "Placental abruption," *Obstetrics and Gynecology*, vol. 108, no. 4, pp. 1005–1016, 2006.

[3] K. E. Francois and M. R. Foley, "Antepartum and post-partum haemorrhage," in *Obstetrics: Normal and Problem Pregnancies*, S. G. Gabbe, J. R. Niebyl, and J. L. Simpson, Eds., pp. 458–466, Churchill Levingstone, New York, NY, USA, 5th edition, 2007.

[4] S. L. Clark, "Placenta previa and abruption," in *Maternal-Fetal Medicine: Principles and Practice*, R. K. Creasy and R. Resnik, Eds., p. 713, WB Saunders Company, Philadelphia, Pa, USA, 5th edition, 2004.

[5] J. P. Neilson, "Interventions for suspected placenta praevia," *Cochrane Database of Systematic Reviews*, no. 2, 2003.

[6] R. Giordano, A. Cacciatore, P. Cignini, R. Vigna, and M. Romano, "Antepartum Haemorrhage," *Journal of Prenatal Medicine*, vol. 4, no. 1, pp. 12–16, 2010.

[7] T. Rosenberg, G. Pariente, R. Sergienko, A. Wiznitzer, and E. Sheiner, "Critical analysis of risk factors and outcome of placenta previa," *Archives of Gynecology and Obstetrics*, vol. 284, no. 1, pp. 47–51, 2011.

[8] J. M. G. Crane, M. C. Van den Hof, L. Dodds, B. A. Armson, and R. Liston, "Maternal complications with placenta previa," *American Journal of Perinatology*, vol. 17, no. 2, pp. 101–105, 2000.

[9] L. N. Nørgaard, A. Pinborg, Ø. Lidegaard, and T. Bergholt, "A Danish national cohort study on neonatal outcome in singleton pregnancies with placenta previa," *Acta Obstetricia et Gynecologica Scandinavica*, vol. 91, no. 5, pp. 546–551, 2012.

[10] C. V. Ananth, J. C. Smulian, and A. M. Vintzileos, "The effect of placenta previa on neonatal mortality: a population-based study in the United States, 1989 through 1997," *The American Journal of Obstetrics and Gynecology*, vol. 188, no. 5, pp. 1299–1304, 2003.

[11] H. M. Salihu, Q. Li, D. J. Rouse, and G. R. Alexander, "Placenta previa: Neonatal death after live births in the United States," *The American Journal of Obstetrics and Gynecology*, vol. 188, no. 5, pp. 1305–1309, 2003.

[12] C. M. Lam, S. F. Wong, K. M. Chow, and L. C. Ho, "Women with placenta praevia and antepartum haemorrhage have a worse outcome than those who do not bleed before delivery," *Journal of Obstetrics and Gynaecology*, vol. 20, no. 1, pp. 27–31, 2000.

[13] N. B. Kyrklund-Blomberg, G. Gennser, and S. Cnattingius, "Placental abruption and perinatal death," *Paediatric and Perinatal Epidemiology*, vol. 15, no. 3, pp. 290–297, 2001.

[14] M. Tikkanen, "Placental abruption: epidemiology, risk factors and consequences," *Acta Obstetricia et Gynecologica Scandinavica*, vol. 90, no. 2, pp. 140–149, 2011.

[15] C. V. Ananth, G. S. Berkowitz, D. A. Savitz, and R. H. Lapinski, "Placental abruption and adverse perinatal outcomes," *Journal of the American Medical Association*, vol. 282, no. 17, pp. 1646–1651, 1999.

[16] M. Tikkanen, O. Riihimäki, M. Gissler et al., "Decreasing incidence of placental abruption in Finland during 1980–2005," *Acta Obstetricia et Gynecologica Scandinavica*, vol. 91, no. 9, pp. 1046–1052, 2012.

[17] C. V. Ananth and A. J. Wilcox, "Placental abruption and perinatal mortality in the United States," *The American Journal of Epidemiology*, vol. 153, no. 4, pp. 332–337, 2001.

[18] M. Tikkanen, T. Luukkaala, M. Gissler et al., "Decreasing perinatal mortality in placental abruption," *Acta Obstetricia et Gynecologica Scandinavica*, vol. 92, no. 3, pp. 298–305, 2013.

[19] S. Rasmussen, L. M. Irgens, P. Bergsjø, and K. Dalaker, "Perinatal mortality and case fatality after placental abruption in Norway 1967–1991," *Acta Obstetricia et Gynecologica Scandinavica*, vol. 75, no. 3, pp. 229–234, 1996.

[20] Central Statistics Agency (CSA), *Ethiopia Demographic and Health Survey 2005*, Addis Ababa, Ethiopia, http://dhsprogram.com/publications/index.cfm.

[21] WHO, *Neonatal and Perinatal Mortality: Country, Regional & Global Estimates*, World Health Organization, Geneva, Switzerland, 2006.

[22] N. van den Broek, "Anaemia and micronutrient deficiencies," *British Medical Bulletin*, vol. 67, pp. 149–160, 2003.

[23] S. A. Siddiqui, G. Tariq, N. Soomro, A. Sheikh, F. Shabih-ul-Hasnain, and K. A. Memon, "Perinatal outcome and near-miss morbidity between placenta previa versus abruptio placentae," *Journal of the College of Physicians and Surgeons Pakistan*, vol. 21, no. 2, pp. 79–83, 2011.

[24] J. M. G. Crane, M. C. van den Hof, L. Dodds, B. A. Armson, and R. Liston, "Neonatal outcomes with placenta previa," *Obstetrics and Gynecology*, vol. 93, no. 4, pp. 541–544, 1999.

[25] S. Shukar-ud-Din, G. Tariq, and N. Soomro, "Abruptio placentae versus placenta previa as a risk factor for preterm labour," *Pakistan Journal Of Surgery*, vol. 26, no. 2, pp. 163–168, 2010.

[26] F. G. Cunningham, K. J. Leneno, S. L. Bloom, J. C. Hauth, L. C. Gilstrap III, and K. D. Wenstrom, *Williams Obstetrics*, McGraw-Hill, New York, NY, USA, 22nd edition, 2005.

[27] R. Kumar and A. Indrayan, "Receiver operating characteristic (ROC) curve for medical researchers," *Indian Pediatrics*, vol. 48, no. 4, pp. 277–287, 2011.

[28] WHO, *Prevention and Management of Severe Anaemia in Pregnancy*, World Health Organization, Geneva, Switzerland, 1993.

12

Clinical Presentation of Preeclampsia and the Diagnostic Value of Proteins and Their Methylation Products as Biomarkers in Pregnant Women with Preeclampsia and Their Newborns

Maria Portelli and Byron Baron (iD)

Centre for Molecular Medicine and Biobanking, Faculty of Medicine and Surgery, University of Malta, Msida MSD2080, Malta

Correspondence should be addressed to Byron Baron; angenlabs@gmail.com

Academic Editor: Fabio Facchinetti

Preeclampsia (PE) is a disorder which affects 1-10% of pregnant women worldwide. It is characterised by hypertension and proteinuria in the later stages of gestation and can lead to maternal and perinatal morbidity and mortality. Other than the delivery of the foetus and the removal of the placenta, to date there are no therapeutic approaches to treat or prevent PE. It is thus only possible to reduce PE-related mortality through early detection, careful monitoring, and treatment of the symptoms. For these reasons the search for noninvasive, blood-borne, or urinary biochemical markers that could be used for the screening, presymptomatic diagnosis, and prediction of the development of PE is of great urgency. So far, a number of biomarkers have been proposed for predicting PE, based on pathophysiological observations, but these have mostly proven to be unreliable and inconsistent between different studies. The clinical presentation of PE and data gathered for the biochemical markers placental growth factor (PlGF), soluble Feline McDonough Sarcoma- (fms-) like tyrosine kinase-1 (sFlt-1), asymmetric dimethylarginine (ADMA), and methyl-lysine is being reviewed with the aim of providing both a clinical and biochemical understanding of how these biomarkers might assist in the diagnosis of PE or indicate its severity.

1. Introduction

Preeclampsia (PE) is a multisystem, pregnancy-specific disorder that is characterised by the development of hypertension and proteinuria (elevated levels of protein in the urine) after 20 weeks of gestation [1]. PE is a leading cause of maternal, perinatal (from the 20th week of gestation to the 4th week after birth), and foetal/neonatal mortality and morbidity worldwide [2, 3].

PE is a very significant disease which complicates from 2% to 5% of pregnancies in Europe and America and can reach up to 10% of pregnancies in developing countries, mainly due to the lack of or inadequacy of emergency care [2]. Also, PE is associated with an increased risk of placental abruption, preterm birth, foetal intrauterine growth restriction (IUGR), acute renal failure, cerebrovascular and cardiovascular complications, disseminated intravascular coagulation, and maternal death [4]. Therefore, the ability to provide an early diagnosis of PE is vital.

2. Clinical Presentation, Diagnosis, and Pathophysiology of PE

Clinically, PE presents as new-onset hypertension in a previously normotensive woman, with systolic and diastolic blood pressure readings of ≥140 and ≥90 mmHg, respectively, on 2 separate occasions that are at least 6 hours apart, together with proteinuria that develops after 20 weeks of gestation [5–7].

This disorder can have an early onset (PE starting before 34 weeks of gestation) or late onset (after 34 weeks of gestation) and can be classified as mild or severe, depending on the severity of the symptoms present [2] (Table 1). In the

TABLE 1: Symptoms presented by patients with mild and severe PE. The diagnosis of any form of PE requires the presentation of both hypertension and proteinuria. This may be accompanied by a multitude of other symptoms if the PE is severe [8, 9].

Symptom	Mild PE	Severe PE
Blood Pressure	Systolic ≥140 mm Hg or diastolic ≥90 mm Hg, over 20 weeks of gestation (in a woman with previously normal blood pressure)	Systolic ≥160 mm Hg or diastolic ≥110 mm Hg (on two occasions at least six hours apart; in a woman on bed rest)
Proteinuria	24-hour urine collection protein ≥0.3 g (urine dipstick test ≥1+)	24-hour urine collection protein ≥5 g (urine dipstick test ≥3+; in two random urine samples collected at least four hours apart)
Others	N.A.	(i) Oliguria (ii) Cerebral or visual disturbances (iii) Pulmonary oedema or cyanosis (iv) Epigastric or right upper quadrant pain (v) Impaired liver function (vi) Thrombocytopenia (vii) Intrauterine growth restriction

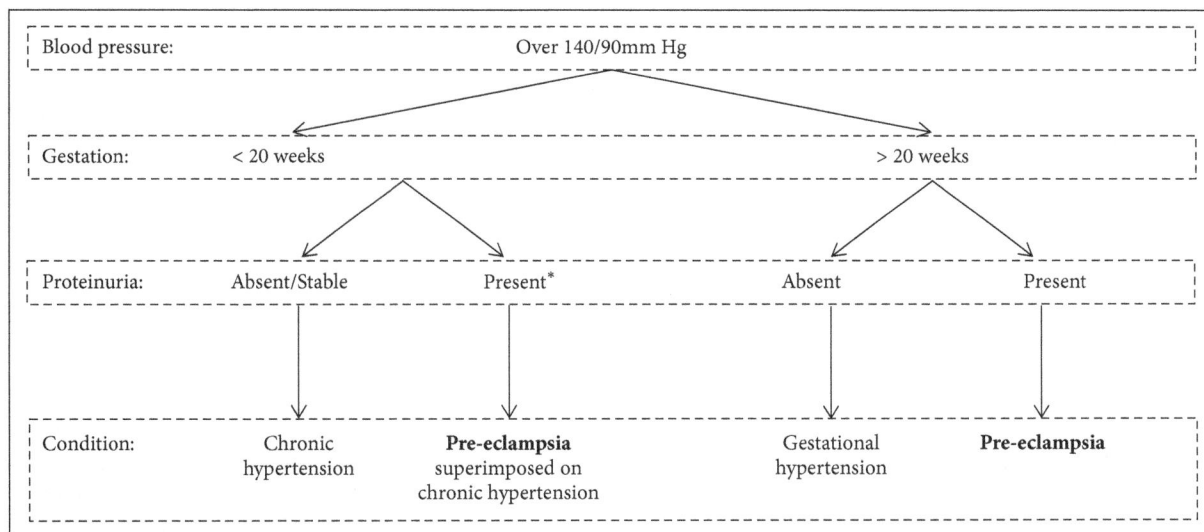

FIGURE 1: Simplified diagnostic information for the distinction of different types of hypertension and preeclampsia. *In the form of new or increased proteinuria, together with development of increasing blood pressure, or HELLP syndrome [9].

case of severe PE, more significant blood pressure elevations and a greater degree of proteinuria are noted. Other symptomatic features of severe PE which may be present include oliguria (less than 500 mL of urine in 24 hours), cerebral or visual disturbances, and pulmonary oedema or cyanosis [8, 9].

Also, the clinical presentation of PE may be either insidious or fulminant since some women may be asymptomatic initially, even after hypertension and proteinuria are noted, while others may present symptoms of severe PE from the start [1]. Finally, this condition may present itself as a maternal disorder only, such that there is normal foetal growth, or else it may lead to intrauterine growth restriction or sudden foetal distress [2].

Hypertensive disorders of pregnancy are the most common complications seen by obstetricians [10] and they are all associated with higher rates of maternal and foetal

mortality and morbidity [11]. This category of disorders includes chronic hypertension, PE, PE superimposed on chronic hypertension, and gestational hypertension [9]. The aetiologies and pathology of these disorders vary, and thus obtaining a diagnosis of PE becomes less difficult if physicians are able to differentiate PE from the other hypertensive disorders of pregnancy (Figure 1).

In chronic hypertension, the elevated blood pressure may predate the pregnancy, be noted before 20 weeks of gestation, or else be present 12 weeks after delivery [9]. This contrasts with PE, which is defined by the presence of elevated blood pressure and proteinuria after 20 weeks of gestation. In severe cases, PE can evolve into eclampsia which is a severe complication that is characterised by new-onset of epileptic seizures (generalised convulsions), due to angiospasms in the brain and brain oedema [13], in a woman with PE [1]. Eclampsia usually occurs in the second half of pregnancy and

Pregnancy-associated factors
● Chromosomal abnormalities
● Hydatidiform mole
● Hydrops fetalis
● Multi-foetal pregnancy
● Oocyte donation or donor insemination
● Structural congenital anomalies
● Urinary tract infection

Pre-eclampsia

Maternally-associated factors
● Age > 20 years or > 35 years
● African ethnicity
● Family history of pre-eclampsia
● Nulliparity
● Prior pre-eclamptic pregnancy
● Specific medical conditions: gestational diabetes, type I diabetes, obesity, chronic hypertension, renal disease, thrombophilias
● Stress

Paternally-associated factors
● First-time father
● Father to a prior pre-eclamptic pregnancy (with a different woman)

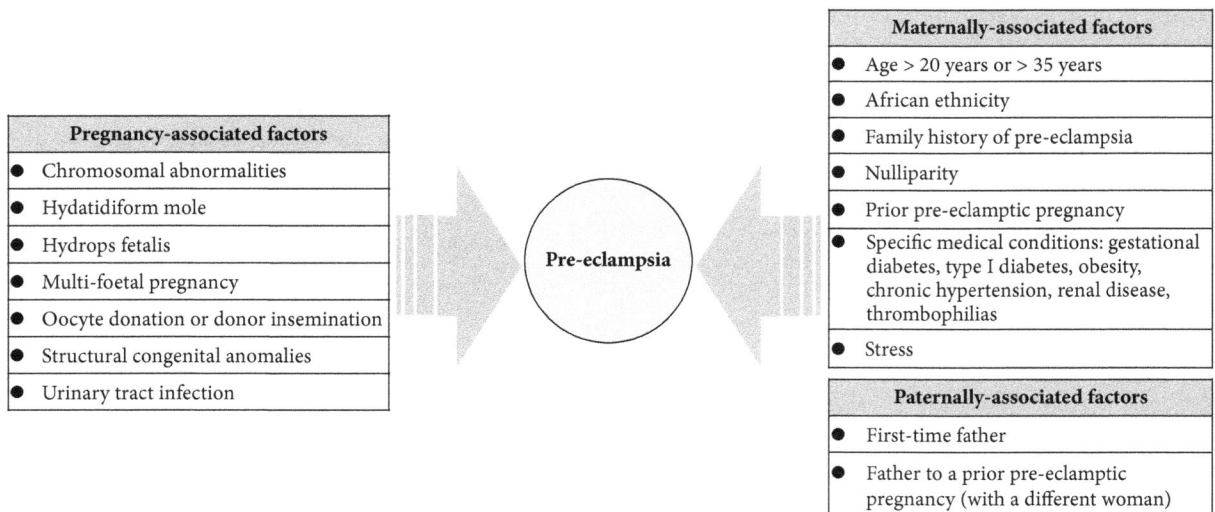

FIGURE 2: Risk factors for PE associated with the pregnancy itself or with specific parental characteristics from both maternal and paternal side [8, 12].

is a significant cause of maternal death, most commonly as a result of cerebral haemorrhage [14].

PE superimposed on chronic hypertension is characterised by new-onset proteinuria (or by a sudden increase in the protein level if proteinuria was already present), an acute increase in blood pressure (assuming proteinuria already exists), or the development of the HELLP (haemolysis, elevated liver enzyme, low platelet count) syndrome [8]. Finally, gestational hypertension can be distinguished from PE since it is characterised by the presence of elevated blood pressure after 20 weeks of gestation, which normalises within 12 weeks after delivery, together with the absence of proteinuria [8].

Medical conditions which have a potential to cause microvascular disease, including diabetes mellitus, chronic hypertension, and vascular and connective tissue disorders, as well as antiphospholipid syndrome and nephropathy, are all risk factors for developing PE. A number of other risk factors for developing PE, which can be associated with the pregnancy itself or with the clinical characteristics of the mother or father of the foetus, are presented in Figure 2 [8, 12, 15].

Although the pathophysiology of PE is not fully understood, problems of placental implantation and the level of trophoblastic invasion, as a consequence of endothelial dysfunction, appear to play a central role in the development and progression of this disorder. During normal pregnancy, cytotrophoblasts derived from the foetus invade and remodel the maternal uterine spiral arteries such that these small diameter, high-resistance arteries are converted into high capacity, low-resistance vessels [16]. This process is completed around midgestation in order to optimise the distribution of the maternal blood and ensure that the developing uteroplacental unit has adequate oxygen and nutrient delivery from the maternal circulation (Ramsey and Donner (1980) as cited in [3]).

PE is thought to evolve in two stages. The first, asymptomatic stage of PE involves impaired trophoblastic invasion

of the decidua (maternal placental bed) that seems to be due to local, abnormal foetomaternal immune interactions within the uterine wall [2, 17, 18]. This abnormal, shallow placentation reduces uteroplacental blood perfusion and consequently leads to local placental hypoxia. This oxidative stress has been shown to further aggravate vascular function in the placenta [19], which consequently leads to insufficient blood perfusion, inflammation, apoptosis, and structural damage [17, 20–23].

In the second stage, placental blood-borne factors released into the maternal circulation from the poorly perfused placenta, together with the aberrant expression of proinflammatory, antiangiogenic, and angiogenic factors, may activate the maternal endothelium and will eventually cause the endothelial dysfunction that leads to the main clinical symptoms of PE: hypertension and proteinuria [14, 24]. It has been noted that the magnitude of defective trophoblastic invasion of the spiral arteries correlates with the severity of PE [25].

Although PE is not preventable, PE-related mortality can be decreased through early detection and careful monitoring of PE [1]. Also, women who have progressive or severe PE should be hospitalised early on to allow close monitoring of both the maternal and foetal health condition.

3. Biomarkers of PE

The search for noninvasive, blood-borne, or urinary biomarkers that could be used to screen for and diagnose this life-threatening disorder of pregnancy is of utmost importance. Such biomarkers could predict the development of PE or assist in its detection, which in turn could have a vital impact on the management of pregnant women and their unborn children [2].

Most significantly, screening pregnant women with the use of biochemical markers for PE could enable presymptomatic diagnosis which will in turn reduce unnecessary suffering and healthcare costs associated with this disorder [26]. By providing an earlier diagnosis, progression of the disorder can be monitored more closely, together with the maternal and foetal health condition, thus allowing for more optimised time for delivery with the aim of reducing the number of premature births or other complications associated with PE [27]. Such biochemical markers may also allow the categorisation of women with PE according to the severity of the symptoms and/or pregnancy outcome which would further improve their clinical management [28].

Numerous biochemical markers for PE, which were selected based on pathophysiological observations noted in cases of PE, such as placental and/or endothelial dysfunction, have been investigated (Table 2). However, the reliability of these markers in predicting PE has been inconsistent between different studies [2]. Consequently, this review will focus on those biochemical markers for PE which appear to be most clinically relevant, alone or in combination, for the diagnosis of PE as well as in their ability to give an indication of the severity of this disorder, namely, placental growth factor (PlGF), soluble Feline McDonough Sarcoma- (fms-) like tyrosine kinase-1 (sFlt-1), and asymmetric dimethylarginine (ADMA), as well as introducing the possibility of screening for methyl-lysine in pregnancy-related proteins.

3.1. Placental Growth Factor (PlGF) and Soluble fms-Like Tyrosine Kinase-1 (sFlt-1).

PlGF belongs to the vascular endothelial growth factor (VEGF) family of proteins and it shares 53% identity with the platelet-derived growth factor-like region of VEGF [29]. Based on this homology with VEGF, PlGF was proposed to be an angiogenic factor [29–31]. In fact, PlGF was seen to possess strong angiogenic and mitogenic properties which are capable of inducing the proliferation, migration, and activation of endothelial cells [32, 33].

The expression of PlGF messenger RNA (mRNA) appears to be restricted to the placenta, trophoblastic tumours, and cultured human endothelial cells [29–31]. Essentially, PlGF is found in high amounts in the placenta, but it is also expressed at a low level under normal physiological conditions in several other organs including heart, lung, skeletal muscle, and adipose tissue [34–40].

The proangiogenic activity of members of the VEGF family of proteins, including PlGF, is achieved through the binding and activation of tyrosine kinase receptors [41, 42]. The most important receptors, which were found to bind the VEGF family of proteins with high affinity, are the fms-like tyrosine kinase receptor (Flt-1, also referred to as VEGF receptor 1, VEGFR1) and kinase domain region (KDR or VEGFR2) [43, 44]. These receptors are made up of a single signal sequence, a transmembrane domain, 7 immunoglobulin-like domains in their extracellular domain (the ligand-binding domain), and an intracellular tyrosine kinase domain [45].

However, it was noted that a cDNA in the endothelial cells of the human umbilical vein in the placenta encodes a truncated form of Flt-1 which is generated through alternative splicing of the mRNA. This soluble isoform of Flt-1 (sFlt-1) lacks the seventh immunoglobulin-like domain, the cytoplasmic domain, and the transmembrane sequence [45].

3.1.1. PlGF and sFlt-1 in Disease States and Pregnancy.

One of the most important properties of vascular endothelial cells is their ability to proliferate and form a network of capillaries through a process termed angiogenesis [33]. In a normal adult, the angiogenic process is tightly regulated and is limited to the endometrium and the ovary during the different phases of the menstrual cycle, and to the heart and skeletal muscles following injury due to prolonged and sustained physical exercise [134]. This process is especially prominent during embryonic development (Ramsey & Donner (1980) and Gilbert (1988) as cited in [33]) since angiogenesis is essential for correct development of the embryo and for postnatal growth [134].

The complex interplay between some members of the VEGF family of proteins, including PlGF, and their cognate receptors, especially Flt-1, is essential for angiogenesis to occur [2]. On the other hand, the soluble splice variant of Flt-1, sFlt-1, is secreted into the circulation and acts as an antiangiogenic factor since it antagonises and neutralises PlGF and VEGF by binding to them and inhibiting their interaction with endothelial receptors on the cell surface [36, 45, 57].

PlGF is present during early embryonic development and throughout all the stages of pregnancy since it is highly expressed by the placenta. It has been suggested that the presence of this proangiogenic factor serves as a control for trophoblast growth and differentiation [31, 37], which in turn implies that PlGF has a role in the invasion of the trophoblast into the maternal decidua [135]. Concurrently, although sFlt-1 is secreted in small amounts by endothelial cells and monocytes, the placenta seems to serve as the major source of sFlt-1 in the circulation during pregnancy. This finding is emphasised by the significant fall in the level of circulating sFlt-1 following the delivery of the placenta [47].

In a normotensive pregnant woman, the level of PlGF in the maternal circulation increases gradually during the first two trimesters and peaks at midgestation, before declining again as the pregnancy comes to term. Alternatively, the sFlt-1 level in normotensive pregnant women remains relatively stable during the first two trimesters, after which it increases steadily until term [45, 47, 53]. This gestational variation can be observed in the results presented in the charts below which were obtained in the Prospective Multicenter Study: Diagnosis of Preeclampsia (Roche Study no. CIM RD000556/X06P006). In this study, the PlGF and sFlt-1 levels were measured in normotensive women from countries across Europe, who had singleton pregnancies and went on to have normal pregnancy outcomes (no PE/HELLP and no IUGR) (Figures 3 and 4).

The levels of these biomarkers have also been investigated in the maternal circulation of patients with PE. There is strong evidence for the reduced occurrence of free, bioactive PlGF, together with higher placental expression of sFlt-1 and, consequently, elevated levels of circulating sFlt-1 in preeclamptic patients during active disease when compared with normotensive pregnant women [46, 47, 50, 53, 55, 67].

In a large cross-sectional study comparing gestational age-matched women with active PE and normotensive pregnancies, PlGF levels were noted to be lower and sFlt-1

TABLE 2: List of proposed serum biomarkers for the detection and diagnosis of PE.

Proposed biomarker	Biological role	Serum level in PE compared to normotensive pregnancy	Type of study	Positive predictive value	References
Soluble fms-like tyrosine kinase 1 (sFlt-1)	Anti-angiogenic factor	Higher	Case-control	No	[24, 46–51]
			Nested case-control	No	[52, 53]
			Cross-sectional case-control	No	[54–56]
			Longitudinal case-control	No	[57, 58]
			Prospective cohort	No	[59, 60]
				Yes	[61]
			Prospective nested case-control	No	[62]
Placental growth factor (PlGF)	Angiogenic factor	Lower	Case-control	No	[24, 46, 48, 50, 51]
				Yes	[63–65]
			Nested case-control	No	[52, 53, 66]
			Cross-sectional case-control	No	[54–56]
			Longitudinal case-control	No	[57, 58, 67]
				Yes	[68]
			Prospective cohort	No	[59, 60]
				Yes	[61]
			Prospective nested case-control	No	[62]
			Prospective longitudinal case-control	No	[69]
			Longitudinal cohort	No	[70]
			Longitudinal cross-sectional	No	[71, 72]
Asymmetric Dimethyl-Arginine (ADMA)	Biochemical degradation product	Higher	Case-control	No	[73–77]
			Longitudinal case-control	No	[78–82]
			Cross-sectional case-control	No	[83, 84]
Soluble Endoglin (sEng)	Modulator of transforming growth factor (TGF)-β signalling	Higher	Longitudinal case-control	No	[58]
			Cross-sectional case-control	No	[85, 86]
			Nested case-control	No	[87, 88]
			Retrospective	No	[89]
			Prospective	No	[90]
			Case-control	No	[91]
Placental Protein 13 (PP-13)	Lysophospholipase activity	Higher	Longitudinal case-control	No	[92, 93]
			Nested case-control	No	[94–98]
			Case-control	No	[99]
P-Selectin	Calcium-dependent receptor	Higher	Cross-sectional case-control	No	[100–105]
				Yes	[106]
			Longitudinal case-control	No	[107]
				Yes	[108]
Adrenomedullin	Vasodilator	Higher	Cross-sectional case-control	No	[109]

TABLE 2: Continued.

Proposed biomarker	Biological role	Serum level in PE compared to normotensive pregnancy	Type of study	Positive predictive value	References
A Disintegrin and Metalloprotease 12 (ADAM12)	Cell-cell and cell-matrix interaction protease	Lower	Retrospective case-control	No	[110]
			Cross-sectional case-control	No	[111, 112]
Pentraxin 3 (PTX3)	Angiogenesis and inflammation factor	Higher	Cross-sectional case-control	No	[113, 114]
Pregnancy-Associated Plasma Protein A (PAPP-A)	Metalloproteinase that cleaves insulin-like growth factor binding proteins (IGFBPs)	Lower	Case-control	Yes	[64]
			Nested case-control	No	[98]
			Cross-sectional case-control	No	[115–118]
			Retrospective cohort	No	[119–122]
			Prospective cohort	No	[123]
Nicotinamide Phospho-ribosyltransferase; Visfatin	Enzyme involved in nicotinamide metabolism	Both	Cross-sectional case-control	No	[124]
Cell free DNA	N.A	Higher	Cross-sectional case-control	No	[125–127]
Cell-free foetal DNA	N.A.	Higher	Cross-sectional case-control	No	[127–129]
			Nested case-control	No	[130, 131]
			Prospective	No	[132, 133]

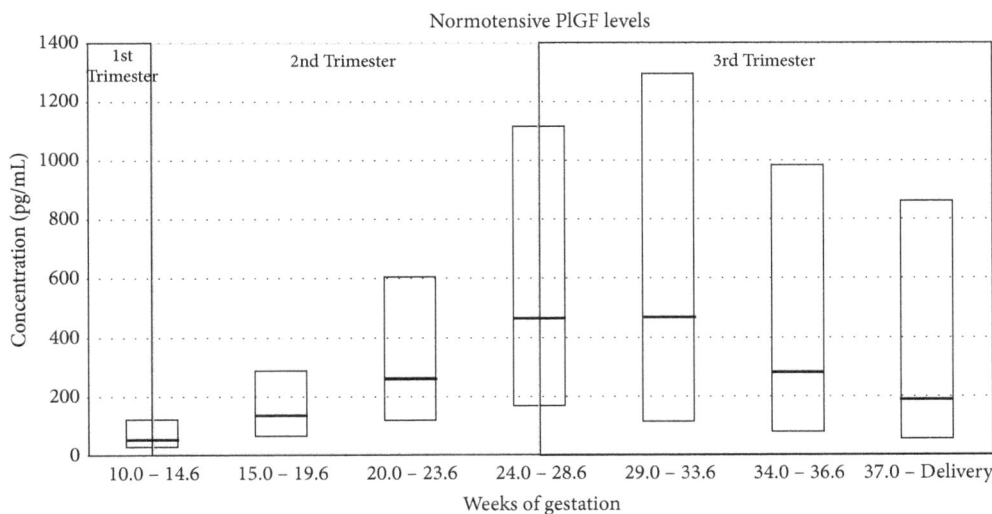

FIGURE 3: PlGF levels (pg/mL) measured in normotensive women during different weeks of gestation (based on data from Roche Study no. CIM RD000556/X06P006).

levels to be higher in the preeclamptic group (mean PlGF level of 137pg/mL versus 669pg/mL; mean sFlt-1 level of 4382pg/mL versus 1643pg/mL) [53]. The decrease in PlGF levels is thought to be due to the increased concentration of circulating sFlt-1 from 33 to 36 weeks of gestation and hence increased binding of PlGF to sFlt-1, rather than the decrease in PlGF caused by reduced production of PlGF [53].

In 2003, Maynard et al. introduced exogenous sFlt-1 into pregnant rats, and remarkably this led to reduced levels of PlGF, hypertension, and proteinuria, symptoms parallel to those observed in patients with PE [47]. This finding led to the idea that the maternal endothelial dysfunction that is noted in preeclamptic patients is caused by the imbalance of the levels of pro- and antiangiogenic factors in the maternal

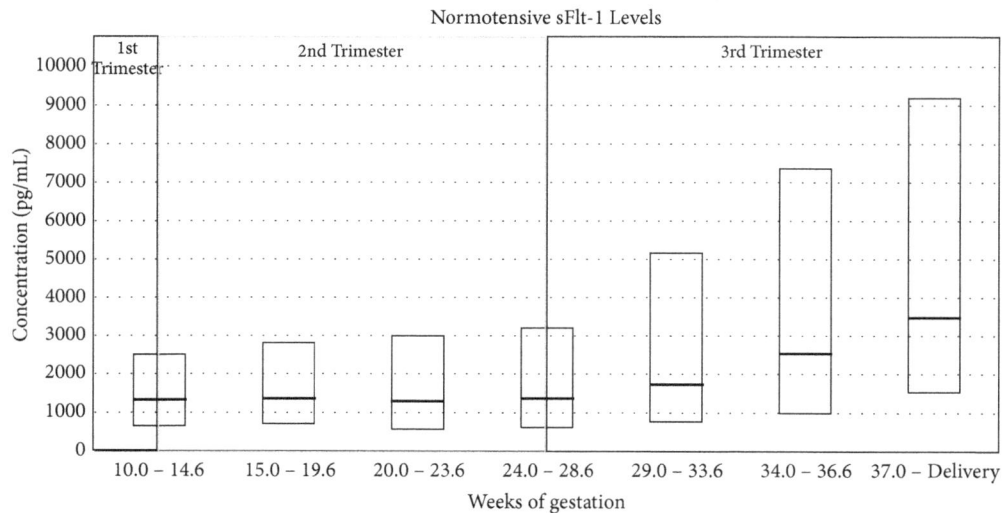

FIGURE 4: sFlt-1 levels (pg/mL) measured in normotensive women during different weeks of gestation (based on data from Roche Study no. CIM RD000556/X06P006).

circulation. There is much supportive evidence suggesting that the antagonism of PlGF by sFlt-1 may be responsible for the endothelial dysfunction in PE [59, 60].

The PlGF deficiency and sFlt-1 excess observed in pre-clamptic patients may also be due to the placental hypoxia that is associated with incomplete remodelling of the maternal spiral arteries. This defective placentation, as a result of incompletely remodelled arteries, offers persistently high resistance to uterine artery blood flow, which may in turn predispose to vascular rupture in the placental bed, especially after the onset of hypertension [136, 137]. However, more evidence is required to determine whether the altered levels of these pro- and antiangiogenic factors are the consequence or the cause of the placentation defect in women with PE.

Studies have shown that the level of maternal PlGF was more significantly reduced in patients with severe symptoms of PE compared to normotensive pregnant women and women with symptoms of mild PE. On the other hand, in the case of maternal sFlt-1 levels, the increased levels were shown to correlate with the severity of PE, with mean sFlt-1 levels ranging from 1.50 ± 0.22ng/mL in normotensive pregnant women to 3.28 ± 0.83ng/mL in women with mild PE and to 7.64 ± 1.5ng/mL in women with severe PE [47, 48]. Furthermore, it has been noted that the variation in PlGF and sFlt-1 is more pronounced in early onset PE when compared to late onset PE as well as in women who had PE and later delivered small for gestational age (SGA) newborns [53, 56]. The results obtained by Levine et al. [53] which show these differences are presented in Figures 5 and 6.

In the study by Levine et al., it was also reported that the increase in sFlt-1 levels in the circulation of patients with PE corresponds to a decrease in free PlGF [53]. Moreover, it was also observed that the alterations in the levels of these factors precede the clinical diagnosis by several weeks. In fact, a significant finding in this study was that the elevated level of sFlt-1 can be detected in the maternal serum 5 weeks before the clinical symptoms of PE appear while the decreased PlGF

level can be detected from 13 to 16 weeks of gestation in women who subsequently develop PE. This finding was later observed by a number of other studies [20, 53, 58, 62–66, 68–72, 138].

These findings have suggested that the measurement of PlGF and sFlt-1 may be used to predict the development of PE several weeks before the clinical onset of symptoms of this disease (Figure 7). The combined measurement of PlGF and sFlt-1 also distinguished women who subsequently developed PE from women who subsequently developed gestational hypertension, delivered SGA newborns, or completed a normal, healthy full term pregnancy [47, 52].

According to some studies, altered levels of sFlt-1 are specific for PE since no changes are detected in women who subsequently delivered SGA newborns or whose pregnancies were complicated by IUGR when compared to normotensive women with normal pregnancy outcomes [51, 58]. However, in a selected group of patients with abnormal uterine perfusion with subsequent IUGR, other studies have detected similar alterations in PlGF and sFlt-1 levels during the second trimester [139].

The combination of sFlt-1 and PlGF values in the form of a ratio, as shown for the Prospective Multicenter Study: Diagnosis of Preeclampsia (Roche Study no. CIM RD000556/X06P006) (Figure 8), has also been used as a predictor of PE. In a prospective study by Rana et al., [61] it was suggested that the ratio of sFlt-1 to PlGF appears to be a better predictor of PE than either measure alone. Kim et al. [24] revealed that the sFlt-1 to PlGF ratio in preeclamptic women was significantly higher when compared to the normal controls since the median value for the log [sFlt-1/PlGF] ratio in preeclamptic women was 1.6 (range 1.0 – 2.9), while the median value in the normotensive controls was 1.2 (range 0.5 – 1.9). In this study, a cut-off value of 1.4 was used since this showed 80.4% sensitivity and 78% specificity, with women having maternal log [sFlt-1/PlGF] ratio values more than 1.4 being at a higher risk of developing PE. Therefore, this ratio is a reliable marker

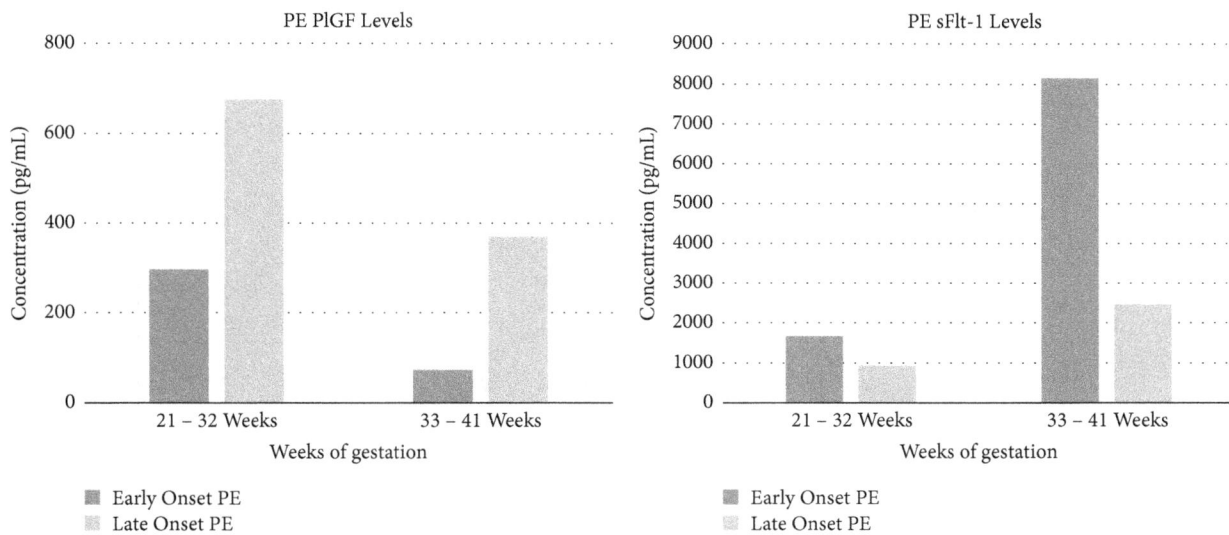

FIGURE 5: PlGF and sFlt-1 results obtained in women with early onset and late onset PE during different gestational periods [53].

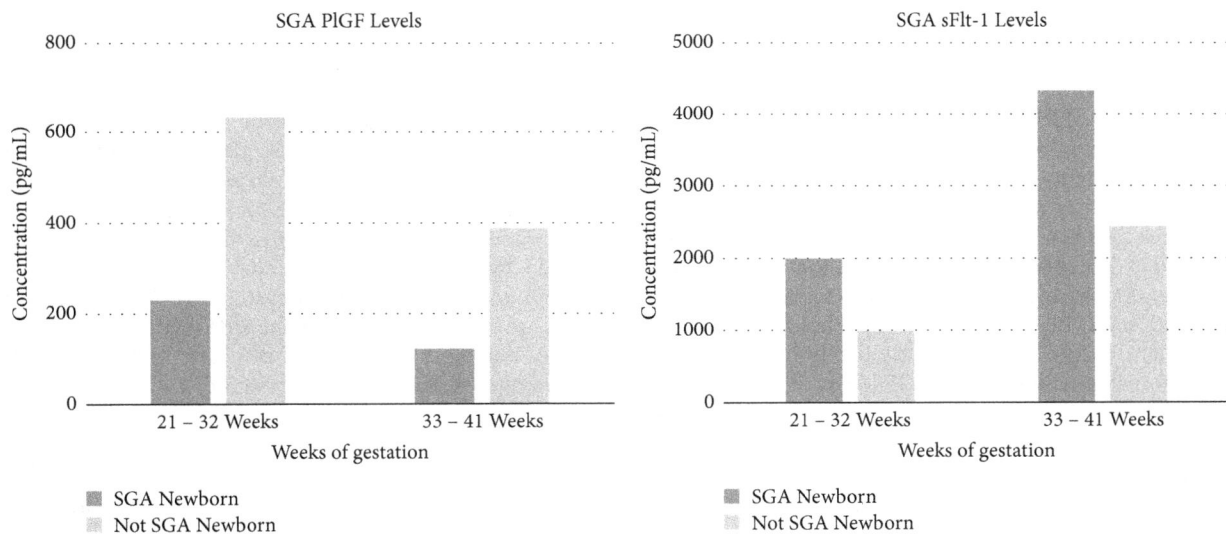

FIGURE 6: PlGF and sFlt-1 results obtained during different gestational periods in women with PE who later delivered small for gestational age (SGA) newborns and those that delivered infants of normal gestational size [53].

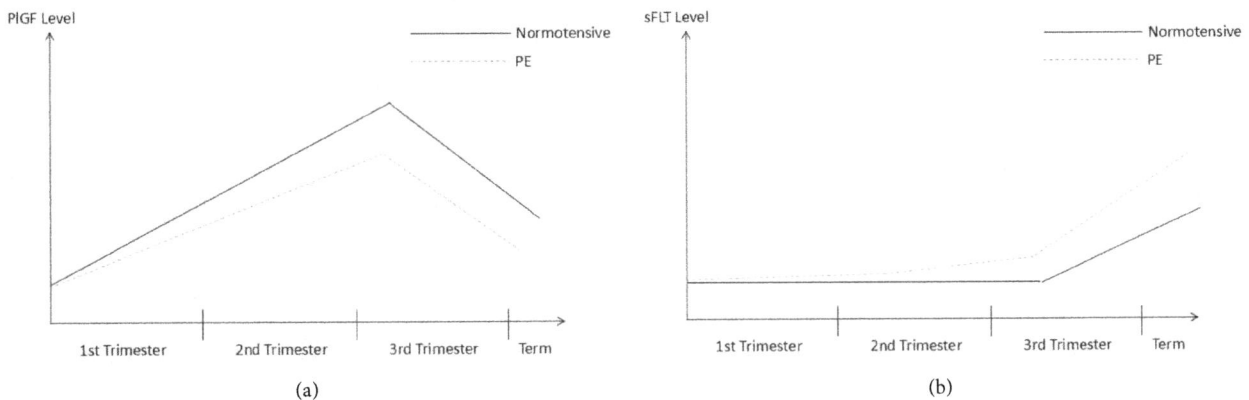

FIGURE 7: Levels of (a) PlGF and (b) sFlt throughout normotensive pregnancy as compared to levels in preeclamptic pregnant women.

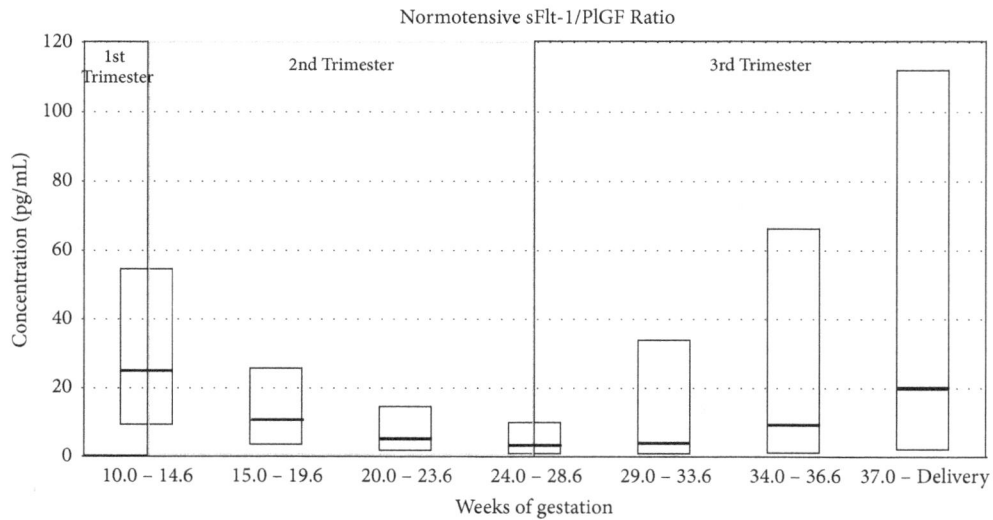

FIGURE 8: PlGF to sFlt-1 ratio (pg/mL) measured in normotensive women during different weeks of gestation (based on data from Roche Study no. CIM RD000556/X06P006).

of overall risk of PE and it may be used to distinguish between normal pregnancy and pregnancy complicated by PE and to define the severity of PE [2, 140].

The measurement of PlGF and sFlt-1 has only rarely been extended to the infants born from preeclamptic pregnancies. In 2005, Staff et al. measured PlGF and sFlt-1 levels in normotensive and preeclamptic pregnant women and their newborns [49]. The results obtained for the mothers reflected the same results obtained by studies mentioned in previous sections, with lower PlGF and higher sFlt-1 levels being noted in the preeclamptic group. In this study, the umbilical samples obtained from all newborns had PlGF levels that were below the concentration of the lowest standard of the ELISA kit used in the study (15.6pg/mL) and thus comparison between the preeclamptic and normotensive control groups could not be achieved. On the other hand, the median sFlt-1 concentration obtained for foetuses born to mothers with PE was found to be significantly higher than the median concentration obtained for those born to normotensive mothers (246 pg/mL, 95% CI for the median 163–255 versus 163 pg/mL, 95% CI for the median 136–201).

At the same time, although sFlt-1 levels were noted to be higher in foetuses born to mothers with PE, the sFlt-1 concentrations measured in umbilical samples were noted to be very low when compared to the maternal sFlt-1 concentrations. This finding suggests that the foetus does not contribute significantly to the elevated maternal sFlt-1 concentration in PE, which further reinforces the assumption that the increase in circulating sFlt-1 concentration in mothers with PE originates primarily from the placenta [49]. This finding is also consistent with the idea that foetuses do not experience hypertension or proteinuria like their preeclamptic mothers because they are not exposed to high concentrations of antiangiogenic factors, including sFlt-1, which, although of placental origin, should be primarily restricted to the maternal vasculature [141].

3.2. Protein Methylation Products. Protein methylation is a posttranslational modification (PTM) that involves the transfer of methyl groups from S-adenosyl-L-methionine (SAM) to a particular protein residue under the control of specific methyltransferase enzymes [142]. This results in the generation of a methylated substrate and the by-product, S-adenosyl-L-homocysteine (SAH), which is then degraded by the enzyme S-adenosylhomocysteine hydrolase to give adenosine and homocysteine [143] (Figure 9). Such PTMs predominantly target the side chains of arginine and lysine, but other amino acid residues, including histidine, asparagine, glutamine, and cysteine, have been shown to serve as minor targets for methylation.

3.2.1. Asymmetric Dimethylarginine (ADMA). Different types of methylarginine are synthesised following arginine methylation, which is a PTM of the nitrogen atom forming part of the guanidino moiety of the arginine (R) group within proteins. Proteins that undergo arginine methylation are involved in a number of different cellular processes, including transcriptional regulation, RNA metabolism, and DNA damage repair [144]. This process involves the addition of one or two methyl groups, derived from S-adenosylmethionine (SAM) [145], to the guanidino nitrogen atom of arginine and is achieved with the help of protein arginine N-methyltransferase enzymes (PRMTs) which belong to a sequence-related family of methyltransferases [146]. The guanidino group of arginine can be methylated in three different ways to give ω-NG-monomethylarginine (MMA), ω-NG,N'G-symmetric dimethylarginine (SDMA), or ω-NG,NG-asymmetric dimethylarginine (ADMA) [144] (Figure 10).

ADMA is eliminated in part by urinary excretion, but it is mainly metabolised via hydrolytic degradation to citrulline and dimethylamine. This metabolic reaction is catalysed by the enzyme NG-dimethylarginine dimethylaminohydrolase

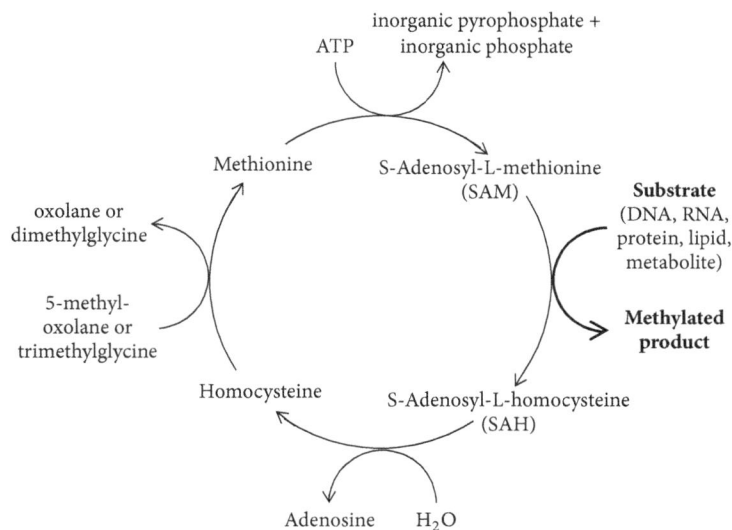

FIGURE 9: The S-adenosyl methionine cycle.

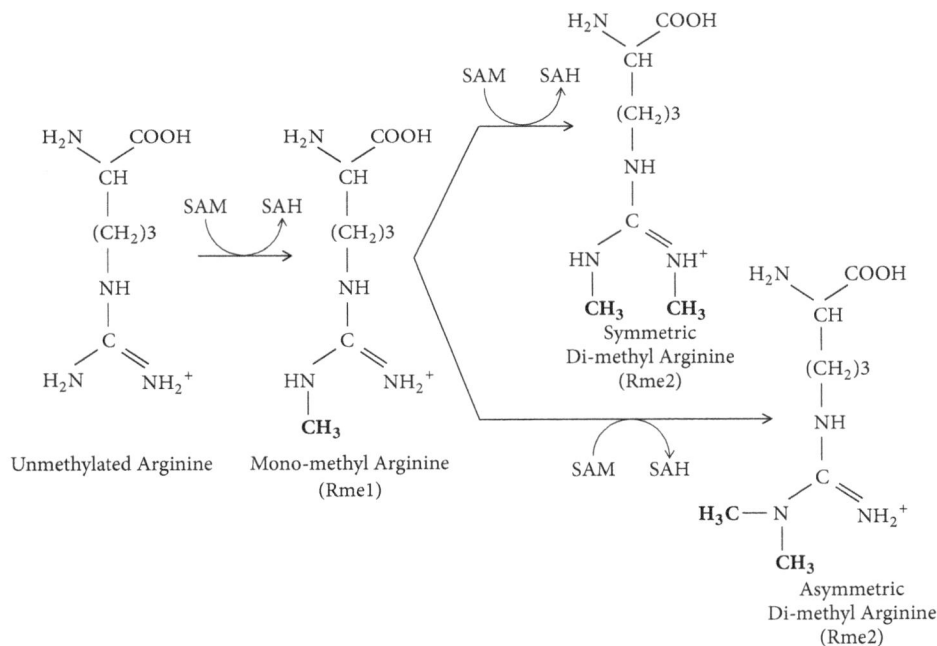

FIGURE 10: Formation of mono-, symmetrical, and asymmetrical dimethylarginine.

(DDAH) [147] (Figure 11). There are 2 isoforms of DDAH: DDAH-1 and DDAH-2. Tissues expressing neuronal nitric oxide synthase (NOS) usually contain DDAH-1, while tissues containing the endothelial isoform of NOS (eNOS) predominantly contain DDAH-2 [148]. Thus, it has been observed that DDAH-1 is found in high levels in the kidneys and liver, whereas DDAH-2 is the most abundant isoform in the endothelium [145].

(1) ADMA in Disease States and Pregnancy. In 1992, it was reported that ADMA is an endogenous competitive inhibitor

of NOS [149]. NOS is responsible for the synthesis of nitric oxide in endothelial cells since it catalyses the conversion of L-arginine to L-citrulline and NO [150]. ADMA is an analogue of L-arginine which is also synthesised and released by endothelial cells.

NO plays multiple roles in the cardiovascular system [144]. It is a potent vasoactive mediator that is released in response to stress [151] and is important in maintaining endothelial homeostasis [145]. Apart from inducing vasodilatation to regulate vascular tone and tissue blood flow [150–152], endothelial NO also inhibits platelet aggregation

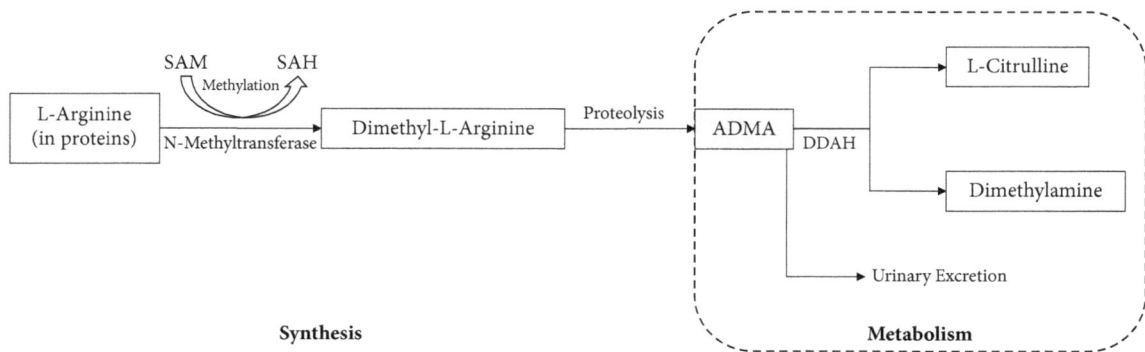

FIGURE 11: Overview of the synthesis and metabolism of ADMA. Synthesis of ADMA involves the methylation of arginine residues with the help of N-methyltransferase (protein arginine N-methyltransferases, PRMTs) which converts the methyl donor S-adenosylmethionine (SAM) to S-adenosylhomocysteine (SAH) followed by proteolytic breakdown of the proteins, which generates ADMA and N-monomethyl-L-arginine (L-NMMA). Elimination of ADMA is partly achieved via urinary excretion. However, ADMA is mainly eliminated through its metabolism to citrulline and dimethylamine by the enzyme dimethylarginine dimethylaminohydrolase (DDAH) [145].

[153], inhibits adhesion of leukocytes and monocytes to the endothelium [154], and inhibits smooth muscle cell proliferation [155].

It has been noted that decreased levels or inhibition of DDAH, which is the enzyme that catalyses the hydrolysis of ADMA, results in higher levels of ADMA in the circulation and causes gradual vasoconstriction [156]. This occurs because the elevated level of ADMA in the circulation results in the reversible inhibition of endogenous NO synthesis which in turn could lead to endothelial dysfunction [157]. The low levels of NO result in increased systemic vascular resistance and blood pressure [75]. High levels of ADMA have been observed in individuals with cardiovascular diseases including atherosclerosis, hypertension, and hypercholesterolaemia and in individuals with chronic renal failure [145]. Conventional cardiovascular risk factors may reduce DDAH activity by increasing oxidative stress, and this will in turn also result in elevated levels of ADMA [148, 158–160].

In a study in 1998 by Holden et al. [73], it was determined that pregnant women have a lower concentration of ADMA in their circulation than nonpregnant women. Their findings revealed that while the mean ADMA concentration in nonpregnant women was 0.82 ± 0.31μmol/L, the mean values of ADMA in pregnant women were in the range of 0.40 ± 0.15 μmol/L in the first trimester, 0.52 ± 0.20μmol/L in the second trimester, and 0.56 ± 0.22μmol/L in the third trimester. A similar observation was later made by Maeda et al. [79] who also noted lower mean ADMA concentrations in pregnant women (0.29 ± 0.05μmol/L in the first and third trimesters and 0.32 ± 0.05μmol/L at term) when compared to mean ADMA levels in nonpregnant women (0.41 ± 0.06μmol/L). At the same time, the results obtained by Holden et al. revealed that although the mean ADMA levels are lower in pregnant women, these tend to increase during the normal gestational period [73]. This finding is not reflected in the results obtained by Maeda et al. since the latter group did not note a change in mean ADMA levels from the first to the third trimester (0.29 ± 0.05μmol/L in the first and third trimesters), with the only increase being noted at full term (0.32 ± 0.05μmol/L at term) [79]. Alternatively, the increase

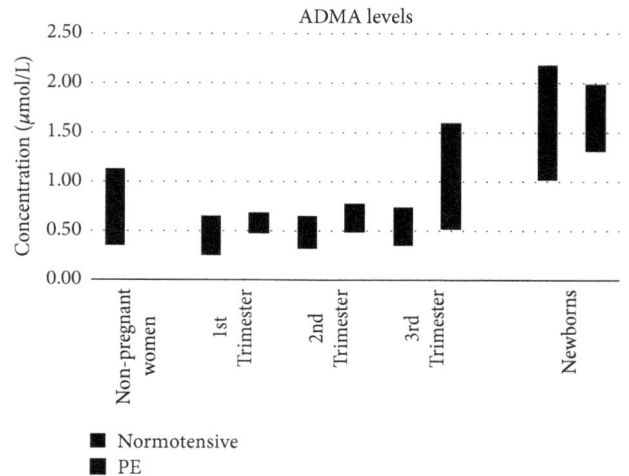

FIGURE 12: Levels of ADMA throughout pregnancy as compared to levels in nonpregnant women.

in mean ADMA levels during pregnancy was observed later on in a study by Rizos et al. in 2012 who showed that the mean ADMA levels in pregnant women increased from 0.51 ± 0.14μmol/L in the first trimester to 0.52 ± 0.13μmol/L in the second trimester and finally to 0.58 ± 0.16μmol/L in the third trimester [81] (Figure 12). Such findings have suggested that ADMA may have a role in vascular dilation and blood pressure regulation during pregnancy [73].

Numerous studies have measured the level of ADMA in pregnant women to determine whether there is a significant difference in ADMA concentrations in the circulation of women with PE when compared to women with uncomplicated pregnancies.

Discrepant findings have been observed. In separate studies in 1998, both Holden et al. [73] and Pettersson et al. [80] observed elevated mean ADMA levels during the third trimester in preeclamptic patients (1.17 ± 0.42μmol/L and 0.55 ± 0.02μmol/L, respectively) when compared to the normotensive pregnant controls during the same gestational

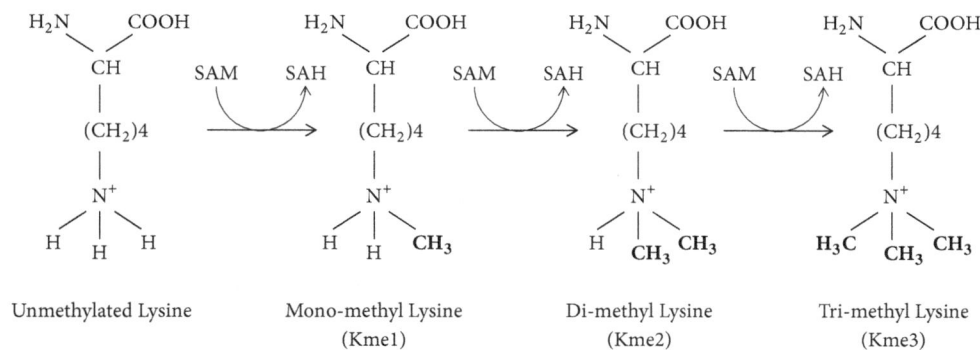

FIGURE 13: Formation of mono-, di-, and trimethyl-lysine.

period ($0.56 \pm 0.22\mu$mol/L and $0.36 \pm 0.01\mu$mol/L, respectively). Similarly, the study by Rizos et al. [81] also showed elevated mean ADMA levels during all three trimesters in preeclamptic patients ($0.58 \pm 0.10\mu$mol/L in the first trimester, $0.63 \pm 0.14\mu$mol/L in the second trimester, and $0.68 \pm 0.11\mu$mol/L in the third trimester) compared to women with uncomplicated pregnancies ($0.51 \pm 0.14\mu$mol/L in the first trimester, $0.52 \pm 0.13\mu$mol/L in the second trimester, and $0.58 \pm 0.16\mu$mol/L in the third trimester). However, in a number of other studies, although the median ADMA levels demonstrated a similar increased trend in preeclamptic patients, these findings were shown not to be statistically significant [74, 76, 77].

Furthermore, elevated ADMA concentrations have been noted in the circulation of pregnant women who went on to develop PE. This increased ADMA concentration was noted prior to the development of clinical signs and symptoms of PE [82, 83], which suggests that ADMA could have a role in the pathogenesis of this condition. Since nitric oxide is known to be important in maintaining both maternal and foetal blood flow and vascular tone and in maintaining the foetomaternal circulation, it has been proposed that elevated levels of ADMA in pregnancy, as well as the consequent decreased levels of NO in the circulation, may contribute to the pathophysiological features of PE [75, 79].

The measurement of ADMA levels in umbilical cord blood samples might be important to explain the regulatory mechanisms of the circulatory system during the perinatal period [84]. However, data regarding the level of ADMA in neonates is limited. In the previously mentioned study by Maeda et al. [79], it was also observed that the ADMA level measured in umbilical blood was significantly higher than the maternal level, which was noted to be highest at term ($1.02 \pm 0.18\mu$mol/L versus $0.32 \pm 0.05\mu$mol/L, respectively). This finding was later observed by Tsukahara et al. [84], who noted that the ADMA levels measured in umbilical blood from control newborns (newborns born to normotensive mothers following uncomplicated pregnancies) were about two times higher than the ADMA levels measured in lactating women, healthy children, and healthy adults ($1.71 \pm 0.47\mu$mol/L versus $0.71 \pm 0.06\mu$mol/L, $0.71 \pm 0.11\mu$mol/L, and $0.52 \pm 0.12\mu$mol/L, respectively).

When comparing ADMA levels measured in umbilical blood of control newborns and newborns born to mothers

with PE, Tsukahara et al. [84] found no significant difference between the two since their respective mean values were $1.71 \pm 0.47\mu$mol/L and $1.66 \pm 0.33\mu$mol/L. However, in a recent study by Gumus et al. [78], the median values for ADMA were noted to be significantly higher in umbilical blood from newborns born to mothers with PE than those from the control newborns (8.344ng/L versus 4.603ng/L). It was also noted that the level of ADMA measured from the umbilical cord blood sample correlated with the severity of the preeclamptic disorder.

3.2.2. Methyl-Lysine. In the case of lysine methylation, specific protein lysine methyltransferases (KMTs) catalyse the transfer of one, two, or three methyl groups from SAM to the epsilon (ε)-amine group of the side chain of a particular lysine residue [142]. This results in the formation of different forms of methylated lysines, namely, monomethyl-, dimethyl-, and trimethyl-lysines, respectively [142] (Figure 13). Some protein KMTs are specific for one or two of these modifications while others may result in the formation of all three derivatives [161]. Thus, it has been shown that these enzymes express product specificity since the type of methyl-lysine that is produced depends on the particular enzyme catalysing the reaction [162].

Nine functional members of the PRMT family have been identified (PRMT1-9) and the specificity of these enzymes for protein substrates varies and is generally much broader than that of KMTs. For instance, it has been shown that PRMT1, 2, 3, 4, 6, and 8 catalyse asymmetric dimethylation of arginine residues while enzyme PRMT5 catalyses symmetric dimethylation and PRMT7 may only catalyse monomethylation [163–165].

Most methyltransferase enzymes are grouped according to their structural features into three large families, namely, seven beta (β) strand [166], SET (suppressor of variegation 3-9 (Su(var)3-9), enhancer of zeste (E(z)), and trithorax (Trx)) domain-containing [167], and SPOUT domain-containing [168] enzymes. However, while all PRMTs belong to the seven β strand family of enzymes, most of the KMTs contain a conserved SET domain [169], which harbours the enzymatic activity of these proteins [170], and hence belong to the SET domain-containing family [171, 172]. Furthermore, an increasing number of enzymes which belong to the seven β

strand family have been shown to catalyse similar methylation reactions [173–176]. Thus, KMTs can be broadly divided according to their enzymatic domain into SET domain-containing and non-SET domain-containing proteins.

The SET domain-containing KMTs have been classified into a number of families according to the sequence motifs surrounding the SET domain. Members of the same family share similar sequence motifs surrounding the SET domain and often also share a higher level of similarity in the SET domain. Seven main families are known and these include the suppressor of variegation (Su(var)) 3-9 (SUV39), SET1, SET2, enhancer of zeste (E(z)), retinoblastoma-interacting zinc-finger protein (RIZ), SET and Myeloid-Nervy-DEAF1 (MYND) domain-containing protein (SMYD), and suppressor of variegation (Su(var)) 4-20 (SUV4-20) families. These families are accompanied by SET7/9 and SET8 (also known as PR-SET7) which are SET domain-containing KMTs but do not fit in with the previously mentioned families [177]. A tabulated list of the KMTs found in humans which belong to each KMTs family, as well as SET7/9 and SET8, together with their properties has been presented by Dillon et al. [177].

Although a large majority of KMTs contain the SET domain, numerous other proteins which do not contain the SET domain, including the disruptor of telomeric silencing (DOT) 1-like (DOT1L) [169, 178] and methyltransferase-like (METTL) family proteins [179], also have lysine methyltransferase activity.

(1) Lysine Methylation in Disease States and Pregnancy. Along the years, numerous KMTs and lysine demethylases (KDMs) have been identified and their activity has been reported to be important in several biological processes, including the regulation of gene expression, cell-cycle progression, DNA replication, and differentiation [180–185]. In normal, healthy states, lysine methylation is tightly controlled and a balance in lysine methylation is maintained by the opposing actions of KMTs and KDMs [186]. At the same time, gene expression patterns must be able to respond to developmental requirements and environmental changes in order to maintain a healthy state [187].

The dysregulation of PTMs in the form of inappropriate expression (inclusion or elimination), as well as mutation of numerous KMTs and KDMs, may be a critical determinant of different diseases, including ageing and cancer [186–191]. In fact, the loss of this appropriate balance in methylation in adult stem cells has been thought to contribute to the decline of tissue function with age [192]. Studies have also shown that aberrant methylation is associated with an increased incidence of various types of cancers and poor survival [193, 194]. For instance, the methyltransferase responsible for histone 3 lysine 27 trimethylation (H3K27me3) is upregulated in prostate cancer [195], breast cancer [196], and lymphomas [197].

The human genome encodes over 200 methyltransferases [198] and although most studies have focused on histone methylation, a number of reports have revealed that these enzymes are also responsible for the regulation of methylation of nonhistone proteins [199]. It has been observed that a number of nonhistone proteins undergo methylation on their lysine residues and this in turn leads to changes in the function and/or stability of these nonhistone proteins [199, 200]. Evidence of lysine methylation-dependent regulation for an ever-increasing number of nonhistone proteins has been reported and in some cases these changes would also be of relevance to stress, hypertension, and PE as described below.

Lysine Methylation of p53. The tumour suppressor protein p53 functions as a sequence-specific transcription factor which regulates important cellular processes including cell-cycle arrest, DNA repair, apoptosis, and senescence in response to stress signals. Under normal conditions, the level of p53 in the cell is maintained low; however, p53 is rapidly stabilised and activated in response to cellular stresses such as DNA damage and hypoxic states [143].

Trophoblast apoptosis in the human placenta has been shown to increase during the gestational period [201]. Furthermore, in pregnancies complicated by PE, dysregulation of cell turnover, which results in increased apoptosis [202–204] and reduced syncytiotrophoblast area [205], has been noted. The impact of exaggerated apoptosis on the placental pathology in cases of PE is unclear; however, this may ultimately prevent the replenishment of the syncytiotrophoblast, promote degeneration of the syncytium, and result in the release of vasoactive or inflammatory factors into the maternal circulation [206]. Since p53 is a vital regulator of the apoptotic pathway, its level has been measured in cases of PE and it has been observed that, at the protein level, the level of p53 is significantly elevated in placentas obtained from pregnancies complicated by PE [207]. This increase in p53 expression was also noted in cases of foetal IUGR [208, 209]. Also, the increase in p53 levels was associated with an increased expression of downstream elements of the apoptotic pathway, including the level of the downstream effector protein p21 [207].

Methylation of p53 by SET7 (KMT7) was the first KMT-mediated methylation of a nonhistone protein reported [210]. Since then, a number of other KMTs, including SET9 (KMT5), SMYD2 (KMT3C), and SET 8 (KMT5A), which methylate p53 at specific C-terminal lysines, together with the lysine-specific demethylase KDM1(LSD1) which mediates p53 demethylation, have also been identified [143] (Figure 14).

P53 undergoes multiple PTMs, including lysine methylation, which regulate its stability, protein-protein interactions, and transcriptional activity. In fact, the transcriptional activity of p53 is enhanced or suppressed depending on the methylation site. Also, the interaction of p53 with its coactivator p53 binding protein 1 (53BP1) to induce apoptosis is mediated through the action of the lysine demethylase KDM1. The balance between methylation and demethylation, in combination with other PTMs, is essential in the response of p53 to cellular stresses since its activity is important in the prevention of tumour formation [143].

Lysine Methylation of Heat Shock Protein (HSP) 70. HSPs are primarily known as intracellular proteins that have molecular chaperone and cytoprotective functions [211] and

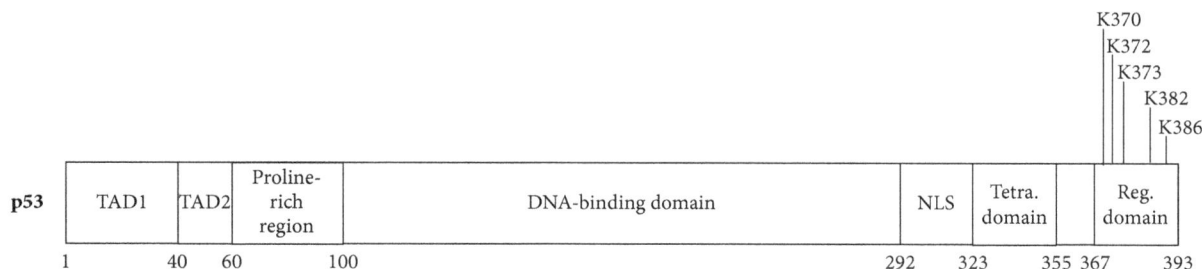

FIGURE 14: p53 lysine methylation sites (based on PhosphoSite data).

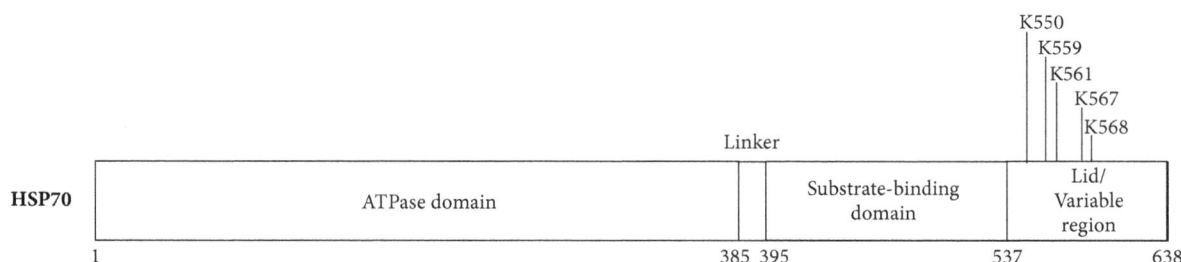

FIGURE 15: HSP70 lysine methylation sites (based on PhosphoSite data).

are essential for cell recovery, survival, and maintenance of homeostasis [212]. HSP70 proteins are ubiquitous, adenosine triphosphate- (ATP-) dependent molecular chaperones which make up one of the most evolutionarily conserved family of proteins [213]. Extracellular HSP70 may contribute to the development of autoimmune disease and may provide an indication of the status of the innate immune system [214–216]. In humans, these proteins are encoded by 13 genes and they are either induced in response to stress (such as heat shock) or constitutively expressed [217]. HSP70 proteins carry out numerous biological processes including protein-protein interactions, protein degradation, and translocation across membranes [218].

HSP70 has been shown to be elevated in cases of PE [212, 219]. Park et al. [220] suggested that increased levels of systemic HSP70 in preeclamptic patients originate from syncytiotrophoblasts and villous endothelial cells of preeclamptic placentas since these were shown to have higher HSP70 proteins levels when compared to placentas from normal, healthy pregnancies. Other studies have also detected higher HSP70 levels in placental tissues of preeclamptic patients [221, 222]. This increase in serum HSP70 reflects systemic inflammation and oxidative stress that is noted in PE [212, 219]. Initially, expression of HSP70 plays a protective role against placental oxidative stress; however, the overexpression of HSP70 may lead to intervillous endothelial dysfunction and may play a role in the pathogenesis of PE [220].

It has been shown that HSP70 can be posttranslationally modified in a number of ways, and numerous methylated lysines have been reported (Figure 15). For instance, it has been reported that the lysine residue K561, which is found in several human HSP70 proteins, can be methylated. Lysine methylation of HSP70 proteins is physiologically significant, especially in tumourigenesis. In particular, dimethylation of

K561 of HSP70 by SETD1A regulates the subcellular localisation of this protein and it promotes the proliferation of cancer cells through its interaction with Aurora Kinase B (AURKB) [143, 223].

Lysine Methylation of Vascular Endothelial Growth Factor Receptor 1 (VEGFR-1) and 2 (VEGFR-2). As was described in previous sections, VEGFR-1 (or Flt-1) and VEGFR-2 are membrane receptors which belong to a receptor tyrosine kinase (RTK) subfamily. VEGRF-1 is able to bind tightly to its ligands, VEGF (including VEGF-A) and PlGF, but has weak tyrosine kinase activity and hence generates an overall weaker signal than other RTKs [224]. Through its interaction with its ligands, VEGFR-1 plays an important role in both physiologic and pathologic angiogenesis, the process by which new blood vessels are formed from preexisting vessels [43, 225, 226]. Angiogenesis is crucial for the normal physiological functions of tissues, but it is also important for the progression of certain diseases, including cancer and inflammation [227, 228].

VEGFR-1 has also been shown to be important in the regulation of vasculogenesis, which is the process by which new blood vessels are formed from precursor cells during early embryogenesis [225]. In 1995, Fong et al. [229] demonstrated that mutant mice which do not express VEGFR-1 (Flt-1-null, Flt-1-/- mice) die in utero due to the uncontrolled growth of vascular endothelial cells and disorganisation of blood vessels, which indicates that VEGFR-1 may have a negative regulatory role in angiogenesis during early embryogenesis.

VEGFR-1, together with its ligand VEGF and the other receptors for VEGF, is expressed throughout the gestational period in the placenta and these are essential for embryonic vascular development [34, 35]. During normal, uncomplicated pregnancies, VEGFR-1 can be primarily detected in

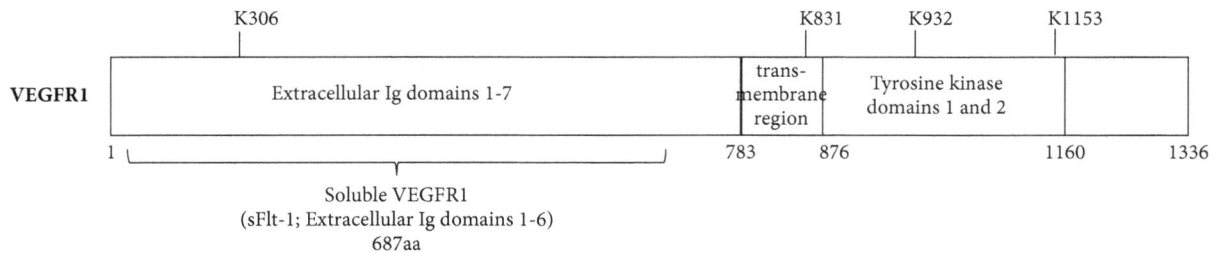

FIGURE 16: VEGFR1 lysine methylation sites (based on PhosphoSite data).

placental syncytiotrophoblasts [230]. Altered levels of VEGF and its receptors during pregnancy can lead to a disruption in angiogenesis which results in placental insufficiency and endothelial dysfunction, both of which are noted in pregnancies complicated by PE [231]. In the study by Helske et al. [230], the expression of VEGFR-1 was seen to be increased in the syncytiotrophoblasts of placentas obtained from a number of cases of PE, but not in all.

VEGFR-1 undergoes methylation at multiple lysine residues and it has been observed that this methylation is important in the regulation of the activity of VEGFR-1 (Figure 16). For instance, it has been shown that VEGFR-1 is a nonhistone target of SMYD3 methyltransferase since lysine 831 of VEGFR-1 is methylated by SMYD3 in vitro [232]. This methylation of VEGFR-1 enhances its kinase activity since lysine 831 is located within the kinase domain of this RTK.

VEGFR-2 is a potent angiogenic RTK, thus making it one of the most important RTKs in endothelial cells [233, 234]. The activity of VEGFR-2 has been noted to be essential in both vasculogenesis and pathological angiogenesis during cancer and ocular neurovascularisation [226].

Consequently, the expression and function of VEGFR-2 are highly regulated since increased angiogenesis plays a significant role in the progression of cancer and other diseases, including age-related macular degeneration, whereas insufficient angiogenesis has been linked to coronary heart disease and delayed wound healing [234]. VEGFR-2 undergoes methylation at multiple lysine residues and it has been shown that this methylation is important in the regulation of VEGFR-2 activity [233]. In fact, Hartsough et al. [233] also determined that methylation of lysine 1043 is essential in controlling the activation of VEGFR-2 since this methylation reaction is important for the tyrosine phosphorylation of this RTK. Consequently, interference of this methylation of VEGFR-2 results in an inability of VEGFR-2 to stimulate angiogenesis.

4. Conclusion

As with all biomarkers, their effectiveness is determined by the ability to diagnose the disease well before the presentation of clinical symptoms, and the advantage is that the changes can be detected through the minimally invasive blood tests, performed as part of the routine checks. So far, PlGF and sFlt-1, alone or in combination, not only have shown promise for the early diagnosis of PE but also have been shown to correlate well to the severity of this condition, with data from

different cohorts being comparable. Similarly, the screening for ADMA has produced interesting trends and can be considered a useful candidate biomarker also based on the knowledge of its role in NO biochemistry. Our laboratory is also interested in exploring lysine methylation in conjunction with the above-mentioned potential biomarkers in order to extend the understanding of the role played by protein methylation in normal and PE biochemistry. Aside from the biomarkers selected, the final aim is to improve pregnancy progression and outcome, as well as to reduce the risks for both mother and foetus. This can only be achieved by unravelling and better understanding the underlying mechanisms leading to the preeclamptic condition.

Conflicts of Interest

The authors declare that there are no conflicts of interest regarding the publication of this article.

References

[1] L. K. Wagner, "Diagnosis and management of preeclampsia," *American Family Physician*, vol. 70, no. 12, pp. 2317–2324, 2004.

[2] S. Grill, C. Rusterholz, R. Zanetti-Dällenbach et al., "Potential markers of preeclampsia - A review," *Reproductive Biology and Endocrinology*, vol. 7, article no. 70, 2009.

[3] A. Reddy, S. Suri, I. L. Sargent, C. W. G. Redman, and S. Muttukrishna, "Maternal circulating levels of activin A, inhibin A, sFlt-1 and endoglin at parturition in normal pregnancy and preeclampsia," *PLoS ONE*, vol. 4, no. 2, Article ID e4453, 2009.

[4] A. P. Mackay, C. J. Berg, and H. K. Atrash, "Pregnancy-Related Mortality from Preeclampsia and Eclampsia," *Obstetrics & Gynecology*, vol. 97, no. 4, pp. 533–538, 2001.

[5] K. Braekke, P. M. Ueland, N. K. Harsem, and A. C. Staff, "Asymmetric dimethylarginine in the maternal and fetal circulation in preeclampsia," *Pediatric Research*, vol. 66, no. 4, pp. 411–415, 2009.

[6] C. W. Redman and I. L. Sargent, "Latest advances in understanding preeclampsia," *Science*, vol. 308, no. 5728, pp. 1592–1594, 2005.

[7] B. SIBAI, G. DEKKER, and M. KUPFERMINC, "Pre-eclampsia," *The Lancet*, vol. 365, no. 9461, pp. 785–799, 2005.

[8] ACOG Committee on Practice Bulletins—Obstetrics, "ACOG practice bulletin. Diagnosis and management of preeclampsia and eclampsia," *Obstetrics & Gynecology*, vol. 99, no. 1, pp. 159–167, 2002.

[9] E. J. Roccella, "Report of the national high blood pressure education program working group on high blood pressure in

pregnancy," *American Journal of Obstetrics & Gynecology*, vol. 183, no. 1, pp. S1–S22, 2000.

[10] S. Grima, M. Vella, and C. Savona-Ventura, "Hypertensive disorders during pregnancy in pre-gestational diabetic women," *Malta Medical Journal*, vol. 22, no. 2, pp. 15–18, 2010.

[11] A. Díaz Pérez, A. Roca Pérez, G. Oñate Díaz, P. Castro Gil, and E. Navarro Quiroz, "Interaction and dynamics of these risk factors in hypertensive disorders of pregnancy: a pilot study," *Salud Uninorte*, vol. 33, no. 1, pp. 27–38, 2017.

[12] G. Dekker and B. Sibai, "Primary, secondary, and tertiary prevention of pre-eclampsia," *The Lancet*, vol. 357, no. 9251, pp. 209–215, 2001.

[13] H. Lipstein, C. C. Lee, and R. S. Crupi, "A current concept of eclampsia," *The American Journal of Emergency Medicine*, vol. 21, no. 3, pp. 223–226, 2003.

[14] E. Nexø, "Clinical biochemistry," *FEBS Letters*, vol. 375, no. 3, pp. 312-313, 1995.

[15] K. Duckitt and D. Harrington, "Risk factors for pre-eclampsia at antenatal booking: systematic review of controlled studies," *British Medical Journal*, vol. 330, no. 7491, p. 565, 2005.

[16] J. P. Warrington, E. M. George, A. C. Palei, F. T. Spradley, and J. P. Granger, "Recent advances in the understanding of the pathophysiology of preeclampsia.," *Hypertension*, vol. 62, no. 4, pp. 666–673, 2013.

[17] T.-H. Hung, J. N. Skepper, D. S. Charnock-Jones, and G. J. Burton, "Hypoxia-reoxygenation: A potent inducer of apoptotic changes in the human placenta and possible etiological factor in preeclampsia," *Circulation Research*, vol. 90, no. 12, pp. 1274–1281, 2002.

[18] N. Soleymanlou, I. Jurisica, O. Nevo et al., "Molecular evidence of placental hypoxia in preeclampsia," *The Journal of Clinical Endocrinology & Metabolism*, vol. 90, no. 7, pp. 4299–4308, 2005.

[19] J. Roberts, "Is oxidative stress the link in the two-stage model of pre-eclampsia?" *The Lancet*, vol. 354, no. 9185, pp. 788-789.

[20] U. D. Anderson, M. G. Olsson, S. Rutardttir et al., "Fetal hemoglobin and α1-microglobulin as first- and early second-trimester predictive biomarkers for preeclampsia," *American Journal of Obstetrics & Gynecology*, vol. 204, no. 6, pp. 520–e5, 2011.

[21] G. J. Burton and E. Jauniaux, "Oxidative stress," *Best Practice & Research Clinical Obstetrics & Gynaecology*, vol. 25, no. 3, pp. 287–299, 2011.

[22] K. May, L. Rosenlöf, M. G. Olsson et al., "Perfusion of human placenta with hemoglobin introduces preeclampsia-like injuries that are prevented by α1-microglobulin," *Placenta*, vol. 32, no. 4, pp. 323–332, 2011.

[23] A. H. Shennan, L. Poston, L. C. Chappell, and P. T. Seed, "Prevention of pre-eclampsia," *The Lancet*, vol. 357, no. 9267, p. 1534, 2001.

[24] S.-Y. Kim, H.-M. Ryu, J.-H. Yang et al., "Increased sFlt-1 to PlGF ratio in women who subsequently develop preeclampsia," *Journal of Korean Medical Science*, vol. 22, no. 5, pp. 873–877, 2007.

[25] R. Madazli, E. Budak, Z. Calay, and M. F. Aksu, "Correlation between placental bed biopsy findings, vascular cell adhesion molecule and fibronectin levels in pre-eclampsia," *BJOG: An International Journal of Obstetrics & Gynaecology*, vol. 107, no. 4, pp. 514–518, 2000.

[26] N. Hadker, S. Garg, C. Costanzo et al., "Financial impact of a novel pre-eclampsia diagnostic test versus standard practice: A decision-analytic modeling analysis from a UK healthcare payer perspective," *Journal of Medical Economics*, vol. 13, no. 4, pp. 728–737, 2010.

[27] U. D. Anderson, M. G. Olsson, K. H. Kristensen, B. Åkerström, and S. R. Hansson, "Review: biochemical markers to predict preeclampsia," *Placenta*, vol. 33, pp. S42–S47, 2012.

[28] P. von Dadelszen, L. A. Magee, and J. M. Roberts, "Subclassification of Preeclampsia," *Hypertension in Pregnancy*, vol. 22, no. 2, pp. 143–148, 2003.

[29] D. Maglione, V. Guerriero, G. Viglietto, P. Delli-Bovi, and M. G. Persico, "Isolation of a human placenta cDNA coding for a protein related to the vascular permeability factor," *Proceedings of the National Acadamy of Sciences of the United States of America*, vol. 88, no. 20, pp. 9267–9271, 1991.

[30] S. Hauser and H. A. Weich, "A heparin-binding form of placenta growth factor (plGF-2) is expressed in human umbilical vein endothelial cells and in placenta," *Growth Factors*, vol. 9, no. 4, pp. 259–268, 1993.

[31] D. Maglione, V. Guerriero, G. Viglietto et al., "Two alternative mRNAs coding for the angiogenic factor, placenta growth factor (PlGF), are transcribed from a single gene of chromosome 14," *Oncogene*, vol. 8, no. 4, pp. 925–931, 1993.

[32] Y. Cao, W.-R. Ji, P. Qi, Å. Rosin, and Y. Cao, "Placenta growth factor: Identification and characterization of a novel isoform generated by RNA alternative splicing," *Biochemical and Biophysical Research Communications*, vol. 235, no. 3, pp. 493–498, 1997.

[33] J. E. Park, H. H. Chen, J. Winer, K. A. Houck, and N. Ferrara, "Placenta growth factor. Potentiation of vascular endothelial growth factor bioactivity, in vitro and in vivo, and high affinity binding to Flt-1 but not to Flk-1/KDR," *The Journal of Biological Chemistry*, vol. 269, no. 41, pp. 25646–25654, 1994.

[34] A. Ahmed, X. F. Li, C. Dunk, M. J. Whittle, D. I. Rushton, and T. Rollason, "Colocalisation of vascular endothelial growth factor and its flt-1 receptor in human placenta," *Growth Factors*, vol. 12, no. 3, pp. 235–243, 1995.

[35] D. E. Clark, S. K. Smith, A. M. Sharkey, and D. S. Charnock-Jones, "Localization of VEGF and expression of its receptors flt and KDR in human placenta throughout pregnancy," *Human Reproduction*, vol. 11, no. 5, pp. 1090–1098, 1996.

[36] D. E. Clark, S. K. Smith, D. Licence, A. L. Evans, and D. S. Charnock-Jones, "Comparison of expression patterns for placenta growth factor, vascular endothelial growth factor (VEGF), VEGF-B and VEGF-C in the human placenta throughout gestation," *Journal of Endocrinology*, vol. 159, no. 3, pp. 459–467, 1998.

[37] A. Khaliq, X. F. Li, M. Shams et al., "Localisation of placenta growth factor (PIGF) in human term placenta," *Growth Factors*, vol. 13, no. 3-4, pp. 243–250, 1996.

[38] M. G. Persico, V. Vincenti, and T. DiPalma, "Structure, Expression and Receptor-Binding Properties of Placenta Growth Factor (PlGF)," in *Vascular Growth Factors and Angiogenesis*, vol. 237 of *Current Topics in Microbiology and Immunology*, pp. 31–40, Springer Berlin Heidelberg, Berlin, Heidelberg, 1999.

[39] G. Viglietto, D. Maglione, M. Rambaldi et al., "Upregulation of vascular endothelial growth factor (VEGF) and downregulation of placenta growth factor (PlGF) associated with malignancy in human thyroid tumors and cell lines," *Oncogene*, vol. 11, no. 8, pp. 1569–1579, 1995.

[40] G. Voros, E. Maquoi, D. Demeulemeester, N. Clerx, D. Collen, and H. R. Lijnen, "Modulation of angiogenesis during adipose

tissue development in murine models of obesity," *Endocrinology*, vol. 146, no. 10, pp. 4545–4554, 2005.

[41] C. De Vries, J. A. Escobedo, H. Ueno, K. Houck, N. Ferrara, and L. T. Williams, "The fms-like tyrosine kinase, a receptor for vascular endothelial growth factor," *Science*, vol. 255, no. 5047, pp. 989–991, 1992.

[42] B. I. Terman, M. Dougher-Vermazen, M. E. Carrion et al., "Identification of the KDR tyrosine kinase as a receptor for vascular endothelial cell growth factor," *Biochemical and Biophysical Research Communications*, vol. 187, no. 3, pp. 1579–1586, 1992.

[43] M. Shibuya, S. Yamaguchi, A. Yamane et al., "Nucleotide sequence and expression of a novel human receptor-type tyrosine kinase gene (flt) closely relatd to the fms family," *Oncogene*, vol. 5, no. 4, pp. 519–524, 1990.

[44] B. I. Terman, M. E. Carrion, E. Kovacs, B. A. Rasmussen, R. L. Eddy, and T. B. Shows, "Identification of a new endothelial cell growth factor receptor tyrosine kinase," *Oncogene*, vol. 6, no. 9, pp. 1677–1683, 1991.

[45] R. L. Kendall and K. A. Thomas, "Inhibition of vascular endothelial cell growth factor activity by an endogenously encoded soluble receptor," *Proceedings of the National Acadamy of Sciences of the United States of America*, vol. 90, no. 22, pp. 10705–10709, 1993.

[46] R. J. Levine and S. A. Karumanchi, "Circulating angiogenic factors in preeclampsia," *Clinical Obstetrics and Gynecology*, vol. 48, no. 2, pp. 372–386, 2005.

[47] S. E. Maynard, J. Y. Min, J. Merchan et al., "Excess placental soluble fms-like tyrosine kinase 1 (sFlt1) may contribute to endothelial dysfunction hypertension, and proteinuria in preeclampsia," *The Journal of Clinical Investigation*, vol. 111, no. 5, pp. 649–658, 2003.

[48] C. J. Robinson, D. D. Johnson, E. Y. Chang, D. M. Armstrong, and W. Wang, "Evaluation of placenta growth factor and soluble Fms-like tyrosine kinase 1 receptor levels in mild and severe preeclampsia," *American Journal of Obstetrics & Gynecology*, vol. 195, no. 1, pp. 255–259, 2006.

[49] A. C. Staff, K. Braekke, N. K. Harsem, T. Lyberg, and M. R. Holthe, "Circulating concentrations of sFlt1 (soluble fms-like tyrosine kinase 1) in fetal and maternal serum during pre-eclampsia," *European Journal of Obstetrics & Gynecology and Reproductive Biology*, vol. 122, no. 1, pp. 33–39, 2005.

[50] V. Tsatsaris, F. Goffin, C. Munaut et al., "Overexpression of the Soluble Vascular Endothelial Growth Factor Receptor in Preeclamptic Patients: Pathophysiological Consequences," *The Journal of Clinical Endocrinology & Metabolism*, vol. 88, no. 11, pp. 5555–5563, 2003.

[51] K.-A. Wathén, E. Tuutti, U.-H. Stenman et al., "Maternal serum-soluble vascular endothelial growth factor receptor-1 in early pregnancy ending in preeclampsia or intrauterine growth retardation," *The Journal of Clinical Endocrinology & Metabolism*, vol. 91, no. 1, pp. 180–184, 2006.

[52] N. A. Bersinger and R. A. Ødegård, "Second- and third-trimester serum levels of placental proteins in preeclampsia and small-for-gestational age pregnancies," *Acta Obstetricia et Gynecologica Scandinavica*, vol. 83, no. 1, pp. 37–45, 2004.

[53] R. J. Levine, S. E. Maynard, C. Qian et al., "Circulating angiogenic factors and the risk of preeclampsia," *The New England Journal of Medicine*, vol. 350, no. 7, pp. 672–683, 2004.

[54] T. Chaiworapongsa, R. Romero, J. Espinoza et al., "Evidence supporting a role for blockade of the vascular endothelial

growth factor system in the pathophysiology of preeclampsia: Young Investigator Award," *American Journal of Obstetrics & Gynecology*, vol. 190, no. 6, pp. 1541–1550, 2004.

[55] J.-Y. Chung, Y. Song, Y. Wang, R. R. Magness, and J. Zheng, "Differential Expression of Vascular Endothelial Growth Factor (VEGF), Endocrine Gland Derived-VEGF, and VEGF Receptors in Human Placentas from Normal and Preeclamptic Pregnancies," *The Journal of Clinical Endocrinology & Metabolism*, vol. 89, no. 5, pp. 2484–2490, 2004.

[56] A.-K. Wikström, A. Larsson, U. J. Eriksson, P. Nash, S. Nordén-Lindeberg, and M. Olovsson, "Placental growth factor and soluble FMS-like tyrosine kinase-1 in early-onset and late-onset preeclampsia," *Obstetrics & Gynecology*, vol. 109, no. 6, pp. 1368–1374, 2007.

[57] T. Chaiworapongsa, R. Romero, Y. M. Kim et al., "Plasma soluble vascular endothelial growth factor receptor-1 concentration is elevated prior to the clinical diagnosis of pre-eclampsia," *The Journal of Maternal-Fetal and Neonatal Medicine*, vol. 17, no. 1, pp. 3–18, 2005.

[58] R. Romero, J. K. Nien, J. Espinoza et al., "A longitudinal study of angiogenic (placental growth factor) and anti-angiogenic (soluble endoglin and soluble vascular endothelial growth factor receptor-1) factors in normal pregnancy and patients destined to develop preeclampsia and deliver a small for gestational age neonate," *The Journal of Maternal-Fetal & Neonatal Medicine*, vol. 21, no. 1, pp. 9–23, 2009.

[59] M. Simon, H.-J. Grone, O. Johren et al., "Expression of vascular endothelial growth factor and its receptors in human renal ontogenesis and in adult kidney," *American Journal of Physiology - Renal Fluid and Electrolyte Physiology*, vol. 268, no. 2, pp. F240–F250, 1995.

[60] M. Simon, W. Röckl, C. Hornig et al., "Receptors of vascular endothelial growth factor/vascular permeability factor (VEGF/VPF) in fetal and adult human kidney: Localization and [125I]VEGF binding sites," *Journal of the American Society of Nephrology*, vol. 9, no. 6, pp. 1032–1044, 1998.

[61] S. Rana, C. E. Powe, S. Salahuddin et al., "Angiogenic factors and the risk of adverse outcomes in women with suspected preeclampsia," *Circulation*, vol. 125, no. 7, pp. 911–919, 2012.

[62] R. Thadhani, W. P. Mutter, M. Wolf et al., "First trimester placental growth factor and soluble fms -like tyrosine kinase 1 and risk for preeclampsia," *The Journal of Clinical Endocrinology & Metabolism*, vol. 89, no. 2, pp. 770–775, 2004.

[63] B. M. Polliotti, A. G. Fry, D. N. Saller Jr., R. A. Mooney, C. Cox, and R. K. Miller, "Second-trimester maternal serum placental growth factor and vascular endothelial growth factor for predicting severe, early-onset preeclampsia," *Obstetrics & Gynecology*, vol. 101, no. 6, pp. 1266–1274, 2003.

[64] L. C. Y. Poon, N. A. Kametas, N. Maiz, R. Akolekar, and K. H. Nicolaides, "First-trimester prediction of hypertensive disorders in pregnancy," *Hypertension*, vol. 53, no. 5, pp. 812–818, 2009.

[65] Y. N. Su, C. N. Lee, W. F. Cheng, W. Y. Shau, S. N. Chow, and F. J. Hsieh, "Decreased maternal serum placenta growth factor in early second trimester and preeclampsia," *Obstetrics & Gynecology*, vol. 97, no. 6, pp. 898–904, 2001.

[66] L. J. Vatten, A. Eskild, T. I. L. Nilsen, S. Jeansson, P. A. Jenum, and A. C. Staff, "Changes in circulating level of angiogenic factors from the first to second trimester as predictors of preeclampsia," *American Journal of Obstetrics & Gynecology*, vol. 196, no. 3, pp. 239–e6, 2007.

[67] D. S. Torry, H.-S. Wang, T.-H. Wang, M. R. Caudle, and R. J. Torry, "Preeclampsia is associated with reduced serum levels of placenta growth factor," *American Journal of Obstetrics & Gynecology*, vol. 179, no. 6 I, pp. 1539–1544, 1998.

[68] R. Akolekar, E. Zaragoza, L. C. Y. Poon, S. Pepes, and K. H. Nicolaides, "Maternal serum placental growth factor at 11 + 0 to 13 + 6 weeks of gestation in the prediction of pre-eclampsia," *Ultrasound in Obstetrics & Gynecology*, vol. 32, pp. 732–773, 2009.

[69] T. Krauss, H. Pauer, and H. G. Augustin, "Prospective analysis of placenta growth factor (PlGF) concentrations in the plasma of women with normal pregnancy and pregnancies complicated by preeclampsia," *Hypertension in Pregnancy*, vol. 23, no. 1, pp. 101–111, 2004.

[70] R. N. Taylor, J. Grimwood, R. S. Taylor, M. T. McMaster, S. J. Fisher, and R. A. North, "Longitudinal serum concentrations of placental growth factor: Evidence for abnormal placental angiogenesis in pathologic pregnancies," *American Journal of Obstetrics & Gynecology*, vol. 188, no. 1, pp. 177–182, 2003.

[71] S. C. Tidwell, H. Ho, W. Chiu, R. J. Torry, and D. S. Torry, "Low maternal serum levels of placenta growth factor as an antecedent of clinical preeclampsia," *American Journal of Obstetrics & Gynecology*, vol. 184, no. 6, pp. 1267–1272, 2001.

[72] M. L. Tjoa, J. M. G. van Vugt, M. A. M. Mulders, R. B. H. Schutgens, C. B. M. Oudejans, and I. J. van Wijk, "Plasma placenta growth factor levels in midtrimester pregnancies," *Obstetrics & Gynecology*, vol. 98, no. 4, pp. 600–607, 2001.

[73] D. P. Holden, S. A. Fickling, G. S. Whitley, and S. S. Nussey, "Plasma concentrations of asymmetric dimethylarginine, a natural inhibitor of nitric oxide synthase, in normal pregnancy and preeclampsia," *American Journal of Obstetrics & Gynecology*, vol. 178, no. 3, pp. 551–556, 1998.

[74] Y. J. Kim, H. S. Park, H. Y. Lee et al., "Reduced L-arginine level and decreased placental eNOS activity in preeclampsia," *Placenta*, vol. 27, no. 4-5, pp. 438–444, 2006.

[75] M. Laskowska and J. Oleszczuk, "Evaluation of ADMA levels in women with pregnancies complicated by severe preeclampsia," *Archives of Perinatal Medicine*, vol. 17, no. 1, pp. 33–36, 2011.

[76] R. Maas, R. H. Böger, E. Schwedhelm et al., "Plasma Concentrations of Asymmetric Dimethylarginine (ADMA) in Colombian Women with Pre-eclampsia [4]," *Journal of the American Medical Association*, vol. 291, no. 7, pp. 823–824, 2004.

[77] M. Noorbakhsh, M. Kianpour, and M. Nematbakhsh, "Serum Levels of Asymmetric Dimethylarginine, Vascular Endothelial Growth Factor, and Nitric Oxide Metabolite Levels in Preeclampsia Patients," *ISRN Obstetrics and Gynecology*, vol. 2013, pp. 1–5, 2013.

[78] E. Gumus, M. A. Atalay, B. Cetinkaya Demir, and E. Sahin Gunes, "Possible role of asymmetric dimethylarginine (ADMA) in prediction of perinatal outcome in preeclampsia and fetal growth retardation related to preeclampsia," *The Journal of Maternal-Fetal and Neonatal Medicine*, vol. 29, no. 23, pp. 3806–3811, 2016.

[79] T. Maeda, T. Yoshimura, and H. Okamura, "Asymmetric dimethylarginine, an endogenous inhibitor of nitric oxide synthase, in maternal and fetal circulation," *J. Soc. Gynecol. Investig*, vol. 10, p. 24, 2003.

[80] A. Pettersson, T. Hedner, and I. Milsom, "Increased circulating concentrations of asymmetric dimethyl arginine (ADMA, an endogenous inhibitor of nitric oxide synthesis, in preeclampsia," *Acta Obstet. Gynecol. Scand*, vol. 77, pp. 808–813, 1998.

[81] D. Rizos, M. Eleftheriades, E. Batakis et al., "Levels of asymmetric dimethylarginine throughout normal pregnancy and in pregnancies complicated with preeclampsia or had a small for gestational age baby," *The Journal of Maternal-Fetal and Neonatal Medicine*, vol. 25, no. 8, pp. 1311–1315, 2012.

[82] P. D. Speer, R. W. Powers, M. P. Frank, G. Harger, N. Markovic, and J. M. Roberts, "Elevated asymmetric dimethylarginine concentrations precede clinical preeclampsia, but not pregnancies with small-for-gestational-age infants," *American Journal of Obstetrics & Gynecology*, vol. 198, no. 1, pp. 112.e1–112.e7, 2008.

[83] M. D. Savvidou, A. D. Hingorani, D. Tsikas, J. C. Frölich, P. Vallance, and K. H. Nicolaides, "Endothelial dysfunction and raised plasma concentrations of asymmetric dimethylarginine in pregnant women who subsequently develop pre-eclampsia," *The Lancet*, vol. 361, no. 9368, pp. 1511–1517, 2003.

[84] H. Tsukahara, N. Ohta, S. Tokuriki et al., "Determination of asymmetric dimethylarginine, an endogenous nitric oxide synthase inhibitor, in umbilical blood," *Metabolism - Clinical and Experimental*, vol. 57, no. 2, pp. 215–220, 2008.

[85] A. Jeyabalan, S. McGonigal, C. Gilmour, C. A. Hubel, and A. Rajakumar, "Circulating and placental endoglin concentrations in pregnancies complicated by intrauterine growth restriction and preeclampsia," *Placenta*, vol. 29, no. 6, pp. 555–563, 2008.

[86] C. J. Robinson and D. D. Johnson, "Soluble endoglin as a second-trimester marker for preeclampsia," *American Journal of Obstetrics & Gynecology*, vol. 197, no. 2, pp. 174.e1–174.e5, 2007.

[87] R. J. Levine, C. Lam, C. Qian et al., "Soluble endoglin and other circulating antiangiogenic factors in preeclampsia," *The New England Journal of Medicine*, vol. 355, no. 10, pp. 992–1005, 2006.

[88] S. Rana, S. A. Karumanchi, R. J. Levine et al., "Sequential changes in antiangiogenic factors in early pregnancy and risk of developing preeclampsia," *Hypertension*, vol. 50, no. 1, pp. 137–142, 2007.

[89] H. Stepan, T. Krämer, and R. Faber, "Maternal plasma concentrations of soluble endoglin in pregnancies with intrauterine growth restriction," *The Journal of Clinical Endocrinology & Metabolism*, vol. 92, no. 7, pp. 2831–2834, 2007.

[90] H. Stepan, A. Geipel, F. Schwarz, T. Krämer, N. Wessel, and R. Faber, "Circulatory soluble endoglin and its predictive value for preeclampsia in second-trimester pregnancies with abnormal uterine perfusion," *American Journal of Obstetrics & Gynecology*, vol. 198, no. 2, pp. 175–e6, 2008.

[91] S. Venkatesha, M. Toporsian, C. Lam et al., "Erratum: Soluble endoglin contributes to the pathogenesis of preeclampsia (Nature Medicine (2006) 12, (642-649))," *Nature Medicine*, vol. 12, no. 7, p. 862, 2006.

[92] O. Burger, E. Pick, J. Zwickel et al., "Placental protein 13 (PP-13): Effects on cultured trophoblasts, and its detection in human body fluids in normal and pathological pregnancies," *Placenta*, vol. 25, no. 7, pp. 608–622, 2004.

[93] B. Huppertz, M. Sammar, I. Chefetz, P. Neumaier-Wagner, C. Bartz, and H. Meiri, "Longitudinal determination of serum placental protein 13 during development of preeclampsia," *Fetal Diagnosis and Therapy*, vol. 24, no. 3, pp. 230–236, 2008.

[94] I. Chafetz, I. Kuhnreich, M. Sammar et al., "First-trimester placental protein 13 screening for preeclampsia and intrauterine growth restriction," *American Journal of Obstetrics & Gynecology*, vol. 197, no. 1, pp. 35.e1–35.e7, 2007.

[95] A. Khalil, N. J. Cowans, K. Spencer, S. Goichman, H. Meiri, and K. Harrington, "First trimester maternal serum placental protein 13 for the prediction of pre-eclampsia in women with a

priori high risk," *Prenatal Diagnosis*, vol. 29, no. 8, pp. 781–789, 2009.

[96] K. H. Nicolaides, R. Bindra, O. M. Turan et al., "A novel approach to first-trimester screening for early pre-eclampsia combining serum PP-13 and Doppler ultrasound," *Ultrasound in Obstetrics & Gynecology*, vol. 27, no. 1, pp. 13–17, 2006.

[97] K. Spencer, N. J. Cowans, I. Chefetz, J. Tal, I. Kuhnreich, and H. Meiri, "Second-trimester uterine artery Doppler pulsatility index and maternal serum PP13 as markers of pre-eclampsia," *Prenatal Diagnosis*, vol. 27, no. 3, pp. 258–263, 2007.

[98] K. Spencer, N. J. Cowans, I. Chefetz, J. Tal, and H. Meiri, "First-trimester maternal serum PP-13, PAPP-A and second-trimester uterine artery Doppler pulsatility index as markers of pre-eclampsia," *Ultrasound in Obstetrics & Gynecology*, vol. 29, no. 2, pp. 128–134, 2007.

[99] R. Romero, J. P. Kusanovic, N. G. Than et al., "First-trimester maternal serum PP13 in the risk assessment for preeclampsia," *American Journal of Obstetrics & Gynecology*, vol. 199, no. 2, pp. 122–e11, 2008.

[100] H. Aksoy, Y. Kumtepe, F. Akçay, and A. K. Yildirim, "Correlation of P-selectin and lipoprotein(a), and other lipid parameters in preeclampsia," *Clinical and Experimental Medicine*, vol. 2, no. 1, pp. 39–43, 2002.

[101] I. Banzola, A. Farina, M. Concu et al., "Performance of a panel of maternal serum markers in predicting preeclampsia at 11-15 weeks' gestation," *Prenatal Diagnosis*, vol. 27, no. 11, pp. 1005–1010, 2007.

[102] F. Bretelle, F. Sabatier, D. Desprez et al., "Circulating microparticles: a marker of procoagulant state in normal pregnancy and pregnancy complicated by preeclampsia or intrauterine growth restriction," *Thrombosis and Haemostasis*, vol. 89, no. 3, pp. 486–492, 2003.

[103] A. Halim, N. Kanayama, E. El Maradny et al., "Plasma P selectin (GMP-140) and glycocalicin are elevated in preeclampsia and eclampsia: Their significances," *American Journal of Obstetrics & Gynecology*, vol. 174, no. 1, pp. 272–277, 1996.

[104] W. Heyl, S. Handt, F. Reister et al., "Elevated soluble adhesion molecules in women with pre-eclampsia," *European Journal of Obstetrics & Gynecology and Reproductive Biology*, vol. 86, no. 1, pp. 35–41, 1999.

[105] C. A. R. Lok, R. Nieuwland, A. Sturk et al., "Microparticle-associated P-selectin reflects platelet activation in preeclampsia," *Platelets*, vol. 18, no. 1, pp. 68–72, 2007.

[106] T. Chaiworapongsa, R. Romero, J. Yoshimatsu et al., "Soluble adhesion molecule profile in normal pregnancy and pre-eclampsia," *The Journal of Maternal-Fetal & Neonatal Medicine*, vol. 12, no. 1, pp. 19–27, 2009.

[107] P. Bosio, S. Cannon, P. McKenna, C. O'Herlihy, R. Conroy, and H. Brady, "Plasma P-selectin is elevated in the first trimester in women who subsequently develop pre-eclampsia," *BJOG: An International Journal of Obstetrics & Gynaecology*, vol. 108, no. 7, pp. 709–715, 2001.

[108] M. E. Chavarría, L. Lara-González, Y. García-Paleta, V. S. Vital-Reyes, and A. Reyes, "Adhesion molecules changes at 20 gestation weeks in pregnancies complicated by preeclampsia," *European Journal of Obstetrics & Gynecology and Reproductive Biology*, vol. 137, no. 2, pp. 157–164, 2008.

[109] A. A. Senna, M. Zedan, G. E. Abd El Salam, and A. I. El Mashad, "Study of plasma adrenomedullin level in normal pregnancy and preclampsia," *The Medscape Journal of Medicine*, vol. 10, no. 2, article no. 29, 2008.

[110] J. Laigaard, T. Sørensen, S. Placing et al., "Reduction of the disintegrin and metalloprotease ADAM12 in preeclampsia," *Obstetrics & Gynecology*, vol. 106, no. 1, pp. 144–149, 2005.

[111] K. H. Nicolaides, L. C. Y. Poon, T. Chelemen, O. Granvillano, and I. Pandeva, "First-trimester maternal serum a disintegrin and metalloprotease 12 (ADAM12) and adverse pregnancy outcome," *Obstetrics & Gynecology*, vol. 112, no. 5, pp. 1082–1090, 2008.

[112] K. Spencer, N. J. Cowans, and A. Stamatopoulou, "ADAM12s in maternal serum as a potential marker of pre-eclampsia," *Prenatal Diagnosis*, vol. 28, no. 3, pp. 212–216, 2008.

[113] I. Cetin, V. Cozzi, F. Pasqualini et al., "Elevated maternal levels of the long pentraxin 3 (PTX3) in preeclampsia and intrauterine growth restriction," *American Journal of Obstetrics & Gynecology*, vol. 194, no. 5, pp. 1347–1353, 2006.

[114] P. Rovere-Querini, S. Antonacci, G. Dell'Antonio et al., "Plasma and tissue expression of the long pentraxin 3 during normal pregnancy and preeclampsia," *Obstetrics & Gynecology*, vol. 108, no. 1, pp. 148–155, 2006.

[115] N. J. Cowans and K. Spencer, "First-trimester ADAM12 and PAPP-A as markers for intrauterine fetal growth restriction through their roles in the insulin-like growth factor system," *Prenatal Diagnosis*, vol. 27, no. 3, pp. 264–271, 2007.

[116] C. Y. T. Ong, A. W. Liao, K. Spencer, S. Munim, and K. H. Nicolaides, "First trimester maternal serum free β human chorionic gonadotrophin and pregnancy associated plasma protein a as predictors of pregnancy complications," *British Journal of Obstetrics and Gynaecology*, vol. 107, no. 10, pp. 1265–1270, 2000.

[117] K. Spencer, N. J. Cowans, and K. H. Nicolaides, "Low levels of maternal serum PAPP-A in the first trimester and the risk of pre-eclampsia," *Prenatal Diagnosis*, vol. 28, no. 1, pp. 7–10, 2008.

[118] Y. Yaron, S. Heifetz, Y. Ochshorn, O. Lehavi, and A. Orr-Urtreger, "Decreased first trimester PAPP-A is a predictor of adverse pregnancy outcome," *Prenatal Diagnosis*, vol. 22, no. 9, pp. 778–782, 2002.

[119] L. Dugoff, J. C. Hobbins, F. D. Malone et al., "First-trimester maternal serum PAPP-A and free-beta subunit human chorionic gonadotropin concentrations and nuchal translucency are associated with obstetric complications: a population-based screening study (the FASTER Trial)," *American Journal of Obstetrics & Gynecology*, vol. 191, no. 4, pp. 1446–1451, 2004.

[120] D. Krantz, L. Goetzl, J. L. Simpson et al., "Association of extreme first-trimester free human chorionic gonadotropin-β, pregnancy-associated plasma protein A, and nuchal translucency with intrauterine growth restriction and other adverse pregnancy outcomes," *American Journal of Obstetrics & Gynecology*, vol. 191, no. 4, pp. 1452–1458, 2004.

[121] K. Spencer, N. J. Cowans, F. Molina, K. O. Kagan, and K. H. Nicolaides, "First-trimester ultrasound and biochemical markers of aneuploidy and the prediction of preterm or early preterm delivery," *Ultrasound in Obstetrics & Gynecology*, vol. 31, no. 2, pp. 147–152, 2008.

[122] N. Tul, S. Pusenjak, J. Osredkar, K. Spencer, and Z Novak-Antolic, "Predicting complications of pregnancy with first-trimester maternal serum free-betahCG, PAPP-A and inhibin-A," *Prenatal Diagnosis*, vol. 23, no. 12, pp. 990–996, 2003.

[123] G. C. Smith, E. J. Stenhouse, J. A. Crossley, D. A. Aitken, A. D. Cameron, and J. M. Connor, "Early Pregnancy Levels of Pregnancy-Associated Plasma Protein A and the Risk of

Intrauterine Growth Restriction, Premature Birth, Preeclampsia, and Stillbirth," *The Journal of Clinical Endocrinology & Metabolism*, vol. 87, no. 4, pp. 1762–1767, 2002.

[124] W. Hu, Z. Wang, H. Wang, H. Huang, and M. Dong, "Serum visfatin levels in late pregnancy and pre-eclampsia," *Acta Obstetricia et Gynecologica Scandinavica*, vol. 87, no. 4, pp. 413–418, 2008.

[125] A. Farina, A. Sekizawa, M. Iwasaki, R. Matsuoka, K. Ichizuka, and T. Okai, "Total cell-free DNA (β-globin gene) distribution in maternal plasma at the second trimester: A new prospective for preeclampsia screening," *Prenatal Diagnosis*, vol. 24, no. 9, pp. 722–726, 2004.

[126] A. Sekizawa, A. Farina, K. Koide et al., "β-globin DNA in maternal plasma as a molecular marker of pre-eclampsia," *Prenatal Diagnosis*, vol. 24, no. 9, pp. 697–700, 2004.

[127] D. W. Swinkels, J. B. De Kok, J. C. M. Hendriks, E. Wiegerinck, P. L. M. Zusterzeel, and E. A. P. Steegers, "Hemolysis, elevated liver enzymes, and low platelet count (HELLP) syndrome as a complication of preeclampsia in pregnant women increases the amount of cell-free fetal and maternal DNA in maternal plasma and serum," *Clinical Chemistry*, vol. 48, no. 4, pp. 650–653, 2002.

[128] Y. M. D. Lo, M. S. C. Tein, T. K. Lau et al., "Quantitative analysis of fetal DNA in maternal plasma and serum: implications for noninvasive prenatal diagnosis," *American Journal of Human Genetics*, vol. 62, no. 4, pp. 768–775, 1998.

[129] X. Y. Zhong, H. Laivuori, J. C. Livingston et al., "Elevation of both maternal and fetal extracellular circulating deoxyribonucleic acid concentrations in the plasma of pregnant women with preeclampsia," *American Journal of Obstetrics & Gynecology*, vol. 184, no. 3, pp. 414–419, 2001.

[130] R. J. Levine, C. Qian, E. S. Leshane et al., "Two-stage elevation of cell-free fetal DNA in maternal sera before onset of preeclampsia," *American Journal of Obstetrics & Gynecology*, vol. 190, no. 3, pp. 707–713, 2004.

[131] R. M. Silver, L. Myatt, J. C. Hauth et al., "Cell-Free Total and Fetal DNA in First Trimester Maternal Serum and Subsequent Development of Preeclampsia," *American Journal of Perinatology*, vol. 34, no. 2, pp. 191–198, 2017.

[132] X. Y. Zhong, W. Holzgreve, and S. Hahn, "The levels of circulatory cell free fetal DNA in maternal plasma are elevated prior to the onset of preeclampsia," *Hypertension in Pregnancy*, vol. 21, no. 1, pp. 77–83, 2002.

[133] N. Leung Tse, Jun. Zhang, K. Tze, Y. S. Lisa, and Y. M. Dennis Lo, *Increased Maternal Plasma Fetal DNA Concentrations in Women Who Eventually Develop Preeclampsia. Clinical Chemistry*, vol. 47, 'Increased Maternal Plasma Fetal DNA Concentrations in Women Who Eventually Develop Preeclampsia.' Clinical Chemistry 47 (1, 137–39, 2001.

[134] S. De Falco, "The discovery of placenta growth factor and its biological activity," *Experimental & Molecular Medicine*, vol. 44, no. 1, p. 1, 2012.

[135] P. Vuorela, E. Hatva, A. Lymboussaki et al., "Expression of vascular endothelial growth factor and placenta growth factor in human placenta," *Biology of Reproduction*, vol. 56, no. 2, pp. 489–494, 1997.

[136] J. Dommisse and A. J. Tiltman, "Placental bed biopsies in placental abruption," *An International Journal of Obstetrics & Gynaecology*, vol. 99, no. 8, pp. 651–654, 1992.

[137] T. K. Eskes, "Abruptio placentae," *European Journal of Obstetrics & Gynecology and Reproductive Biology*, vol. 75, no. 1, pp. 63–70, 1997.

[138] R. Thadhani, J. L. Ecker, W. P. Mutter et al., "Insulin Resistance and Alterations in Angiogenesis: Additive Insults That May Lead to Preeclampsia," *Hypertension*, vol. 43, no. 5, pp. 988–992, 2004.

[139] H. Stepan, A. Unversucht, N. Wessel, and R. Faber, "Predictive value of maternal angiogenic factors in second trimester pregnancies with abnormal uterine perfusion," *Hypertension*, vol. 49, no. 4, pp. 818–824, 2007.

[140] C. S. Buhimschi, E. R. Norwitz, E. Funai et al., "Urinary angiogenic factors cluster hypertensive disorders and identify women with severe preeclampsia," *American Journal of Obstetrics & Gynecology*, vol. 192, no. 3, pp. 734–741, 2005.

[141] A. C. Staff, K. Braekke, G. M. Johnsen, S. A. Karumanchi, and N. K. Harsem, "Circulating concentrations of soluble endoglin (CD105) in fetal and maternal serum and in amniotic fluid in preeclampsia," *American Journal of Obstetrics & Gynecology*, vol. 197, no. 2, pp. 176–e6, 2007.

[142] B. C. Smith and J. M. Denu, "Chemical mechanisms of histone lysine and arginine modifications," *Biochimica et Biophysica Acta (BBA) - Gene Regulatory Mechanisms*, vol. 1789, no. 1, pp. 45–57, 2009.

[143] A. Scoumanne and X. Chen, "Protein methylation: A new mechanism of p53 tumor suppressor regulation," *Histology and Histopathology*, vol. 23, no. 9, pp. 1143–1149, 2008.

[144] M. T. Bedford and S. Richard, "Arginine methylation: an emerging regulator of protein function," *Molecular Cell*, vol. 18, no. 3, pp. 263–272, 2005.

[145] L. Sibal, S. C. Agarwal, P. D. Home, and R. H. Boger, "The role of asymmetric dimethylarginine (ADMA) in endothelial dysfunction and cardiovascular disease," *Current Cardiology Reviews*, vol. 6, no. 2, pp. 82–90, 2010.

[146] S. G. Clarke, "Protein methylation at the surface and buried deep: Thinking outside the histone box," *Trends in Biochemical Sciences*, vol. 38, no. 5, pp. 243–252, 2013.

[147] T. Ogawa, M. Kimoto, and K. Sasaoka, "Occurrence of a new enzyme catalyzing the direct conversion of NG,NG-dimethyl-L-arginine to L-citrulline in rats," *Biochemical and Biophysical Research Communications*, vol. 148, no. 2, pp. 671–677, 1987.

[148] A. Ito, P. S. Tsao, S. Adimoolam, M. Kimoto, T. Ogawa, and J. P. Cooke, "Novel mechanism for endothelial dysfunction: Dysregulation of dimethylarginine dimethylaminohydrolase," *Circulation*, vol. 99, no. 24, pp. 3092–3095, 1999.

[149] P. Vallance, A. Leone, A. Calver, J. Collier, and S. Moncada, "Accumulation of an endogenous inhibitor of nitric oxide synthesis in chronic renal failure," *The Lancet*, vol. 339, no. 8793, pp. 572–575, 1992.

[150] M. S. Goligorsky, "Endothelial cell dysfunction: can't live with it, how to live without it," *American Journal of Physiology-Renal Physiology*, vol. 288, no. 5, pp. F871–F880, 2005.

[151] J. P. Cooke, E. Rossitch Jr., N. A. Andon, J. Loscalzo, and V. J. Dzau, "Flow activates an endothelial potassium channel to release an endogenous nitrovasodilator," *The Journal of Clinical Investigation*, vol. 88, no. 5, pp. 1663–1671, 1991.

[152] R. F. Furchgott and J. V. Zawadzki, "The obligatory role of endothelial cells in the relaxation of arterial smooth muscle by acetylcholine," *Nature*, vol. 288, no. 5789, pp. 373–376, 1980.

[153] A. Wolf, C. Zalpour, G. Theilmeier et al., "Dietary L-arginine supplementation normalizes platelet aggregation in hypercholesterolemic humans," *Journal of the American College of Cardiology*, vol. 29, no. 3, pp. 479–485, 1997.

[154] P. Kubes, M. Suzuki, and D. N. Granger, "Nitric oxide: an endogenous modulator of leukocyte adhesion," *Proceedings of the National Acadamy of Sciences of the United States of America*, vol. 88, no. 11, pp. 4651–4655, 1991.

[155] R. H. Böger, "Asymmetric dimethylarginine, an endogenous inhibitor of nitric oxide synthase, explains the "L-arginine paradox" and acts as a novel cardiovascular risk factor," *Journal of Nutrition*, vol. 134, no. 10, pp. 2842S–2847S, 2004.

[156] R. J. MacAllister, H. Parry, M. Kimoto et al., "Regulation of nitric oxide synthesis by dimethylarginine dimethylaminohydrolase," *British Journal of Pharmacology*, vol. 119, no. 8, pp. 1533–1540, 1996.

[157] M. C. Stühlinger, R. K. Oka, E. E. Graf et al., "Endothelial Dysfunction Induced by Hyperhomocyst(e)inemia: Role of Asymmetric Dimethylarginine," *Circulation*, vol. 108, pp. 933–938, 2003.

[158] K. Y. Lin, A. Ito, T. Asagami et al., "Impaired nitric oxide synthase pathway in diabetes mellitus: role of asymmetric dimethylarginine and dimethylarginine dimethylaminohydro-lase," *Circulation*, vol. 106, no. 8, pp. 987–992, 2002.

[159] M. Weis, T. N. Kledal, K. Y. Lin et al., "Cytomegalovirus Infection Impairs the Nitric Oxide Synthase Pathway: Role of Asymmetric Dimethylarginine in Transplant Arteriosclerosis," *Circulation*, vol. 109, no. 4, pp. 500–505, 2004.

[160] M. C. Stühlinger, P. S. Tsao, J.-H. Her, M. Kimoto, R. F. Balint, and J. P. Cooke, "Homocysteine impairs the nitric oxide synthase pathway: role of asymmetric dimethylarginine," *Circulation*, vol. 104, no. 21, pp. 2569–2575, 2001.

[161] J.-F. Couture, L. M. A. Dirk, J. S. Brunzelle, R. L. Houtz, and R. C. Trievel, "Structural origins for the product specificity of SET domain protein methyltransferases," *Proceedings of the National Acadamy of Sciences of the United States of America*, vol. 105, no. 52, pp. 20659–20664, 2008.

[162] X. Zhang and T. C. Bruice, "Enzymatic mechanism and product specificity of SET-domain protein lysine methyltransferases," *Proceedings of the National Acadamy of Sciences of the United States of America*, vol. 105, no. 15, pp. 5728–5732, 2008.

[163] M. T. Bedford and S. G. Clarke, "Protein arginine methylation in mammals: who, what, and why," *Molecular Cell*, vol. 33, no. 1, pp. 1–13, 2009.

[164] Y. Yang and M. T. Bedford, "Protein arginine methyltransferases and cancer," *Nature Reviews Cancer*, vol. 13, no. 1, pp. 37–50, 2013.

[165] C. I. Zurita-Lopez, T. Sandberg, R. Kelly, and S. G. Clarke, "Human protein arginine methyltransferase 7 (PRMT7) is a type III enzyme forming ω-NG-monomethylated arginine residues," *The Journal of Biological Chemistry*, vol. 287, no. 11, pp. 7859–7870, 2012.

[166] H. L. Schubert, R. M. Blumenthal, and X. Cheng, "Many paths to methyltransfer: A chronicle of convergence," *Trends in Biochemical Sciences*, vol. 28, no. 6, pp. 329–335, 2003.

[167] P. A. del Rizzo and R. C. Trievel, "Substrate and product specificities of SET domain methyltransferases," *Epigenetics*, vol. 6, no. 9, pp. 1059–1067, 2011.

[168] K. L. Tkaczuk, S. Dunin-Horkawicz, E. Purta, and J. M. Bujnicki, "Structural and evolutionary bioinformatics of the SPOUT superfamily of methyltransferases," *BMC Bioinformatics*, vol. 8, article 73, 2007.

[169] Q. Feng, H. Wang, H. H. Ng et al., "Methylation of H3-lysine 79 is mediated by a new family of HMTases without a SET domain," *Current Biology*, vol. 12, no. 12, pp. 1052–1058, 2002.

[170] C. Qian and M.-M. Zhou, "SET domain protein lysine methyltransferases: structure, specificity and catalysis," *Cellular and Molecular Life Sciences*, vol. 63, no. 23, pp. 2755–2763, 2006.

[171] T. C. Petrossian and S. G. Clarke, "Uncovering the human methyltransferasome," *Molecular & Cellular Proteomics*, vol. 10, no. 1, 2011.

[172] V. M. Richon, D. Johnston, C. J. Sneeringer et al., "Chemogenetic Analysis of Human Protein Methyltransferases," *Chemical Biology & Drug Design*, vol. 78, no. 2, pp. 199–210, 2011.

[173] S. Kernstock, E. Davydova, M. Jakobsson et al., "Lysine methylation of VCP by a member of a novel human protein methyltransferase family," *Nature Communications*, vol. 3, article no. 1038, 2012.

[174] R. Magnani, L. M. A. Dirk, R. C. Trievel, and R. L. Houtz, "Calmodulin methyltransferase is an evolutionarily conserved enzyme that trimethylates Lys-115 in calmodulin," *Nature Communications*, vol. 1, no. 4, 2010.

[175] A. T. Nguyen and Y. Zhang, "The diverse functions of Dot1 and H3K79 methylationanh," *Genes & Development*, vol. 25, no. 13, pp. 1345–1358, 2011.

[176] K. J. Webb, Q. Al-Hadid, C. I. Zurita-Lopez, B. D. Young, R. S. Lipson, and S. G. Clarke, "The ribosomal L1 protuberance in yeast is methylated on a lysine residue catalyzed by a seven-β-strand methyltransferase," *The Journal of Biological Chemistry*, vol. 286, no. 21, pp. 18405–18413, 2011.

[177] S. C. Dillon, X. Zhang, R. C. Trievel, and X. Cheng, "The SET-domain protein superfamily: Protein lysine methyltransferases," *Genome Biology*, vol. 6, no. 8, article no. 227, 2005.

[178] T. Shimazu, J. Barjau, Y. Sohtome, M. Sodeoka, and Y. Shinkai, "Selenium-based S-adenosylmethionine analog reveals the mammalian seven-beta-strand methyltransferase METTL10 to be an EF1A1 lysine methyltransferase," *PLoS ONE*, vol. 9, no. 8, Article ID e105394, 2014.

[179] P. Cloutier, M. Lavallée-Adam, D. Faubert, M. Blanchette, and B. Coulombe, "A Newly Uncovered Group of Distantly Related Lysine Methyltransferases Preferentially Interact with Molecular Chaperones to Regulate Their Activity," *PLoS Genetics*, vol. 9, no. 1, Article ID e1003210, 2013.

[180] J. C. Black, C. Van Rechem, and J. R. Whetstine, "Histone lysine methylation dynamics: establishment, regulation, and biological impact," *Molecular Cell*, vol. 48, no. 4, pp. 491–507, 2012.

[181] J. C. Eissenberg and A. Shilatifard, "Histone H3 lysine 4 (H3K4) methylation in development and differentiation," *Developmental Biology*, vol. 339, no. 2, pp. 240–249, 2010.

[182] R. A. Greenberg, "Histone tails: Directing the chromatin response to DNA damage," *FEBS Letters*, vol. 585, no. 18, pp. 2883–2890, 2011.

[183] T. Kouzarides, "Chromatin modifications and their function," *Cell*, vol. 128, no. 4, pp. 693–705, 2007.

[184] A. Nottke, M. P. Colaiácovo, and Y. Shi, "Developmental roles of the histone lysine demethylases," *Development*, vol. 136, no. 6, pp. 879–889, 2009.

[185] M. T. Pedersen and K. Helin, "Histone demethylases in development and disease," *Trends in Cell Biology*, vol. 20, no. 11, pp. 662–671, 2010.

[186] J. C. Black and J. R. Whetstine, "Tipping the lysine methylation balance in disease," *Biopolymers*, vol. 99, no. 2, pp. 127–135, 2013.

[187] E. L. Greer and Y. Shi, "Histone methylation: a dynamic mark in health, disease and inheritance," *Nature Reviews Genetics*, vol. 13, no. 5, pp. 343–357, 2012.

[188] R. A. Copeland, M. P. Moyer, and V. M. Richon, "Targeting genetic alterations in protein methyltransferases for personalized cancer therapeutics," *Oncogene*, vol. 32, no. 8, pp. 939–946, 2013.

[189] S. Hake, A. Xiao, and C. Allis, "Linking the epigenetic 'language' of covalent histone modifications to cancer," *British Journal of Cancer*, vol. 90, no. 4, pp. 761–769, 2004.

[190] H. Ü. Kaniskan and J. Jin, "Chemical probes of histone lysine methyltransferases," *ACS Chemical Biology*, vol. 10, no. 1, pp. 40–50, 2015.

[191] R. A. Varier and H. T. M. Timmers, "Histone lysine methylation and demethylation pathways in cancer," *Biochimica et Biophysica Acta (BBA) - Reviews on Cancer*, vol. 1815, no. 1, pp. 75–89, 2011.

[192] E. A. Pollina and A. Brunet, "Epigenetic regulation of aging stem cells," *Oncogene*, vol. 30, no. 28, pp. 3105–3126, 2011.

[193] M. Albert and K. Helin, "Histone methyltransferases in cancer," *Seminars in Cell & Developmental Biology*, vol. 21, no. 2, pp. 209–220, 2010.

[194] P. Chi, C. D. Allis, and G. G. Wang, "Covalent histone modifications-miswritten, misinterpreted and mis-erased in human cancers," *Nature Reviews Cancer*, vol. 10, no. 7, pp. 457–469, 2010.

[195] S. Varambally, S. M. Dhanasekaran, M. Zhou et al., "The polycomb group protein EZH2 is involved in progression of prostate cancer," *Nature*, vol. 419, no. 6907, pp. 624–629, 2002.

[196] C. G. Kleer, Q. Cao, S. Varambally et al., "EZH2 is a marker of aggressive breast cancer and promotes neoplastic transformation of breast epithelial cells," *Proceedings of the National Acadamy of Sciences of the United States of America*, vol. 100, no. 20, pp. 11606–11611, 2003.

[197] H. P. J. Visser, M. J. Gunster, H. C. Kluin-Nelemans et al., "The Polycomb group protein EZH2 is upregulated in proliferating, cultured human mantle cell lymphoma," *British Journal of Haematology*, vol. 112, no. 4, pp. 950–958, 2001.

[198] R. Chen, Y. Tan, M. Wang et al., "Development of glycoprotein capture-based label-free method for the high-throughput screening of differential glycoproteins in hepatocellular carcinoma," *Molecular ##hssm###38; Cellular Proteomics*, vol. 10, no. 7, Article ID M110.006445, 2011.

[199] R. Hamamoto, V. Saloura, and Y. Nakamura, "Critical roles of non-histone protein lysine methylation in human tumorigenesis," *Nature Reviews Cancer*, vol. 15, no. 2, pp. 110–124, 2015.

[200] S. Ko, J. Ahn, C. S. Song, S. Kim, K. Knapczyk-Stwora, and B. Chatterjee, "Lysine methylation and functional modulation of androgen receptor by set9 methyltransferase," *Molecular Endocrinology*, vol. 25, no. 3, pp. 433–444, 2011.

[201] S. C. Smith, P. N. Baker, and E. M. Symonds, "Placental apoptosis in normal human pregnancy," *American Journal of Obstetrics & Gynecology*, vol. 177, no. 1, pp. 57–65, 1997.

[202] A. D. Allaire, K. A. Ballenger, S. R. Wells, M. J. McMahon, and B. A. Lessey, "Placental apoptosis in preeclampsia," *Obstetrics & Gynecology*, vol. 96, no. 2, pp. 271–276, 2000.

[203] A. E. P. Heazell, H. R. Buttle, P. N. Baker, and I. P. Crocker, "Altered expression of regulators of caspase activity within trophoblast of normal pregnancies and pregnancies complicated by preeclampsia," *Reproductive Sciences*, vol. 15, no. 10, pp. 1034–1043, 2008.

[204] D. N. Leung, S. C. Smith, K. To, D. S. Sahota, and P. N. Baker, "Increased placental apoptosis in pregnancies complicated by preeclampsia," *American Journal of Obstetrics & Gynecology*, vol. 184, no. 6, pp. 1249-1250, 2001.

[205] B. Huppertz and J. C. P. Kingdom, "Apoptosis in the trophoblast—role of apoptosis in placental morphogenesis," *Journal of the Society for Gynecologic Investigation*, vol. 11, no. 6, pp. 353–362, 2004.

[206] A. N. Sharp, A. E. Heazell, I. P. Crocker, and G. Mor, "Placental Apoptosis in Health and Disease," *American Journal of Reproductive Immunology*, vol. 64, no. 3, pp. 159–169, 2010.

[207] A. N. Sharp, A. E. P. Heazell, D. Baczyk et al., "Preeclampsia is associated with alterations in the p53-pathway in villous trophoblast," *PLoS ONE*, vol. 9, no. 1, Article ID e87621, 2014.

[208] T. Hung, S. Chen, L. Lo et al., "Increased Autophagy in Placentas of Intrauterine Growth-Restricted Pregnancies," *PLoS ONE*, vol. 7, no. 7, p. e40957, 2012.

[209] R. Levy, S. D. Smith, K. Yusuf et al., "Trophoblast apoptosis from pregnancies complicated by fetal growth restriction is associated with enhanced p53 expression," *American Journal of Obstetrics & Gynecology*, vol. 186, no. 5, pp. 1056–1061, 2002.

[210] S. Chuikov, J. K. Kurash, J. R. Wilson et al., "Regulation of p53 activity through lysine methylation," *Nature*, vol. 432, no. 7015, pp. 353–360, 2004.

[211] J. Oyake, M. Otaka, T. Matsuhashi et al., "Over-expression of 70-kDa heat shock protein confers protection against monochloramine-induced gastric mucosal cell injury," *Life Sciences*, vol. 79, no. 3, pp. 300–305, 2006.

[212] S. Jirecek, M. Hohlagschwandtner, C. Tempfer, M. Knöfler, P. Husslein, and H. Zeisler, "Serum levels of heat shock protein 70 in patients with preeclampsia: A pilot-study," *Wiener Klinische Wochenschrift*, vol. 114, no. 15-16, pp. 730–732, 2002.

[213] J. Hageman, M. A. W. H. van Waarde, A. Zylicz, D. Walerych, and H. H. Kampinga, "The diverse members of the mammalian HSP70 machine show distinct chaperone-like activities," *Biochemical Journal*, vol. 435, no. 1, pp. 127–142, 2011.

[214] E. L. Davies, M. M. F. V. G. Bacelar, M. J. Marshall et al., "Heat shock proteins form part of a danger signal cascade in response to lipopolysaccharide and GroEL," *Clinical & Experimental Immunology*, vol. 145, no. 1, pp. 183–189, 2006.

[215] X. Luo, X. Zuo, B. Zhang et al., "Release of heat shock protein 70 and the effects of extracellular heat shock protein 70 on the production of IL-10 in fibroblast-like synoviocytes," *Cell Stress and Chaperones*, vol. 13, no. 3, pp. 365–373, 2008.

[216] D. G. Millar, K. M. Garza, B. Odermatt et al., "Hsp70 promotes antigen-presenting cell function and converts T-cell tolerance to autoimmunity in vivo," *Nature Medicine*, vol. 9, no. 12, pp. 1469–1476, 2003.

[217] H. H. Kampinga, J. Hageman, M. J. Vos et al., "Guidelines for the nomenclature of the human heat shock proteins," *Cell Stress and Chaperones*, vol. 14, no. 1, pp. 105–111, 2009.

[218] H. H. Kampinga and E. A. Craig, "The HSP70 chaperone machinery: J proteins as drivers of functional specificity," *Nature Reviews Molecular Cell Biology*, vol. 11, no. 8, pp. 579–592, 2010.

[219] A. Fukushima, H. Kawahara, and C. Isurugi, "Changes in serum levels of heat shock protein 70 in preterm delivery and preeclampsia," *Journal of Obstetrics and Gynaecology Research*, vol. 31, no. 1, pp. 72–77, 2005.

[220] J. K. Park, T. G. Kang, M. Y. Kang et al., "Increased NFAT5 expression stimulates transcription of Hsp70 in preeclamptic placentas," *Placenta*, vol. 35, no. 2, pp. 109–116, 2014.

[221] F. Barut, A. Barut, B. Dogan Gun et al., "Expression of heat shock protein 70 and endothelial nitric oxide synthase in placental tissue of preeclamptic and intrauterine growth-restricted pregnancies," *Pathology - Research and Practice*, vol. 206, no. 9, pp. 651–656, 2010.

[222] Y. Liu, N. Li, L. You, X. Liu, H. Li, and X. Wang, "HSP70 is associated with endothelial activation in placental vascular diseases," *Molecular Medicine*, vol. 14, no. 9-10, pp. 561–566, 2008.

[223] H.-S. Cho, T. Shimazu, G. Toyokawa et al., "Enhanced HSP70 lysine methylation promotes proliferation of cancer cells through activation of Aurora kinase B," *Nature Communications*, vol. 3, article 1072, 2012.

[224] A. Sawano, T. Takahashi, S. Yamaguchi, M. Aonuma, and M. Shibuya, "Flt-1 but not KDR/Flk-1 tyrosine kinase is a receptor for placenta growth factor, which is related to vascular endothelial growth factor," *Cell Growth & Differentiation*, vol. 7, no. 2, pp. 213–221, 1996.

[225] N. Ferrara and R. S. Kerbel, "Angiogenesis as a therapeutic target," *Nature*, vol. 438, no. 7070, pp. 967–974, 2005.

[226] N. Rahimi, "Vascular endothelial growth factor receptors: Molecular mechanisms of activation and therapeutic potentials," *Experimental Eye Research*, vol. 83, no. 5, pp. 1005–1016, 2006.

[227] D. Hanahan and J. Folkman, "Patterns and emerging mechanisms of the angiogenic switch during tumorigenesis," *Cell*, vol. 86, no. 3, pp. 353–364, 1996.

[228] W. Risau, "Mechanisms of angiogenesis," *Nature*, vol. 386, no. 6626, pp. 671–674, 1997.

[229] G.-H. Fong, J. Rossant, M. Gertsenstein, and M. L. Breitman, "Role of the Flt-1 receptor tyrosine kinase in regulating the assembly of vascular endothelium," *Nature*, vol. 376, no. 6535, pp. 66–70, 1995.

[230] S. Helske, P. Vuorela, O. Carpén, C. Hornig, H. Weich, and E. Halmesmäki, "Expression of vascular endothelial growth factor receptors 1, 2 and 3 in placentas from normal and complicated pregnancies," *Molecular Human Reproduction*, vol. 7, no. 2, pp. 205–210, 2001.

[231] Y. Zhou, M. McMaster, K. Woo et al., "Vascular endothelial growth factor ligands and receptors that regulate human cytotrophoblast survival are dysregulated in severe preeclampsia and hemolysis, elevated liver enzymes, and low platelets syndrome," *The American Journal of Pathology*, vol. 160, no. 4, Article ID 62567, pp. 1405–1423, 2002.

[232] M. Kunizaki, R. Hamamoto, F. P. Silva et al., "The lysine 831 of vascular endothelial growth factor receptor 1 is a novel target of methylation by SMYD3," *Cancer Research*, vol. 67, no. 22, pp. 10759–10765, 2007.

[233] E. J. Hartsough, R. D. Meyer, V. Chitalia et al., "Lysine methylation promotes VEGFR-2 activation and angiogenesis," *Science Signaling*, vol. 6, no. 304, Article ID ra104, 2013.

[234] N. Rahimi and C. E. Costello, "Emerging roles of post-translational modifications in signal transduction and angiogenesis," *Proteomics*, vol. 15, no. 2-3, pp. 300–309, 2015.

Physiologic Course of Female Reproductive Function: A Molecular Look into the Prologue of Life

Joselyn Rojas, Mervin Chávez-Castillo, Luis Carlos Olivar, María Calvo, José Mejías, Milagros Rojas, Jessenia Morillo, and Valmore Bermúdez

Endocrine-Metabolic Research Center, "Dr. Félix Gómez", Faculty of Medicine, University of Zulia, Maracaibo 4004, Zulia, Venezuela

Correspondence should be addressed to Joselyn Rojas; rojas.joselyn@gmail.com

Academic Editor: Sam Mesiano

The genetic, endocrine, and metabolic mechanisms underlying female reproduction are numerous and sophisticated, displaying complex functional evolution throughout a woman's lifetime. This vital course may be systematized in three subsequent stages: prenatal development of ovaries and germ cells up until *in utero* arrest of follicular growth and the ensuing interim suspension of gonadal function; onset of reproductive maturity through puberty, with reinitiation of both gonadal and adrenal activity; and adult functionality of the ovarian cycle which permits ovulation, a key event in female fertility, and dictates concurrent modifications in the endometrium and other ovarian hormone-sensitive tissues. Indeed, the ultimate goal of this physiologic progression is to achieve ovulation and offer an adequate environment for the installation of gestation, the consummation of female fertility. Strict regulation of these processes is important, as disruptions at any point in this evolution may equate a myriad of endocrine-metabolic disturbances for women and adverse consequences on offspring both during pregnancy and postpartum. This review offers a summary of pivotal aspects concerning the physiologic course of female reproductive function.

1. Introduction

Historically, the phenomenon of human reproduction has awakened great interest. One of its first scientific descriptions, authored by Hippocrates, dates back to the fifth century BC, suggesting generation of new beings to stem from the union of the male's ejaculate and the female's menstrual bleeding. More than two millennia after, we now know that reproduction derives from a complex succession of biologic events, where the union of the gametes, spermatozoa and oocytes, plays a fundamental role [1].

In their earliest stage, gametes originate from specific cells that abandon their somatic lineage to differentiate into primordial germ cells (PGC), key components in reproduction [2]. In female humans, the ovary represents an essential structural support for the development of PGC throughout their evolution [3]. Once they have matured into primordial follicles, a stage reached before birth, and once the subject has reached puberty, folliculogenesis begins, a series of cellular changes necessary for maturation and preparation for a second wave of structural and functional modifications inherent to the ovarian cycle, which in turn finalizes with the crucial event in female fertility: ovulation [4]. In ensemble, these processes permit generation of new life, reproduction.

Indeed, female reproductive physiology entails intricate interactions among hormonal, metabolic-energetic, genetic-epigenetic, and intra- and extraovarian factors, which in coordination modulate the successive development of the female gamete [5]. Disruptions in any of these components may lead to infertility, an alarming problem in women's global health, currently affecting 48.5 million females aged 20–44 years [6]. Moreover, alterations of female reproductive physiology often bear implications in other organ systems, as in the classical example of polycystic ovary syndrome [7]. Beyond the physical and mental implications in women [8], these alterations may also reflect on the ulterior health of their potential offspring [9]. Due to this profound impact in female well-being and their progeny, this review aims to describe the physiological and molecular phenomena implicated in female fertility.

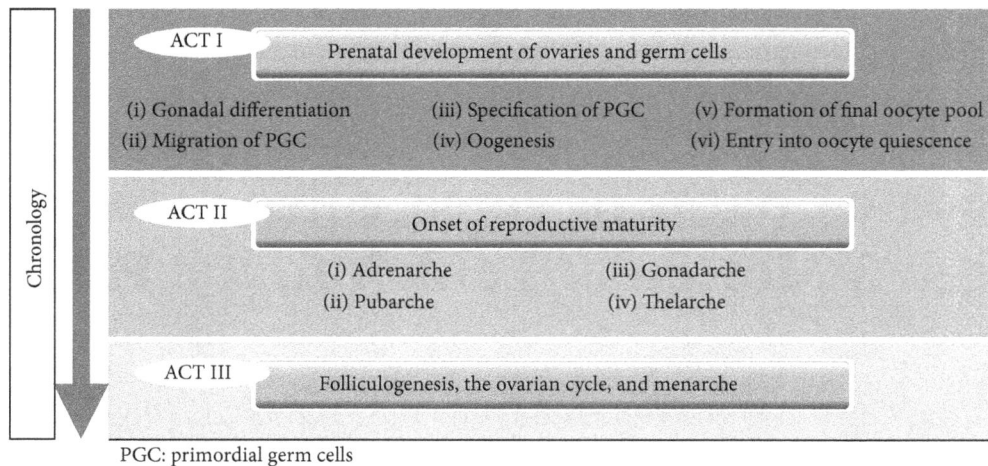

PGC: primordial germ cells

FIGURE 1: Main events in the physiologic life course of female reproductive function.

TABLE 1: Approximate values for serum levels of various endocrine mediators at distinct stages in the physiologic life course of female reproductive function.

Stage	LH (IU/L)[a]	FSH (IU/L)[a]	Estradiol (pg/mL)[a]	DHEAS (μg/dL)[a]	Testosterone (ng/dL)[a]	Leptin (ng/mL)	IGF-I (μg/dL)
Prepubertal	>0.3	<4	<10	5–40	<20	0.5–11.7[b]	115–208[d]
Premenarchal	≤12	1–12	<50	35–130	13–44	1.6–12.6[c]	232–363[e]
Postmenarchal (early follicular phase)	2–11	1–12	20–85	75–255	15–59	5.8–19.2[c]	251–440[e]
Postmenarchal (midcycle)	≤85	≤19	≤350	—	—	—	—

LH: luteinizing hormones; FSH: Follicle-Stimulating Hormone; DHEAS: dehydroepiandrosterone sulfate.
[a]Bordini and Rosenfield [91].
[b]Ellis and Nicolson [228].
[c]Bandini et al. [229].
[d]Yüksel et al. [230].
[e]Zumbado et al. [10].

2. Overview of Female Reproductive Function: Fertility as a Three-Act Theatre Piece

The ovary goes through a wide array of structural and functional modifications throughout a female's life, in order to provide reproductive potential [4]. Figure 1 chronologically summarizes the principal events in this timeline. These processes are subject to regulation by multiple endocrine signals, as reflected in the ample fluctuations in gonadotropin, sex hormone, and other mediators' serum concentrations throughout various stages of life (Table 1). Nonetheless, these molecules are only selected representatives from the abundance of mediators from many interconnected and overlapping neuroendocrine regulation systems, where both reproductive and metabolic signals are integrated [10].

Much like a theatrical play, this sequence may be schematized in three elemental parts or "acts": (1) the setup: embryonic origin and *in utero* development of the ovary, and infantile quiescence; (2) the buildup: ovarian and adrenal reactivation in puberty and neuroendocrine cues initiating sexual maturation; and (3) the climax: molecular mechanisms in folliculogenesis and the normal ovarian cycle.

3. Act I: The Setup—Prenatal Development of Ovaries and Germ Cells

In mammals, the prenatal period is a critical stage for the functional development of all organ systems. Within the female reproductive sphere, it comprises sexual differentiation, according to the chromosomal load inherited in syngamy, and formation of the future female gametes (Figure 2), both coordinated by successive genetic interactions [11].

3.1. Gonadal Differentiation. Gametes, spermatozoa and secondary oocytes, are haploid cells responsible for generation of offspring through fecundation, which culminates in the formation of a single cell, the zygote, whose genome proceeds from the conjugation of its predecessors' genomes. From this pivotal step, zygotes inherit a pair of sex chromosomes (XX or XY) which will drive the transformation of this cellular unit into a multicellular organism with a sex-specific phenotype [12]. Once the embryo has attained the definitive organization of germ layers, the urogenital ridge, a thickening of coelomic epithelium superimposed on the anterior portion of the mesonephros, becomes the gonadal primordium and

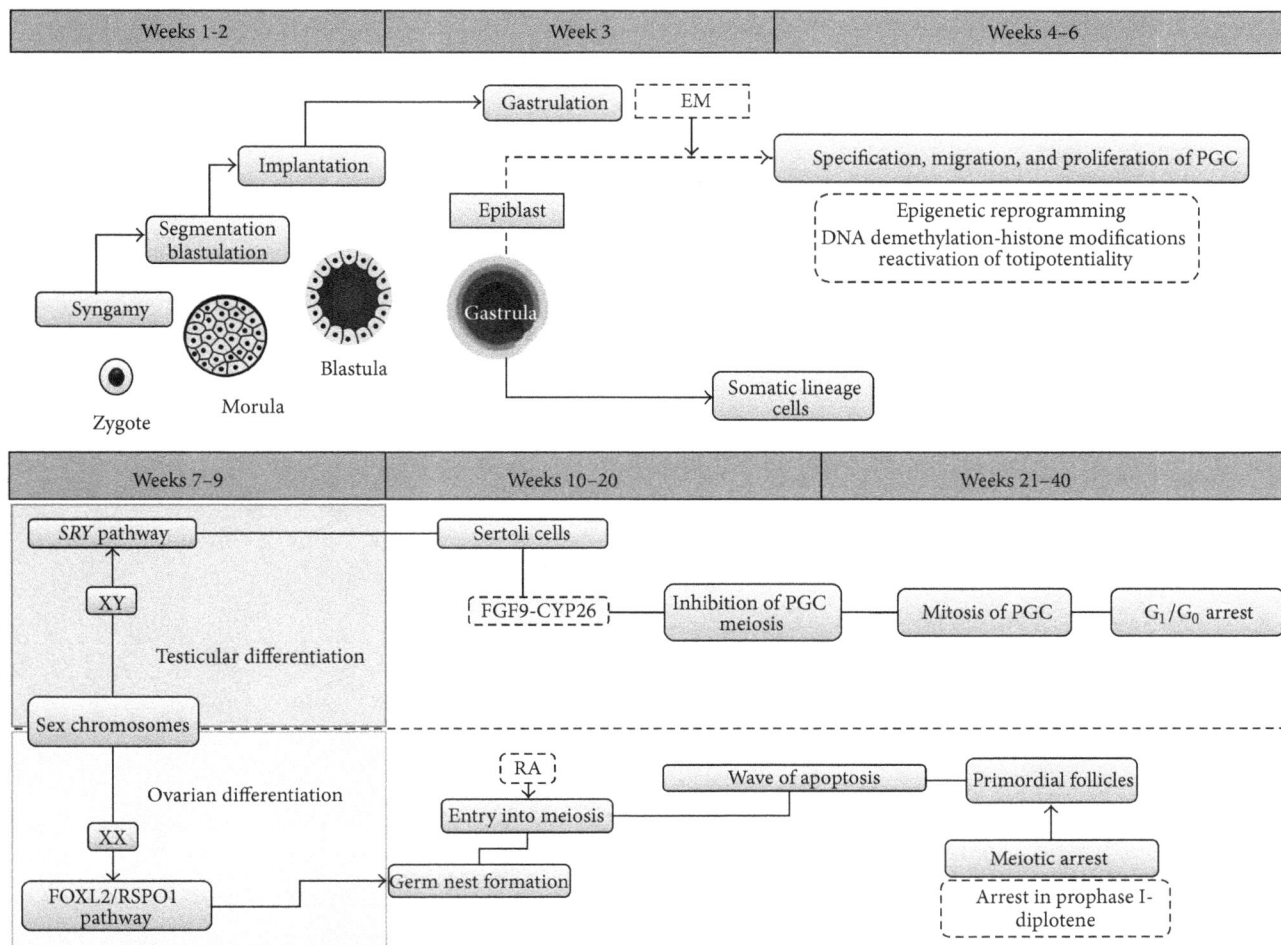

FIGURE 2: Overview of gonadal differentiation and germ cell development. CYP26: retinoic acid hydroxylases; EM: extraembryonic mesoderm; FGF9: fibroblast growth factor-9; PGC: primordial germ cells. RA: retinoic acid. Syngamy yields a single totipotent cell, the zygote, which subsequently undergoes several proliferative and reorganizational processes. After *gastrulation*, arrangement into a three-layered embryonic structure, has occurred, nascent PGC undergo induction into pluripotent cells, *specification*, by EM. PGC also begin *migration* towards their final residence, the gonadal ridges, whilst simultaneously suffering epigenetic reprogramming essential for reactivation of totipotentiality. Afterwards, according to the sex chromosome load, both PGC and gonads undergo *differentiation*. In XY subjects, *SRY* induces differentiation of Sertoli cells, which thereafter drive testicular differentiation. Likewise, FGF9 and RA hydroxylases inhibit meiosis in these PGC, instead favoring mitosis and then cell cycle arrest until puberty. In contrast, in XX individuals it is FOXL2/RSPO1 signaling in ovarian primordia that drives development of female gonads and germ nest formation. RA then induces entry into meiosis and proliferation. These cells later suffer a wave of apoptosis which determines the final pool of primordial follicles, which remain arrested in meiosis I until puberty.

the chief site for PGC development [13]. In beings with XY sex chromosome load, the *SRY* transcription factor binds to a promoter of *Sox9*, the Testis-Specific Enhancer of Sox9 Core Element (TESCO), which drives differentiation of Sertoli cells and in turn propels testicular formation. In absence of a Y chromosome, the undifferentiated or bipotential gonad does not express this gene, nor are its downstream mechanisms triggered, leading to formation of an ovary, the so-called standard process [14].

Although this description reflects the traditional approach to these phenomena as a "standard" or passive process, it is currently known to be a complex, active chain of events involving coordinated expression of a myriad of genes [15, 16]. Among these, the *FOXL2* transcription factor

appears to play an important role by antagonizing *Sox9* activity [17]. Additionally, ovarian differentiation pathways involve R-spondin homolog 1 (RSPO1), a protein secreted in gonadal primordia increasing Wnt4 signaling which regulates β-catenin activity. This mediator can then translocate to the nucleus and interact with Hepatocyte Nuclear Factor 1 Homeobox A (HNF1A) to regulate transcriptional activity and cell adhesion in the ovary in formation [18].

3.2. Specification and Migration of Primordial Germ Cells. PGC experience an extensive and complex succession of cellular transformations in order to become viable gametes ready for fecundation (Figure 3). Among embryonic cells, those who eventually evolve into PGC appear very early

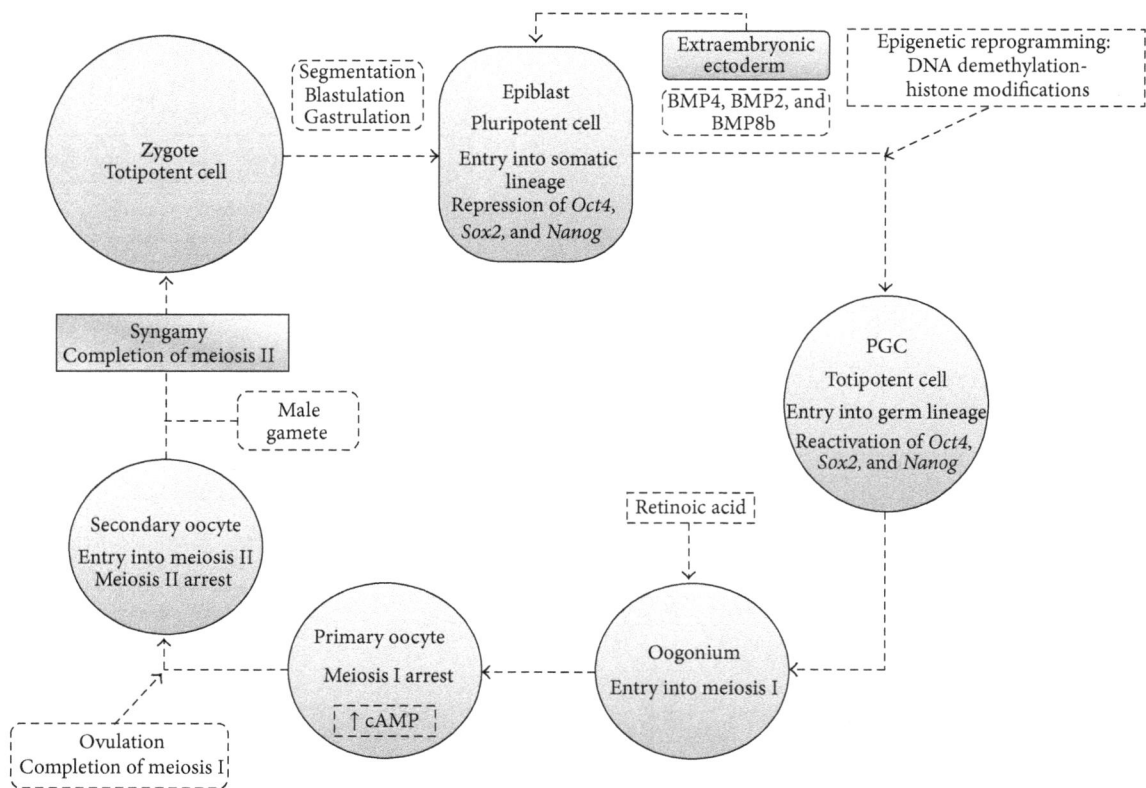

FIGURE 3: Cellular stages and signaling in female germ cell development. Syngamy produces a single totipotent cell, the zygote, which evolves through various structural stages. After gastrulation, extraembryonic ectoderm induces some epiblastic cells into pluripotency and entry into somatic lineage. These later undergo epigenetic reprogramming to regain totipotentiality and become primordial germ cells. These migrate to the gonadal ridges and suffer intense mitosis, becoming oogonia, which are then induced by retinoic acid to enter meiosis I. Primary oocytes are then arrested in this division and appear to survive until ovulation due to elevated intracellular cAMP levels. With ovulation, meiosis I is completed and meiosis II begins in secondary oocytes. Nonetheless, this division is only fulfilled if union with a male gamete occurs, which ultimately leads to formation of a zygote.

and must transition from the somatic to the germ lineage and reactivate their totipotentiality by effacing their progenitor imprinting, which constitute *specification* [19]. These processes require intense genetic and epigenetic reprogramming which happens simultaneously to these cells' *migration* towards the urogenital ridge (Figure 4) [20].

Circa day 6 after fecundation in mice, approximately the fourth-fifth week in humans [21], extraembryonic ectoderm subjects a small quantity of epiblastic cells from the primitive embryonic ectoderm to high levels of Bone Morphogenetic Protein 4 (BMP4) [22]. This induces expression of the *Prdm1* gene (PRD1-BF1 and RIZ domain-1) which codes for the B Lymphocyte-Induced Maturation Protein 1 (BLIMP1), which appears to be an important "switch" in transition to the germ lineage [23, 24]. LIN28 cooperates in this process by inhibiting Let7, a *Prdm1* repressor [25], and allowing expression of Stella, an early marker of PGC [26]. Loss of expression of various genes related to somatic development is also seen, such as *evx1*, *tbx1*, and *mesp1*, which are associated with development of ectodermic and mesodermic structures [27].

Roughly in day 8.5, between the fifth and eighth week in humans [21], these nascent PGC begin expressing genes

typical of pluripotent cells such as *Oct4*, *Nanog*, and *Sox2* [28] and begin their migration towards the gonadal primordia [29]. Specific genetic programming coordinates the proliferation, survival, and migration of these cells. Molecules related to PGC migration include chemoattractants such as Stromal-Derived Factor (SDF1/CXCL12) [30] and Stem Cell Factor/c-Kit Ligand (SCF/KITL) [31], which bind to specific receptors expressed in the surface of PGC [32, 33]. Wnt3A is a glycoprotein which also appears to intervene in PGC migration and proliferation, presumably through stabilization of β-catenin [34].

Another molecular determinant of pluripotentiality in nascent PGC is expression of DNMT3 and DNMT4, families of DNA methyltransferases which mediate methylation of cytosine mainly in "CpG" (Cytosine-phosphate-Guanine) sequences, originating 5-methylcytosine (5mC) sites important for genomic imprinting [35]. These genomic stamps must be erased to achieve the totipotentiality inherent to fully specified PGC [36]. This demethylation is an active phenomenon that occurs around day 11.5 in mice, sixth-seventh week in humans [21], where TET1, TET2, and TET3, enzymes from the Methylcytosine Dioxygenase Ten-Eleven Translocation (TET) family, catalyze this process with oxidation of 5mC

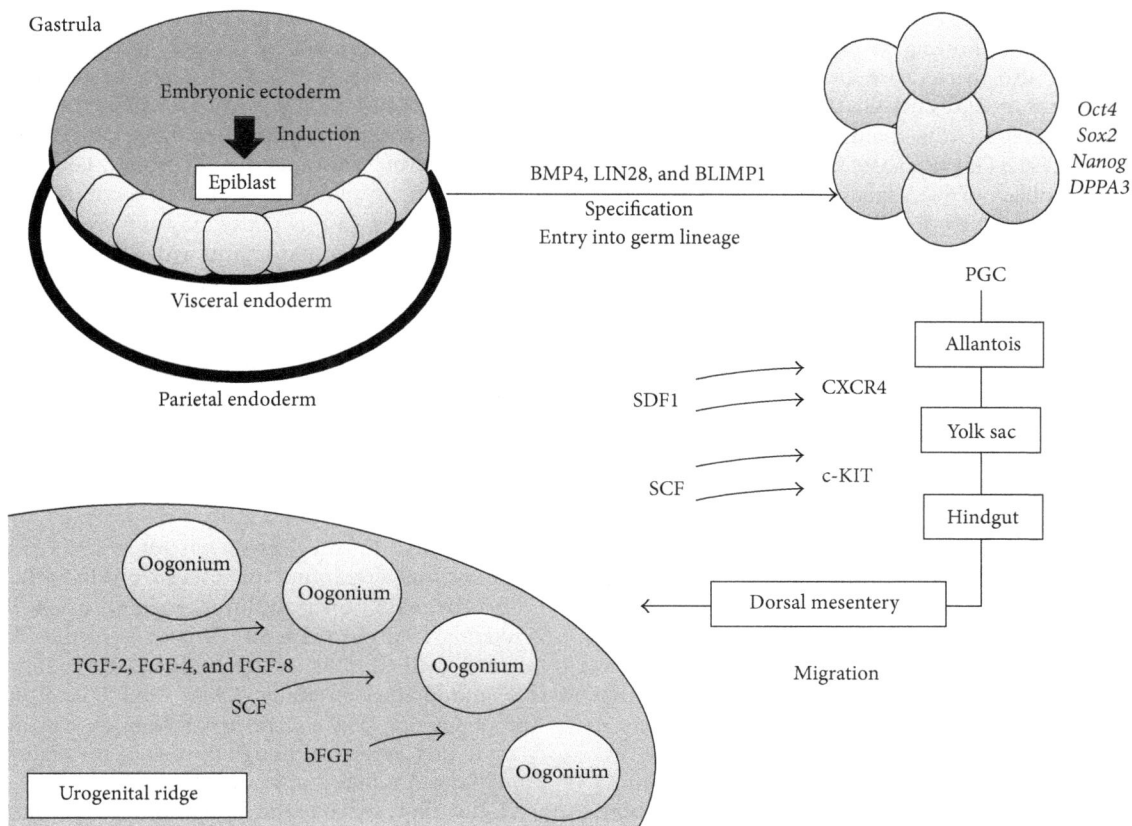

FIGURE 4: Factors controlling specification and migration of primordial germ cells. bFGF: basic fibroblast growth factor; FGF: fibroblast growth factor; PGC: primordial germ cells; SCF: Stem Cell Factor; SDF1: stromal cell-derived factor. Formation of fully competent gonads demands the presence of PGC in the genital primordia, which in turn requires the fulfillment of two fundamental processes. (1) *Specification*: PGC stem from a small group of cells which are subjected to induction by the extraembryonic ectoderm, via intense BMP4 signaling, which induces expression of BLIMP1 in these cells. The main factors controlling specification are the expression of pluripotent genes, for example, *Oct4*, *Sox2*, and *Nanog*, and thorough epigenetic reprogramming. In addition, BLIMP1 and LIN28 allow expression of DPPA3 (Stella), which mediates protection of maternal imprinting in PGC. (2) *Migration*: PGC initially reside with the epiblast in the gastrula in the posterior end of the primitive streak, which will later become the extraembryonic mesoderm. Then, PGC migrate through the allantois and reside temporarily in the yolk sac. These cells then migrate caudally through the hindgut towards the dorsal mesentery and then the urogenital ridges, their definitive location. The principal factors regulating this process are SDF1 and SCF, which bind to CXCR4 and c-KIT, respectively, mediating chemotaxis and survival of PGC.

through iron- and 2-oxoglutarate-dependent mechanisms [37, 38].

Notably, these epigenetic changes do not affect maternal-origin genome in the embryoblast; therefore, methylation of various genes is maintained, generating epigenetic asymmetry in these loci in comparison to the paternal-origin genome [39]. The Developmental Pluripotency-Associated Protein 3 (DPPA3) or Stella factor, a 159-amino acid protein expressed in preimplantation embryos, embryonic stem cells, and PGC, appears to be the "molecular shield" of these loci. Stella is able to block TET3 activity on 5mC of the maternal-origin genome, and some paternal loci [39]. This selectivity derives from differential recognition of histones. The maternal genome is predominantly associated with demethylated H3 histones (H3K9me2), which are Stella binding targets [40]. This union appears to cause conformational disposition which impede TET3 activity on 5mC [38]. In consequence, Stella possesses a preservative effect on PGC imprinting [41].

In parallel, nascent PGC undergo histone modifications, presumably a mass substitution of histones mediated by HIRA and NAP1, as a sort of "repairing" required for restitution of totipotentiality [28]. Completion of this genetic-epigenetic reprogramming and localization of PGC in gonadal primordia mark the end of the specification and migration processes, respectively [11], which happen approximately in the sixth-seventh weeks in humans [42]. Cells that do not complete or deviate from either process suffer apoptosis due to a lack of prosurvival signals [43].

3.3. Oogenesis: Mitosis, Meiosis, and Meiotic Arrest. Once the genome has been reorganized, PGC continue abundant mitosis in gonadal primordia, leading to production of a great amount of cells, now denominated gonocytes, or oogonia in females, a process known as *oogenesis*. Sexual identity of gonocytes depends heavily on signals from their microenvironment. At this point, gonocyte expression of DAZL, an ARN-binding protein, is necessary not only to silence somatic genetic programming associated with markers of pluripotency, but also to facilitate an adequate response to these microenvironmental cues in the gonadal primordia [44, 45]. In this respect, the main messengers in ovarian primordia are SCF/KITL [46], basic fibroblast growth factor (bFGF), and fibroblast growth factors 2, 4, and 8 [47, 48]. In this scenario, around weeks 10–20 oogonia form cysts or transitory germ cell nests or clusters derived from multiple mitotic divisions that do not fully complete cytokinesis [49]. These nests are masses of approximately 16 germ cells which are interconnected by cytoplasmic bridges and enveloped by somatic cells that appear to be essential for the functional integrity of gametes [50].

Nevertheless, the fundamental event in oogenesis is induction of meiosis, destined to produce a haploid genome, necessary for syngamy [51]. This process begins roughly in weeks 11–13 in humans [52], with adjacent mesonephros-secreted retinoic acid (RA) as a key trigger [53]. Indeed, this molecule induces expression of the Stimulated by Retinoic Acid 8 (Strat8) protein in premeiotic germ cells, mediated by RXR nuclear receptors [54, 55]. Despite detailed downstream mechanisms remaining unclear, Strat8 signaling appears to downregulate synthesis of *Nanos2*, an inhibitor of meiosis through posttranscriptional modification of key mediators in this process [56, 57]. In addition, DAZL may exert a permissive role for RA signaling [58]. Epigenetic reprogramming appears to be a required step for initiation of meiosis, as both PGC and oogonia are subjected to high RA concentrations in the gonadal interstitium, yet only the latter enter meiosis [2].

In contrast, RA also participates in male sexual development, yet its effects are not seen until puberty, with male germ cells remaining arrested in G_0/G_1 until this stage, when meiosis is favored in this gender [55]. To this end, during *in utero* life and throughout infancy, RA is degraded by hydroxylases, CYP26B1 and CYP26C1, expressed in Sertoli cells [59]. Secretion of fibroblast growth factor-9 by Sertoli cells also contributes to inhibition of meiosis by upregulation *Nanos2* [57, 60], and by aiding in differentiation of Leydig cells [61].

In females, formation of germ cell nests and induction of meiosis occur simultaneously. By week 20, these clusters begin rupturing as some cells die through apoptosis, destabilizing the cystic structure. At this point, outlying somatic cells begin invading the nest and surround oocytes, defining the structure of primordial follicles [62, 63]. On the other hand, meiotic division encompasses two successive cycles, meiosis I and meiosis II, each with four phases: Prophase, Metaphase, Anaphase, and Telophase [64]. Oocytes advance through Prophase I and are arrested at the diplotene, where they remain quiescent awaiting induction of gonadotropin-dependent maturation at puberty, when they will obtain primary oocyte status [65]. This state is maintained by the Maturation Promoting Factor (MPF) complex, which consists of a catalytic subunit, the cyclin-dependent kinase 1 (CDK1), and a regulatory subunit, cyclin B1 (CB1) [66, 67]. CDK1 exhibits two regulatory sites that may be phosphorylated by WEE1/MYT1, inhibiting its activity [68, 69], whereas dephosphorylation by CDC25A permits progress through

meiosis I [70]. This is facilitated by the constantly elevated levels of cAMP present in oocytes, which allow activation of Protein Kinase A (PKA), leading to reinforcement of WEE1/MYT1 and inhibition of CDC25A [69]. These high cAMP concentrations appear to originate from a constitutively activated stimulatory G protein-coupled receptor which supplies requirements of this second messenger [71]. Oocytes arrested in this phase may survive for years owing to their decondensed chromatin which facilitates gene transcription, as well as bidirectional communication with the surrounding somatic cells, which provide nourishment [72].

3.4. Programmed Cell Death: Formation of the Definitive Oocyte Pool. Two-thirds of all primordial oocytes suffer programmed cell death, in a phenomenon denominated "apoptotic wave," considered a cellular "quality control" mechanism [73]. This is presumed to occur through the intrinsic apoptosis pathway, activated by two potential triggers: (a) suppression of prosurvival signals for oocytes [74] and (b) chromosomal alterations stemming from flaws in Prophase I [73]. The main prosurvival messengers are SCF/KITL [75], Leukemia Inhibitory Factor [76], and insulin-like growth factor I (IGF-I) [77], which induce expression of apoptosis modulatory proteins Bcl-XL, Bcl-2, and Bcl-w [78]. Autophagy may play a secondary role as another form of cell death in this context, although the causal correlation for each kind of death remains unknown [79].

Cells that survive the apoptotic wave constitute the final pool of primordial follicles available for the entirety of the female's reproductive life [80, 81]. Primary oocytes remain quiescent until puberty, when, with each iteration of the ovarian cycle, a luteinizing hormone (LH) surge will resume meiosis [82]. Indeed, female humans are born with approximately 1-2 million primordial follicles [83]. This reserve gradually wanes throughout the female's lifetime, as follicles abandon this pool due to either death or entry into folliculogenesis [84].

4. Act II: The Buildup—Onset of Reproductive Maturity

Puberty is the process through which male and female children become young adults, comprehending several events: (a) maturation of gametogenesis; (b) adrenarche, the onset of adrenal androgen synthesis and secretion; (c) pubarche, the appearance of pubic hair; (d) gonadarche, maturation of the hypothalamus-hypophysis-gonadal axis (HHGA), with gonadal sexual steroid synthesis and secretion; and, exclusively in females, (e) thelarche, onset of mammary development and (f) menarche, onset of ovulation and menstrual bleeding. Although the chronological order of these phenomena is widely variable, in conjunction, they allow for acquisition of full reproductive potential [85, 86].

The age at which each of these events occurs is highly variable and subject to a myriad of environmental and genetic factors [87]. For example, the National Health and Nutrition Examination Survey (NHANES III) found Caucasian girls to experience thelarche at a mean age of 10.4 years, whereas in their African American peers, the mean was 9.5 years [88].

Likewise, it tends to happen earlier in Mexican American girls and latest among Asian Americans [89]. These distinct patterns are also seen worldwide amongst different ethnical backgrounds [87, 90]. Nonetheless, most frequently, the-larche tends to be followed by pubarche, roughly 1–1.5 years afterwards, and menarche usually follows approximately 2.5 years after thelarche [91].

In recent years, onset of puberty appears to have transitioned to younger ages by 1-2 years; hypotheses explaining this shift encompass both extrinsic and intrinsic factors [92]. Regarding the former, endocrine-disrupting chemicals with estrogenic and antiestrogenic activity, such as polybrominated biphenyls and dichlorodiphenyltrichloroethane (DDT), are known to be powerful inductors of precocious puberty [93]. On the other hand, nutritional status appears to be the paramount intrinsic regulator of puberty onset parallel to genetic factors: girls with higher body mass index tend to display thelarche, pubarche, and even menarche much earlier, between 8 and 9.5 years of age; and conversely, low weight and malnutrition can significantly delay this process [94]. The following sections describe the molecular principles dictating the onset of puberty and its individual components.

4.1. Neuroendocrine Regulation of Sex Hormone Synthesis throughout Life.

Although the HHGA is essential in reproductive function, it is active in stages as early as fetal development. Indeed, the fetal testicle begins functioning during the first half of gestation, firstly driven by human chorionic gonadotropin (hCG) and then by LH stimulation following the development of the hypothalamus-hypophysis portal system around weeks 11-12, with testicular androgens being key for male sexual differentiation [95]. In contrast, though the fetal ovary displays scarce steroidogenic activity with CYP11A1 and CYP17A1, this organ is considered to be functionally quiescent regarding hormone synthesis throughout in utero life and infancy, only accomplishing significant estrogenic synthesis at puberty; nevertheless, mechanisms underlying this latency remain unknown [96].

However, both genders appear to undergo a process described as the "newborn's miniature puberty," a significant surge in HHGA activity after birth, presumably due to the relieving of GnRH secretion inhibition by maternal estrogen. This peak persists for roughly 12 months in females, where it manifests as moderate mammary development, and approximately 6 months in males, where it entails hyperplasia of Leydig and Sertoli cells, and a modest increase in size of external genital organs [91, 97].

This occurrence is succeeded by the "juvenile pause," where secretion of GnRH, and consequently gonadal steroids, returns to quiescence as a result of full development of neural structures regulating this hypothalamic center [85]. This scenario underlines the pivotal role of GnRH pulsatile secretion as a "master switch" for maturation of the HHGA. In turn, this secretion pattern is subject to modulation by interactions of both inhibitory and excitatory neuroendocrine and synaptic systems on GnRH-secreting cells, amidst numerous endogenous and exogenous environmental signals. Dominance of excitatory signals permits this pulsatile

pattern, leading to maturation of gonadal steroidogenesis: gonadarche [85, 97].

Glutamate and γ-amino-butyric acid (GABA) are the key excitatory and inhibitory hypothalamic neurotransmitters regarding puberty onset, respectively. A decrease in GABAergic tone, with a corresponding rise in glutamatergic tone, appears to be the fundamental process in this scenario [98]. The underlying trigger to this shift may be the expression of estrogen and progesterone receptors in glutamatergic and GABAergic neurons, which are absent previous to puberty, yet the stimuli for this sensitization to sex hormones remain incompletely understood [99]. Proposed mechanisms include a regulatory role for allopregnanolone, which appears to modify glutamate and GABA secretion, as well as modulate NMDA and GABA receptor expression in hypothalamic neurons [100], and an inhibitory effect by endogenous opioids, as suggested by precocious puberty induced by administration of naloxone [101].

Decreased GABAergic tone has been observed to be accompanied by a critical increase in kisspeptin signaling [102]. Kisspeptin, a hypothalamic neuropeptide coded by the Kiss1 gene, has long been known to be crucial in sexual development, with mutations of the GPR54 gene, which codes its receptor, being associated with a loss of reproductive function in both humans and mice [103, 104]. Hypothalamic disposition of kisspeptinergic neurons varies by species [105]; in humans, they have been located in both the arcuate nucleus (AN) and anteroventral periventricular nucleus (AVPV), most densely in the former [106]. During puberty, kisspeptin and GPR54 expression is upregulated in both nuclei, accompanied with greater GnRH secretion [107, 108]. In addition, kisspeptinergic signaling may be amplified by sex hormone-induced reorganization of neuronal projections in the hypothalamus [109].

Nonetheless, kisspeptinergic neurons in the AN and AVPV respond differently to sex steroid signaling: in the AVPV, sex hormones appear to favor LH secretion, completing a positive feedback circuit with the ovary that results in potentiation of gonadal steroid release, which may be especially important in the preovulatory LH wave [110]. On the other hand, stimulation of AN kisspeptinergic neurons appears to reduce LH secretion, suggesting a regulatory role [111].

These neuronal pathways are also subject to another level of regulation themselves: various signals reflective of the overall metabolic status are integrated into a modulatory "somatometer" [112]. These signals include leptin, glucose, and insulin levels, among many others [113]. Indeed, reproduction is an evolutionarily costly process in terms of energy expenditure and investment, and therefore, an optimal metabolic-energetic milieu is required for initiation of these phenomena [112].

Notoriously, leptin appears to mediate the impact of adipose depots on puberty onset. Leptin is a proteic adipokine secreted by both visceral and subcutaneous adipose tissue and participates not only in reproductive but also in immune and metabolic physiology [114]. Leptin may circulate freely or bind to its soluble receptor (sOB-R), which limits its availability for membrane receptors [115]. Approximately

40% of kisspeptinergic neurons in the AN express leptin membrane receptors [116], representing the fundamental link between adipose tissue and sexual development. In consonance, these elements act as sensors of energy storage, by facilitating GnRH pulsatile secretion in the presence of sufficient adipose tissue [117]. In addition, leptin also directly favors FSH and LH secretion [86]. Furthermore, expression of sOB-R appears to be inverse to adiposity and DHEAS levels, thus contributing to the role of obesity as an accelerator of puberty [118], and outlining a possible synergic mechanism between adrenarche and leptin for gonadarche induction.

Conversely, females with scarce body or intense physical activity often display disrupted GnRH secretion patterns [119]. Similarly, patients with anorexia nervosa frequently exhibit low gonadotropin and estradiol levels [120] associated with lower leptin concentrations in cerebrospinal fluid [121] and greater levels of circulating sOB-R [122]. Moreover, delay of puberty has been described as an adaptive mechanism in the face of scant energetic reserves, such as that seen in malnutrition and other conditions [123].

Notwithstanding this critical part of leptin in modulation of the HHGA, its role does not appear to be absolute, as leptin alone has been shown to fail to normalize LH secretion in animal models of caloric restriction-induced hypoleptinemia [124]. Thus, integration of other stimuli is also important. To this end, insulin appears to contribute by various pathways. Insulin appears to directly exert a positive, dose-dependent effect on GnRH secretion, as well as an inhibitory effect on GABAergic and neuropeptide Y-secreting neurons, both of which would suppress GnRH expression and secretion [125]. Insulin also has an indirect influence by regulating appetite in other hypothalamic centers [126].

Maturation of the HHGA is accompanied by the appearance of secondary sexual traits, propelled by sex steroids. In females, estrogens are key for the structural and functional development of the mammary glands. Estrogen receptor α is expressed in epithelial terminal ductolobular cells and is the main driver of mammary development during puberty, whereas the β isoform is found in myoepithelial cells, fibroblasts, and adipocytes in the breasts, yet it is considered to play a secondary role [127]. In breast tissue, estrogenic signaling appears to trigger paracrine and juxtacrine mediator secretion from epithelial cells, which in turn favor cell proliferation in neighboring cells [128].

Metabolic-energetic modulation is also implicated in breast development: both Growth Hormone (GH) and IGF-I, of both local and systemic origin, intervene much like estradiol, promoting expression of various growth factors [129], amongst which amphiregulin may be the most prominent as it amplifies all proliferative signals by potentiating local growth factor expression, permitting accelerated development of mammary glands during puberty [130].

4.2. Adrenarche and Pubarche: Role of Adrenal Androgens. *Adrenarche* entails maturation of the *zona reticularis* (ZR), the innermost layer of the adrenal cortex, accompanied by an increase in adrenal androgen synthesis and secretion, specifically 19-carbon DHEA and DHEAS, and apparition of

androgen-dependent hair, *pubarche*, its fundamental clinical manifestation [131].

In contrast to the salient role adrenal androgens serve during fetal life, where they are key precursors for augmented estrogen synthesis during gestation [132], their significance concerning adult reproductive function remains unclear. Indeed, the onsets of adrenarche and gonadarche are largely independently regulated, and adrenarche does not appear to be necessary for gonadarche to take place [133], although premature maturation of the HHGA in subjects with congenital adrenal hyperplasia suggests the existence of a currently unelucidated link [134].

Likewise, the unequivocal mechanisms underlying the initiation of adrenarche are also unclear. Intrinsic and autonomous modifications in adrenal structure and function may be one of the key phenomena in this aspect: after birth, the fetal zone of the adrenal gland devolves, allowing for an expansion of the neocortex, with well-defined *zona fasciculata* and *zona glomerulosa*, yet scarce ZR-like cells [135]. This shift is associated with an acute decrease in DHEA and DHEAS synthesis. This adrenal architecture persists during infancy, with only sparse ZR-like islets until adrenarche, where the ZR acquires its adult configuration. Nonetheless, the molecular mechanisms underlying this timeline remain cryptic [136].

Regarding hormonal signals for adrenarche, ACTH is not considered a trigger as its serum levels do not change during this event, although it appears to play a permissive role, as individuals with ACTH receptor mutations fail to undergo adrenarche [137]. Alternative proteolytic derivatives of proopiomelanocortin, the precursor of ACTH, have also been proposed, yet results have been inconclusive [138]. Likewise, CRH may be able to prompt DHEA synthesis, but the relative impact of CRH versus ACTH activity in this scenario is undiscerned [139].

Finally, metabolic status may also be an important regulator of adrenarche. This influence appears to begin as early as *in utero*, where low birth weight might trigger adrenal hyperfunction at adrenarche, with reports of an inverse relationship between birth weight and DHEAS levels, independent of cortisol levels [140]. Similarly, *in vitro* treatment of fetal adrenal cells with insulin, IGF-I, and IGF-II has been linked with significant increases in DHEAS synthesis [140], as well as augmented sensitivity to ACTH signaling, with greater CYP17A1 and 3βHSD2 expression [141]. In addition, leptin may mediate the impact of obesity in this event: it has proved to increase CYP17A1 activity *in vitro* [142], although its significance *in vivo* during adrenarche is undetermined [143].

Regardless of the initiating signals, the fundamental characteristic of adrenarche is an increase in adrenal androgen levels (Figure 5). This augmentation stems from the coordinated interactions of CYP11A1 and CYP17A1 mainly, alongside 3βHSD2 and SULT2A1 [131]. Firstly, CYP11A1 acts in consonance with StAR signaling, both stimulated by ACTH, driving quantitative upregulation of adrenal steroidogenesis [144]. On the other hand, CYP17A1 exhibits dual function, exhibiting both 17α-hydroxylase and 17,20-lyase activity on 21-carbon steroids, which leads to formation of 19-carbon

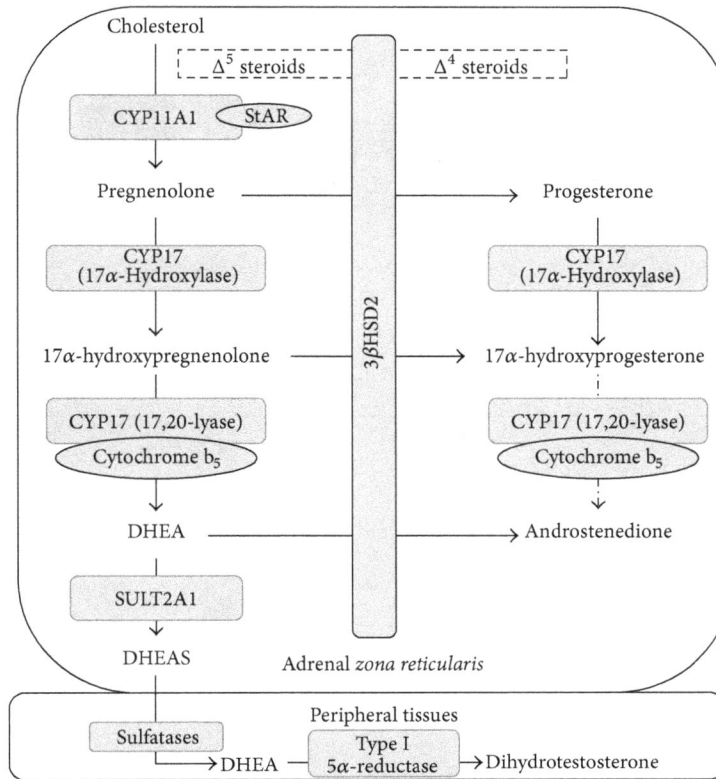

FIGURE 5: Steroidogenesis pathways and regulation in the adrenal *zona reticularis*. 3βHSD2: 3β-hydroxysteroid dehydrogenase 2; CYP11A1: cholesterol side-chain cleavage enzyme; CYP17: 17α-hydroxylase/17,20 lyase; DHEA: dehydroepiandrosterone; DHEAS: dehydroepiandrosterone sulfate; StAR: Acute Steroidogenic Regulatory Protein. After CYP11A1 acts on cholesterol, pregnenolone may undergo both functions of CYP17 (17α-hydroxylation and 17,20-lyation, the latter with cytochrome b$_5$ as a cofactor), rendering DHEA as a product. DHEA synthesis is favored in the *zona reticularis* because the 17,20-lyase function acts preferentially on Δ^5 steroids, whose production is potentiated in adrenarche due to 3βHSD2 underexpression. Additionally, upregulated SULT2A1 expression augments DHEA sulfonation, preventing conversion to other metabolites. DHEAS is secreted and reconverted to DHEA by sulfatases in peripheral tissues, where it also undergoes type 5α-reductase catalysis and then exerts its effects.

molecules, such as DHEA [145]. Whereas its 17α-hydroxylase activity displays comparable efficacy in both Δ^4 and Δ^5 steroids, its 17,20-lyase activity shows predilection for Δ^5 substrates. Therefore, DHEA is the main product of this enzyme, with 17α-hydroxypregnenolone as an intermediary metabolite, from which DHEAS and androstenedione are obtained [146]. During adrenarche, the ZR displays increased expression of not only CYP17A1, but also cytochrome b$_5$, a hemoprotein required for the 17,20-lyase function of CYP17A1. This cofactor is preferentially colocalized with CYP17A1 in the ZR, with lesser expression in other zones, partly explaining the absence of a significant increment in glucocorticoid synthesis during adrenarche [147].

Additionally, 3βHSD2 does not participate in the DHEA pathway but plays an indirect synergic role. This enzyme catalyzes the conversion of Δ^5 steroids to their Δ^4 homologues [145]. By unknown mechanisms, this enzyme is downregulated in the ZR during adrenarche, resulting in potentiated DHEA production down the Δ^5 pathway [131]. Lastly, SULT2A1 is upregulated in adrenarche, thus assuring that metabolites continue down the pathway for Δ^5 steroids,

as sulfonation impedes activity by CYP17A1 and 3βHSD2, ultimately favoring DHEAS synthesis in the ZR [148].

Although DHEAS is biologically inactive, it may be reconverted to DHEA by sulfatases in peripheral tissues and subsequently converted to dihydrotestosterone, an active androgen, by 5α-reductase. This step is essential, as it exponentially multiplies its bioactivity in comparison to the weaker adrenal androgens [149]. The key manifestation of adrenarche is pubarche, the development of androgen-dependent hair in the pubic, axillar, and pectoral areas, as well as facial hair in males. Moreover, development of cutaneous apocrine glands originates a characteristic body odor [137].

5. Act III: The Climax—Folliculogenesis and the Ovarian Cycle

Once histologic and functional maturity is attained by the components of the HHGA, the ovarian cycle begins, involving a series of endocrine interactions oriented to the expulsion of oocytes, *ovulation*, which, owing to parallel

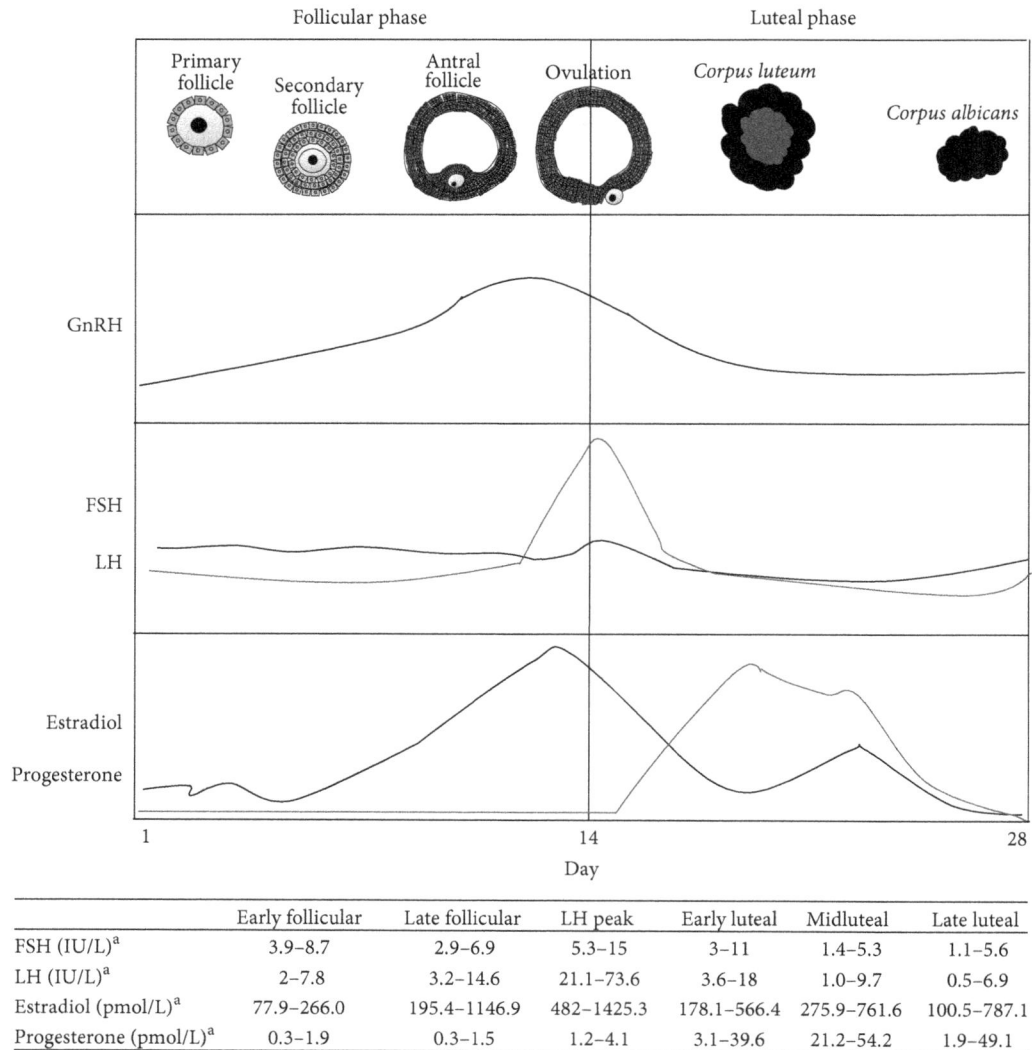

FIGURE 6: Evolution of the ovarian follicle and hormonal levels throughout the ovarian cycle. FSH: Follicle-Stimulating Hormone; GnRH: Gonadotropin-Releasing Hormone; LH: luteinizing hormone. [a]Stricker et al. [151]. The first day of the ovarian cycle, GnRH levels commence a progressive rise, which is accompanied by FSH and, to a lesser extent, LH secretion. Ovarian stimulation by gonadotropins leads to a gradual increase in estradiol levels, which towards midcycle induce a LH peak. This LH acme triggers ovulation and thus begins formation of the *corpus luteum*. This tissue will then progressively achieve a peak in progesterone secretion and then gradually decline as gonadotropin levels drop and the *corpus luteum* degenerates into the *corpus albicans,* marking the end of the luteal phase, and the beginning of a new cycle.

modifications in the endometrium, offer the necessary support for implantation, thus acting coordinately to assure female fertility [150, 151]. The ovarian cycle comprises two phases, follicular and luteal (Figure 6), each with distinct endocrine profiles hereby summarized.

5.1. The Follicular Phase: Preparing for Ovulation. Ovarian follicles are the fundamental morphophysiologic units of the ovaries, as they represent the main endocrine and reproductive compartment in this organ. Primordial follicles present at birth may either perish, as part of ovarian senescence, or enter folliculogenesis (FG) [152]. FG encompasses a succession of cell changes required for maturation of ovarian follicles, in preparation for ovulation [153].

Starting from primordial follicles, that is, oocytes surrounded only by a monolayer of squamous granulosa cells (GC), this sequential development depicts 4 typical stages: primary, secondary, and tertiary or Graafian follicles [153] (Figure 7). The first structural shift in FG involves transformation of squamous GC into cuboidal cells, which define the primary follicle [154]. Afterwards, at least two layers of cuboidal GC exist in secondary follicles, which also exhibit upregulated FSH, estrogen, and androgen receptor expression [155], as well as an additional layer of somatic cells, theca cells (TC), in the external surface of the basal lamina [19]. The latter determines cell polarity and aids in control of proliferation and differentiation [156].

These early modifications appear to be FSH-independent and rely on intraovarian mechanisms [157]. Peptides such

Primordial follicle	Primary follicle	Secondary follicle	Graafian follicle
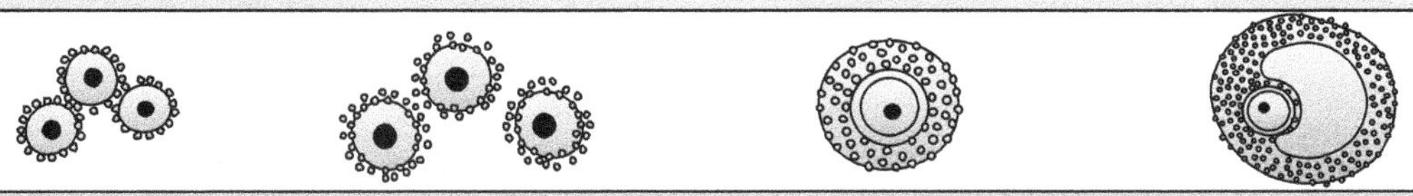			
Structural evolution			
PO surrounded by a single layer of squamous follicular cells. Approximate diameter: 25 μm	PO surrounded by the *zona pellucid* (mucopolysaccharides secreted by GC) and a layer of cuboidal GC	PO surrounded by multiple layers of cuboidal GC, plus internal and external layers of TC	GC proliferate and produce fluid, forming the antrum and defining periantral GC, while GC around the PO are organized into the *corona radiata, cumulus oophorus,* and *membrana,* from innermost to outermost layer. Approximate diameter: 150 μm
Functional aspects			
Formed around week 20 *in utero,* constituting the definitive lifetime pool of follicles. PO remain arrested in meiosis I until ovulation	Gonadotropin-independent stage: cuboidal shift driven by intraovarian stimuli	Gonadotropin-dependent stage: upregulated expression of FSH and estrogen receptors in GC. Internal TC synthesize androgens which may be then aromatized by GC	Structurally and functionally prepared for ovulation. The *corona radiata* and *cumulus oophorus* exit the follicle with the oocyte during ovulation

GC: granulosa cells
PO: primary oocytes
TC: theca cells

FIGURE 7: Follicular stages in folliculogenesis.

as bFGF, IGF-I, Epidermal Growth Factor, and Growth Differentiation Factor-9 (GDF-9) are important in this respect, as they are expressed by oocytes during FG, promoting differentiation and proliferation of GC, stimulating development of TC, inhibiting differentiation into luteocytes, and promoting estradiol secretion [158]. GDF-9 appears to be the principal driver of these effects until entry into the antral stage [159]. Likewise, anti-Müllerian hormone, a member of the Transforming Growth Factor-β (TGF-β) family, is a powerful inhibitor of follicular growth, governing entry of primordial follicles into FG [159].

Later events depend on FSH and, secondarily, LH signaling [160], including hyperplasia an hypertrophy of GC and TC, as well as the apparition of estrogen-rich fluid-filled spaces among GC, due to the osmotic gradient produced by the hyaluronan and chondroitin sulfate molecules present in GC, as well as upregulation of aquaporins and remodeling of intercellular junctions [161]. The additive effect of these changes facilitates a rapid increase in follicular volume and coalescence of these spaces, leading to formation of the antrum, which defines Graafian follicles [162].

Selection of a dominant follicle is paramount in order to preserve the integrity of the ovarian cycle [163]. Complex endocrine interplay underlies this aspect: around the middle of the follicular phase, the progressive increase in circulating FSH levels induces expression of LH receptors and aromatase in ovarian follicles [159]. In consequence, estradiol secretion by GC increases, leading to suppression of FSH secretion, marking a transition from FSH- to LH-dependent

stimulation [164]. This shift hinges on the "rescue" of the dominant follicle from all other FSH-recruited follicles in development which will subsequently suffer atresia. The LH-rescued follicle is also prepared to respond to the LH peak later in the ovarian cycle [153].

Activins and inhibins are important regulators of dominant follicle growth [165]. These messengers belong to the TGF-β family [166] and as such are active as dimers: activins are constituted by two β subunits, βA, βB, βC, or βD; the most widely studied are activin A (a βA-βA homodimer), activin B (a βB-βB homodimer), and activin AB (a βA-Bb heterodimer) [167]. On the other hand, inhibins are comprised of an α subunit disulfide linked to one of the activins β, yielding two heterodimers: inhibin A (α-βA), or inhibin B (α-βB) [168]. Both activins and inhibins are synthesized in ovarian follicles, as well as hypophyseal gonadotropic cells and placental tissue, among others [169].

Activins directly intervene in follicular development in two principal manners: (a) extraovarian effects, by favoring FSH synthesis at the hypophysis, and (b) intraovarian autocrine signaling by GC, self-stimulating proliferation, and upregulation of aromatase and FSH receptor expression in these cells within the dominant follicle [170]. Preferential induction of aromatase expression by IGF-II in CG of the dominant follicle may play a secondary role in this scenario [171]. Once the antral stage is reached, activins also upregulate LH receptor expression in TC, essential for the LH-mediated rescue of the dominant follicle [172]. Additionally, activins appear to attenuate LH-induced androgen secretion in TC

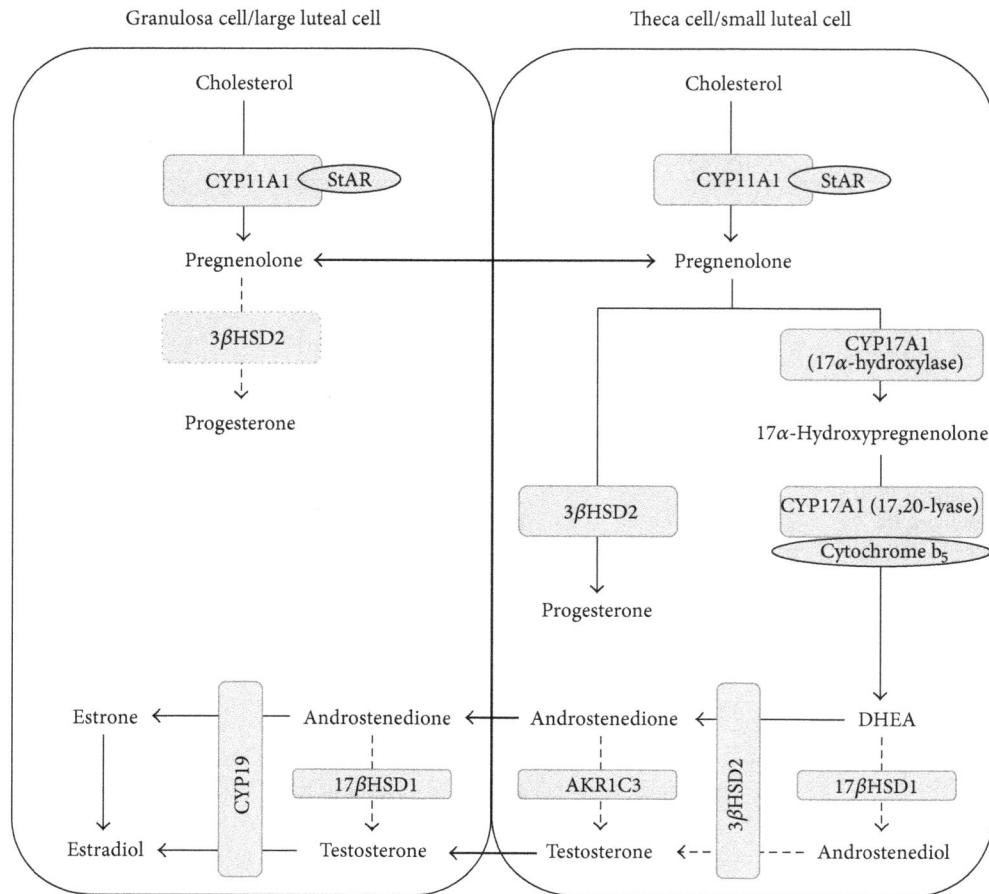

FIGURE 8: Ovarian steroidogenic pathways. Solid lines are major pathways. Dashed lines are minor pathways. Dotted line represents route only available after luteinization. Double lines represent intercellular steroid traffic. Underlined steroids are major secretion products. 3βHSD2: 3-β-hydroxysteroid dehydrogenase 2; 17βHSD1: 17-β-hydroxysteroid dehydrogenase 1; AKR1C3: aldo-keto reductase family 1 member C3; CYP11A1: cholesterol side-chain cleavage enzyme; CYP17A1: 17α-hydroxylase/17,20 lyase; CYP19: aromatase; DHEA: dehydroepiandrosterone; StAR: Acute Steroidogenic Regulatory Protein.

[173]. Activin signaling is regulated by follistatin, an autocrine monomeric glycoprotein also secreted by GC, which binds to activin and blocks its receptor-binding residues [174].

As the follicular phase transpires and the dominant follicle increases in size and estrogen synthesis, activin levels drop and inhibin levels rise [175]. Inhibins are also released by GC and are particularly relevant during the antral stage, as they enhance androgen production by TC, which are necessary substrates for subsequent aromatization [176]. Moreover, inhibins also seem to directly interfere with growth of all nondominant follicles [170, 173].

Because steroid hormones are the key hormonal products of the ovarian cycle with fundamental effects both systemically and in the ovary, ovarian steroidogenesis is tightly regulated [145]. Indeed, in ovarian follicles, steroid metabolism is compartmentalized between GC and TC during the follicular phase (Figure 8), both of which possess prominent smooth endoplasmic reticula and abundant lipid vesicles, typical features of steroidogenic cells [177]. GC express CYP11A1, CYP19, and 17βHSD1, while TC express

CYP17A1 and scant levels of CYP11A1. Therefore, the preliminary product of GC is pregnenolone following cleavage of the cholesterol side-chain by CYP11A1, which diffuses to TC to be converted chiefly to androstenedione by CYP17A1. This androgen returns to GC to finalize the enzymatic pathway towards estradiol, the key steroid hormone product during the follicular phase [145].

Estrogens induce uterine modifications parallel to these ovarian events, inducing endometrial proliferation with intense mitotic activity in its epithelium and stroma, resulting in a near triplication of endometrial thickness, accompanied with elongation and coiling of spiral arteries [178, 179].

5.2. Ovulation: The Big Bang in Female Fertility. Shortly before midcycle, estrogen concentrations reach their peak, resulting in a LH wave critical for ovulation. This acme is achieved due to recruitment of a promoter region in *Kiss1* by estrogen receptor α isoforms in kisspeptinergic neurons in the AVPV, thus upregulating kisspeptin synthesis and secretion, which in turn boosts GnRH and LH secretion and ultimately raises ovarian estrogen secretion, thus completing a positive feedback circuit [180].

The resulting elevation in LH levels promotes progesterone secretion and augments plasminogen activator in GC [181, 182], leading to increased tissue plasmin which activates collagenases and stimulates TNF release by TC, thus enhancing collagenolysis by inducing expression of matrix metalloproteinases. The integrated effect of these mechanisms is the weakening of follicular walls on their apical side [183]. Additionally, TNF potentiates local prostaglandin synthesis [184]; and LH drives follicular angiogenesis and vascular remodeling, primarily through induction of vascular endothelial growth factors [185], resulting in plasma transudation to the inside of follicles, with follicular swelling. In consonance, follicular wall degeneration and swelling finalize in ovulation: follicular rupture, with expulsion of the oocyte and antral fluid [186].

Preceding ovulation, the oocyte must resume meiosis I and progress through meiosis II. Oocytes quiescent in Prophase I possess an intact nuclear envelope, in a stage known as germinal vesicle, whose rupture is an early sign of recommencement of meiosis [69]. Because the LH surge is associated with this breakdown, yet no LH receptors are present in oocytes, indirect mechanisms are suspected to convey this signaling from GC and TC to oocytes, yet remaining obscure [187]. Nonetheless, the key outcome is a decrease in intracellular cAMP, which may be due to (a) increased cGMP concentration with activation of phosphodiesterase 3A, thus favoring cAMP degradation [188]; (b) activation of inhibitory G proteins [189]; or (c) disruption of stimulatory G protein-coupled receptors [190]. Lower cAMP levels result in relief of PKA-mediated inactivation of CDC25B, which is then free to inhibit WEE1/MYT1 activity, thus allowing MPF to promote cell division [69]. This division is unequal, leading to formation of a polar body much smaller than the oocyte. Indeed, asymmetric spindle pole attachment leads to cortical activation of CDC42 during Anaphase, which determines the surface of forming polar body [191]. This process is aided by a RhoA-based contractile ring whose constriction contributes to localization of one spindle pole and one set of chromosomes into the CDC42 budding compartment [192].

Once meiosis I is completed, the oocyte immediately enters meiosis II, where cytostatic factor maintains MPF in a stable state, allowing inhibition of the Anaphase-promoting complex/cyclosome (APC/C) and therefore halting progress through the cell cycle in Metaphase II, thus preventing parthenogenetic activation and development of an embryo without paternal genomic contribution [193]. These characteristics define the secondary oocyte, whose cell cycle only continues with syngamy, when the spermatozoon triggers a calcium-calmodulin Protein Kinase II-mediated disinhibition of APC/C [193, 194]. This occurs due to proteosomal degradation of cyclin B 26S subunit, resuming meiosis II with transition from Metaphase to Anaphase [195].

5.3. The Luteal Phase: A Time Window for Implantation. After ovulation, *luteinization* occurs in the ovaries, a conglomerate of architectural and physiologic changes aimed to offer support for the newly released oocyte. Although these changes

are intensified after ovulation, they begin approximately 36 hours before ovulation, driven by the LH surge typical of this time, which in turn obeys increased GnRH pulses [196]. Furthermore, preovulatory luteinization is essential for follicular rupture, as it entails induction of COX-2 expression in GC undergoing luteinization, with increased production of PGE2 [197]. In turn, this mediator promotes synthesis of tissue plasminogen activator (tPA), favoring fibrinolysis and oocyte release [198].

After follicular rupture, this tissue undergoes thorough reorganization, with formation of the *corpus luteum* and mitotic arrest of its constituent cells. Steroidogenic cells suffer phenotypical modifications: TC become small luteal cells (SLC); and GC become large luteal cells (LLC) [199]. SLC retain the androgenic synthesis capacity of TC, and LLC keep aromatase expression as seen in GC. However, LLC begin expressing 3βHSD2, allowing progesterone secretion from both cell types, although it is greater in LLC (Figure 8) [200]. Although in SLC progesterone synthesis is directly induced by LH, via PKA activation and StAR phosphorylation [201], in LLC it appears to depend on PGE2 for PKA activation [202]; yet LLC also seem to require lower levels of cAMP for this event in comparison to SLC [203]. Additionally, SLC appear to express 5α-reductase, 5β-reductase, and 3α-hydroxysteroid oxidoreductase, the key enzymes for allopregnanolone synthesis [204], a neurosteroid important for modulation of estrous behavior [205].

These rearrangements of steroidogenic cells are concomitant with extensive angiogenesis in order to offer nutrition to this tissue, driven by local neutrophil- and macrophage-secreted messengers [206]. These include VEGF-4, which acts through delta-like ligand-4/notch signaling [207], and nestin, a filamentous protein associated with *de novo* development of capillaries [208]. Nitric oxide is another fundamental regulator, which, depending on the ovarian microenvironment and under regulation of prostaglandin F2α, may act as either a luteotropic or luteolytic agent through modulation of angiogenesis [209].

These events lead to the elevated progesterone synthesis and secretion typical of this phase, which in turn is oriented to setting an optimal stage for implantation, thus maintaining the functional correlation between the ovarian uterine cycles [210]. These effects include augmented secretion of glycogen and mucus and greater tortuosity of spiral arteries [211]. Likewise, invasion by immune cells is increased, chiefly by NK cells, macrophages, and T cells, which reach their peak during this phase and are destined to regulate trophoblastic invasion and angiogenesis [212, 213].

Increased levels of sex hormones also constitute early signals for luteolysis, by lowering hypophyseal gonadotropin secretion through negative feedback [210]. At a cellular level, both the extrinsic, Fas/Fas-L-dependent [213], and intrinsic apoptosis pathways seem to be involved. Regarding the latter, luteocytes possess numerous prosurvival signals such as LH, leptin, and glucocorticoids, which suppress expression of intrinsic proapoptotic proteins such as Bax and cIAP-2 [214], whereas luteocyte stress can activate the p53 pathway [215]. Ultimately, luteolysis finalizes with hyalinization of the *corpus luteum* as luteocytes die, originating the *corpus albicans*. This process implicates synthesis of extracellular matrix by ovarian fibroblasts [216], whilst the eventual resorption of these remnants, and the consequent restitution of preovulatory ovarian architecture, depends on activity by local macrophages and myofibroblasts [217].

6. Resolution: Concluding Remarks

After ovulation, the course of female reproductive function pivots fundamentally on the presence of fecundation. Indeed, if absent, the *corpus luteum* will swiftly degenerate, prompting the reinitiation of the ovarian cycle and the beginning of menstrual bleeding. On the other hand, the presence of an adequately implanted zygote in the endometrium will prompt the decidual reaction, an increase in endometrial secretion and stromal edema [218]. These modifications allow for adequate syncytiotrophoblast development, which, in turn, is able to grant maintenance to the corpus luteum via hCG secretion, representing one of the first of many endocrine modifications inherent to gestation [219].

Under healthy conditions, the ovarian cycle periodically gives rise to this bifurcation until menopause, the natural cessation of the ovaries' primary function: folliculogenesis and the ovarian cycle [220]. Early stages of this transition feature briefer cycles, owing to shorter follicular phases with smaller-sized follicles [221]. This phenomenon appears to be due chiefly to a decrease in inhibin B and AMH synthesis, which leads to augmented FSH release and thus increased estrogen synthesis. In turn, this would facilitate earlier triggering of the LH surge [222]. Secretion patterns of the latter and GnRH are also altered, with a decline in pulse frequency [223], in association with disruptions of the neural networks modulating GnRH release [224]. In consonance with reduced signaling by inhibin B and AMH, increased expression of proapoptotic genes in oocytes propels accelerated depletion of follicle reserve until its eventual exhaustion [225]. In this scenario, there is a significant decline in circulating estradiol levels, as only extraovarian sources of this hormone remain active, in particular, adipose tissue [226]. Lower estrogen levels entail a broad range of multisystemic changes in physiology [220]. Indeed, menopause, the "curtain call" of female reproductive function, is a well-recognized risk factor for cardiovascular disease and osteoporosis, among many other disorders [227].

Further understanding of the molecular mechanisms underlying female fertility is required in order to provide better management to the multiple disturbances which may occur within its complex regulatory systems, as these have consequences on global female health beyond the reproductive sphere.

Abbreviations

17βHSD1: 17-β-Hydroxysteroid dehydrogenase 1
3βHSD2: 3-β-Hydroxysteroid dehydrogenase 2
5mC: 5-Methylcytosine
ACTH: Adrenocorticotropic hormone
AN: Arcuate nucleus
AVPV: Anteroventral periventricular nucleus
bFGF: Basic fibroblast growth factor
cAMP: Cyclic adenosine monophosphate
CRH: Corticotropin-releasing hormone
CYP11A1: Cholesterol side-chain cleavage enzyme
CYP17A1: 17α-Hydroxylase/17,20-lyase
CYP19: Aromatase
DHEA: Dehydroepiandrosterone
DHEAS: Dehydroepiandrosterone sulfate
FG: Folliculogenesis
FSH: Follicle-Stimulating Hormone
GABA: γ-Amino-butyric acid
GC: Granulosa cells
GH: Growth Hormone
GnRH: Gonadotropin-Releasing Hormone
hCG: Human chorionic gonadotropin
HHGA: Hypothalamus-hypophysis-gonadal axis
IGF-I: Insulin-like growth factor I
IGF-II: Insulin-like growth factor II
LH: Luteinizing hormone
LLC: Large luteal cells
MPF: Maturation Promoting Factor
PGC: Primordial germ cells
PKA: Protein Kinase A
RA: Retinoic acid
SLC: Small luteal cells
SULT2A1: DHEA sulfotransferase
SCF/KITL: Stem Cell Factor/c-Kit Ligand
StAR: Acute Steroidogenic Regulatory Protein
TC: Theca cells
ZR: Zona reticularis.

Conflict of Interests

The authors declare that there is no conflict of interests regarding the publication of this paper.

References

[1] R. Yanagimachi, "Fertilization studies and assisted fertilization in mammals: their development and future," *Journal of Reproduction and Development*, vol. 58, no. 1, pp. 25–32, 2012.

[2] C. M. Spiller, J. Bowles, and P. Koopman, "Regulation of germ cell meiosis in the fetal ovary," *International Journal of Developmental Biology*, vol. 56, no. 10–12, pp. 779–787, 2012.

[3] T. Toloubeydokhti, O. Bukulmez, and N. Chegini, "Potential regulatory functions of MicroRNAs in the ovary," *Seminars in Reproductive Medicine*, vol. 26, no. 6, pp. 469–478, 2008.

[4] A. R. Baerwald, G. P. Adams, and R. A. Pierson, "Ovarian antral folliculogenesis during the human menstrual cycle: a review," *Human Reproduction Update*, vol. 18, no. 1, Article ID dmr039, pp. 73–91, 2012.

[5] D. A. Dumesic and D. H. Abbott, "Implications of polycystic ovary syndrome on oocyte development," *Seminars in Reproductive Medicine*, vol. 26, no. 1, pp. 53–61, 2008.

[6] M. N. Mascarenhas, S. R. Flaxman, T. Boerma, S. Vanderpoel, and G. A. Stevens, "National, regional, and global trends in infertility prevalence since 1990: a systematic analysis of 277 health surveys," *PLoS Medicine*, vol. 9, no. 12, Article ID e1001356, 2012.

[7] J. Rojas, M. Chávez, L. Olivar et al., "Polycystic ovary syndrome, insulin resistance, and obesity: navigating the pathophysiologic labyrinth," *International Journal of Reproductive Medicine*, vol. 2014, Article ID 719050, 17 pages, 2014.

[8] V. L. Souter, J. L. Hopton, G. C. Penney, and A. A. Templeton, "Survey of psychological health in women with infertility," *Journal of Psychosomatic Obstetrics and Gynecology*, vol. 23, no. 1, pp. 41–49, 2002.

[9] C. Dupont, D. R. Armant, and C. A. Brenner, "Epigenetics: definition, mechanisms and clinical perspective," *Seminars in Reproductive Medicine*, vol. 27, no. 5, pp. 351–357, 2009.

[10] M. Zumbado, O. P. Luzardo, P. C. Lara et al., "Insulin-like growth factor-I (IGF-I) serum concentrations in healthy children and adolescents: Relationship to level of contamination by DDT-derivative pesticides," *Growth Hormone and IGF Research*, vol. 20, no. 1, pp. 63–67, 2010.

[11] G. D. Hodgen, "Neuroendocrinology of the normal menstrual cycle," *The Journal of Reproductive Medicine*, vol. 34, supplement 1, pp. 68–75, 1989.

[12] D. Wilhelm, S. Palmer, and P. Koopman, "Sex determination and gonadal development in mammals," *Physiological Reviews*, vol. 87, no. 1, pp. 1–28, 2007.

[13] M. Ikawa, N. Inoue, A. M. Benham, and M. Okabe, "Fertilization: a sperm's journey to and interaction with the oocyte," *The Journal of Clinical Investigation*, vol. 120, no. 4, pp. 984–994, 2010.

[14] C.-F. Liu, C. Liu, and H. H.-C. Yao, "Building pathways for ovary organogenesis in the mouse embryo," *Current Topics in Developmental Biology*, vol. 90, pp. 263–290, 2010.

[15] R. P. Piprek, "Molecular and cellular machinery of gonadal differentiation in mammals," *International Journal of Developmental Biology*, vol. 54, no. 5, pp. 779–786, 2010.

[16] R. P. Piprek, "Molecular mechanisms underlying female sex determination—antagonism between female and male pathway," *Folia Biologica*, vol. 57, no. 3-4, pp. 105–113, 2009.

[17] A. Biason-Lauber, "WNT4, RSPO1, and FOXL2 in sex development," *Seminars in Reproductive Medicine*, vol. 30, no. 5, pp. 387–395, 2012.

[18] D. Schmidt, C. E. Ovitt, K. Anlag et al., "The murine winged-helix transcription factor Foxl2 is required for granulosa cell differentiation and ovary maintenance," *Development*, vol. 131, no. 4, pp. 933–942, 2004.

[19] M. A. Edson, A. K. Nagaraja, and M. M. Matzuk, "The mammalian ovary from genesis to revelation," *Endocrine Reviews*, vol. 30, no. 6, pp. 624–712, 2009.

[20] S. Seisenberger, S. Andrews, F. Krueger et al., "The dynamics of genome-wide DNA methylation reprogramming in mouse primordial germ cells," *Molecular Cell*, vol. 48, no. 6, pp. 849–862, 2012.

[21] S. Gkountela, Z. Li, J. J. Vincent et al., "The ontogeny of cKIT$^+$ human primordial germ cells proves to be a resource for human germ line reprogramming, imprint erasure and *in vitro* differentiation," *Nature Cell Biology*, vol. 15, no. 1, pp. 113–122, 2013.

[22] Y. Ying, X. Qi, and G.-Q. Zhao, "Induction of primordial germ cells from pluripotent epiblast," *The Scientific World Journal*, vol. 26, no. 2, pp. 801–810, 2002.

[23] Y. Ohinata, H. Ohta, M. Shigeta, K. Yamanaka, T. Wakayama, and M. Saitou, "A signaling principle for the specification of the germ cell lineage in mice," *Cell*, vol. 137, no. 3, pp. 571–584, 2009.

[24] Y. Ohinata, B. Payer, D. O'Carroll et al., "Blimp1 is a critical determinant of the germ cell lineage in mice," *Nature*, vol. 436, no. 7048, pp. 207–213, 2005.

[25] J. A. West, S. R. Viswanathan, A. Yabuuchi et al., "A role for Lin28 in primordial germ-cell development and germ-cell malignancy," *Nature*, vol. 460, no. 7257, pp. 909–913, 2009.

[26] M. M. Mikedis and K. M. Downs, "STELLA-positive subregions of the primitive streak contribute to posterior tissues of the mouse gastrula," *Developmental Biology*, vol. 363, no. 1, pp. 201–218, 2012.

[27] W. Wei, T. Qing, X. Ye et al., "Primordial germ cell specification from embryonic stem cells," *PLoS ONE*, vol. 3, no. 12, Article ID e4013, 2008.

[28] P. Hajkova, K. Ancelin, T. Waldmann et al., "Chromatin dynamics during epigenetic reprogramming in the mouse germ line," *Nature*, vol. 452, no. 7189, pp. 877–881, 2008.

[29] M. De Felici, "Germ stem cells in the mammalian adult ovary: considerations by a fan of the primordial germ cells," *Molecular Human Reproduction*, vol. 16, no. 9, Article ID gaq006, pp. 632–636, 2010.

[30] T. Ara, Y. Nakamura, T. Egawa et al., "Impaired colonization of the gonads by primordial germ cells in mice lacking a chemokine, stromal cell-derived factor-1 (SDF-1)," *Proceedings of the National Academy of Sciences of the United States of America*, vol. 100, no. 9, pp. 5319–5323, 2003.

[31] A. M. Zama, F. P. Hudson III, and M. A. Bedell, "Analysis of hypomorphic Kitl^{Sl} mutants suggests different requirements for KITL in proliferation and migration of mouse primordial germ cells," *Biology of Reproduction*, vol. 73, no. 4, pp. 639–647, 2005.

[32] D. Farini, G. La Sala, M. Tedesco, and M. De Felici, "Chemoattractant action and molecular signaling pathways of Kit ligand on mouse primordial germ cells," *Developmental Biology*, vol. 306, no. 2, pp. 572–583, 2007.

[33] T. Takeuchi, Y. Tanigawa, R. Minamide, K. Ikenishi, and T. Komiya, "Analysis of SDF-1/CXCR4 signaling in primordial germ cell migration and survival or differentiation in *Xenopus laevis*," *Mechanisms of Development*, vol. 127, no. 1-2, pp. 146–158, 2010.

[34] T. Kimura, T. Nakamura, K. Murayama et al., "The stabilization of β-catenin leads to impaired primordial germ cell development via aberrant cell cycle progression," *Developmental Biology*, vol. 300, no. 2, pp. 545–553, 2006.

[35] M. Saitou, S. Kagiwada, and K. Kurimoto, "Epigenetic reprogramming in mouse pre-implantation development and primordial germ cells," *Development*, vol. 139, no. 1, pp. 15–31, 2012.

[36] M. A. Surani and P. Hajkova, "Epigenetic reprogramming of mouse germ cells toward totipotency," *Cold Spring Harbor Symposia on Quantitative Biology*, vol. 75, pp. 211–218, 2010.

[37] J. Kang, S. Kalantry, and A. Rao, "PGC7, H3K9me2 and Tet3: regulators of DNA methylation in zygotes," *Cell Research*, vol. 23, no. 1, pp. 6–9, 2013.

[38] T.-P. Gu, F. Guo, H. Yang et al., "The role of Tet3 DNA dioxygenase in epigenetic reprogramming by oocytes," *Nature*, vol. 477, no. 7366, pp. 606–612, 2011.

[39] T. Nakamura, Y. Arai, H. Umehara et al., "PGC7/Stella protects against DNA demethylation in early embryogenesis," *Nature Cell Biology*, vol. 9, no. 1, pp. 64–71, 2007.

[40] F. Santos, A. H. Peters, A. P. Otte, W. Reik, and W. Dean, "Dynamic chromatin modifications characterise the first cell cycle in mouse embryos," *Developmental Biology*, vol. 280, no. 1, pp. 225–236, 2005.

[41] M. S. Bartolomei and A. C. Ferguson-Smith, "Mammalian genomic imprinting," *Cold Spring Harbor Perspectives in Biology*, vol. 3, no. 7, 2011.

[42] T. G. Baker, "A quantitative and cytological study of germ cells in human ovaries," *Proceedings of the Royal Society of London B: Biological Sciences*, vol. 158, pp. 417–433, 1963.

[43] S.-R. Chen, Q.-S. Zheng, Y. Zhang, F. Gao, and Y.-X. Liu, "Disruption of genital ridge development causes aberrant primordial germ cell proliferation but does not affect their directional migration," *BMC Biology*, vol. 11, article 22, 2013.

[44] N. Reynolds, B. Collier, K. Maratou et al., "Dazl binds in vivo to specific transcripts and can regulate the pre-meiotic translation of Mvh in germ cells," *Human Molecular Genetics*, vol. 14, no. 24, pp. 3899–3909, 2005.

[45] M. E. Gill, Y.-C. Hu, Y. Lin, and D. C. Page, "Licensing of gametogenesis, dependent on RNA binding protein DAZL, as a gateway to sexual differentiation of fetal germ cells," *Proceedings of the National Academy of Sciences of the United States of America*, vol. 108, no. 18, pp. 7443–7448, 2011.

[46] I. Godin, R. Deed, J. Cooke, K. Zsebo, M. Dextert, and C. C. Wylie, "Effects of the steel gene product on mouse primordial germ cells in culture," *Nature*, vol. 352, no. 6338, pp. 807–809, 1991.

[47] J. L. Resnick, M. Ortiz, J. R. Keller, and P. J. Donovan, "Role of fibroblast growth factors and their receptors in mouse primordial germ cell growth," *Biology of Reproduction*, vol. 59, no. 5, pp. 1224–1229, 1998.

[48] E. Kawase, K. Hashimoto, and R. A. Pedersen, "Autocrine and paracrine mechanisms regulating primordial germ cell proliferation," *Molecular Reproduction and Development*, vol. 68, no. 1, pp. 5–16, 2004.

[49] M. De Cuevas, M. A. Lilly, and A. C. Spradling, "Germline cyst formation in *Drosophila*," *Annual Review of Genetics*, vol. 31, pp. 405–28, 1997.

[50] M. E. Pepling, "From primordial germ cell to primordial follicle: mammalian female germ cell development," *Genesis*, vol. 44, no. 12, pp. 622–632, 2006.

[51] J. Kimble, "Molecular regulation of the mitosis/meiosis decision in multicellular organisms," *Cold Spring Harbor Perspectives in Biology*, vol. 3, no. 8, Article ID a002683, 2011.

[52] M. Garcia, A. J. J. Dietrich, L. Freixa, A. C. G. Vink, M. Ponsa, and J. Egozcue, "Development of the first meiotic prophase stages in human fetal oocytes observed by light and electron microscopy," *Human Genetics*, vol. 77, no. 3, pp. 223–232, 1987.

[53] J. Bowles, D. Knight, C. Smith et al., "Retinoid signaling determines germ cell fate in mice," *Science*, vol. 312, no. 5773, pp. 596–600, 2006.

[54] Y.-J. Choi, J.-W. Yoon, C.-W. Pyo, J.-A. Kim, S.-H. Bae, and S.-S. Park, "A possible role of STRA8 as a transcriptional factor," *Genes & Genomics*, vol. 32, no. 6, pp. 521–526, 2010.

[55] M. D. Griswold, C. A. Hogarth, J. Bowles, and P. Koopman, "Initiating meiosis: the case for retinoic acid," *Biology of Reproduction*, vol. 86, no. 2, article 35, 2012.

[56] E. L. Anderson, A. E. Baltus, H. L. Roepers-Gajadien et al., "Stra8 and its inducer, retinoic acid, regulate meiotic initiation in both spermatogenesis and oogenesis in mice," *Proceedings of the National Academy of Sciences of the United States of America*, vol. 105, no. 39, pp. 14976–14980, 2008.

[57] F. Barrios, D. Filipponi, M. Pellegrini et al., "Opposing effects of retinoic acid and FGF9 on Nanos2 expression and meiotic entry of mouse germ cells," *Journal of Cell Science*, vol. 123, no. 6, pp. 871–880, 2010.

[58] Y. Lin, M. E. Gill, J. Koubova, and D. C. Page, "Germ cell-intrinsic and -extrinsic factors govern meiotic initiation in mouse embryos," *Science*, vol. 322, no. 5908, pp. 1685–1687, 2008.

[59] G. Duester, "Retinoic acid synthesis and signaling during early organogenesis," *Cell*, vol. 134, no. 6, pp. 921–931, 2008.

[60] R. Saba, Y. Kato, and Y. Saga, "NANOS2 promotes male germ cell development independent of meiosis suppression," *Developmental Biology*, vol. 385, no. 1, pp. 32–40, 2014.

[61] L. DiNapoli and B. Capel, "SRY and the standoff in sex determination," *Molecular Endocrinology*, vol. 22, no. 1, pp. 1–9, 2008.

[62] C. Tingen, A. Kim, and T. K. Woodruff, "The primordial pool of follicles and nest breakdown in mammalian ovaries," *Molecular Human Reproduction*, vol. 15, no. 12, Article ID gap073, pp. 795–803, 2009.

[63] M. E. Pepling and A. C. Spradling, "Mouse ovarian germ cell cysts undergo programmed breakdown form primordial follicles," *Developmental Biology*, vol. 234, no. 2, pp. 339–351, 2001.

[64] A. S. Wilkins and R. Holliday, "The evolution of meiosis from mitosis," *Genetics*, vol. 181, no. 1, pp. 3–12, 2009.

[65] K. T. Jones, "Meiosis in oocytes: predisposition to aneuploidy and its increased incidence with age," *Human Reproduction Update*, vol. 14, no. 2, pp. 143–158, 2008.

[66] D. Adhikari and K. Liu, "The regulation of maturation promoting factor during prophase I arrest and meiotic entry in mammalian oocytes," *Molecular and Cellular Endocrinology*, vol. 382, no. 1, pp. 480–487, 2014.

[67] M. Godet, A. Dametoy, S. Mouradian, B. B. Rudkin, and P. Durand, "Key role for cyclin-dependent kinases in the first and second meiotic divisions of rat spermatocytes," *Biology of Reproduction*, vol. 70, no. 4, pp. 1147–1152, 2004.

[68] M. Malumbres and M. Barbacid, "Mammalian cyclin-dependent kinases," *Trends in Biochemical Sciences*, vol. 30, no. 11, pp. 630–641, 2005.

[69] P. Solc, R. M. Schultz, and J. Motlik, "Prophase I arrest and progression to metaphase I in mouse oocytes: comparison of resumption of meiosis and recovery from G2-arrest in somatic cells," *Molecular Human Reproduction*, vol. 16, no. 9, Article ID gaq034, pp. 654–664, 2010.

[70] P. Solc, A. Saskova, V. Baran, M. Kubelka, R. M. Schultz, and J. Motlik, "CDC25A phosphatase controls meiosis I progression in mouse oocytes," *Developmental Biology*, vol. 317, no. 1, pp. 260–269, 2008.

[71] L. M. Mehlmann, Y. Saeki, S. Tanaka et al., "The G$_s$-linked receptor GPR3 maintains meiotic arrest in mammalian oocytes," *Science*, vol. 306, no. 5703, pp. 1947–1950, 2004.

[72] K. Sugiura, Y.-Q. Su, F. J. Diaz et al., "Oocyte-derived BMP15 and FGFs cooperate to promote glycolysis in cumulus cells," *Development*, vol. 134, no. 14, pp. 2593–2603, 2007.

[73] M. De Felici, F. G. Klinger, D. Farini, M. L. Scaldaferri, S. Iona, and M. Lobascio, "Establishment of oocyte population in the fetal ovary: primordial germ cell proliferation and oocyte programmed cell death," *Reproductive BioMedicine Online*, vol. 10, no. 2, pp. 182–191, 2005.

[74] A. M. Lobascio, F. G. Klinger, M. L. Scaldaferri, D. Farini, and M. De Felici, "Analysis of programmed cell death in mouse fetal oocytes," *Reproduction*, vol. 134, no. 2, pp. 241–252, 2007.

[75] K. J. Hutt, E. A. McLaughlin, and M. K. Holland, "KIT/KIT ligand in mammalian oogenesis and folliculogenesis: Rroles

in rabbit and murine ovarian follicle activation and oocyte growth," *Biology of Reproduction*, vol. 75, no. 3, pp. 421–433, 2006.

[76] M. Pesce, M. G. Farrace, M. Piacentini, S. Dolci, and M. De Felici, "Stem cell factor and leukemia inhibitory factor promote primordial germ cell survival by suppressing programmed cell death (apoptosis)," *Development*, vol. 118, no. 4, pp. 1089–1094, 1993.

[77] B. C. Jee, J. H. Kim, D. H. Park, H. Youm, C. S. Suh, and S. H. Kim, "In vitro growth of mouse preantral follicles: effect of animal age and stem cell factor/insulin-like growth factor supplementation," *Clinical and Experimental Reproductive Medicine*, vol. 39, no. 3, pp. 107–113, 2012.

[78] M.-R. Kim and J. L. Tilly, "Current concepts in Bcl-2 family member regulation of female germ cell development and survival," *Biochimica et Biophysica Acta*, vol. 1644, no. 2-3, pp. 205–210, 2004.

[79] M. De Felici, A. M. Lobascio, and F. G. Klinger, "Cell death in fetal oocytes: many players for multiple pathways," *Autophagy*, vol. 4, no. 2, pp. 240–242, 2008.

[80] N. Fulton, S. J. Martins da Silva, R. A. L. Bayne, and R. A. Anderson, "Germ cell proliferation and apoptosis in the developing human ovary," *Journal of Clinical Endocrinology and Metabolism*, vol. 90, no. 8, pp. 4664–4670, 2005.

[81] W. E. Roudebush, W. J. Kivens, and J. M. Mattke, "Biomarkers of ovarian reserve," *Biomarker Insights*, vol. 3, pp. 259–268, 2008.

[82] L. M. Mehlmann, R. R. Kalinowski, L. F. Ross, A. F. Parlow, E. L. Hewlett, and L. A. Jaffe, "Meiotic resumption in response to luteinizing hormone is independent of a G_i family G protein or calcium in the mouse oocyte," *Developmental Biology*, vol. 299, no. 2, pp. 345–355, 2006.

[83] A. Perheentupa and I. Huhtaniemi, "Aging of the human ovary and testis," *Molecular and Cellular Endocrinology*, vol. 299, no. 1, pp. 2–13, 2009.

[84] Q. Li, X. Geng, W. Zheng, J. Tamg, B. Xu, and Q. Shi, "Current understanding of ovarian aging," *Science China Life Sciences*, vol. 55, no. 8, pp. 659–669, 2012.

[85] C. M. Burt Solorzano and C. R. McCartney, "Obesity and the pubertal transition in girls and boys," *Reproduction*, vol. 140, no. 3, pp. 399–410, 2010.

[86] B. Bordini and R. L. Rosenfield, "Normal pubertal development: part I: the endocrine basis of puberty," *Pediatrics in Review*, vol. 32, no. 6, pp. 223–229, 2011.

[87] A.-S. Parent, G. Teilmann, A. Juul, N. E. Skakkebaek, J. Toppari, and J.-P. Bourguignon, "The timing of normal puberty and the age limits of sexual precocity: variations around the world, secular trends, and changes after migration," *Endocrine Reviews*, vol. 24, no. 5, pp. 668–693, 2003.

[88] NHANES III, *NHANES III Reference Manuals and Reports (CD-ROM). Analytic and Reporting Guidelines: The Third National Health and Nutrition Examination Survey (1988–94)*, National Center for Health Statistics, Centers for Disease Control and Prevention, Hyattsville, Md, USA, 1997.

[89] G. Schoeters, E. Den Hond, W. Dhooge, N. Van Larebeke, and M. Leijs, "Endocrine disruptors and abnormalities of pubertal development," *Basic and Clinical Pharmacology and Toxicology*, vol. 102, no. 2, pp. 168–175, 2008.

[90] C. Macías-Tomei, M. López-Blanco, I. Espinoza, and M. Vasquez-Ramirez, "Pubertal development in caracas upper-middle-class boys and girls in a longitudinal context," *American Journal of Human Biology*, vol. 12, no. 1, pp. 88–96, 2000.

[91] B. Bordini and R. L. Rosenfield, "Normal pubertal development: part II: clinical aspects of puberty," *Pediatrics in Review*, vol. 32, no. 7, pp. 281–292, 2011.

[92] G. M. Buck Louis, L. E. Gray Jr., M. Marcus et al., "Environmental factors and puberty timing: expert panel research needs," *Pediatrics*, vol. 121, supplement 3, pp. S192–S207, 2008.

[93] S. Özen and Ş. Darcan, "Effects of environmental endocrine disruptors on pubertal development," *Journal of Clinical Research in Pediatric Endocrinology*, vol. 3, no. 1, pp. 1–6, 2011.

[94] R. L. Rosenfield, R. B.Lipton, and M. L. Drum, "Thelarche, pubarche, and menarche attainment in children with normal and elevated body mass index," *Pediatrics*, vol. 123, no. 1, pp. 84–88, 2009.

[95] I. Huhtaniemi, "Endocrine function and regulation of the fetal and neonatal testis," *International Journal of Developmental Biology*, vol. 33, no. 1, pp. 117–123, 1989.

[96] I. Huhtaniemi, "Molecular aspects of the ontogeny of the pituitary-gonadal axis," *Reproduction, Fertility and Development*, vol. 7, no. 5, pp. 1025–1035, 1995.

[97] M. M. Grumbach, "The neuroendocrinology of human puberty revisited," *Hormone Research*, vol. 57, no. 2, pp. 2–14, 2002.

[98] E. Terasawa, "Role of GABA in the mechanism of the onset of puberty in non-human primates," *International Review of Neurobiology*, vol. 71, pp. 113–129, 2005.

[99] K. K. Thind and P. C. Goldsmith, "Expression of estrogen and progesterone receptors in glutamate and GABA neurons of the pubertal female monkey hypothalamus," *Neuroendocrinology*, vol. 65, no. 5, pp. 314–324, 1997.

[100] F. A. Giuliani, C. Escudero, S. Casas et al., "Allopregnanolone and puberty: modulatory effect on glutamate and GABA release and expression of 3α-hydroxysteroid oxidoreductase in the hypothalamus of female rats," *Neuroscience*, vol. 243, pp. 64–75, 2013.

[101] S. R. Ojeda, C. Dubay, A. Lomniczi et al., "Gene networks and the neuroendocrine regulation of puberty," *Molecular and Cellular Endocrinology*, vol. 324, no. 1-2, pp. 3–11, 2010.

[102] S. R. Ojeda, C. Roth, A. Mungenast et al., "Neuroendocrine mechanisms controlling female puberty: new approaches, new concepts," *International Journal of Andrology*, vol. 29, no. 1, pp. 256–263, 2006.

[103] S. Funes, J. A. Hedrick, G. Vassileva et al., "The KiSS-1 receptor GPR54 is essential for the development of the murine reproductive system," *Biochemical and Biophysical Research Communications*, vol. 312, no. 4, pp. 1357–1363, 2003.

[104] S. B. Seminara, S. Messager, E. E. Chatzidaki et al., "The *GPR54* gene as a regulator of puberty," *The New England Journal of Medicine*, vol. 349, no. 17, pp. 1614–1627, 2003.

[105] X. d'Anglemont de Tassigny and W. H. Colledge, "The role of Kisspeptin signaling in reproduction," *Physiology*, vol. 25, no. 4, pp. 207–217, 2010.

[106] A. M. Rometo, S. J. Krajewski, M. L. Voytko, and N. E. Rance, "Hypertrophy and increased kisspeptin gene expression in the hypothalamic infundibular nucleus of postmenopausal women and ovariectomized monkeys," *Journal of Clinical Endocrinology and Metabolism*, vol. 92, no. 7, pp. 2744–2750, 2007.

[107] M. Shahab, C. Mastronardi, S. B. Seminara, W. F. Crowley, S. R. Ojeda, and T. M. Plant, "Increased hypothalamic GPR54 signaling: a potential mechanism for initiation of puberty in primates," *Proceedings of the National Academy of Sciences of the United States of America*, vol. 102, no. 6, pp. 2129–2134, 2005.

[108] V. M. Navarro, J. M. Castellano, R. Fernández-Fernández et al., "Developmental and hormonally regulated messenger ribonucleic acid expression of KiSS-1 and its putative receptor, GPR54, in rat hypothalamus and potent luteinizing hormone-releasing activity of KiSS-1 peptide," *Endocrinology*, vol. 145, no. 10, pp. 4565–4574, 2004.

[109] J. Roa, E. Aguilar, C. Dieguez, L. Pinilla, and M. Tena-Sempere, "New frontiers in kisspeptin/GPR54 physiology as fundamental gatekeepers of reproductive function," *Frontiers in Neuroendocrinology*, vol. 29, no. 1, pp. 48–69, 2008.

[110] J. T. Smith, H. M. Dungan, E. A. Stoll et al., "Differential regulation of KiSS-1 mRNA expression by sex steroids in the brain of the male mouse," *Endocrinology*, vol. 146, no. 7, pp. 2976–2984, 2005.

[111] S. M. Popa, D. K. Clifton, and R. A. Steiner, "A KiSS to remember," *Trends in Endocrinology and Metabolism*, vol. 16, no. 6, pp. 249–250, 2005.

[112] T. M. Plant, V. L. Gay, G. R. Marshall, and M. Arslan, "Puberty in monkeys is triggered by chemical stimulation of the hypothalamus," *Proceedings of the National Academy of Sciences of the United States of America*, vol. 86, no. 7, pp. 2506–2510, 1989.

[113] M. S. Smith, "Estrus and menstrual cycles: neuroendocrine control," *Encyclopedia of Neuroscience*, pp. 1–5, 2009.

[114] V. Van Harmelen, S. Reynisdottir, P. Eriksson et al., "Leptin secretion from subcutaneous and visceral adipose tissue in women," *Diabetes*, vol. 47, no. 6, pp. 913–917, 1998.

[115] A. Lammert, W. Kiess, A. Bottner, A. Glasow, and J. Kratzsch, "Soluble leptin receptor represents the main leptin binding activity in human blood," *Biochemical and Biophysical Research Communications*, vol. 283, no. 4, pp. 982–988, 2001.

[116] J. T. Smith, B. V. Acohido, D. K. Clifton, and R. A. Steiner, "KiSS-1 neurones are direct targets for leptin in the ob/ob mouse," *Journal of Neuroendocrinology*, vol. 18, no. 4, pp. 298–303, 2006.

[117] R. S. Ahima, J. Dushay, S. N. Flier, D. Prabakaran, and J. S. Flier, "Leptin accelerates the onset of puberty in normal female mice," *The Journal of Clinical Investigation*, vol. 99, no. 3, pp. 391–395, 1997.

[118] V. P. Sepilian, J. R. Crochet, and M. Nagamani, "Serum soluble leptin receptor levels and free leptin index in women with polycystic ovary syndrome: relationship to insulin resistance and androgens," *Fertility and Sterility*, vol. 85, no. 5, pp. 1441–1447, 2006.

[119] G. Á. Martos-Moreno, J. A. Chowen, and J. Argente, "Metabolic signals in human puberty: effects of over and undernutrition," *Molecular and Cellular Endocrinology*, vol. 324, no. 1-2, pp. 70–81, 2010.

[120] B. Couzinet, J. Young, S. Brailly, Y. Le Bouc, P. Chanson, and G. Schaison, "Functional hypothalamic amenorrhoea: a partial and reversible gonadotrophin deficiency of nutritional origin," *Clinical Endocrinology*, vol. 50, no. 2, pp. 229–235, 1999.

[121] C. Mantzoros, J. S. Flier, M. D. Lesem, T. D. Brewerton, and D. C. Jimerson, "Cerebrospinal fluid leptin in anorexia nervosa: correlation with nutritional status and potential role in resistance to weight gain," *Journal of Clinical Endocrinology and Metabolism*, vol. 82, no. 6, pp. 1845–1851, 1997.

[122] J. Argente, I. Barrios, J. A. Chowen, M. K. Sinha, and R. V. Considine, "Leptin plasma levels in healthy Spanish children and adolescents, children with obesity, and adolescents anorexia nervosa and bulimia nervosa," *Journal of Pediatrics*, vol. 131, no. 6, pp. 833–838, 1997.

[123] M. T. Muñoz and J. Argente, "Anorexia nervosa in female adolescents: endocrine and bone mineral density disturbances," *European Journal of Endocrinology*, vol. 147, no. 3, pp. 275–286, 2002.

[124] C. True, M. A. Kirigiti, P. Kievit, K. L. Grove, and M. S. Smith, "Leptin is not the critical signal for kisspeptin or luteinising hormone restoration during exit from negative energy balance," *Journal of Neuroendocrinology*, vol. 23, no. 11, pp. 1099–1112, 2011.

[125] F. P. Pralong, "Insulin and NPY pathways and the control of GnRH function and puberty onset," *Molecular and Cellular Endocrinology*, vol. 324, no. 1-2, pp. 82–86, 2010.

[126] M. Gamba and F. P. Pralong, "Control of GnRH neuronal activity by metabolic factors: the role of leptin and insulin," *Molecular and Cellular Endocrinology*, vol. 254-255, pp. 133–139, 2006.

[127] B. Hómez, "Hormonas en la mama: de la fisiología a la enfermedad. Revisión," *Revista Venezolana de Endocrinología y Metabolismo*, vol. 6, no. 2, pp. 9–14, 2008.

[128] E. Anderson, "Progesterone receptors—animal models and cell signaling in breast cancer: the role of oestrogen and progesterone receptors in human mammary development and tumorigenesis," *Breast Cancer Research*, vol. 4, no. 5, pp. 197–201, 2002.

[129] J. McBryan, J. Howlin, S. Napoletano, and F. Martin, "Amphiregulin: role in mammary gland development and breast cancer," *Journal of Mammary Gland Biology and Neoplasia*, vol. 13, no. 2, pp. 159–169, 2008.

[130] H. Macias and L. Hinck, "Mammary gland development," *Wiley Interdisciplinary Reviews: Developmental Biology*, vol. 1, no. 4, pp. 533–557, 2012.

[131] J. C. Havelock, R. J. Auchus, and W. E. Rainey, "The rise in adrenal androgen biosynthesis: adrenarche," *Seminars in Reproductive Medicine*, vol. 22, no. 4, pp. 337–347, 2004.

[132] J. Kaludjerovic and W. E. Ward, "The interplay between estrogen and fetal adrenal cortex," *Journal of Nutrition and Metabolism*, vol. 2012, Article ID 837901, 12 pages, 2012.

[133] B. M. Nathan and M. R. Palmert, "Regulation and disorders of pubertal timing," *Endocrinology and Metabolism Clinics of North America*, vol. 34, no. 3, pp. 617–641, 2005.

[134] T. M. K. Völkl, L. Öhl, M. Rauh, C. Schöfl, and H. G. Dörr, "Adrenarche and puberty in children with classic congenital adrenal hyperplasia due to 21-hydroxylase deficiency," *Hormone Research in Paediatrics*, vol. 76, no. 6, pp. 400–410, 2011.

[135] J. Bocian-Sobkowska, W. Woźniak, and L. K. Malendowicz, "Postnatal involution of the human adrenal fetal zone: stereologic description and apoptosis," *Endocrine Research*, vol. 24, no. 3-4, pp. 969–973, 1998.

[136] H. Ishimoto and R. B. Jaffe, "Development and function of the human fetal adrenal cortex: a key component in the feto-placental unit," *Endocrine Reviews*, vol. 32, no. 3, pp. 317–355, 2011.

[137] R. J. Auchus and W. E. Rainey, "Adrenarche-physiology, biochemistry and human disease," *Clinical Endocrinology*, vol. 60, no. 3, pp. 288–296, 2004.

[138] S. H. Mellon, J. E. Shively, and W. L. Miller, "Human proopiomelanocortin-(79–96), a proposed androgen stimulatory hormone, does not affect steroidogenesis in cultured human fetal adrenal cells," *Journal of Clinical Endocrinology and Metabolism*, vol. 72, no. 1, pp. 19–22, 1991.

[139] R. Smith, S. Mesiano, E.-C. Chan, S. Brown, and R. B. Jaffe, "Corticotropin-releasing hormone directly and preferentially stimulates dehydroepiandrosterone sulfate secretion by human

fetal adrenal cortical cells," *Journal of Clinical Endocrinology and Metabolism*, vol. 83, no. 8, pp. 2916–2920, 1998.

[140] K. K. Ong, N. Potau, C. J. Petry et al., "Opposing influences of prenatal and postnatal weight gain on adrenarche in normal boys and girls," *Journal of Clinical Endocrinology and Metabolism*, vol. 89, no. 6, pp. 2647–2651, 2004.

[141] C. Fottner, D. Engelhardt, and M. M. Weber, "Regulation of steroidogenesis by insulin-like growth factors (IGFs) in adult human adrenocortical cells: IGF-I and, more potently, IGF-II preferentially enhance androgen biosynthesis through interaction with the IGF-I receptor and IGF-binding proteins," *Journal of Endocrinology*, vol. 158, no. 3, pp. 409–417, 1998.

[142] A. Biason-Lauber, M. Zachmann, and E. J. Schoenle, "Effect of leptin on CYP17 enzymatic activities in human adrenal cells: new insight in the onset of adrenarche," *Endocrinology*, vol. 141, no. 4, pp. 1446–1454, 2000.

[143] D. L'Allemand, S. Schmidt, V. Rousson, G. Brabant, T. Gasser, and A. Grüters, "Associations between body mass, leptin, IGF-I and circulating adrenal androgens in children with obesity and premature adrenarche," *European Journal of Endocrinology*, vol. 146, no. 4, pp. 537–543, 2002.

[144] Y. Xing, C. R. Parker, M. Edwards, and W. E. Rainey, "ACTH is a potent regulator of gene expression in human adrenal cells," *Journal of Molecular Endocrinology*, vol. 45, no. 1, pp. 59–68, 2010.

[145] W. L. Miller and R. J. Auchus, "The molecular biology, biochemistry, and physiology of human steroidogenesis and its disorders," *Endocrine Reviews*, vol. 32, no. 1, pp. 81–151, 2011.

[146] M. K. Akhtar, S. L. Kelly, and M. A. Kaderbhai, "Cytochrome b$_5$ modulation of 17α hydroxylase and 17–20 lyase (CYP17) activities in steroidogenesis," *Journal of Endocrinology*, vol. 187, no. 2, pp. 267–274, 2005.

[147] S. Dharia, A. Slane, M. Jian, M. Conner, A. J. Conley, and C. R. Parker Jr., "Colocalization of P450c17 and cytochrome b5 in androgen-synthesizing tissues of the human," *Biology of Reproduction*, vol. 71, no. 1, pp. 83–88, 2004.

[148] T. Suzuki, H. Sasano, J. Takeyama et al., "Developmental changes in steroidogenic enzymes in human postnatal adrenal cortex: immunohistochemical studies," *Clinical Endocrinology*, vol. 53, no. 6, pp. 739–747, 2000.

[149] F. Labrie, V. Luu-The, C. Labrie, G. Pelletier, and M. El-Alfy, "Intracrinology and the skin," *Hormone Research*, vol. 54, no. 5-6, pp. 218–229, 2000.

[150] M. Mihm, S. Gangooly, and S. Muttukrishna, "The normal menstrual cycle in women," *Animal Reproduction Science*, vol. 124, no. 3-4, pp. 229–236, 2011.

[151] R. Stricker, R. Eberhart, M.-C. Chevailler, F. A. Quinn, P. Bischof, and R. Stricker, "Establishment of detailed reference values for luteinizing hormone, follicle stimulating hormone, estradiol, and progesterone during different phases of the menstrual cycle on the Abbott ARCHITECT analyzer," *Clinical Chemistry and Laboratory Medicine*, vol. 44, no. 7, pp. 883–887, 2006.

[152] O. Salha, N. Abusheikha, and V. Sharma, "Dynamics of human follicular growth and in-vitro oocyte maturation," *Human Reproduction Update*, vol. 4, no. 6, pp. 816–832, 2000.

[153] A. R. Baerwald, G. P. Adams, and R. A. Pierson, "Ovarian antral folliculogenesis during the human menstrual cycle: a review," *Human Reproduction Update*, vol. 18, no. 1, pp. 73–91, 2012.

[154] F. Sánchez and J. Smitz, "Molecular control of oogenesis," *Biochimica et Biophysica Acta—Molecular Basis of Disease*, vol. 1822, no. 12, pp. 1896–1912, 2012.

[155] J. K. Findlay and A. E. Drummond, "Regulation of the FSH receptor in the ovary," *Trends in Endocrinology and Metabolism*, vol. 10, no. 5, pp. 183–188, 1999.

[156] H. F. Irving-Rodgers, S. Morris, R. A. Collett et al., "Phenotypes of the ovarian follicular basal lamina predict developmental competence of oocytes," *Human Reproduction*, vol. 24, no. 4, pp. 936–944, 2009.

[157] M. Mihm and A. C. O. Evans, "Mechanisms for dominant follicle selection in monovulatory species: a comparison of morphological, endocrine and intraovarian events in cows, mares and women," *Reproduction in Domestic Animals*, vol. 43, no. 2, pp. 48–56, 2008.

[158] W. Miller, D. Geller, and M. Rosen, "Ovarian and adrenal androgen biosynthesis and metabolism," in *Androgen Excess Disorders in Women*, Contemporary Endocrinology, pp. 19–33, Springer, 2007.

[159] S. Jonard and D. Dewailly, "The follicular excess in polycystic ovaries, due to intra-ovarian hyperandrogenism, may be the main culprit for the follicular arrest," *Human Reproduction Update*, vol. 10, no. 2, pp. 107–117, 2004.

[160] G. F. Erickson and S. Shimasaki, "The physiology of folliculogenesis: the role of novel growth factors," *Fertility and Sterility*, vol. 76, no. 5, pp. 943–949, 2001.

[161] R. J. Rodgers and H. F. Irving-Rodgers, "Formation of the ovarian follicular antrum and follicular fluid," *Biology of Reproduction*, vol. 82, no. 6, pp. 1021–1029, 2010.

[162] G. F. Erickson, D. A. Magoffin, C. A. Dyer, and C. Hofeditz, "The ovarian androgen producing cells: a review of structure/function relationships," *Endocrine Reviews*, vol. 6, no. 3, pp. 371–399, 1985.

[163] A. J. Zeleznik, "The physiology of follicle selection," *Reproductive Biology and Endocrinology*, vol. 2, no. 1, article 31, 2004.

[164] S. J. Roseff, M. L. Bangah, L. M. Kettel et al., "Dynamic changes in circulating inhibin levels during the luteal-follicular transition of the human menstrual cycle," *The Journal of Clinical Endocrinology & Metabolism*, vol. 69, no. 5, pp. 1033–1039, 1989.

[165] W.-Y. Son, M. Das, E. Shalom-Paz, and H. Holzer, "Mechanisms of follicle selection and development," *Minerva Ginecologica*, vol. 63, no. 2, pp. 89–102, 2011.

[166] K. Miyazono, Y. Kamiya, and M. Morikawa, "Bone morphogenetic protein receptors and signal transduction," *Journal of Biochemistry*, vol. 147, no. 1, pp. 35–51, 2010.

[167] T. B. Thompson, R. W. Cook, S. C. Chapman, T. S. Jardetzky, and T. K. Woodruff, "Beta A versus beta B: is it merely a matter of expression?" *Molecular and Cellular Endocrinology*, vol. 225, no. 1-2, pp. 9–17, 2004.

[168] G. R. Aleman-Muench and G. Soldevila, "When versatility matters: activins/inhibins as key regulators of immunity," *Immunology and Cell Biology*, vol. 90, no. 2, pp. 137–148, 2012.

[169] A. S. McNeilly, "Diagnostic applications for inhibin and activins," *Molecular and Cellular Endocrinology*, vol. 359, no. 1-2, pp. 121–125, 2012.

[170] P. G. Knight, L. Satchell, and C. Glister, "Intra-ovarian roles of activins and inhibins," *Molecular and Cellular Endocrinology*, vol. 359, no. 1-2, pp. 53–65, 2012.

[171] A. El-Roeiy, X. Chen, V. J. Roberts, D. LeRoith, C. T. Roberts Jr., and S. S. C. Yen, "Expression of insulin-like growth factor-I (IGF-I) and IGF-II and the IGF-I, IGF-II, and insulin receptor genes and localization of the gene products in the human ovary," *Journal of Clinical Endocrinology and Metabolism*, vol. 77, no. 5, pp. 1411–1418, 1993.

[172] J. K. Findlay, "An update on the roles of inhibin, activin, and follistatin as local regulators of folliculogenesis," *Biology of Reproduction*, vol. 48, no. 1, pp. 15–23, 1993.

[173] P. G. Knight and C. Glister, "TGF-β superfamily members and ovarian follicle development," *Reproduction*, vol. 132, no. 2, pp. 191–206, 2006.

[174] T. B. Thompson, T. F. Lerch, R. W. Cook, T. K. Woodruff, and T. S. Jardetzky, "The structure of the follistatin: activin complex reveals antagonism of both type I and type II receptor binding," *Developmental Cell*, vol. 9, no. 4, pp. 535–543, 2005.

[175] C. Glister, N. P. Groome, and P. G. Knight, "Bovine follicle development is associated with divergent changes in activin-A, inhibin-A and follistatin and the relative abundance of different follistatin isoforms in follicular fluid," *Journal of Endocrinology*, vol. 188, no. 2, pp. 215–225, 2006.

[176] C. Glister, L. Satchell, and P. G. Knight, "Changes in expression of bone morphogenetic proteins (BMPs), their receptors and inhibin co-receptor betaglycan during bovine antral follicle development: inhibin can antagonize the suppressive effect of BMPs on thecal androgen production," *Reproduction*, vol. 140, no. 5, pp. 699–712, 2010.

[177] J. M. Young and A. S. McNeilly, "Theca: the forgotten cell of the ovarian follicle," *Reproduction*, vol. 140, no. 4, pp. 489–504, 2010.

[178] P. G. Groothuis, H. H. N. M. Dassen, A. Romano, and C. Punyadeera, "Estrogen and the endometrium: lessons learned from gene expression profiling in rodents and human," *Human Reproduction Update*, vol. 13, no. 4, pp. 405–417, 2007.

[179] J. G. Bromer, T. S. Aldad, and H. S. Taylor, "Defining the proliferative phase endometrial defect," *Fertility and Sterility*, vol. 91, no. 3, pp. 698–704, 2009.

[180] J. Tomikawa, Y. Uenoyama, M. Ozawa et al., "Epigenetic regulation of *Kiss1* gene expression mediating estrogen-positive feedback action in the mouse brain," *Proceedings of the National Academy of Sciences of the United States of America*, vol. 109, no. 20, pp. E1294–E1301, 2012.

[181] J. A. Jackson, S. A. Tischkau, P. Zhang, and J. M. Bahr, "Plasminogen activator production by the granulosa layer is stimulated by factor(s) produced by the theca layer and inhibited by the luteinizing hormone surge in the chicken," *Biology of Reproduction*, vol. 50, no. 4, pp. 812–819, 1994.

[182] R. Reich, R. Miskin, and A. Tsafriri, "Follicular plasminogen activator: involvement in ovulation," *Endocrinology*, vol. 116, no. 2, pp. 516–521, 1985.

[183] W. J. Murdoch and A. C. McDonnel, "Roles of the ovarian surface epithelium in ovulation and carcinogenesis," *Reproduction*, vol. 123, no. 6, pp. 743–750, 2002.

[184] M. Brannstrom, N. Bonello, L. J. Wang, and R. J. Norman, "Effects of tumour necrosis factor alpha (TNF alpha) on ovulation in the rat ovary," *Reproduction, Fertility and Development*, vol. 7, no. 1, pp. 67–73, 1995.

[185] R. Gómez, C. Simón, J. Remohí, and A. Pellicer, "Administration of moderate and high doses of gonadotropins to female rats increases ovarian vascular endothelial growth factor (VEGF) and VEGF receptor-2 expression that is associated to vascular hyperpermeability," *Biology of Reproduction*, vol. 68, no. 6, pp. 2164–2171, 2003.

[186] D. L. Russell and R. L. Robker, "Molecular mechanisms of ovulation: co-ordination through the cumulus complex," *Human Reproduction Update*, vol. 13, no. 3, pp. 289–312, 2007.

[187] X.-R. Peng, A. J. W. Hsueh, P. S. LaPolt, L. Bjersing, and T. Ny, "Localization of luteinizing hormone receptor messenger ribonucleic acid expression in ovarian cell types during follicle development and ovulation," *Endocrinology*, vol. 129, no. 6, pp. 3200–3207, 1991.

[188] R. P. Norris, W. J. Ratzan, M. Freudzon et al., "Cyclic GMP from the surrounding somatic cells regulates cyclic AMP and meiosis in the mouse oocyte," *Development*, vol. 136, no. 11, pp. 1869–1878, 2009.

[189] R. R. Kalinowski, L. A. Jaffe, K. R. Foltz, and A. F. Giusti, "A receptor linked to a Gi-family G-protein functions in initiating oocyte maturation in starfish but not frogs," *Developmental Biology*, vol. 253, no. 1, pp. 139–149, 2003.

[190] L. M. Mehlmann, T. L. Z. Jones, and L. A. Jaffe, "Meiotic arrest in the mouse follicle maintained by a Gs protein in the oocyte," *Science*, vol. 297, no. 5585, pp. 1343–1345, 2002.

[191] C. Ma, H. A. Benink, D. Cheng et al., "Cdc42 activation couples spindle positioning to first polar body formation in oocyte maturation," *Current Biology*, vol. 16, no. 2, pp. 214–220, 2006.

[192] X. Zhang, C. Ma, A. L. Miller, H. A. Katbi, W. M. Bement, and X. J. Liu, "Polar body emission requires a RhoA contractile ring and Cdc42-mediated membrane protrusion," *Developmental Cell*, vol. 15, no. 3, pp. 386–400, 2008.

[193] J. S. Oh, A. Susor, K. Schindler, R. M. Schultz, and M. Conti, "Cdc25A activity is required for the metaphase II arrest in mouse oocytes," *Journal of Cell Science*, vol. 126, no. 5, pp. 1081–1085, 2013.

[194] J. S. Oh, A. Susor, and M. Conti, "Protein tyrosine kinase Wee1B is essential for metaphase II exit in mouse oocytes," *Science*, vol. 332, no. 6028, pp. 462–465, 2011.

[195] H.-Y. Chang, P. C. Jennings, J. Stewart, N. M. Verrills, and K. T. Jones, "Essential role of protein phosphatase 2A in metaphase II arrest and activation of mouse eggs shown by okadaic acid, dominant negative protein phosphatase 2A, and FTY720," *The Journal of Biological Chemistry*, vol. 286, no. 16, pp. 14705–14712, 2011.

[196] C. A. Christian and S. M. Moenter, "The neurobiology of pre-ovulatory and estradiol-induced gonadotropin-releasing hormone surges," *Endocrine Reviews*, vol. 31, no. 4, pp. 544–577, 2010.

[197] M. Gaytán, C. Bellido, C. Morales, J. E. Sánchez-Criado, and F. Gaytán, "Effects of selective inhibition of cyclooxygenase and lipooxygenase pathways in follicle rupture and ovulation in the rat," *Reproduction*, vol. 132, no. 4, pp. 571–577, 2006.

[198] N. Markosyan and D. M. Duffy, "Prostaglandin E2 acts via multiple receptors to regulate plasminogen-dependent proteolysis in the primate periovulatory follicle," *Endocrinology*, vol. 150, no. 1, pp. 435–444, 2009.

[199] A. Bachelot and N. Binart, "Corpus luteum development: lessons from genetic models in mice," *Current Topics in Developmental Biology*, vol. 68, pp. 49–84, 2005.

[200] M. F. Smith, E. W. McIntush, and G. W. Smith, "Mechanisms associated with corpus luteum development," *Journal of Animal Science*, vol. 72, no. 7, pp. 1857–1872, 1994.

[201] G. D. Niswender, "Molecular control of luteal secretion of progesterone," *Reproduction*, vol. 123, no. 3, pp. 333–339, 2002.

[202] R. G. Richards, J. E. Gadsby, and G. W. Almond, "Differential effects of LH and PGE2 on progesterone secretion by small and large porcine luteal cells," *Journal of Reproduction and Fertility*, vol. 102, no. 1, pp. 27–34, 1994.

[203] C. J. Smith and R. Sridaran, "The steroidogenic response of large and small luteal cells to dibutyryl Camp and 25-OH-cholesterol," in *Growth Factors and the Ovary*, pp. 375–379, Springer US, 1989.

[204] U. Ottander, I. S. Poromaa, E. Bjurulf, Å. Skytt, T. Bäckström, and J. I. Olofsson, "Allopregnanolone and pregnanolone are produced by the human corpus luteum," *Molecular and Cellular Endocrinology*, vol. 239, no. 1-2, pp. 37–44, 2005.

[205] A. R. Genazzani, M. A. Palumbo, A. A. De Micheroux et al., "Evidence for a role for the neurosteroid allopregnanolone in the modulation of reproductive function in female rats," *European Journal of Endocrinology*, vol. 133, no. 3, pp. 375–380, 1995.

[206] K. Shirasuna, T. Shimizu, M. Matsui, and A. Miyamoto, "Emerging roles of immune cells in luteal angiogenesis," *Reproduction, Fertility and Development*, vol. 25, no. 2, pp. 351–361, 2013.

[207] C. M. García-Pascual, R. C. Zimmermann, H. Ferrero et al., "Delta-like ligand 4 regulates vascular endothelial growth factor receptor 2-driven luteal angiogenesis through induction of a tip/stalk phenotype in proliferating endothelial cells," *Fertility and Sterility*, vol. 100, no. 6, pp. 1768–1776, 2013.

[208] J. Mokrý, D. Čížková, S. Filip et al., "Nestin expression by newly formed human blood vessels," *Stem Cells and Development*, vol. 13, no. 6, pp. 658–664, 2004.

[209] Y. S. Weems, E. Lennon, T. Uchima et al., "Is nitric oxide luteolytic or antiluteolytic?" *Prostaglandins & Other Lipid Mediators*, vol. 78, no. 1–4, pp. 129–138, 2005.

[210] S. M. Hawkins and M. M. Matzuk, "Menstrual cycle: basic biology," *Annals of the New York Academy of Sciences*, vol. 1135, pp. 10–18, 2008.

[211] A. Lindaman, A. Dowden, and N. Zavazava, "Soluble HLA-G molecules induce apoptosis in natural killer cells," *American Journal of Reproductive Immunology*, vol. 56, no. 1, pp. 68–76, 2006.

[212] A. Gutiérrez, R. Donato, and A. Mindlin, "Aspectos inmunológicos del embarazo normal," *Archivos de Alergia e Inmunología Clínica*, vol. 37, no. 3, pp. 92–95, 2006.

[213] S. A. Roughton, R. R. Lareu, A. H. Bittles, and A. M. Dharmarajan, "Fas and Fas ligand messenger ribonucleic acid and protein expression in the rat corpus luteum during apoptosis-mediated luteolysis," *Biology of Reproduction*, vol. 60, no. 4, pp. 797–804, 1999.

[214] M. Das, O. Djahanbakhch, B. Hacihanefioglu et al., "Granulosa cell survival and proliferation are altered in polycystic ovary syndrome," *Journal of Clinical Endocrinology and Metabolism*, vol. 93, no. 3, pp. 881–887, 2008.

[215] A. Amsterdam, R. Sasson, I. Keren-Tal et al., "Alternative pathways of ovarian apoptosis: death for life," *Biochemical Pharmacology*, vol. 66, no. 8, pp. 1355–1362, 2003.

[216] G. R. Focchi, M. J. Simões, E. C. Baracat, and G. R. de Lima, "Morphological and morphometrical features of the corpus albicans in the course of the postmenopausal period," *Bulletin de l'Association des Anatomistes*, vol. 79, no. 244, pp. 15–18, 1995.

[217] R. V. Joel and A. G. Foraker, "Fate of the corpus albicans: a morphologic approach," *American Journal of Obstetrics & Gynecology*, vol. 80, pp. 314–316, 1960.

[218] L. A. Salamonsen, E. Dimitriadis, R. L. Jones, and G. Nie, "Complex regulation of decidualization: a role for cytokines and proteases. A review," *Placenta*, vol. 24, supplement 1, pp. S76–S85, 2003.

[219] A. E. Schindler, "Endocrinology of pregnancy: consequences for the diagnosis and treatment of pregnancy disorders," *Journal of Steroid Biochemistry and Molecular Biology*, vol. 97, no. 5, pp. 386–388, 2005.

[220] H. G. Burger, "The endocrinology of the menopause," *Maturitas*, vol. 23, no. 2, pp. 129–136, 1996.

[221] N. Santoro, B. Isaac, G. Neal-Perry et al., "Impaired folliculogenesis and ovulation in older reproductive aged women," *Journal of Clinical Endocrinology and Metabolism*, vol. 88, no. 11, pp. 5502–5509, 2003.

[222] H. G. Burger, G. E. Hale, L. Dennerstein, and D. M. Robertson, "Cycle and hormone changes during perimenopause: the key role of ovarian function," *Menopause*, vol. 15, part 1, no. 4, pp. 603–612, 2008.

[223] J. E. Hall, H. B. Lavoie, E. E. Marsh, and K. A. Martin, "Decrease in gonadotropin-releasing hormone (GnRH) pulse frequency with aging in postmenopausal women," *Journal of Clinical Endocrinology and Metabolism*, vol. 85, no. 5, pp. 1794–1800, 2000.

[224] J. L. Downs and P. M. Wise, "The role of the brain in female reproductive aging," *Molecular and Cellular Endocrinology*, vol. 299, no. 1, pp. 32–38, 2009.

[225] Y. Morita and J. L. Tilly, "Oocyte apoptosis: like sand through an hourglass," *Developmental Biology*, vol. 213, no. 1, pp. 1–17, 1999.

[226] C. Stocco, "Tissue physiology and pathology of aromatase," *Steroids*, vol. 77, no. 1-2, pp. 27–35, 2012.

[227] D. E. R. Warburton, C. W. Nicol, S. N. Gatto, and S. S. D. Bredin, "Cardiovascular disease and osteoporosis: balancing risk management," *Vascular Health and Risk Management*, vol. 3, no. 5, pp. 673–689, 2007.

[228] K. J. Ellis and M. Nicolson, "Leptin levels and body fatness in children: effects of gender, ethnicity, and sexual development," *Pediatric Research*, vol. 42, no. 4, pp. 484–488, 1997.

[229] L. G. Bandini, A. Must, E. N. Naumova et al., "Change in leptin, body composition and other hormones around menarche—a visual representation," *Acta Paediatrica*, vol. 97, no. 10, pp. 1454–1459, 2008.

[230] B. Yüksel, M. N. Özbek, N. Ö. Mungan et al., "Serum IGF-1 and IGFBP-3 levels in healthy children between 0 and 6 years of age," *Journal of Clinical Research in Pediatric Endocrinology*, vol. 3, no. 2, pp. 84–88, 2011.

Reference Ranges of Amniotic Fluid Index in Late Third Trimester of Pregnancy: What Should the Optimal Interval between Two Ultrasound Examinations Be?

Shripad Hebbar, Lavanya Rai, Prashant Adiga, and Shyamala Guruvare

Department of Obstetrics and Gynaecology, Kasturba Medical College, Manipal University, Manipal 576 104, India

Correspondence should be addressed to Shripad Hebbar; drshripadhebbar@yahoo.co.in

Academic Editor: Sinuhe Hahn

Background. Amniotic fluid index (AFI) is one of the major and deciding components of fetal biophysical profile and by itself it can predict pregnancy outcome. Very low values are associated with intrauterine growth restriction and renal anomalies of fetus, whereas high values may indicate fetal GI anomalies, maternal diabetes mellitus, and so forth. However, before deciding the cut-off standards for abnormal values for a local population, what constitutes a normal range for specific gestational age and the ideal interval of testing should be defined. *Objectives.* To establish reference standards for AFI for local population after 34 weeks of pregnancy and to decide an optimal scan interval for AFI estimation in third trimester in low risk antenatal women. *Materials and Methods.* A prospective estimation of AFI was done in 50 healthy pregnant women from 34 to 40 weeks at weekly intervals. The trend of amniotic fluid volume was studied with advancing gestational age. Only low risk singleton pregnancies with accurately established gestational age who were available for all weekly scan from 34 to 40 weeks were included in the study. Women with gestational or overt diabetes mellitus, hypertensive disorders of the pregnancy, prelabour rupture of membranes, and congenital anomalies in the foetus and those who delivered before 40 completed weeks were excluded from the study. For the purpose of AFI measurement, the uterine cavity was arbitrarily divided into four quadrants by a vertical and horizontal line running through umbilicus. Linear array transabdominal probe was used to measure the largest vertical pocket (in cm) in perpendicular plane to the abdominal skin in each quadrant. Amniotic fluid index was obtained by adding these four measurements. Statistical analysis was done using SPSS software (Version 16, Chicago, IL). Percentile curves (5th, 50th, and 95th centiles) were constructed for comparison with other studies. Cohen's *d* coefficient was used to examine the magnitude of change at different time intervals. *Results.* Starting from 34 weeks till 40 weeks, 50 ultrasound measurements were available at each gestational age. The mean (standard deviation) of AFI values (in cms) were 34 W: 14.59 (1.79), 35 W: 14.25 (1.57), 36 W: 13.17 (1.56), 37 W: 12.48 (1.52), 38 W: 12.2 (1.7), and 39 W: 11.37 (1.71). The 5th percentile cut-off was 8.7 cm at 40 weeks. There was a gradual decline of AFI values as the gestational age approached term. Significant drop in AFI was noted at two-week intervals. AFI curve generated from the study varied significantly when compared with already published data, both from India and abroad. *Conclusion.* Normative range for AFI values for late third trimester was established. Appreciable changes occurred in AFI values as gestation advanced by two weeks. Hence, it is recommended to follow up low risk antenatal women every two weeks after 34 weeks of pregnancy. The percentile curves of AFI obtained from the present study may be used to detect abnormalities of amniotic fluid for our population.

1. Introduction

The ultimate goal of antepartum surveillance program is to improve perinatal outcome and to decrease intrauterine fetal demise besides prevention of maternal morbidity and mortality [1, 2]. A fetus in distress should be identified at the earliest so that timely delivery will not only salvage the fetus but also prevent long term neurological impairments such as injury to fetal central nervous system [3]. Though it is said that such an event is more common in high risk pregnancies, the fetuses belonging to low risk mothers are not totally immune [4]. There are definite guidelines for frequency of antenatal testing for high risk pregnant women, but what constitutes an ideal screening program for low risk pregnancies is still unknown [5].

Amniotic fluid assessment by ultrasound is one of the important tools in assessing the fetal health in all risk categories especially beyond the period of viability [6]. Though there are several ways [7] to assess quantity of amniotic fluid ranging from clinical palpation to measurement of single deepest vertical pocket [8], amniotic fluid index (AFI) by four-quadrant technique as described by Phelan et al. [9] in 1987 and among them AFI is popular and reliable method of quantifying amniotic fluid till today. AFI is one of the essential components of fetal biophysical profile (BPP) and its values correlate well with adequacy of fetal renal perfusion. Normally it peaks at 32 to 34 weeks of gestation and thereafter there is a gradual reduction in amniotic fluid due to increase in concentrating capacity of fetal kidneys [10]. However, a drastic reduction in its quantity may indicate underlying placental insufficiency, which has definite implications on growing fetus. The values between 8 and 25 are considered to be normal, 5–8 low normal, and less than 5 oligoamnios [11]. At values less than 5, there is higher incidence of perinatal morbidity and mortality and many a time immediate delivery is the only way out [12, 13]. Hence it is very important to scan the patient to note such a trend periodically during antenatal visits. AFI is the fifth parameter in traditional five-point biophysical profile and second parameter in rapid two-point modified BPP (the other one being NST) [14]. Though there is no definite said protocol for identifying compromised fetus, many believe that biweekly nonstress test and AFI assessment should be offered to all women at risk [15]. But what constitutes an ideal frequency of AFI monitoring for low risk pregnancy is still unknown. Frequent monitoring adds to the cost and maternal anxiety and optimizing the ultrasound examinations is the need of the day.

The present study is an effort to examine the quantum of decrease in AFI in the third trimester and interval of scanning to detect a significant change, thereby formulating guidelines for antenatal ultrasound examinations in low risk women.

2. Aims and Objectives

The purpose of the present investigation is

(1) to study the pattern of change in AFI on weekly basis from 34 weeks till delivery;

(2) to constitute reference ranges of AFI from 34 to 40 weeks of gestation;

(3) to find the time interval by which there is a significant fall in AFI, which will help obstetrician to plan an ideal protocol for antenatal ultrasound examination in the third trimester.

3. Materials and Methods

This was a prospective observational study conducted at the Department of Obstetrics and Gynaecology, Kasturba Medical College, Manipal, from January 2012 to December 2012. Institutional ethical committee approval was obtained prior to study. Inclusion criteria were low risk singleton pregnancy, starting gestational age of 34 weeks, reliable last menstrual period and dates correlated and confirmed by comparison with first trimester CRL (Crown Rump Length). Once initial criteria were met, those who were subsequently diagnosed to have abnormalities of liquor volume due to conditions such as hypertensive disorders, gestational diabetes, and placental insufficiency were excluded from the study, so as to obtain normative data. Only those patients who delivered at 40 weeks were included in the study as we wanted longitudinal data till term. The final study subjects were 50 low risk pregnant women who underwent serial scans at weekly interval starting from 34 weeks till term.

The subjects belonged to the local population consisting mainly of Tuluva, Billava, Bunt, Koraga, Kulala, Devadiga, Konkanis, Shivalli Brahmins, Bayri Muslim, and Catholic communities, the spoken language mainly being Kannada, Tulu, and Konkani. The women were medium built, the average height was of 152 to 156 cms, and prepregnancy weight was between 45 and 50 kg.

The ultrasound examination was carried out after instructing the patient to empty her bladder. The examinations were performed with a convex 3.5 MHz probe (Philips HD11XE ultrasound equipment). The patient was asked to lie down in supine position. Uterus was arbitrarily divided into four quadrants using linea nigra as a vertical line and a transverse line passing through umbilicus, as described by Phelan et al. [9]. The transducer was placed in each of these quadrants in sagittal plane perpendicular to patient's abdomen and maximum depth of amniotic fluid was calculated in centimeters excluding the cord loops and small fetal parts. Caution was exercised to avoid excessive pressure on the transducer as it can alter AFI measurements. The values of all four quadrants were added to obtain the final amniotic fluid index (AFI).

3.1. Sample Size Estimation. Khadilkar et al. [16] from the Department of Obstetrics and Gynaecology, Grant Medical College, Mumbai, conducted a prospective, cross sectional study in low risk healthy pregnant subjects to obtain a gestational reference range for AFI among Indian women. They noted that the mean and standard deviation of AFI (cm) at 34 weeks of gestation was 14.2 and 2.4, respectively. We hypothesised that a difference of 1.5 cm in the mean AFI would be significantly different from the normal values and accordingly estimated sample size to show a desired level of power of 90% and level of significance 0.05, by using the formula,

$$n = \left(\frac{(z\alpha + z\beta)\,\sigma}{\mu 1 - \mu 0} \right)^2, \tag{1}$$

where $z\alpha = 1.96$ (critical value that divides the central 95% of z distribution from 5% in the tails), $z\beta = 1.28$ (critical value that separates the lower 10% of distribution from upper 90%), σ = standard deviation, and $\mu 1 - \mu 0$ = difference of two means.

Accordingly it was estimated that 27 patients are required and we decided to recruit 50 patients to have satisfactory results.

TABLE 1: AFI values from 34 to 40 weeks; mean, standard deviation, and percentile values (all in centimeters).

Gestational age	Mean	Standard deviation	5th percentile	10th percentile	50th percentile	90th percentile	95th percentile
34 weeks	14.59	1.79	11.7	12.0	14.6	17.0	17.3
35 weeks	14.25	1.57	11.1	11.8	14.2	16.2	16.4
36 weeks	13.17	1.56	10.6	11.0	13.2	15.3	15.7
37 weeks	12.48	1.52	10.1	10.2	12.6	14.7	15.1
38 weeks	12.20	1.70	9.8	10.0	12.1	14.4	14.7
39 weeks	11.37	1.71	8.8	9.1	11.4	14.0	14.4
40 weeks	10.99	1.55	8.7	8.8	10.8	13.5	13.7

4. Statistical Methods

Data was analyzed using SPSS version 16 for windows (SPSS Inc., Chicago, IL, USA). Descriptive analysis was performed to obtain mean, standard deviation, and percentile values for AFI from 34 to 40 weeks. Microsoft Excel 2010 was used to plot percentile values (5th, 50th, and 95th) across various gestational ages. A polynomial regression analysis of 3rd order was used to find the best fit. The decline in AFI value was calculated at weekly interval and the magnitude of change was analyzed by effect size estimation (Cohen d coefficient) [17].

The formula for Cohen's d is given as follows:

$$d = \frac{M_1 - M_2}{\sqrt{\left(s_1^2 + s_2^2\right)/2}}, \qquad (2)$$

where M_1 and M_2 are the means and s_1 and s_2 are the standard deviations of two groups.

5. Results

Of the 50 patients who were recruited for the study and were between the age of 22 to 28 years, more than half (32 patients, 64%) were primigravidae and 18 (36%) were multigravidae. None of them had any antenatal complications. All of them delivered at around 39+ to 40 weeks. 16 (32%) patients required caesarean delivery for obstetric indication such as failed induction, cephalopelvic disproportion, and fetal distress in labour. The mean (standard deviation) birth weight of the neonates (measured in kg) was 2.83 (0.34), with 1st minute APGAR score (mean and standard deviation) of 8.48 (1.09) and 5th minute APGAR was 8.72 (1.01). As mentioned in methodology, we have excluded those who delivered before term as we required AFI from 34 weeks to 40 weeks of gestation for analysis purpose.

Table 1 describes the descriptive data for AFI. The AFI values differed throughout the gestation and there was a gradual decline in the values as pregnancy advanced. The 5th, 50th, and 95th percentiles ranged from 11.7, 14.6, and 17.3, respectively, at 34 weeks to 8.7, 10.8, and 13.7, respectively, at 40 weeks. It is interesting to note that all the values were within 8 to 25 cm range (which is accepted and established normal range for AFI values worldwide). The maximum value of AFI in any single patient was 17.6 cm and minimum 8.5 cm in our series of low risk antenatal pregnant women. If minimum (5th centile) and maximum (95th centile) are considered as normal range, it was noted that the corresponding values too

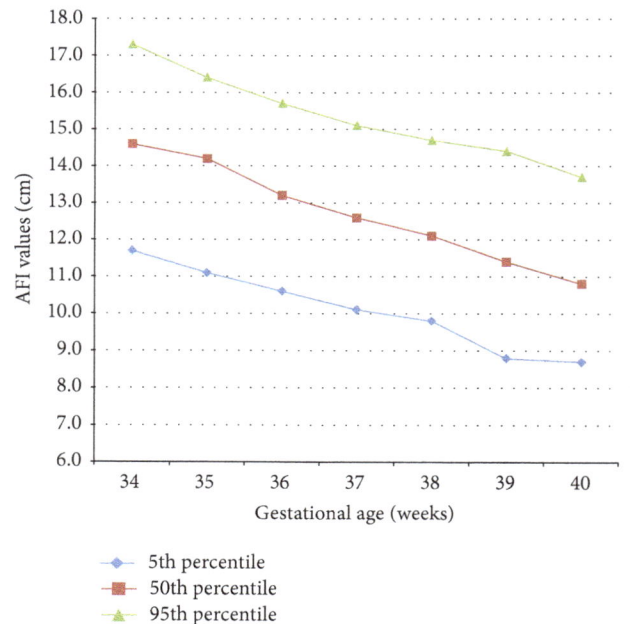

FIGURE 1: Graphical representation of AFI centiles at various gestational ages.

were different at different gestational ages; the more advanced the gestational age, the lesser the values. These changes are graphically represented in Figure 1.

We used difference in mean values of one week to the next week to evaluate the decreasing trend of amniotic fluid from 34 to 40 weeks of gestation (Table 2). Dark shaded area indicates cells where calculations are not required as they are the same weeks or previous weeks. It can be seen that many cells have the values less than 1, but still the difference may be calculated statistically significant if ordinary statistical tests such as paired t test were applied and hence we have used Cohen's test which very well detects the magnitude of change.

Table 3 indicates Cohen's d values for week to week comparison and it can be seen that not much change was seen in immediate week, but changes became significant when the interval between two scans was more than 2 weeks or more in most of the comparisons. Hence from this table there is substantial evidence that liquor volume decreases significantly over the period of 14 days more in low risk antenatal women.

Reference Ranges of Amniotic Fluid Index in Late Third Trimester of Pregnancy: What Should...

127

TABLE 2: Mean change in AFI (cm) values at different intervals.

From	To					
	35 weeks	36 weeks	37 weeks	38 weeks	39 weeks	40 weeks
34 weeks	0.34	1.42	2.12	2.39	3.22	3.61
35 weeks	*	1.08	1.77	2.05	2.88	3.26
36 weeks	*	*	0.7	0.97	1.8	2.19
37 weeks	*	*	*	0.27	1.1	1.49
38 weeks	*	*	*	*	0.83	1.22
39 weeks	*	*	*	*	*	0.39

*Comparison not done.

TABLE 3: Cohen d coefficients of effect size at different intervals.

From	To					
	35 weeks	36 weeks	37 weeks	38 weeks	39 weeks	40 weeks
34 weeks	0.21	0.85	1.29	1.38	1.86	2.18
35 weeks	#	0.7	1.16	1.27	1.77	2.12
36 weeks	#	#	0.46	0.6	1.11	1.42
37 weeks	#	#	#	0.17	0.69	0.98
38 weeks	#	#	#	#	0.49	0.76
39 weeks	#	#	#	#	#	0.24

0.2–0.49 small effect, 0.5–0.8 medium effect, and >0.8 large effect.
#Comparison not done.

Our results indicated that from 34 weeks onwards there is a gradual reduction in AFI. Using polynomial regression analysis, we have established reference standards for AFI ranges from 34 to 40 weeks (Figure 2). The regression analysis further showed that there was a good degree of correlation between GA (gestational age) and AFI (R^2 = 0.89 to 0.95; $P < 0.005$).

The following equations were derived by third degree polynomial regression using **y** (AFI in cm) as dependent variable and **x** (gestation age in weeks) as independent variable, where Y^{5th}, Y^{50th}, and Y^{95th} indicate 5th, 50th, and 95th centile values for AFI and GA indicates gestational age in weeks:

$$Y^{5th} = (-84.8833337026) + (9.46507939511 \times GA)$$
$$+ \left(-0.289285715099 \times GA^2\right)$$
$$+ \left(0.0027777777851 \times GA^3\right),$$

$$Y^{50th} = (-283.684761575) + (26.1987698144 \times GA)$$
$$+ \left(-0.748571427845 \times GA^2\right) \quad (3)$$
$$+ \left(0.00694444443791 \times GA^3\right),$$

$$Y^{95th} = (-212.166667464) + (20.6884921284 \times GA)$$
$$+ \left(-0.598809525566 \times GA^2\right)$$
$$+ \left(0.00555555557137 \times GA^3\right).$$

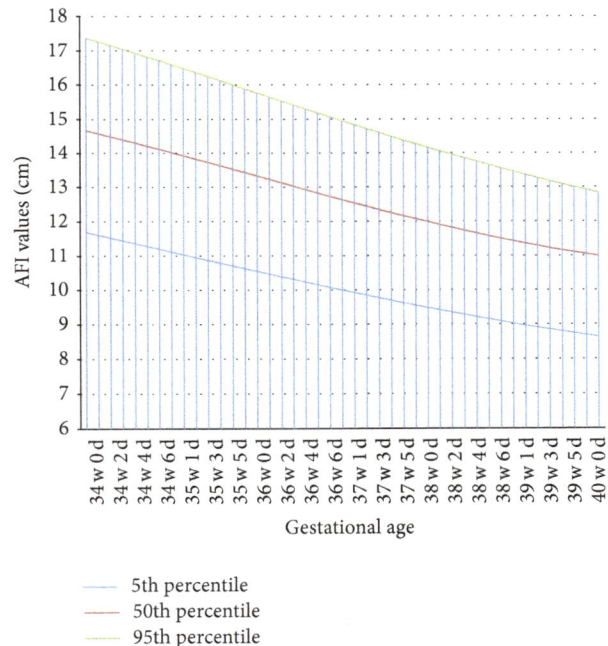

FIGURE 2: Curve of AFI values (5th, 50th, and 95th centiles) from 34 to 40 weeks following smoothing procedure from polynomial regression of 3rd degree.

6. Discussion

Amniotic fluid production and regulation is a complex and dynamic process involving the fetus, placenta, and mother.

TABLE 4: Values of AFI (in cm) by different authors.

Authors	AFI values	34 W	35 W	36 W	37 W	38 W	39 W	40 W
Khadilkar et al. 2003 [16]	5th centile	7.6	7.4	7.2	7.0	6.8	6.1	5.9
	50th centile	14.2	13.8	13.5	12.8	12.2	11.5	11.3
	95th centile	19	18.5	18.3	18.2	17.6	16.8	16.6
Hinh and Ladinsky 2005 [22]	Mean (St. Dev)	13.7 (3.1)	12.6 (2.2)	11.1 (2.6)	12.1 (2.4)	11.4 (2.1)	11.8 (1.7)	11.0 (1.0)
	Min	8.5	8.6	7.1	6.7	6.3	8.4	9.4
	Max	18.8	16.8	16.3	15.9	15.4	14.8	12.7
MacHado et al. 2007 [23]	10th centile	10.2	9.7	9.1	8.4	7.7	7	6.2
	50th centile	14.4	14.1	13.9	13.5	13.2	12.8	12.4
	90th centile	19.5	19.4	19.3	19.1	18.9	18.6	18.3
Birang 2008 [24]	Mean (St. Dev)	13.8 (1.18)	12.9 (0.60)	12.7 (1.55)	12.8 (0.84)	12.8 (0.89)	12.8 (1.19)	12.5 (0.98)
	5th centile	8.3	7.3	7.1	7.1	7.1	7.0	6.6
	95th centile	23.7	23.2	22.8	22.1	20	18.7	18
Singh et al. 2013 [25]	Mean	17.1	16.9	16.3	16.2	15.7	15.3	14.8
	5th centile	11.0	10	9.7	10.1	9.9	8.1	8.8
	95th centile	24.5	24.1	24.8	24.2	24.1	23.7	18
Present study	Mean	14.59 (1.79)	14.25 (1.57)	13.17 (1.56)	12.48 (1.52)	12.2 (1.7)	11.37 (1.71)	10.99 (1.55)
	5th centile	11.7	11.1	10.6	10.1	9.8	8.8	8.7
	95th centile	17.3	16.4	15.7	15.1	14.7	14.4	13.7

Amniotic fluid volume gradually increases till 32–34 weeks of gestation and thereafter there is a gradual reduction till term [18, 19]. The critical AFI range of 8 to 25 cm signifies fetal well-being and the deviation from this range is associated with increase in fetal and maternal complications due to oligoamnios and polyhydramnios. The third trimester AFI values are proportionate to fetal urine production [20, 21] and hence in normal range indicate good placental perfusion and fetal nutrient and oxygen transfer. Hence monitoring the AFI has become a standard of antenatal care.

There is wide variation in reference standards for mean AFI values according to population, race, and geography. Table 4 compares our finding with that of other authors [16, 22–25]. We have also graphically interpreted findings in the other studies (either mean or 50th percentile values) in Figure 3. However, it is noticeable that majority of the studies agree that from 34 weeks onward there is a gradual fall in AFI values. The two studies [16, 25] are from India, but the reported AFI range has a wide range. This may be because their observations were based upon retrospective cross sectional data. It is noticeable that AFI reference values published by Singh et al. are 2 to 3 cm more than all other series at all gestational ages; we presume this may be because the study was done in Indraprastha Apollo Hospital, New Delhi, where patients from very high socioeconomic status are catered. Khadilkar et al. reported their findings from patients attending antenatal clinic of Grant Medical College, Bombay, and our findings too match with their data. Hence, it can be opined that AFI standards have to be defined for specific populations in order to eliminate bias resulting from socioeconomic groups, geographical locations, race, and so forth. However, it must be noted that almost all authors have reported a steady decline in AFI values with the advancing gestational age, except Birang et al. from Iran. Their series

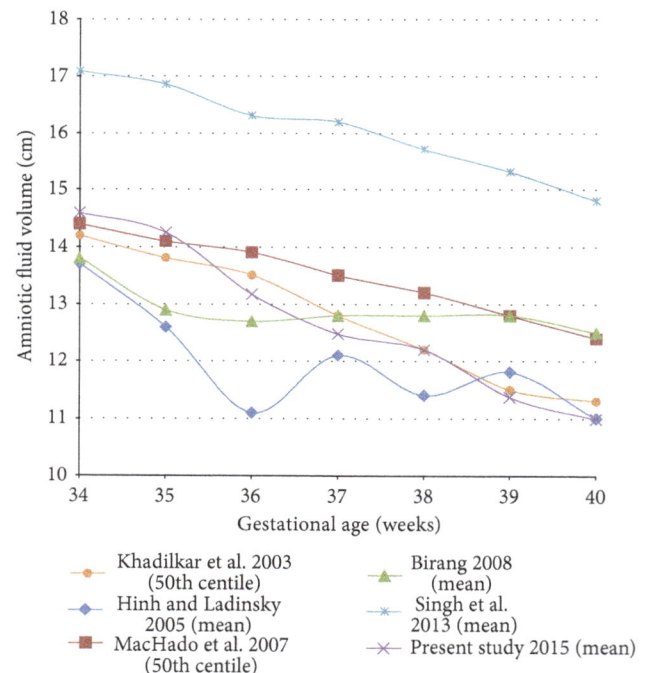

FIGURE 3: Comparison of AFI values at different gestational ages in various studies.

included retrospective cross sectional data and the number differed from minimum of 12 observations at 35 weeks to maximum of 68 observations at 39 weeks. This might be the reason for their finding of rapid fall of AFI from 34 to 35 weeks, plateauing between 37 and 39 weeks and once again slow fall at 40 weeks. Such observations indicate weakness of cross sectional cohort, as the same patients are not followed up sequentially.

Amniotic fluid once thought to be a stagnant pool with approximate turn over time of twenty-four hours. In high risk pregnancies complicated by chronic placental insufficiency liquor is known to drastically reduce in a shorter time and it has been recommended to perform AFI estimation once in three days or at times even frequently depending upon other fetal well-being surveillance tools such as Doppler assessment of fetal circulation. However, there is no universal consensus regarding the frequency of AFI estimation in low risk antenatal women. Hence, it is important to determine a critical interval at which the fall in AFI becomes clinically significant.

We have not used statistical significance test (involving estimation of *P* value) such as *paired t test* for comparing AFI values at different gestational ages, as these tests tend to give significant *P* values even when a minor variation exists in the means of two groups. When sample size is sufficiently large, even the fractional differences are likely to be reported as significant *P* values, hence giving meaningless interpretations. Instead, we have calculated effect size estimate (Cohen *d*) to quantify the changes in the AFI over a period of time.

Effect size is a simple measure for quantifying the difference between two groups or the same group over time, on a common scale. There are several methods mentioned in the literature to calculate the effect sizes (Cohen 1988 [17], Rosenthal and Rosnow 1991 [26], Partial Eta squared Richardson 2011 [27]) and so forth. However, we have used Cohen's *d* estimate as described by Cohen 1988, to calculate effect sizes as this method is easy, simple to understand and can be applied to any measured outcome in scientific study.

From our statistical analysis, we have found that there is no much decrease in AFI at interval of one week, but thereafter the differences become large and significant. Hence, it appears that when the liquor is within normal range, the chances of fetal jeopardy are unlikely to occur within next week; one can safely repeat the AFI after 2 weeks. At the time of estimation of AFI, one can also perform other tests for foetal well-being such as documentation of gross foetal body movements, foetal tone, and foetal breathing movements to be assured that foetus is not hypoxic. In addition, interval biometry may be done at whenever required to quantify satisfactory foetal growth. In the absence of any maternal or foetal risk factors, we are of the opinion that AFI estimation once in fortnight is good enough to ensure satisfactory pregnancy outcome.

7. Conclusions

We have established not only gestational specific normative AFI reference standards for late third trimester (34 to 40 weeks) for our local population but also magnitude of change in AFI values at weekly interval by quantitative analysis using effect size statistics. Strength of present study is that it is based on longitudinal data of normal healthy pregnant women and percentile curves obtained can be used to define what constitutes normal range of AFI for low risk antenatal patients. Though our results are based on required number of patients

by sample size determination, larger number of subjects if studied may yield robust reference curves for AFI and identify extreme values to define what constitutes oligo- or polyhydramnios. The same study can be extended to high risk pregnancies such as preeclampsia, chronic hypertension, multiple gestation, and intrauterine growth restriction, in order to determine the frequency of liquor testing for these cohorts.

Conflict of Interests

The authors have no conflict of interests to declare.

References

[1] L. Yeo, M. G. Ross, and A. M. Vintzileos, "Antepartum and intra-partum surveillance of the fetus and the amniotic fluid," in *Clinical Obstetrics: The Fetus & Mother*, pp. 586–606, John Wiley & Sons, 3rd edition, 2008.

[2] R. Liston, D. Sawchuck, and D. Young, "Fetal health surveillance: antepartum and intrapartum consensus guideline," *Journal of Obstetrics and Gynaecology Canada*, vol. 29, supplement 4, no. 9, pp. S3–S56, 2007.

[3] A. A. Baschat, R. M. Viscardi, B. Hussey-Gardner, N. Hashmi, and C. Harman, "Infant neurodevelopment following fetal growth restriction: Relationship with antepartum surveillance parameters," *Ultrasound in Obstetrics & Gynecology*, vol. 33, no. 1, pp. 44–50, 2009.

[4] G. Heller, B. Misselwitz, and S. Schmidt, "Early neonatal mortality, asphyxia related deaths, and timing of low risk births in Hesse, Germany, 1990–8: observational study," *British Medical Journal*, vol. 321, no. 7256, pp. 274–275, 2000.

[5] F. A. Manning, "Antepartum fetal testing: a critical appraisal," *Current Opinion in Obstetrics and Gynecology*, vol. 21, no. 4, pp. 348–352, 2009.

[6] P. Nash, "Amniotic fluid index," *Neonatal Network*, vol. 32, no. 1, pp. 46–49, 2013.

[7] E. A. Dubil, "Amniotic fluid as a vital sign for fetal wellbeing," *AJUM*, vol. 16, no. 2, pp. 62–70, 2013.

[8] A. F. Nabhan and Y. A. Abdelmoula, "Amniotic fluid index versus single deepest vertical pocket as a screening test for preventing adverse pregnancy outcome," *The Cochrane Database of Systematic Reviews*, no. 3, Article ID CD006593, 2008.

[9] J. P. Phelan, M. O. Ahn, C. V. Smith, S. E. Rutherford, and E. Anderson, "Amniotic fluid index measurements during pregnancy," *Journal of Reproductive Medicine for the Obstetrician and Gynecologist*, vol. 32, no. 8, pp. 601–604, 1987.

[10] M. H. Beall, J. P. H. M. van den Wijngaard, M. J. C. van Gemert, and M. G. Ross, "Amniotic fluid water dynamics," *Placenta*, vol. 28, no. 8-9, pp. 816–823, 2007.

[11] J. P. Phelan, C. V. Smith, P. Broussard, and M. Small, "Amniotic fluid volume assessment with the four-quadrant technique at 36–42 weeks' gestation," *Journal of Reproductive Medicine*, vol. 32, no. 7, pp. 540–542, 1987.

[12] S. Iqbal and A. Noreen, "Low amniotic fluid index as a predictor of perinatal outcome in low risk pregnancies at term," *Pakistan Journal of Medical and Health Sciences*, vol. 4, no. 3, pp. 270–271, 2010.

[13] E. G. Voxman, S. Tran, and D. A. Wing, "Low amniotic fluid index as a predictor of adverse perinatal outcome," *Journal of Perinatology*, vol. 22, no. 4, pp. 282–285, 2002.

[14] J. G. Lalor, B. Fawole, Z. Alfirevic, and D. Devane, "Biophysical profile for fetal assessment in high risk pregnancies," *The Cochrane Database of Systematic Reviews*, no. 1, Article ID CD000038, 2008.

[15] C. Signore, R. K. Freeman, and C. Y. Spong, "Antenatal testing-a reevaluation: executive summary of a Eunice Kennedy Shriver National Institute of Child Health and Human Development wrkshop," *Obstetrics and Gynecology*, vol. 113, no. 3, pp. 687–701, 2009.

[16] S. S. Khadilkar, S. S. Desai, S. M. Tayade, and C. N. Purandare, "Amniotic fluid index in normal pregnancy: an assessment of gestation specific reference values among Indian women," *Journal of Obstetrics and Gynaecology Research*, vol. 29, no. 3, pp. 136–141, 2003.

[17] J. Cohen, *Statistical Power Analysis for the Behavioral Sciences*, Lawrence Earlbaum Associates, Hillsdale, NJ, USA, 2nd edition, 1988.

[18] R. A. Brace and E. J. Wolf, "Normal amniotic fluid volume changes throughout pregnancy," *The American Journal of Obstetrics and Gynecology*, vol. 161, no. 2, pp. 382–388, 1989.

[19] T. R. Moore and J. E. Cayle, "The amniotic fluid index in normal human pregnancy," *American Journal of Obstetrics & Gynecology*, vol. 162, no. 5, pp. 1168–1173, 1990.

[20] E. F. Magann, A. T. Sandlin, and S. T. Ounpraseuth, "Amniotic fluid and the clinical relevance of the sonographically estimated amniotic fluid volume: oligohydramnios," *Journal of Ultrasound in Medicine*, vol. 30, no. 11, pp. 1573–1585, 2011.

[21] S. M. Lee, S. K. Park, S. S. Shim, J. K. Jun, J. S. Park, and H. C. Syn, "Measurement of fetal urine production by three-dimensional ultrasonography in normal pregnancy," *Ultrasound in Obstetrics and Gynecology*, vol. 30, no. 3, pp. 281–286, 2007.

[22] N. D. Hinh and J. L. Ladinsky, "Amniotic fluid index measurements in normal pregnancy after 28 gestational weeks," *International Journal of Gynecology & Obstetrics*, vol. 91, no. 2, pp. 132–136, 2005.

[23] M. R. MacHado, J. G. Cecatti, F. Krupa, and A. Faundes, "Curve of amniotic fluid index measurements in low-risk pregnancy," *Acta Obstetricia et Gynecologica Scandinavica*, vol. 86, no. 1, pp. 37–41, 2007.

[24] S. Birang, "Ultrasonographic assessment of normal amniotic fluid index in a group of Iranian women," *Iranian Journal of Radiology*, vol. 5, no. 1, pp. 31–34, 2008.

[25] C. Singh, T. Tayal, R. Gupta, A. P. Sharma, D. Khurana, and A. Kaul, "Amniotic fluid index in healthy pregnancy in an Indian population," *International Journal of Gynecology and Obstetrics*, vol. 121, no. 2, pp. 176–177, 2013.

[26] R. Rosenthal and R. L. Rosnow, *Essentials of Behavioral Research: Methods and Data Analysis*, McGraw Hill, New York, NY, USA, 2nd edition, 1991.

[27] J. T. E. Richardson, "Eta squared and partial eta squared as measures of effect size in educational research," *Educational Research Review*, vol. 6, no. 2, pp. 135–147, 2011.

15

Prevalence and Factors Associated with Teenage Pregnancy, Northeast Ethiopia, 2017

Yohannes Ayanaw Habitu [ID],[1] Anteneh Yalew,[2] and Telake Azale Bisetegn[3]

[1]*Department of Reproductive Health, College of Medicine and Health Sciences, University of Gondar, Gondar, Ethiopia*
[2]*Wogedi District Health Office, Wogedi, South Wollo Zone, Northeast Ethiopia, Ethiopia*
[3]*Department of Health Communication and Behavioural Sciences, Institute of Public Health, College of Medicine and Health Sciences, University of Gondar, Gondar, Ethiopia*

Correspondence should be addressed to Yohannes Ayanaw Habitu; yohaneshabitu@gmail.com

Academic Editor: Olav Lapaire

Introduction. Though teen age pregnancy had poor maternal and perinatal health outcomes, its magnitude and determinants are not well understood. Therefore, the aim of this study was to assess the prevalence and associated factors of teenage pregnancy in Wogedi, northeast Ethiopia. *Methods*. A community-based cross-sectional study was conducted among 514 teenagers in Wogedi, northeast Ethiopia, from April to May 2017. Data were collected using a structured questionnaire, entered, and analyzed appropriately. Odds ratios with 95% confidence interval and P-values were computed using appropriate logistic regression models to determine the presence and strength of associations between the dependent and independent variables. *Results*. The prevalence of teenage pregnancy in Wogedi was 28.6% (95% CI: 24.9, 32.5). Age (AOR=2.10; 95% CI: 1.55, 2.88), rural residence (AOR=3.93; 95% CI: 1.20, 12.83), contraceptive nonuse (AOR=10.62; 95% CI: 5.28, 21.36), and parental marital status (divorce) (AOR=1.98; 95%CI: 1.13, 3.93) were found to have statistically significant associations with teenage pregnancy. *Conclusions*. There is high prevalence of teenage pregnancy in the area. Age, residence, contraceptive nonuse, and parental divorce were found to have a statistically significant association. Strengthening contraceptive use by giving special attention to rural dwellers and showing the consequences of divorce to the community are strongly recommended.

1. Introduction

Adolescent pregnancy is defined as a pregnancy in girls 10–19 years of age. It is estimated that about 16 million girls 15–19 years old give birth each year, contributing nearly 11% of all births worldwide [1]. Although adolescent fertility rates are falling globally, approximately 18 million girls under the age of 20 give birth each year [2]. Two million of these births are from girls under 15 years of age [2]. More than 90% of these births occur in low and middle-income countries [1–3]. Most teenage pregnancies and childbirths take place in west and central Africa, east and southern Africa, South Asia, Latin America, and the Caribbeans [2].

Different pieces of literature show that the prevalence of teenage pregnancy varies across regions of the world. In the Asia Pacific regions, it ranges up to 43% in Bangladesh [4] and from 11.1% [5] to 47.3% in Nepal [6]. In Jordan, the prevalence

is 25% [7]. The prevalence of teenage pregnancy also varies in Africa; for instance, in Nigeria, it ranges from 6.2% in Niger Delta state [8] to 49% in Abia State [9]. In South Africa [10], East Africa (Kenya) [11], Assossa (Ethiopia) [12], and Sudan [13], it ranges from 2.3 to 19.2%, 31%, 20.4%, and 31%, respectively.

Currently about 17% of the adolescents between 15 and 19 years in Ethiopia are married [14] and the median age of women at first sexual intercourse is now 16.6 years [14]. There is a low contraceptive prevalence rate (CPR) (7.5%) among all female adolescents of 15-19 years; CPR is higher among currently married (31.9%) and sexually active unmarried adolescents (59%) of the same age [14]. In addition, 20.5% of female adolescents 15-19 years face unmet needs for family planning and 52.5% total demand for same [14].

Teenage pregnancy is very common in Ethiopia, and it is an important demographic factor making the country the second most populous in Africa, with a total population of around 102 million in 2016 [15]. According to the EDHS 2016 finding, the prevalence of teenage pregnancy is 13% [14]. It varies depending on residence, urban 5%, and rural 15% [14]. Moreover, disparities are seen across regions, with the highest 23% in Afar, 8% in Amhara, and the lowest 3% in Addis Ababa [14].

Literature showed different sociodemographic, cultural, and other individual factors were associated with teenage pregnancy. Approximately 90% of teenage pregnancies in the developing world are of girls who are married, owing to their high exposure to sex and pressure to conceive quickly after marriage [8, 16–18]. As a result, the majority (75%) of married teenage pregnancies are planned [1, 17]. Employment status [6, 9, 18, 19], poverty [2, 6, 14, 20–22], marital status [9, 12, 18, 23], type of occupation [12, 21], culture [9, 11], peer pressure [11, 20, 22, 24], early marriage [25], forced marriage [20], rape [26], and the need for a dowry [20] were factors associated with teenage pregnancy in recorded literature.

Studies have shown that teenage pregnancy has poor maternal and perinatal health outcomes [1, 2, 8, 27]. Complications during pregnancy and childbirth are the second cause of death for 15-19-year-old girls globally [1]. Every year, some 3 million girls aged 15 to 19 undergo unsafe abortions [1]. Babies born to adolescent mothers face a substantially high risk of dying than those born to women aged 20 to 24[1, 25]. School dropout [14, 20, 22, 25], poverty [2, 25], high rate of marriage [8], pregnancy-induced hypertension [27–30], and induced abortion [1, 20] are some of the consequences of adolescent pregnancy on the mother. Preterm delivery [19, 27, 29–31], low birth weight [5, 19, 27, 29–32], stillbirth [5, 27, 31], and high fetal and neonatal mortality [19, 27, 29, 30, 32] are some of the consequences of teenage pregnancy for the fetus.

The limited studies conducted in the world as well as in Ethiopia have tried to show the prevalence and factors associated with teenage pregnancy, but most of the studies were done using secondary data (health facility-based studies). Hence, due to the poor data recording system of our country, we may not get appropriate information from health facilities. Moreover, research results from health facilities lack representativeness to the general population. Therefore, this study was conducted to show the prevalence and determinants of teenage pregnancy in Wegedi, northeast Ethiopia, 2017, by using primary data.

2. Materials and Methods

2.1. Study Design and Setting. This community-based cross-sectional study was conducted in Wogedi from April to May 2017. Wogedi, one of the districts in South Wollo zone, is 192 km to the west of Dessie. According to the national census report of 2007, the projected population of Wogedi for the year 2016 was 152,719 of whom 26.5% were adolescents 15-19 years of age [33]. Wogedi has 35 kebeles (lowest administrative units), two district health offices, five health centers, and thirty-two health posts [33].

2.2. Source and Study Population. All female adolescents 15-19 years of age in the selected kebeles of Wogedi were the source population of the study.

2.3. Inclusion Criteria. Female adolescents 15-19 years of age.

2.4. Sample Size and Sampling Procedure. The sample size was calculated using the single population proportion formula with the following assumptions. The proportion of teenage pregnancy among 15-19 years of age females in Ethiopia (20.4%) [34] was taken from the previous study with a 5% margin of error and 95% confidence interval. Lastly, by considering a 10% nonresponse rate, and a design effect of 2, the final sample size obtained was 542. A multistage sampling technique was employed in order to select study units. First, out of the 35 kebeles, six were selected randomly, to represent 20% of the district population. Then, to each selected kebele, we allocated the sample size by considering the proportional allocation technique. Finally, study units were randomly selected at the household level using the lottery method.

2.5. Study Variables

2.5.1. Dependent Variable. Teenage pregnancy.

2.5.2. Independent Variables. Sociodemographic variables, like age, sex, marital status, education, occupation, and income were considered. History of sexual and reproductive health, like age at first sexual intercourse, early marriage, contraceptive use, perception on teenage pregnancy, family income, family education, peer pressure, and casual sex assessed.

2.6. Operational Definition. Teenage pregnancy: pregnancy in adolescents 15-19 years who believe that they are pregnant and confirmed by a health care providers.

2.7. Data Collection Instruments and Procedures. Data were collected using a pretested, structured, interviewer-administered questionnaire which was first prepared in English and translated into Amharic (the local language) by a language expert. Then, the Amharic version was again translated back to English to check for consistency. The structured, interviewer-administered questionnaire was adapted from the WHO (Illustrative-questionnaire for interview survey with young people developed by John Cleland) standard tool which was developed to assess the sexual and reproductive health of adolescents and youth. Appropriate modifications were made to fit with the local set up. In addition we conducted a pretest and we have made some simple analysis to see if we can address the desired objectives or not, from the results of the pretest. Moreover, some language corrections and rearrangements on the order of questions were made to keep the logical flow of the questions, based on the comments from the pretest we got. Four data collectors, with Bachelor's degrees in nursing and data collection experience were recruited. One supervisor, with a master's of public health was employed. The supervisor and data collectors were females chosen in order to minimize participant discomfort. A one day training was given to data collectors and the supervisor to help them know the objective and the relevance of the study and the rights of the respondents either to participate or decline.

2.8. Data Management. Data manually checked by the investigators were entered and cleaned using EPI info data version 7 and exported to SPSS version 20 for further analysis. Descriptive statistics like frequencies, percentages, and means were computed. Bivariable analyses were carried out to examine the relationship between teenage pregnancy and each explanatory variable. All explanatory variables that were statistically significant at the Bivariable model at <0.2 p-value were included in the multivariate logistic regression model to see the real determinants of teenage pregnancy. Adjusted odds ratios with a 95% confidence interval were computed, and variables with a p-value <0.05 in the Multivariate Model were considered as statistically significant.

2.9. Ethical Considerations. Ethical approval was obtained from the Institutional Review Board (IRB) of the Institute of Public Health, College of Medicine and Health Sciences, the University of Gondar (IRB reference number: IPH/2471/2017). Participants were informed about the objective of the study and the fact that the confidentiality of their responses will be insured by excluding personal identifiers and carefully securing the questionnaire in such a way that it is accessed only by the investigators.

3. Results

3.1. Sociodemographic Characteristics of Respondents. A total of 514 female adolescents 15-19 years of age were included in the study with a response rate of 95%. The majority, 157 (30.5%), of the respondents were 19 years old, with the median Inter Quartile Range of 3 years. More than half, 270 (52.5%), of the respondents were Orthodox Christians. Three hundred seventeen, (61.7%), attended primary school, and more than half, 271 (52.7%), were married. Nearly half, 253 (49.2%), of the respondents were students, and 251 (48.8%) earned less than Birr 1500 per month (Table 1).

3.2. Sexual and Reproductive Health Characteristics of Participants. This study showed that 337 (65.6%) of the respondents had sexual intercourse and that 130 (38.6%) started it before 15 years of age. Out of those who had sex, 156 (46.3%), used contraceptives. The proportion of teenage pregnancy among respondents in Wogedi was 147 (28.6%) with a 95% CI (24.9, 32.5). The study also indicated that the majority of the pregnancies, 93 (63.3%), were unplanned, and 54 (36.7%) of the teenagers were unhappy about their pregnancy. Moreover, 36 (24.5%) were pregnant at the time of the survey (Table 2).

The major reason mentioned by 65% of the respondents for exposure to pregnancy was marriage, followed by 20% who were exposed for nonuse of contraceptives.

3.3. Factors Associated with Teenage Pregnancy. Age, religion, educational status, marital status, occupation, living arrangement, parent's age, parents' religion, parents' marital status, parents' monthly income, and contraceptive nonuse were variables with P-values of less than 0.2 in the Bivariable Logistic regression. All variables with less than 0.2 P-values were fitted in to the multivariate logistic regression model

TABLE 1: Sociodemographic characteristics of teenagers in Wogedi, northeast Ethiopia, 2017.

Variables	Frequency (N=514)	Percent
Age in years		
15	86	16.7
16	83	16.2
17	76	14.8
18	112	21.8
19	157	30.5
Religion		
Muslim	244	47.5
Orthodox	270	52.5
Marital status		
Married	205	39.9
Divorced	63	12.3
Widowed	3	0.6
Single	243	47.2
Educational status		
College	5	1.0
Secondary (9-12)	101	19.6
Primary (1-8)	317	61.7
Unable to read and write	91	17.7
Occupation		
Farmer	173	33.7
Housewife	39	7.6
Merchant	18	3.5
Daily laborer	31	6.0
Student	253	49.2
Live with		
Alone	16	3.1
Husband	164	31.9
Parent	334	65.0
Expected household income		
<1500	251	48.8
1501-7500	244	47.5
>7500	19	3.7

after adjusting for possible confounders. In the multivariate logistic regression model, age, residence, contraceptive nonuse, and parents' marital status were identified as statistically significant variables.

Increase in age is significantly associated with teenage pregnancy (AOR=2.10; CI: 1.55, 2.88). Teenagers from rural settings were more likely to be pregnant than students (AOR=3.93; 95% CI: 1.20, 12.83). This study also showed that contraceptive nonuse was found to be significantly associated with teenage pregnancy. Respondents who did not use contraceptives were ten times (AOR=10.62; 95%CI: 5.28, 21.36) more likely to be pregnant than their counterparts.

Teenagers from divorced parents were nearly two times more exposed to teenage pregnancy as compared to those who were from married parents (AOR=1.98; 95%CI: 1.13, 3.93) (Table 3).

TABLE 2: Sexual and reproductive health characteristics of teenagers in Wogedi, northeast Ethiopia, 2017.

Variable	Frequency	Percent
Ever had sex (N=514)		
No	177	34.4
Yes	337	65.6
Age at first sex (N=337)		
13-15	130	38.6
16-18	205	60.8
>18	2	0.6
Contraceptive use (N=337)		
No	181	53.7
Yes	156	46.3
Reasons for contraceptive non-use (N=181)		
Do not have accesses	17	9.4
Do not have knowledge	68	37.6
Family influence	81	44.8
Due to divorce	8	4.4
Wants to be pregnant	7	3.8
Ever had pregnancy (N=514)		
No	367	71.4
Yes	147	28.6
Currently pregnant (N=147)		
No	111	75.5
Yes	36	24.5
Conditions of pregnancy (N=147)		
Planned	54	36.7
Unplanned	93	63.3
Feeling about the pregnancy (N=147)		
Happy	58	39.5
Unhappy	64	43.5
Nothing	25	17.0
Outcomes of pregnancy (N=111)		
Delivered (Live Birth)	97	87.4
Aborted	14	12.6

4. Discussion

The prevalence of teenage pregnancy extremely varies in the world. Some of the reasons for these differences could be variations in sociodemographic, cultural, sexual, and reproductive health characteristics of adolescents. This study explored the prevalence of teenage pregnancy and its associated factors in Wogedi district, northeast Ethiopia. The study showed that the prevalence of teenage pregnancy was 28.6% (95% CI: 24.9, 32.5). Factors associated with it were increase in age, farming occupation, contraceptive nonuse, and parents' marital status (divorce).

This finding is similar with those of studies conducted in Sudan, 31% [13], Kenya, 31% [11], Jordan, 25% [7], and Turkey, 29% [35]. This similarity could be due to the presence of some related sociodemographic, cultural, and individual adolescent characteristics in the current and those studies. For instance, the proportion of married adolescents in the Kenya

study was similar to that of the current study. Moreover, there was a similarity in the culture of early marriage in the current and the other studies.

This finding is higher than the 13.0% national report on teenage pregnancy [14]. The possible reason may be that the EDHS study includes all settlements, like urban and rural areas, whereas the current study was conducted in one of the rural districts in Amhara Region, where there is a high prevalence of early marriage. In the region, the median age at first marriage is 16.2 years, and the median age at first sex 15.8 years, the lowest in the country [14]. All these factors may contribute to the high prevalence of teenage pregnancy in the current study as compared to the national one.

This finding is higher than those of studies conducted in Niger Delta state of Nigeria 6.2% [8], and Assosa 20.4% [12]. The variation could be due to the presence of some sociodemographic, cultural, sexual, and reproductive characteristics of participants in the other and the current study. For instance, the proportion of marriage in the Niger Delta state was 27.7% [8], lower than that of the current study 39.9%. Shreds of evidence showed that as the proportion of marriage increased, the probability of exposure to pregnancy also increased [36]. In addition, the proportion of participants who had secondary or more education was higher in the Niger Delta state study (46.0%) [8] compared to the current study (20.6%). Evidence showed that as the educational level of girls increased, the chance of exposure to pregnancy decreased [14]. Compared to marriage in the current study (39.9%), the proportion of marriage was lower in the Assosa study 20.7% [12]. In addition, the proportion of participants who could not read and write was lower in the Assosa study (3.4%) [12] compared to that of the current study (17.7%). Moreover, the proportion of contraceptive use was higher (69.5%) in the Assosa study [12] compared to the present study (46.3%). Different scientific researchers showed contraceptive use decreased the prevalence of teenage pregnancy [36].

This finding is lower than those of studies conducted in Abia State of Nigeria (49.0%) [9] and the Cape Coast Municipality in Nepal (47.3%) [6]. This difference could be due to some social, cultural, and individual characteristics of participants and the time gap among the studies. For instance, in the Abia study, the proportion of participants who had no formal education (28.5%) [9] was more than that of the current study which represented 17.7%. Moreover, the proportion of study participants who were unemployed (75.8%) was higher in Abia State study [9] compared to that of the present study (49.2%). The possible explanation for these may be unemployed adolescents may have poorer access to contraceptives; hence, the chance of getting pregnancy increased. In the study conducted in Cape Coast Municipality, Nepal, the proportion of participants who had no formal education (30.2%) [6], was higher compared to that of the current study (17.7%). Furthermore, the proportion of participants who had secondary education and above (2.1%) [6] was less in the Nepal study compared to that of the present study (20.6%). Besides, the proportion of contraceptive use in the Nepal study 11.1% [6] was less than that of the present study (53.7%).

TABLE 3: Bivariable and multivariable logistic regression analysis showing factors associated with teenage pregnancy in Wogedi, northeast Ethiopia, 2017.

Variable	Teenage pregnancy		Crude OR (95% CI)	Adjusted OR (95% CI)
	Yes	No		
Age (Mean =17.33 years with SD=1.47)	147	367	2.60 (2.12,3.20)	**2.10 (1.55,2.88)**∗∗
Marital status				
Married	111	94	30.7 (14.9, 41.0)	2.16 (0.59, 4.80)
Divorced	24	39	16 .0 (6.9, 36.1)	1.38 (0.37, 5.00)
Widowed	3	0	-	-
Single	9	234	1	1
Educational level				
College	2	3	0.5 (0.08, 3.13)	3.00 (0.28, 6.1)
Secondary	4	97	0.03 (0.01, 0.09)	0.87 (0.42, 1.78)
Primary	89	228	0.29 (0.18, 0.47)	0.41 (0.10, 1.67)
Unable to read and write	52	39	1	1
Occupation				
Farmer	91	82	30.00 (14.5,62.3)	**3.93 (1.20,12.83)**∗
House wife	28	11	69.01 (26.3,80.0)	4.23 (0.94,19.01)
Merchant	12	6	54.22 (16.5,77.0)	4.26 (0.75, 6.13)
Daily laborer	7	24	7.91 (2.73, 23.1)	1.42 (0.31, 6.57)
Student	9	244	1	1
Live with				
Alone	11	5	16.62 (5.43, 20.04)	3.24 (0.55, 8.83)
Husband	97	67	10.91 (6.93,17.01)	2.26 (0.81, 6.28)
Parents	39	295	1	1
Monthly income				
<1500	81	170	0.65 (0.25, 1.69)	2.59 (0.69, 9.61)
1501-7500	58	186	0.42 (0.16, 1.12)	1.33 (0.36, 4.96)
>7500	8	11	1	1
Parent age				
30-49	95	265	0.7 (0.46, 1.04)	0.96 (0.49, 1.86)
>49	52	102	1	1
Parents' marital status				
Divorced	7	29	2.2 (0.72, 6.90)	**1.98 (1.13, 3.93)**∗
Widowed	14	36	2.42 (0.91, 6.32)	1.54 (0.12, 18.95)
Married	126	302	1	1
Contraceptive use				
No	117	64	7.6 (4.65, 12.67)	**10.62 (5.28, 21.36)**∗∗
Yes	30	126	1	1

∗Significant at a p-value less than 0.05 and ∗∗significant at a p-value less than 0.001; SD: Standard Deviation.

In this study, as respondents' age increased by one year, the odds of being pregnant increased by 2.1%. This finding is in line with that of national study in Ethiopia [14], Kenya [11], and Abia State [9]. As age increases, teenagers will have more exposure to sex and their chance of being married will also increase to procreate children.

Teenagers from rural setups were four times more likely to have pregnancy compared to student respondents. This finding is consistent with that of a study conducted in South Asia [37]. This might be so because teenagers from the rural areas are less educated and have limited access to contraceptives. Besides, rural communities are pronatalists compared to educated people [14].

Contraceptive nonusers were nearly eleven times more likely to be pregnant compared to those who used contraceptives. Other studies are in line with this finding in that the prevalence of teenage pregnancy increased among contraceptive nonusers [18, 20, 36]. It has been evidenced that as the proportion of contraceptive nonusers increased the proportion of pregnancy increased [36].

Teenagers from divorced parents were nearly two times more exposed to teenage pregnancy compared to adolescents from married parents (AOR=1.98; 95%CI: 1.13, 3.93). This is due to the existence of low parental control and communication about sexual and reproductive issues among divorced parents compared to married ones. These lead to increased early sexual debut and risky sexual behaviors among adolescents from divorced parents, and all these expose them to teenage pregnancy [38–40]. Since the study design employed is a cross-sectional, causality may not be inferred. Social desirability bias is one of the potential biases, which may affect the results of this study. To minimize the effect of social desirability bias we recruited data collectors who have no close contact with the respondents.

5. Conclusions

This study showed that there is a high prevalence of teenage pregnancy in the area. Increased age, rural residence, contraceptive nonuse, and parental marital status (divorce) were found to have a statistically significant association with teenage pregnancy. Strengthening contraceptive service promotion and provision for teenagers by giving special attention to rural ones and showing the consequences of divorce in the community are strongly recommended.

Abbreviations

AOR: Adjusted odds ratio
CI: Confidence interval
COR: Crude Odds Ratio
CPR: Contraceptive prevalence rate
EDHS: Ethiopian Demographic Health Survey
SPSS: Statistical Package for Social Science.

Disclosure

Anteneh Yalew is Principal Investigator.

Conflicts of Interest

The authors declare that they have no conflicts of interest in this work.

Authors' Contributions

Yohannes Ayanaw Habitu, Anteneh Yalew, and Telake Azale Bisetegn were involved in study conception, design, coordination, data collection, data analysis, interpretation, and write-up. Yohannes Ayanaw Habitu prepared the manuscript. All authors read and approved the final manuscript.

Acknowledgments

The authors would like to acknowledge all the study participants for participation in the study, the data collectors, supervisors, and authorities of Wogedi district, University of Gondar, and Institute of Public Health for ethical approval.

References

[1] WHO, "Adolescent pregnancy fact sheet," 2014.

[2] UNFPA, "Motherhood in Childhood, Facing the challenge of adolescent pregnancy, state of world population," 2013.

[3] WHO, *Guidelines on Preventing Early Pregnancy and Poor Reproductive Outcome Among Adolescents in Developing Countries*, WHO, Geneva, 2011.

[4] E. Presler-Marshall and N. Jones, "Charting the future, Empowering girls to prevent early pregnancy," 2012.

[5] L. Lama, P. Rijal, S. Budathoki, and A. D. Shrestha, "Profile of neonates born to adolescent mothers at Nepal," *Nepal Medical College journal*, vol. 14, no. 4, pp. 294–297, 2012.

[6] F. Dagadu, *The Magnitude and Determinants of Teenage Pregnancy in the Cape Coast Municipality*, University of Ghana, Accra, Ghana, 1997.

[7] S. Ziadeh, "Obstetric outcome of teenage pregnancies in north Jordan," *Archives of Gynecology and Obstetrics*, vol. 265, no. 1, pp. 26–29, 2001.

[8] O. Ayuba Gani, "Outcome of teenage pregnancy in the Niger Delta of Nigeria," *Ethiopian journal of health sciences*, vol. 22, no. 1, pp. 45–50, 2012.

[9] U. M. Nwosu, "Contemporary factors of teenage pregnancy in rural communities of Abia state, Nigeria," *International Journal Of Community Medicine And Public Health*, vol. 4, no. 2, pp. 588–592, 2017.

[10] G. Mchunu, K. Peltzer, B. Tutshana, and L. Seutlwadi, "Adolescent pregnancy and associated factors in South Africa," *African health science*, vol. 12, no. 4, pp. 426–434, 2012.

[11] M. Were, "Determinants of teenage pregnancies: The case of Busia District in Kenya," *Economics & Human Biology*, vol. 5, no. 2, pp. 322–339, 2007.

[12] B. Assefa, M. Abiyou, and G. Yeneneh, "Assessment of the magnitude of teenage pregnancy and its associated factors among teenage females visiting Assosa General Hospital," *Ethiopian Medical Journal*, vol. 53, p. 53, 2015.

[13] G. K. Adam, E. M. Elhassan, A. M. Ahmed, and I. Adam, "Maternal and perinatal outcome in teenage pregnancies in Sudan," *International Journal of Gynecology and Obstetrics*, vol. 105, no. 2, pp. 170-171, 2009.

[14] Central Statistical Agency and The DHS Program ICF, *The DHS Program ICF Rockville M, USA Ethiopian Demographic and Health Survey*, vol. 201, CSA and ICF, Addis Ababa, Ethiopia and Rockville, MD, USA, 2017.

[15] Agency CI, "The World Fact Book, Country population Comparison," 2016.

[16] A. Erulkar, "Adolescence lost: The realities of child marriage," *Journal of Adolescent Health*, vol. 52, no. 5, pp. 513-514, 2013.

[17] E. Presler-Marshal and N. Jones, *Charting The Future: Empowering Girls to Prevent Early Pregnancy*, ODI and save the children, London, UK, 2012.

[18] T. Alemayehu, J. Haider, and D. Habte, "Determinants of adolescent fertility in Ethiopia," *Ethiopian Journal of Health Development*, vol. 24, no. 1, pp. 30–38, 2010.

[19] H. U. Ezegwui, L. C. Ikeako, and F. Ogbuefi, "Obstetric outcome of teenage pregnancies at a tertiary hospital in Enugu, Nigeria," *Nigerian Journal of Clinical Practice*, vol. 15, no. 2, pp. 147–150, 2012.

[20] G. Vincent and F. M. Alemu, "Factors contributing to, and effects of, teenage pregnancy in Juba," *South Sudan Medical Journal*, vol. 9, no. 2, pp. 28–31, 2016.

[21] O. E. Amoran, "A comparative analysis of predictors of teenage pregnancy and its prevention in a rural town in Western Nigeria.," *International Journal for Equity in Health*, vol. 11, article no. 37, 2012.

[22] C. Gyan, "The effects of teenage pregnancy on the educational attainment of girls at Chorkor, a suburb of Accra," *Journal of Educational and Social Research*, vol. 3, no. 3, p. 53, 2013.

[23] R. Gideon, "Factors Associated with Adolescent Pregnancy and Fertility in Uganda: Analysis of the 2011 Demographic and Health Survey Data," *The Social Science Journal*, vol. 2, no. 1, p. 7, 2013.

[24] K. Mwaba, "Perceptions of teenage pregnancy among South African adolescents," *Health SA Gesondheid*, vol. 5, no. 3, pp. 30–34, 2000.

[25] E. Presler-Marshall and N. Jones, "Charting the future: Empowering girls to prevent early pregnancy," 2012.

[26] A. de Haan, "Teenage Pregnancy and Motherhood in Merkato Slums in Ethiopia: Perspectives of Teenagers and Implications for Sexual," 2010.

[27] G. Qazi, "Obstetric characteristics and complications of teenage pregnancy," *Journal of Postgraduate Medical Institute*, vol. 25, no. 2, pp. 134–138, 2011.

[28] I. Goonewardene and R. Waduge, "Adverse effects of teenage pregnancy," *Ceylon Medical Journal*, vol. 50, no. 3, 2009.

[29] T. Ganchimeg, E. Ota, N. Morisaki et al., "Pregnancy and childbirth outcomes among adolescent mothers: a World Health Organization multicountry study," *BJOG: An International Journal of Obstetrics and Gynaecology*, vol. 121, pp. 40–48, 2014.

[30] A. Kumar, T. Singh, S. Basu, S. Pandey, and V. Bhargava, "Outcome of teenage pregnancy," *The Indian Journal of Pediatrics*, vol. 74, no. 10, pp. 927–931, 2007.

[31] E. Kovavisarach, S. Chairaj, K. Tosang, S. Asavapiriyanont, and U. Chotigeat, "Outcome of teenage pregnancy in Rajavithi Hospital," *Journal of the Medical Association of Thailand*, vol. 93, no. 1, pp. 1–8, 2010.

[32] G. Woldemichael, "Teenage Childbearing and its Health Consequences on the Mother and Child in Eritrea," *Journal of the Eritrean Medical Association*, vol. 1, no. 1, 2010.

[33] office Wwfaed, "Socio-demographic profile of wogedi woreda for the year 2016/2017," 2017.

[34] B. Assefa, "Assessment of the magnitude of teenage pregnancy and its associated factors among teenage females," *Ethiopian Medical Journal*, 2015.

[35] S. Canbaz, A. T. Sunter, C. E. Cetinoglu, and Y. Peksen, "Obstetric outcomes of adolescent pregnancies in Turkey," *Advances in Therapy*, vol. 22, no. 6, pp. 636–641, 2005.

[36] J. Bongaarts, "The fertility-inhibiting effects of the intermediate fertility variables.," *Studies in Family Planning*, vol. 13, no. 6-7, pp. 179–189, 1982.

[37] D. R. Acharya, R. Bhattarai, and A. Poobalan, "Factors associated with teenage pregnancy in South Asia," 2014.

[38] R. D. Day, "The Transition to First Intercourse among Racially and Culturally Diverse Youth," *Journal of Marriage and Family*, vol. 54, no. 4, p. 749, 1992.

[39] B. J. Ellis, J. E. Bates, K. A. Dodge et al., "Does Father Absence Place Daughters at Special Risk for Early Sexual Activity and Teenage Pregnancy?" *Child Development*, vol. 74, no. 3, pp. 801–821, 2003.

[40] R. L. Flewelling and K. E. Bauman, "Family Structure as a Predictor of Initial Substance Use and Sexual Intercourse in Early Adolescence," *Journal of Marriage and Family*, vol. 52, no. 1, p. 171, 1990.

16

Naegele Forceps Delivery and Association between Morbidity and the Number of Forceps Traction Applications

Naoki Matsumoto, Toshifumi Takenaka, Nobuyuki Ikeda, Satoshi Yazaki, and Yuichi Sato

Department of Obstetrics and Gynecology, Tatedebari Sato Hospital, 96 Wakamatsucho, Takasaki, Gunma 370-0836, Japan

Correspondence should be addressed to Naoki Matsumoto; research@matsumotoc.org

Academic Editor: Fabio Facchinetti

Objective. To present the method of Naegele forceps delivery clinically practiced by the lead author, its success rate, and morbidity and to evaluate the relationship between morbidity and the number of forceps traction applications. *Methods.* Naegele forceps delivery was performed when the fetal head reached station +2 cm, the forceps were applied in the maternal pelvic application, and traction was slowly and gently performed. In the past two years, Naegele forceps delivery was attempted by the lead author in 87 cases, which were retrospectively reviewed. *Results.* The numbers of traction applications were one in 64.7% of cases, two in 24.7%, and three or more in 10.7%. The success rate was 100%. No severe morbidity was observed in mothers or neonates. Neonatal facial injury occurred most commonly in cases with fetal head malrotation, elevated numbers of traction applications, and maternal complications. Umbilical artery acidemia most commonly occurred in cases with nonreassuring fetal status. The significant crude odds ratio for three or more traction applications was 20 in cases with malrotation. *Conclusion.* Naegele forceps delivery has a high success rate, but multiple traction applications will sometimes be required, particularly in cases with malrotation. Malrotation and elevated numbers of traction applications may lead to neonatal head damage.

1. Introduction

Recently, the very high rate of cesarean delivery has been a topic of discussion and is considered a problem that should be solved [1]. In 2011, the cesarean delivery rate was 33% of all births in the United States [2]. With the increasing rate of cesarean delivery, the rate of operative vaginal deliveries has decreased during the past 20 years [2]. In Japan, the overall rate of cesarean delivery in 2011 was 19% [3] and that at high-level medical facilities was 34% [4]. In operative vaginal delivery, the rate of forceps delivery has decreased more than that of vacuum extraction [5]. In Japanese high-level medical facilities, the rates of cesarean, vacuum, and forceps delivery are 20%, 6%, and 1%, respectively, among all deliveries except for planned cesarean deliveries [4].

Thus, forceps delivery has become a minor obstetrical method in management of labor and delivery. However, the lead author considers that forceps delivery is his first-choice method in the operative vaginal deliveries. Forceps delivery has a higher success rate than vacuum extraction [6] and affords robust reliability for an experienced operator. Nonetheless, the author always bears in mind the potential risks of forceps. Therefore, he applies the forceps sufficiently in a gentle and slow manner to avoid undue maternal and neonatal morbidity. Sometimes multiple traction applications are needed. Some obstetricians believe that forceps delivery should be completed by one forceps' traction application [7]. However, no recent study has assessed the correlation between morbidity and the number of forceps traction applications.

The aim of this study was to present the method of Naegele forceps delivery clinically practiced by the lead author and its success rate and morbidity and moreover to evaluate the relationship between morbidity and other factors including the number of forceps traction applications.

2. Methods

2.1. Delivery Procedures with Naegele Forceps. Naegele forceps are most commonly used for forceps delivery in Japan. They have adequate pelvic and cephalic curves for nonrotational forceps delivery and fenestrated blades that permit firmer grasp of the fetal head [5]. Furthermore, Japanese obstetricians commonly use Naegele forceps modified and ameliorated for the Japanese women, which are called UTokyo Naegele forceps. They have lighter weight (417 g), shorter length (35 cm), and thinner blades than the original. Indications, prerequisites, and precautions for forceps delivery that were stipulated in the guidelines for obstetrical practice in Japan [8] were followed. In principle, forceps delivery was performed when the leading point of the fetal head reached or nearly reached station +2 cm over the ischial spine. The measurement of the station was performed based on internal digital examination in the dorsal position. The station was determined as the distance on the pelvic axis from the ischial spine to the leading point of the fetal head. Before application of forceps delivery, fetal head rotation and spine position were checked by internal digital examination as well as abdominal (sometimes with transperineal) ultrasonography. Based on this assessment, fetal head malrotation was diagnosed and classified as the occiput transverse position (with rotation greater than 45 degrees) or occiput posterior position. On the decision of forceps delivery, verbal informed consent was obtained. The option of primary cesarean delivery without trial of operative vaginal delivery was presented to the patient especially when the forceps trial was considered to have a possibility of failure and relatively high risk of maternal and neonatal morbidity. Rotation with Kielland rotational forceps was attempted when it was considered that it might effectively improve malrotation. In this study, it was attempted in three cases. Effective improvement of malrotation was obtained in one case, which was excluded from this study, but not in the other two cases, which were followed by Naegele forceps delivery and were included in this study. Naegele forceps were applied in the maternal pelvic application. After articulation of the forceps, the operator (the lead author) suspended the hooks on the first and middle fingers and placed the handles on the palm of his right hand with an underhand grip. He did not usually hold the handles. To feel the exact progression and to avoid sudden emergence, the tips of the fingers of the left hand were placed on the fetal head. To avoid falling, he adopted a fighter's stance with a wide stance and slightly bent knees. Before genuine traction, test traction was applied to check the forceps grip, fetal head movement, and feeling of fetal descent. Except in urgent situations, forceps traction was applied slowly and gently in synchrony with contractions and pushing efforts to avoid undue maternal and neonatal damage and forceps slipoff. Traction was directed, as per principle, along the axis of the birth canal with no rotational movement. Episiotomy (midline or mediolateral) was performed if necessary. The forceps were disarticulated when the operator considered

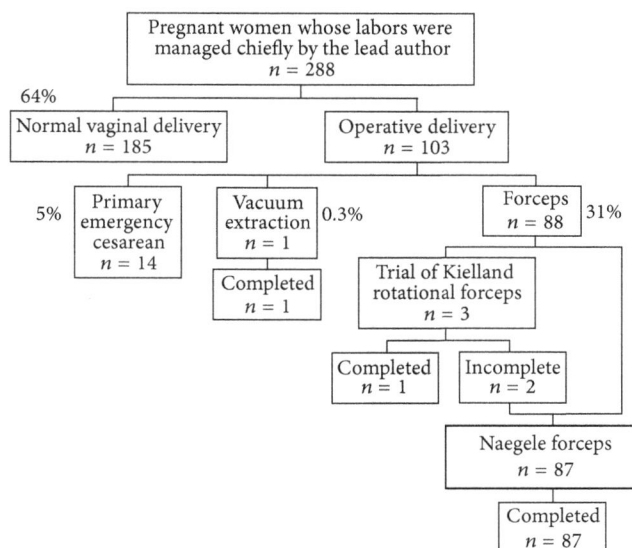

FIGURE 1: Mode of delivery of 288 term pregnant women with live singleton pregnancies and cephalic presentation whose labor and delivery were managed chiefly by the lead author.

the fetal head would not recede. The operator dictated a midwife to support the delivery by perineal protection when required. Forceps application was halted when the operator felt no evidence of progressive descent with three traction applications at most.

2.2. Study Design. The study period was the past two years from July 2012 to June 2014. In this period, 288 term pregnant women with live singleton pregnancies and cephalic presentation were managed chiefly by the lead author. In 87 of these cases, Naegele forceps delivery was attempted and successfully completed (Figure 1). We retrospectively reviewed the 87 cases and obtained patient characteristic factors, parturition outcomes, and short-term (during a period of one month after delivery) maternal and neonatal morbidity outcomes from the medical records.

The relationships between characteristic factors and morbidity were assessed by Fisher's exact test. The five morbidity outcomes considered were as follows: maternal anal sphincter injuries, acute postpartum urinary retention lasting over 24 h, dehiscence or maternal injuries except for perineal lacerations, neonatal facial injuries, and umbilical artery acidemia. Anal sphincter injuries were defined as third- or fourth-degree perineal lacerations. Acute postpartum urinary retention was defined as a postvoid residual volume of >100 mL. Neonatal facial injuries were defined as forceps marks with bruising or skin lacerations. Umbilical artery acidemia was defined as acidemia with umbilical artery pH <7.2. The relationship between characteristic factors and the number of traction applications was assessed by calculation of crude odds ratios for two or more and three or more traction applications.

The study protocol was approved by the ethical review board of the hospital. Two-tailed *P* values and confidence intervals were calculated using univariate methods including

Fisher's exact test and univariate logistic regression. P values of <0.05 were considered statistically significant.

3. Results

The characteristics of 87 patients on whom Naegele forceps delivery was performed are presented in Table 1. The proportion of nulliparas in the study group (82.8%) was larger than that in the normal vaginal delivery group (35.1%) in the same period. Maternal complications included gestational diabetes mellitus (11.5%), pregnancy-induced hypertension (10.3%), and psychiatric disorders (4.6%). One case with a previous cesarean history was managed for a trial of labor after cesarean. Fetal head malrotation was diagnosed in 14 (16.1%) cases before forceps delivery, including seven cases each of occiput transverse and occiput posterior position. The numbers of forceps traction applications were one in 64.7% of cases, two in 24.7%, and three or more in 10.7%. The maximum number of traction applications was six. Uterine fundal pressure maneuvers were required only in two (2.3%) cases. The median and maximum traction-to-delivery times were 2 min and 13 min, respectively.

No forceps failure and no slipoff were experienced in the study period, so that the success rate was 100%. No case of shoulder dystocia occurred. Morbidity associated with the forceps deliveries is presented in Table 2. No severe morbidity was seen in the mothers or neonates during short-term observation. Maternal anal sphincter injuries occurred in 35.6%. All cases of anal sphincter injury were appropriately examined and repaired using absorbable sutures without leading to severe problems. Acute postpartum urinary retention lasting over 24 h was seen in 13.8% of cases. All of these cases were eventually resolved by passive catheter bladder drainage. Eight (66.7%) of these cases were resolved within 48 h after delivery. The longest duration to resolution of urinary retention was eight days after delivery. Dehiscence and maternal injuries except for perineal lacerations were seen in five cases (5.7%). They included two cases of pudendal hematoma, two cases of pubic symphysis pain, and one case of wound abscess, which were all resolved in a short period. Neonatal facial injuries were seen in 18.4% of cases. All were mild, and no treatment was indicated. Concerning umbilical artery acidemia, no severe acidemia and no severe neonatal asphyxia were seen. Apgar scores (at 1 and/or 5 min) lower than 7 were not observed.

The relationships between patient characteristic factors and morbidity are described in Table 3. No significant relationship was observed between any of these factors and maternal morbidity. Neonatal facial injury occurred most commonly in cases with malrotation, elevated numbers of traction applications, and maternal complications. Umbilical artery acidemia occurred most commonly in cases with chief indication of nonreassuring fetal status.

Figure 2 shows the crude odds ratios for two or more and three or more traction applications. Significant odds ratios for two or more traction applications were 5.5, 3.3, and 2.9 in cases with malrotation, augmentation, and station of ≤+2, respectively. Significant odds ratios for three or more traction applications were 20 in cases with malrotation.

TABLE 1: Characteristics of the 87 pregnant women on whom Naegele forceps delivery was performed.

Factors	Median	Range	n	%
Gestational age at delivery (weeks)	39 5/7	37 3/7–41 4/7		
Early term (37 0/7–38 6/7 weeks)			19	21.8
Full term (39 0/7–40 6/7 weeks)			56	64.4
Late term (41 0/7 weeks and after)			12	13.8
Age (years)	32	19–40		
Parity				
Nullipara			72	82.8
Para 1			11	12.6
Para 2			4	4.6
Maternal complications			37	42.5
Maternal height (cm)	158	147–170		
Maternal weight at labor (kg)	59.6	44.7–91.8		
Maternal BMI at labor (kg/m²)	24.2	18.6–34.8		
Neonatal birth weight (g)	3036	2072–3926		
Augmentation			48	55.2
Epidural analgesia			18	20.7
Episiotomy			35	40.2
Midline			24	27.6
Mediolateral			11	12.6
Fetal head malrotation			14	16.1
Chief indication				
Prolonged second stage			51	58.6
Nonreassuring fetal status			33	37.9
Severe PIH			3	3.4
Station (cm)				
+1			2	2.4
+2			41	47.7
+3			30	34.9
≥+4			13	15.1
Missing			1	
Numbers of forceps traction applications				
1			55	64.7
2			21	24.7
3			5	5.9
4			2	2.4
5			1	1.2
6			1	1.2
Missing			2	
Uterine fundal pressure maneuver			2	2.3
Traction-to-delivery intervals (min)	2	0–13		

BMI: body mass index; PIH: pregnancy-induced hypertension.

4. Discussion

All cases were successfully delivered by the Naegele forceps delivery according to the lead author's method as mentioned

TABLE 2: Morbidity associated with Naegele forceps deliveries.

Morbidity	n	%
Maternal morbidity		
Postpartum hemorrhage >500 mL	5	5.7
Blood transfusion	1	1.1
Perineal laceration		
None	0	0.0
1st degree	2	2.3
2nd degree	54	62.1
3rd degree	26	29.9
4th degree	5	5.7
Acute postpartum urinary retention lasting over 24 h	12	13.8
Dehiscence and maternal injury except for perineal lacerations	5	5.7
Neonatal morbidity		
Facial injuries	16	18.4
Cephalohematoma	3	3.4
Umbilical artery acidemia		
Umbilical artery pH: 7.10–7.19	8	9.2
Umbilical artery pH: <7.1	0	0.0
Neonatal intensive care unit admission	1	1.1

in the Methods. The forceps delivery was completed with one forceps' traction application in approximately two-thirds of the cases, within two in nearly 90%, and within three in 95%. Malrotation is associated with traction applied three times or more. Malrotation and elevated numbers of forceps traction applications were both related to the occurrence of neonatal facial injury. No severe morbidity was seen in mothers and neonates in the short-term observation.

All the cases were successfully delivered and no forceps failure or slipoff was seen. The success rate of operative vaginal delivery will vary with the chosen type of instrument. In a meta-analysis, O'Mahony et al. [6] reported that forceps delivery was less likely (with risk ratio 0.65) to fail to achieve a vaginal delivery with the chosen instrument than vacuum extraction. In a large-scale retrospective cohort study, Ben-Haroush et al. [9] reported that the failure rates of forceps and vacuum extraction were 1.3% and 10.0%, respectively. Even in cases with failed vacuum extraction, the failure rate of subsequent forceps was 3.5%. Generally, forceps delivery is considered to have a higher success rate than vacuum extraction [6, 10–13]. However, the success rates of operative vaginal delivery will vary with other factors including range of indication, approval for subsequent forceps after failed vacuum extraction, and the operator's proficiency and preference [14].

In this study, forceps delivery was completed with one traction application in approximately two-thirds of cases, within two in nearly 90%, and within three in 95%. In a trial with vacuum extraction, excessive numbers of pulls are considered to increase the risk of neonatal morbidity [10–13]. The guidelines for obstetrical practice in Japan [8]

recommend five or fewer pulls in vacuum extraction. In contrast, excessive numbers of forceps traction applications are rarely discussed. There are no recent studies and no recommendations concerning the allowable maximum number of forceps traction applications. Not only in vacuum extraction but also in forceps delivery, multiple traction applications will sometimes be required in cases of dystocia, particularly with fetal head malrotation. In the present study, malrotation seems to be the strongest predictive factor to elevate the number of forceps traction applications. Fetal head malrotation and elevated numbers of forceps traction applications are both risk factors for neonatal facial injury. In the present study, the neonatal facial injuries were mild; therefore, our results may be insufficient to discuss the association between forceps delivery and severe neonatal injuries. However, we believe that our results imply a potential risk for severe neonatal head damage in cases with malrotation and/or elevated numbers of traction applications. Careful attention to the risk factors is thus required.

The rate of maternal anal sphincter injury in forceps deliveries is considered to be approximately 30% [11]. However, the rate will vary with facility and practitioner. Hirsch et al. [15] reported historically two anal sphincter injury rates in their level III teaching hospital. After they promulgated a recommendation to reduce the occurrence of high-degree perineal laceration, the rate of anal sphincter injury with operative vaginal delivery declined from 41% to 26% and that with forceps declined from 40% to 28%. The present lead author usually performs forceps delivery with priority given to delayed disarticulation for smooth fetal head expulsion and midline episiotomy for reducing postsuture pain when episiotomy is needed. There may still be room for measures to reduce the occurrence of anal sphincter injury. Operative vaginal delivery is associated with the occurrence of postpartum urinary retention [16]. Symptoms are brief and are typically resolved within 24 to 48 h of passive catheter bladder drainage [5].

In their large-scale retrospective cohort study, Werner et al. [17] reported that forceps delivery had a lower risk of adverse neonatal outcomes including cephalohematoma, low Apgar score, and neurologic complications and posed a higher risk of facial nerve palsy than did vacuum extraction. In their meta-analysis, O'Mahony et al. [6] reported that facial injury was more likely with forceps but cephalohematoma was more likely with vacuum. Sequential use of vacuum and forceps is associated with increased risk of both maternal and neonatal injury [18]. Relatively low neonatal morbidity and high success rate are the chief reasons for the lead author's choice of forceps for the first-choice instrument.

The management of cases with occiput transverse position is clinically indeterminate. Recently, some researchers have reevaluated the value of Kielland rotational forceps delivery for fetal head malrotation [19, 20]. The lead author uses the method only for cases with deep occiput transverse position, which presents a relatively wide gap within the birth canal to accommodate insertion of the blades of the Kielland forceps and its rotational maneuvering. In cases of dystocia, particularly with malrotation, nonrotational forceps delivery poses a risk of rare and sometimes severe outcomes such

TABLE 3: Relationship between patient characteristics and morbidity.

Factors	Maternal anal sphincter injury ($n = 31$)		Acute postpartum urinary retention lasting over 24 h ($n = 12$)		Dehiscence and maternal injury except for perineal lacerations ($n = 5$)		Neonatal facial injuries ($n = 16$)		Umbilical artery acidemia ($n = 8$)	
	%	P	%	P	%	P	%	P	%	P
Gestational age at delivery										
Early term (37 0/7-38 6/7 weeks)	35.7		16.7		5.3		25.0		10.5	
Full term (39 0/7-40 6/7 weeks)	31.6	0.85	12.5	0.73	7.1	>0.99	26.3	0.56	8.9	>0.99
Late term (41 0/7 weeks and after)	41.7		16.7		0.0		16.7		8.3	
Maternal age										
≥35 years	48.0	0.15	11.3	0.31	4.0	>0.99	12.0	0.54	4.0	0.43
<35 years	30.7		20.8		6.5		21.0		11.3	
Parity										
Nullipara	37.5	0.56	12.7	0.44	6.9	0.39	20.8	0.29	9.3	>0.99
Multipara	26.7		20.0		0.0		6.7		6.7	
Maternal complications										
Yes	27.0	0.15	16.7	0.55	2.7	0.30	32.4	0.005*	5.4	0.46
No	42.0		12.0		8.0		8.0		12.0	
Maternal height										
<155 cm	36.0	>0.99	12.0	>0.99	8.0	0.63	28.0	0.22	4.0	0.43
≥155 cm	35.5		14.8		4.8		14.5		11.3	
Maternal BMI at labor										
≥29 kg/m²	50.0	0.46	37.5	0.064	0.0	>0.99	12.5	1	0.0	>0.99
<29 kg/m²	34.6		10.4		6.4		19.2		10.3	
Neonatal birth weight										
≥3500 g	35.7	>0.99	7.1	0.70	0.0	0.59	21.4	0.72	7.1	>0.99
<3500 g	35.6		15.3		6.9		17.8		9.6	
Augmentation										
Yes	43.8	0.12	10.3	0.54	6.3	>0.99	25.0	0.099	6.3	0.46
No	25.6		17.0		5.1		10.3		12.8	
Epidural analgesia										
Yes	38.9	0.79	22.2	0.27	1.1	0.28	22.2	0.74	5.6	>0.99
No	34.8		11.8		4.4		17.4		10.1	
Episiotomy										
Yes	40.0	0.51	5.7	0.12	8.6	0.39	20.0	0.79	2.9	0.14
No	32.7		19.6		3.9		17.3		13.5	
Fetal head malrotation										
Yes	42.9	0.56	7.1	0.69	0.0	0.59	64.3	<0.001*	7.1	>0.99
No	34.3		15.3		6.9		9.6		9.6	
Station										
≤+2 cm	27.9	0.26	14.3	>0.99	4.7	>0.99	20.9	0.79	11.6	0.71
>+2 cm	41.9		14.0		7.0		16.3		7.0	
Chief indication										
Prolonged second stage	43.1		16.0		5.9		23.5		2.0	
Nonreassuring fetal status	24.2	0.11	12.1	0.85	3.0	>0.99	6.1	0.053	26.9	0.0053*
Severe PIH†	33.3		0.0		0.0		66.7		0.0	
Numbers of forceps traction applications										
1	34.5		16.7		7.3		7.3		5.5	
2	42.9	0.58	14.3	0.58	4.8	>0.99	19.0	<0.001*	14.3	0.14
≥3	22.2		0.0		0.0		88.9		22.2	

Percentages mean proportions of the morbidity in each factor. P values were calculated using Fisher's exact test.
BMI: body mass index; PIH: pregnancy-induced hypertension.
*Statistically significant.
†Chief indication of severe PIH was excluded from the statistical test because of the lack of the cases ($n = 3$).

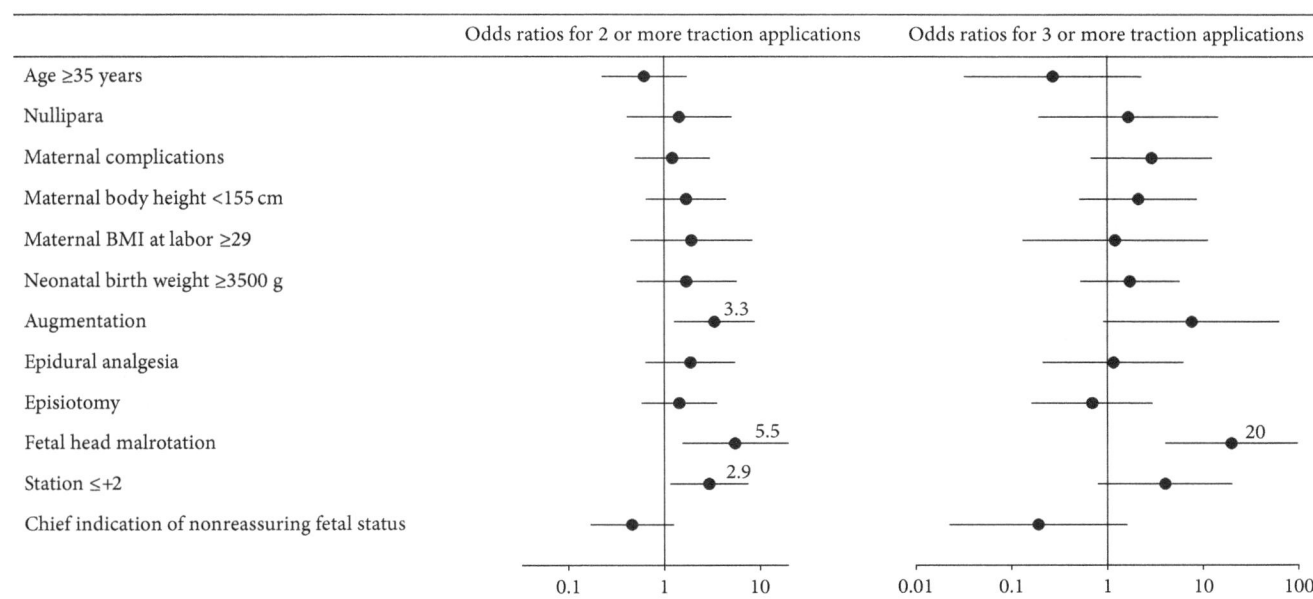

FIGURE 2: Crude odds ratios for two or more and three or more traction applications. Horizontal bars indicate 95% confidence intervals. BMI: body mass index.

as facial nerve palsy [21], depressed skull fracture [22], and corneal abrasion [23]. If the Kielland rotational forceps can be used in the given situation, using it prior to Naegele forceps may reduce the risk of neonatal head damage. The lead author suggests four important points that a forceps operator should recognize: accurate diagnosis of fetal head position including rotation and station, gentle traction, anticipation of potential risks in each case before forceps trial, and decisiveness for halting the forceps trial if descent is not detected.

As described here, the lead author gives priority to forceps delivery for operative vaginal delivery. In the author's opinion, particularly for the fetus and neonates, excessive stress can be avoided not only in cases with successful forceps delivery but also in cases with failed forceps delivery, as compared to cases with vacuum extraction. The reasons are relatively short traction-to-delivery time, no need of uterine fundal pressure maneuvers, and even in failure cases the possibility of an early decision to halt the forceps trial. Excessive pulls of vacuum extraction with uterine fundal pressure maneuvers may lead to infant cerebral palsy and uterine rupture [24]. We hope that the value of forceps delivery will be rerecognized and that many obstetric residents will be given the chance of training in the method and technique of forceps delivery.

Disclosure

The summary of this report was presented at the 67th Academic Conference of the Japan Society of Obstetrics and Gynecology, Yokohama, Japan, 2015.

Conflict of Interests

The authors have no conflict of interests to declare.

References

[1] A. B. Caughey, A. G. Cahill, J. M. Guise, and D. J. Rouse, "Safe prevention of the primary cesarean delivery," *American Journal of Obstetrics & Gynecology*, vol. 210, no. 3, pp. 179–193, 2014.

[2] J. A. Martin, B. E. Hamilton, S. J. Ventura, M. J. K. Osterman, and T. J. Mathews, "Births: final data for 2011," *National Vital Statistics Reports*, vol. 62, no. 1, pp. 1–69, 2013.

[3] K. Ishikawa, T. Sugihara, T. Ikeda, and R. Miyazaki, "Recent trends in cesarean delivery rates in Japan," *Journal of Japan Society of Perinatal and Neonatal Medicine*, vol. 49, no. 1, pp. 383–387, 2013 (Japanese).

[4] N. Unno, H. Masuzaki, N. Kanayama, T. Kubo, K. Fujimori, and Y. Matsuda, "Annual report of perinatology committee," *Acta Obstetrica et Gynaecologica Japonica*, vol. 65, no. 6, pp. 1377–1419, 2013 (Japanese).

[5] "Operative vaginal delivery," in *Williams Obstetrics*, F. G. Cunningham, K. J. Leveno, S. L. Bloom et al., Eds., pp. 574–586, McGraw-Hill, New York, NY, USA, 24th edition, 2014.

[6] F. O'Mahony, G. J. Hofmeyr, and V. Menon, "Choice of instruments for assisted vaginal delivery," *Cochrane Database of Systematic Reviews*, no. 11, Article ID CD005455, 2010.

[7] N. Miyasaka and T. Aso, "Forceps delivery," *Acta Obstetrica et Gynaecologica Japonica*, vol. 54, no. 7, pp. N186–N191, 2002 (Japanese).

[8] H. Minakami, Y. Hiramatsu, M. Koresawa et al., "Guidelines for obstetrical practice in Japan: Japan Society of Obstetrics and Gynecology (JSOG) and Japan Association of Obstetricians and Gynecologists (JAOG) 2011 edition," *The Journal of Obstetrics and Gynaecology Research*, vol. 37, no. 9, pp. 1174–1197, 2011.

[9] A. Ben-Haroush, N. Melamed, B. Kaplan, and Y. Yogev, "Predictors of failed operative vaginal delivery: a single-center experience," *American Journal of Obstetrics & Gynecology*, vol. 197, no. 3, pp. 308.e1–308.e5, 2007.

[10] American College of Obstetricians and Gynecologists (ACOG), *ACOG Practice Bulletin No. 17: Operative Vaginal Delivery*, American College of Obstetricians and Gynecologists (ACOG), Washington, DC, USA, 2000.

[11] Y. M. Cargill, C. J. MacKinnon, M. Y. Arsenault et al., "Guidelines for operative vaginal birth," *Journal of Obstetrics and Gynaecology Canada*, vol. 26, no. 8, pp. 747–761, 2004.

[12] Royal College of Obstetricians and Gynaecologists (RCOG), *Green-Top Guideline No. 26: Operative Vaginal Delivery*, Royal College of Obstetricians and Gynaecologists (RCOG), London, UK, 2011.

[13] C. Vayssiere, G. Beucher, O. Dupuis et al., "Instrumental delivery: clinical practice guidelines from the French College of Gynaecologists and Obstetricians," *European Journal of Obstetrics & Gynecology and Reproductive Biology*, vol. 159, no. 1, pp. 43–48, 2011.

[14] E. R. Yeomans, "Operative vaginal delivery," *Obstetrics and Gynecology*, vol. 115, no. 3, pp. 645–653, 2010.

[15] E. Hirsch, E. I. Haney, T. E. J. Gordon, and R. K. Silver, "Reducing high-order perineal laceration during operative vaginal delivery," *The American Journal of Obstetrics and Gynecology*, vol. 198, no. 6, pp. 668.e1–668.e5, 2008.

[16] F. E. M. Mulder, M. A. Schoffelmeer, R. A. Hakvoort et al., "Risk factors for postpartum urinary retention: a systematic review and meta-analysis," *BJOG: An International Journal of Obstetrics & Gynaecology*, vol. 119, no. 12, pp. 1440–1446, 2012.

[17] E. F. Werner, T. M. Janevic, J. Illuzzi, E. F. Funai, D. A. Savitz, and H. S. Lipkind, "Mode of delivery in nulliparous women and neonatal intracranial injury," *Obstetrics and Gynecology*, vol. 118, no. 6, pp. 1239–1246, 2011.

[18] C. Gardella, M. Taylor, T. Benedetti, J. Hitti, and C. Critchlow, "The effect of sequential use of vacuum and forceps for assisted vaginal delivery on neonatal and maternal outcomes," *American Journal of Obstetrics & Gynecology*, vol. 185, no. 4, pp. 896–902, 2001.

[19] S. J. Stock, K. Josephs, S. Farquharson et al., "Maternal and neonatal outcomes of successful Kielland's rotational forceps delivery," *Obstetrics and Gynecology*, vol. 121, no. 5, pp. 1032–1039, 2013.

[20] N. Tempest, A. Hart, S. Walkinshaw, and D. K. Hapangama, "A re-evaluation of the role of rotational forceps: retrospective comparison of maternal and perinatal outcomes following different methods of birth for malposition in the second stage of labour," *BJOG: An International Journal of Obstetrics and Gynaecology*, vol. 120, no. 10, pp. 1277–1284, 2013.

[21] K. Al Tawil, N. Saleem, H. Kadri, M. T. Rifae, and H. Tawakol, "Traumatic facial nerve palsy in newborns: is it always iatrogenic?" *American Journal of Perinatology*, vol. 27, no. 9, pp. 711–713, 2010.

[22] O. Dupuis, R. Silveira, C. Dupont et al., "Comparison of 'instrument-associated' and 'spontaneous' obstetric depressed skull fractures in a cohort of 68 neonates," *American Journal of Obstetrics and Gynecology*, vol. 192, no. 1, pp. 165–170, 2005.

[23] M. A. Honig, J. Barraquer, H. D. Perry, J. L. Riquelme, and W. R. Green, "Forceps and vacuum injuries to the cornea: histopathologic features of twelve cases and review of the literature," *Cornea*, vol. 15, no. 5, pp. 463–472, 1996.

[24] Japan Council for Quality Health Care, *The Japan Obstetric Compensation System for Cerebral Palsy: The 4th Report about the Prevention of Recurrence*, Japan Council for Quality Health Care, Tokyo, Japan, 2014, (Japanese).

17

Utilization of Antenatal Care Services in Dalit Communities in Gorkha, Nepal

Mamata Sherpa Awasthi (ID),[1] **Kiran Raj Awasthi** (ID),[2] **Harish Singh Thapa**,[3] **Bhuvan Saud** (ID),[1,4] **Sarita Pradhan**,[5] **and Roshani Agrawal Khatry**[5]

[1]*Department of Nursing, Janamaitri Foundation Institute of Health Sciences, Hattiban, Lalitpur, Nepal*
[2]*Save the Children, Malaria Program, Nepal*
[3]*Department of Pharmacy, Janamaitri Foundation Institute of Health Sciences, Hattiban, Lalitpur, Nepal*
[4]*Department of Medical Laboratory Technology, Janamaitri Foundation Institute of Health Sciences, Hattiban, Lalitpur, Nepal*
[5]*Department of Nursing, Lalitpur Nursing Campus, Sanepa, Lalitpur, Nepal*

Correspondence should be addressed to Mamata Sherpa Awasthi; link2mamata@gmail.com
and Kiran Raj Awasthi; kiran.awasthi@savethechildren.org

Academic Editor: Luca Marozio

Background and Objective. Antenatal care (ANC) is one of the main components of maternal health. Utilization of safe motherhood is deprived in women who belong to low-caste groups like Dalit of Nepal. Low socioeconomic status, poor knowledge and awareness on obstetric complications, lack of decision-making autonomy, and limited health care options lead to underutilization of existing maternal health care service. The aim of this study was to ascertain the utilization of antenatal care services in terms of ANC visits with health personnel, receiving recommended period of iron tablets, consumption of antihelminthes and number of Tetanus Toxoid (TT) vaccines taken among child bearing women in Dalit community. *Materials and Methods.* Descriptive cross-sectional research design was used to conduct the study of 150 child bearing women of reproductive age (15-49 years) having at least one child up to three years of age in a Dalit community of Gorkha from March 2015 to March 2016. The data was collected from each mother by conducting face to face interview with each household by using a questionnaire. *Result.* The study revealed that mean age at marriage of respondents was 17.7 years and mean age at first pregnancy was 18 years. 44.6% of respondents experienced complication during last pregnancy, labour, and postpartum period in their last pregnancy. 59.3% of respondents stated that neighbors, relatives, and traditional healers were the best first contact person during health problem of women. 76.0% of respondents had attended antepartum visit during their last pregnancy whereas 24.0% of respondents did not attend any antepartum clinic. 68.3% of the mothers had consumed Iron/Folates within 45 days after delivery. Only 30.0% of respondents received antihelminthes (albendazole) while 70.0% of respondents had received TT Vaccines during their last pregnancy. Age, type of family, and education of the mothers were significantly associated with utilization of antenatal care services. *Conclusion.* Even though there is reasonable good utilization rate of antenatal service, the study revealed that low education and awareness among mothers, low socioeconomic condition, early marriage and pregnancy, inappropriate antenatal health check-up, and cultural taboos were significant factors affecting the satisfactory utilization of services among the Dalit community. Hence, there is a need to emphasize on raising awareness of Dalit mothers for receiving available prenatal services.

1. Introduction

Maternal mortality is one of the major causes of death among women of reproductive age in developing countries. The annual number of maternal deaths was estimated 303,000 in 2015. Globally, maternal death accounted to be approximately 99% deaths in developing regions [1]. Despite Antenatal care (ANC) being one of the four major initiatives of the Safe Motherhood Initiative, its relative contribution to improving the maternal health morbidity and mortality still is uncertain and debatable. Nonetheless some of the ANC procedures have been found to be beneficial [2]. World Health Organization (WHO) recommends a four-visit ANC schedule for low risk pregnancies [3]. During these visits, the components of

ANC suggested in Nepal include iron supplementation, blood and urine tests, at least two Tetanus Toxoid (TT) injections, blood pressure measurement, intestinal parasite drugs, and health education related to pregnancy and detection of the problems that make the pregnancy high risk one [4, 5]. It is difficult to predict which expectant mother will develop pregnancy related complications that is why it is essential that all pregnant women must have an access to high quality obstetric care throughout their pregnancies. Maternal complications and poor perinatal outcome are usually associated with other factors like nonutilization of antenatal and delivery care services and poor socioeconomic condition of the family. Unwanted outcomes are seen in those mothers who have not done ANC registration compared to registered one [6].

In Nepal, utilization of maternal health services depends on the Socio Economic Status (SES) of women. Higher SES women in terms of education level, wealth and urban residence utilize better health care services including maternity care [7]. Dalits are defined as untouchables and marginalized groups within the Hindu caste system. Often the social, economic, and health status and political conditions among these population are lowest compared to other groups in Nepal [8]. Women from Dalit community suffer from not only discrimination based on their gender but also caste identity and consequent economic deprivation [9]. Dalit women face numerous barriers in accessing maternal healthcare services due to their lower status in the society and, in Nepal, women with disabilities and women from Dalit caste groups are with low rates of maternal health service utilization [10, 11].

A study done in Bara district in the same community found that 41.6% of mothers did not receive any antenatal checkup while only 28.0% completed all four ANC visits, more than 55.0% had not taken vaccine, and 48.3% had not taken folic acid during pregnancy period [12]. Based on the Dalit women's status in the country, it is therefore necessary to identify the gaps in the utilization of antenatal health care services so that the condition of Dalit women, particularly their awareness and utilization of antenatal health can be improved. Therefore, the present study will help to investigate the status of ANC services, i.e., ANC visits with health personnel, receiving days of iron tablets and number of TT vaccines taken during last pregnancy in Dalit community in rural area health care facilities.

2. Materials and Methods

Quantitative descriptive cross-sectional design was adopted to find out the utilization of antenatal care services among child bearing women of reproductive age (15-49 years) having at least one child up to three years of age in a Dalit community between March 2015 to March 2016 in wards one, two, and three in Gorkha municipality, a hilly district in central Nepal. A list of households having child bearing women with child up to 3 years from these wards where predominantly Dalit communities resided was obtained from Female Community Health Volunteers (FCHV). A total number of 150 child bearing women having at least one child up to 3 years of age were considered for this research.

Pretesting of the instrument was done in 16 (10%) of child bearing women having a child up to 3 years in ward number 8 Tanchintar of Godawari where Dalit community were predominant. Permission from the concerned authorities was obtained by submitting a written request letter to the local Village development committee. Selected child bearing women having child up to 3 years were interviewed from each household. The confidentiality of respondent was maintained through code numbers in questionnaire. Each respondent was informed that she had right to withdraw from the study at any time without prejudice to her care. An informal verbal consent was obtained from each of them prior to conducting the face to face interview for data collection. The duration of interview was about 40-50 minutes which was mentioned prior to conducting the interview.

3. Data Analysis

The collected data was analyzed by using Statistical Package for Social Science (SPSS) 20 version. Descriptive statistics such as frequency, percentage, mean, standard deviation, and inferential statistics (chi-square test) was used to measure the association between different variables and utilization of antenatal care services in the Dalit community.

4. Results

Table 1 shows the sociodemographic characteristics of the women. Out of the total women in the study 51.4% of respondents were of age group of less than or equal to 25 years while 73.3% of the respondents had married at an age of less than or equal to 18 years while the mean age of marriage was 17.7. A total of 84.7% of the respondents had become pregnant for the first time at an age of less than or equal to 20 years with the mean age of pregnancy being 18 years. Out of these mothers 7.3% of them had given birth more than four times. It was found that 75.3% of respondents belonged to a nuclear family (not living with their inlaws) while the rest of them live in joint families (couple living with their inlaws). The results showed that 68% of the decision makers in the family were husbands. In this study all of the respondents were Hindus. Primary level of education was completed by only 44.7% of the respondents where as 26.6% of respondents were illiterate. Nearly half of the mothers were housewives and worked at home.

As illustrated in Table 2, 76.0% of respondents had attended an ANC clinic out of which a further 72.8% of had undergone four or more ANC visits. It was observed that 51.8% of the respondents had their first ANC visit in the fourth or later months of pregnancy. All of the respondents who visited hospital for antepartum care attended a government hospital. Table 2 depicts that 24.0% of respondents did not attend any antepartum care. The main reasons for not attending an antepartum clinic by 38.9% of mothers were due to inadequate knowledge regarding obstetric complication and availability of free safe motherhood services across the public hospitals. Furthermore, 27.7% of the respondents indicated that that they did not face any problem/complication

TABLE 1: Respondents' characteristics.

Items	Frequency	Percentage
Age (in Years)		
<=25	77	51.4
26-30	59	39.3
31=>	14	9.3
Mean ±SD =	25.8±3.6	
Age at Marriage (in Years)		
<=18	110	73.3
19=+	40	26.7
Mean ±SD =	17.7±1.7	
Age at First Pregnancy(in Years)		
<=20	127	84.7
20=+	23	15.3
Mean ±SD =	18±1.7	
Number of Pregnancies		
One Time	39	26.0
Two Times	51	34.0
Three Times	49	32.7
Four or more Times	11	7.3
Type of family		
Nuclear Family	113	75.3
Joint Family	37	24.7
Decision Maker of the family		
Husband		
Father-in-Law	26	17.4
Mother-in-Law	11	7.3
Husband	102	68.0
Self	11	7.3
Religion		
Hindu	150	100.0
Education level		
Illiterate	40	26.6
Primary level	67	44.7
Secondary level	36	24.0
Higher secondary level	7	4.7
Occupation		
House-maker	74	49.4
Business	8	5.3
Service	7	4.7
Daily wages	53	35.3
Agriculture	8	5.3

during their pregnancy; therefore did not feel the need of any ANC care, while the remaining 16.7% cited lack of time due to household choirs, field work, and traditional views of their inlaws that pregnancy based on their personal experiences as the main reasons for not undergoing the predelivery checkups.

As shown in Table 3, 82.0% of respondents had consumed Iron/Folates out of which 68.3% of them had consumed Iron/Folates up to 45 days postdelivery. Only 30.0% of respondents received antihelminthes (albendazole). The reason for not taking antihelminthes in 85.9% of the mothers was due to the fact that they had not been prescribed by the health facility. This could be because the hospital health care providers were not aware of prescribing antihelminthes during pregnancy or may have been due to stock out of the medicines in their facility. In addition to this, it was observed that a majority of respondents had attended antepartum care in a nearby government hospital. A total of 70% mothers had received TT Vaccines and among them 65.7% received both the recommended doses during the period of their pregnancy.

Table 4 indicates that around two third of respondents utilized antenatal care services well whereas 39.3% of respondents had poor utilization of antenatal care services.

The association between sociodemographic variables and utilization of antenatal care services has been illustrated in Table 5. It was observed that 88.3% of the respondents aged less than 25 years utilized antenatal care services more suggestive of a statistically significant association between age of mother and utilization of antenatal care services. Furthermore, the results also illustrated that 76.4% of literate mothers underwent safe motherhood practices. This high percentage indicates a significant relationship between educational status and utilization of antenatal care services at 95% level of confidence ($p < 0.05$). Mothers from nuclear families were strongly associated with utilization of antenatal care services 95% level of confidence ($p < 0.05$) compared to those that live in joint families. Age at marriage and age at first pregnancy of respondents were not found to be statistically significant to utilization of the Safe Motherhood Practices.

5. Discussion

The current study showed that the mean age of the mothers was 25.8 (SD, 3.6). A total of 73.3% of respondents got married at an age of less than or equal to 18 years with a mean age of marriage among all respondents at 17.7 years (SD, 1.7). It was noted that 84.7% of the respondents became pregnant before they were 20 years which is similar to the findings of the study done at Bara district of Nepal among a similar Dalit community where 53.3% were married between the age of 15 and 19 years [12]. The results of another study conducted among similar group in Rupandehi of Nepal also showed early pregnancy among 72.55 of the women, which further adds weight to the fact that women from Dalit castes are predisposed to a higher risk of obstetric complications including higher mortality rates [13, 14]. This result pinpoints the fact that majority of women from the lower castes especially the Dalits get married before the legal age of marriage (i.e.18 years) and become pregnant before the age of reproductive maturity. This could be attributed to poor economic status and strong sociocultural beliefs instilled within the community. Early marriage and childbearing age plays a significant role in reproductive health and utilization of maternal health care practices. Studies have proven that pregnancy at an early age could lead to miscarriage and even bring about unwanted complications during and after

TABLE 2: ANC visits for pregnancy checkups.

Item	Frequency	Percentage (%)
ANC Visits		
Yes	114	76.0
No	36	24.0
Number of ANC visit during last pregnancy(n=114)		
Once	8	7.0
Two times	4	3.5
Three times	19	16.7
Four times or more	83	72.8
Month of ANC visit for first time(n=114)		
2nd month of pregnancy	24	21.1
3rd month of pregnancy	31	27.1
4th and later month of pregnancy	59	51.8
Place of antenatal visit for check up during last pregnancy(n=114)		
Government	114	100.0
If not visited, reason for not visit health centre for antepartum care(n=36)		
Lack of Knowledge	14	38.9
Lack of time	6	16.7
Traditional View of in laws	6	16.7
Not having any problem during pregnancy	10	27.7

TABLE 3: Respondents' utilization of medicines during antepartum period.

Items	Frequency	Percentage (%)
Consumption of Iron/Foliate		
Yes	123	82.0
No	27	18.0
If yes, duration of iron/foliate tablets consumed(n=123)		
until delivery	39	31.7
up to 45days after delivery	84	68.3
Intake of anti-helminthes (n=150)		
Yes	45	30.0%
No	92	61.3%
Don't remember(Unsure)	13	8.7%
Reason for not taking Anti-helminthes (n=92)		
Not prescribed	79	85.9%
No Antepartum Visit	13	14.1%
TT Vaccine (n=150)		
Yes	105	70.0
No	45	30.0
Number of TT vaccine		
Received (n=105)		
One dose or booster	36	34.3%
Two doses	69	65.7%

TABLE 4: Overall utilization of antenatal care services.

Item	Frequency	Percentage
Utilization of Antenatal Care Services		
Poor Utilization (up to 50%)	59	39.3
Good Utilization (above 50%)	101	60.7

pregnancy as a woman at such an early age would not be having a mature body structure [15].

With regards to education level of the respondents, secondary level of education was completed by only 24.0% of the respondents whereas 26.7% of respondents were illiterate. Educated mothers are more aware of their health and development of the family. The literacy rate of Dalit females is quite low compared to the national female literacy rate which

TABLE 5: Association between sociodemographic variables and utilization of antenatal care services.

Demographic Variables	Utilization of Antenatal Care Services		Total	χ^2	P Value
	Poor Utilization	Good Utilization			
Age					
Up to 25 years	9(11.7%)	68(88.3%)	77	50.674	**0.001**
Above 25years	50(68.5%)	23(31.5%)	73		
Educational status					
Illiterate	33(82.5%)	7(17.5%)	40	42.594	**0.001**
Literate	26(23.6%)	84(76.4%)	110		
Age at Marriage					
Up to 18 Years	46(41.8%)	64(58.2%)	110	1.067	0.302
Above 18 Years	13(32.5%)	27(67.5%)	40		
Age at first pregnancy					
Up to 19 years	52(40.9%)	75(59.1%)	127	0.901	0.342
Above 19 years	7(30.4%)	16(69.5%)	23		
Type of Family					
Nuclear	33(29.2%)	80(70.8%)	113	19.700	**0.001**
Joint	26(70.3%)	11(29.7%)	37		

is 57.4% according to 2011 census [16]. It was noted that almost half of the respondents 49.3% were housewives. The husbands were the main decision makers in the household (68.0%), followed by the father in laws 17.3% whereas only a few number of respondents took their own decisions on healthcare. Women have little preference in the family; hence they have to rely on their husband and family members (mostly inlaws) to take any decision. It is even more important for the women to make their own choices and decisions based on the adequate information of the services they use as per their personal, family, and social needs. Studies have revealed that both economic status and social dynamics regarding distribution of power between spouses have an influence on the use of maternal health services [17]. In our study, around 75.0% of the respondents belonged to a joint family. This was slightly higher compared to a similar study done in the Mid-Western region of the country where 58.2% of the mothers belonged to a joint family [18]. It is often seen that a good marital relationship between spouses exists when they live in nuclear families and for those women living in joint families better relation with their mother in laws results in better utilization rates of the ANC services during pregnancy [19].

In this study, 40.7% of the respondents stated that the first person of contact during pregnancy related issues, childbirth and postpartum period were health workers while 59.3% of respondents identified others such as neighbors, relatives and traditional healers as their immediate contact with the preference more on the later. This help seeking behavior could be attributed to various factors including their availability, cost effectiveness, and deep rooted traditional and cultural values in the society. In rural areas, people put their faith and prefer to seek care from traditional healers, a social behavior that has been passed down to them across generations from their ancestors [20].

With regards to antenatal health check-up during their latest pregnancy, 76.0% of respondents had attended antepartum visit in their last pregnancy, a figure that is higher than national statistics (NDHS, 2011) average of 58.3% [21]. Similar results were seen in studies from Lalitpur and Ilam districts of Nepal where majority of the women attended ANC in the last pregnancy. Around 79.0% of the women in Lalitpur and 95.0% in Ilam underwent ANC visits during the last episode of pregnancy [22, 23]. Despite the provision of free maternal health care services provided by Government of Nepal across all government hospitals, 24.0% of respondents did not attend any antepartum care. This finding is similar to the study done in hilly area of Nepal where 21.1% did not attend any ANC visit [22]. The reason for not attending antepartum clinic was due to the lack of knowledge regarding obstetric complication and free delivery services among 38.9% of the respondents followed by 27.7% of the women experiencing no complications during their pregnancy. Similarly, 16.7% cited lack of time due to household choirs and incumbent traditional views within the family as the reason for the low service utilization. During the interview process the several factors that led to underutilization of ANC services included a lower SES of the women in the community as well as the persistent traditional belief that pregnancy was a natural phenomenon which did not require additional health checkup like their in-laws during their pregnancies. It was found that the mothers-in-laws were not supportive and did not encourage the ANC checkups as the pregnant women were expected to carry out the daily household choirs.

Despite the Government of Nepal launching a Safe Motherhood Initiative Program to promote utilization of institutional delivery services which includes free delivery care with 4 ANC visit incentives for women, complete ANC visit is still quite low. Our study revealed that among 114 respondents who attended ANC visits, 7.0% of them visited

ANC once, 3.5% visited twice, 16.7% visited thrice, and the remaining majority 72.8% percent of them completed all four ANC visits. This finding is consistent with the study done in Nepal where that 70.0% of mothers underwent four antenatal visits, 14.0% did 3 antenatal visits 13.7% with 2 antenatal visits, and 2.1% had a single antenatal visit [24]. Furthermore, among the 114 respondents who attended first ANC visit at a health facility, 51.9% of the respondents had their first antenatal visit at 4 months or later. Similarly, 27.1% of respondents had an antepartum visit in the third month of pregnancy while 21.0% of respondents had their first ANC visit during the second month of pregnancy. Among them who had done their ANC visit, all of the respondent had visited a government hospital. In contrast to this, present study revealed that 56.0% were registered for ANC in the first trimester of pregnancy, whereas only 1.0% were registered in the third trimester. They were registered at different level of health services, i.e., 1.8% in subhealth posts, 28.0% in PHCs, 34.3% in a Zonal hospital, and 35.9% in private nursing homes [24]. This variation must have resulted from the existing good and free maternal and child health services developed for pregnant mother across all public health facilities in the country.

Among the participants, it was observed that 82.0% of the mothers had consumed Iron/Foliates out of which a further 68.3% of them had consumed the tablets up to 45 days after delivery. The study also revealed that only one third of respondents received an anti-helminths (albendazole). Around 70.0% of respondents had received TT Vaccines out of which only 65.7% of respondents received both doses with the remaining mothers either receiving a single or a booster dose of the TT Vaccine during their pregnancy. This finding is lower than National Family Health Survey (NFHS-3) of India average of 73.6% scheduled caste receiving two or more doses and 1.5% receiving a single dose of TT injection during their pregnancy [25]. This finding was similar to another study which showed TT immunization of expecting mothers with 62.3% receiving 2 doses and 37.7% receiving a single or booster dose [24]. In this study, among 92 respondents that did not receive anti-helminths, 85.9% stated that they had not been prescribed the same by the health person. This could be due to the lack of adequate supply of free Anti-helminths medicine across public health facilities or also could be attributed to the lack of knowledge on prescribing the anti-helminths among the health workers.

Our study revealed that 60.7% of the mothers utilized the existing ANC care services well whereas the remaining 39.3% of the respondents showed poor utilization of antenatal care services. While assessing the sociodemographic determinants, it was observed that age (p=0.001), education levels of respondents (p=0.001), and type of family of respondents (p =0.001) were strongly associated with utilization of the ANC services; however, age at marriage (p=0.302) and age at first pregnancy (p=0.342) did not affect the utilization of ANC services among women. This result illustrates that 76.4% of educated women, 88.3% of women below 25 years of age, and 70.8% of them from nuclear families utilized antenatal health care services more than respondents who were illiterate and above 25 years of age and lived in a joint family. This could

be attributed to lack of time from household activities and pressure from in laws to the mothers of Dalit communities. Younger mothers (less than age 20) are more likely to receive antenatal care from a skilled provider than older mothers (age 35-49) [21]. Other studies have also reflected how educated mothers often seek more ANC services than those that are not literate [26, 27]. Therefore the 2001 Nepal Demographic and Health Survey study in its recommendation outlined the emphasis on better maternal education to help improve the greater utilization of maternal health care services among women in Nepal [28]. It is important to focus on education of the women from the lower caste groups such as Dalits as the dropout rates in these communities is very high [29, 30]. It is also necessary to provide more emphasis to uplift the awareness levels of Dalit mothers for receiving available prenatal services [31].

Several factors such as lower SES and low level of awareness on ANC are inversely related to overall quality of health among women including safe motherhood practices especially among marginalized Dalit population [12].

6. Conclusion

Antenatal care is an essential component of safe motherhood. The study revealed that the overall utilization of antenatal health services was good as almost two third of the mothers utilize it, while more than one third of them had poor utilization of antenatal care services. Regardless of free safe motherhood services in government hospital and high utilization rate of maternal health care services utilization of all four ANC visits, consumption of iron tablet, anti-helminthes and administration of TT vaccine during their last pregnancy was considerably low among the women in the Dalit community. The study also revealed that educational status of mothers, age and type of family played a significant role in underutilization of ANC services among the women from lower castes. The study identifies the need to hence look at the significant factors associated with utilization of the available free safe motherhood services across all public health facilities especially among Dalit communities and to address this prioritized intensive awareness programs and behavioral change interventions on maternal health and socioeconomical development for women in Dalit communities should be planned. Community engagement and social awareness could play a very crucial role to help promote maternal health thereby impacting the overall maternal health of these women in the future. The policy-makers should also advocate for prioritizing accessibility and such awareness raising activities targeting underserved communities such as the Dalit women residing in rural hard to reach areas.

List of Abbreviations

ANC: Antenatal care
TT: Tetanus Toxoid
SES: Socio Economic Status
SPSS: Statistical Package for Social Science
FCHV: Female Community Health Volunteers
WHO: World Health Organization.

Conflicts of Interest

There are no conflicts of interest regarding the manuscript.

Authors' Contributions

Mamata Sherpa Awasthi and Kiran Raj Awasthi are responsible for the overall design, data analysis, and drafting of the paper. Bhuvan Saud contributed to drafting the manuscript as per the template. Harish Singh Thapa, Sarita Pradhan, and Roshani Agrawal Khatry provided critical comments on the draft. All authors have read and approved the final manuscript. Authors Mamata Sherpa Awasthi and Kiran Raj Awasthi have equal contributions.

References

[1] World Health Organization, "Trends in maternal mortality: 1990 to 2015: estimates by WHO, UNICEF, UNFPA, World Bank Group and the United Nations Population Division," 2015, http://www.afro.who.int/sites/default/files/2017-05/trends-in-maternal-mortality-1990-to-2015.pdf.

[2] A. A. A. Ali, M. M. Osman, A. O. Abbaker, and I. Adam, "Use of antenatal care services in Kassala, eastern Sudan," *BMC Pregnancy and Childbirth*, vol. 10, no. 1, article 67, 2010.

[3] World Health Organization, "WHO recommendations on antenatal care for a positive pregnancy experience," 2016, http://apps.who.int/iris/bitstream/handle/10665/250796/9789241549912-eng.pdf?sequence=1.

[4] Ministry of Health and Population, "Annual report Department of Health Services 2066/67 (2009/2010)," 2011, http://dohs.gov.np/wpcontent/uploads/Annual_Report_2066_67.pdf.

[5] Y. R. Paudel, T. Jha, and S. Mehata, "Timing of First Antenatal Care (ANC) and Inequalities in Early Initiation of ANC in Nepal," *Frontiers in Public Health*, vol. 5, article 242, 2017.

[6] A. T. Owolabi, A. O. Fatusi, O. Kuti, A. Adeyemi, S. O. Faturoti, and P. O. Obiajuwa, "Maternal complications and perinatal outcomes in booked and unbooked Nigerian mothers," *Singapore Medical Journal*, vol. 49, no. 7, pp. 526–531, 2008.

[7] Y. R. Baral, K. Lyons, J. Skinner, and E. R. van Teijlingen, "Maternal health services utilisation in Nepal: progress in the new millennium?" *Health Science Journal*, vol. 6, no. 4, pp. 618–633, 2012.

[8] D. R. Dahal, Y. B. Gurung, B. Acharya, K. Hemchuri, and D. Swarnakar, "National Dalit Strategy Report Part I Situational Analysis of Dalits in Nepal," Tech. Rep., National Planning Commission HMG, Kathmandu, Nepal, 2002.

[9] N. S. Sabharwal and W. Sonalkar, "Dalit Women in India: at the crossroads of gender, class and caste," *Global Justice: Theory Practice Rhetoric*, vol. 8, no. 1, 2015.

[10] J. P. Pandey, M. R. Dhakal, S. Karki, P. Poudel, and M. S. Pradhan, *Maternal and Child Health in Nepal: The Effects of Caste, Ethnicity, and Regional Identity: Further Analysis of the 2011 Nepal Demographic and Health Survey*, Kathmandu, Nepal, 2013.

[11] J. Morrison, M. Basnet, B. Budhathoki et al., "Disabled women's maternal and newborn health care in rural Nepal: A qualitative study," *Midwifery*, vol. 30, no. 11, pp. 1132–1139, 2014.

[12] S. Pasad, "Safe Motherhood Practice in Dalit Community," *Academic Voices: A Multidisciplinary Journal*, vol. 2, no. 1, pp. 63–68, 2013.

[13] H. R. Devkota, A. Clarke, S. Shrish, and D. N. Bhatta, "Does women's caste make a significant contribution to adolescent pregnancy in Nepal? A study of Dalit and non-Dalit adolescents and young adults in Rupandehi district," *BMC Women's Health*, vol. 18, no. 1, article 23, 2018.

[14] R. W. Blum and W. H. Gates Sr, "Girlhood not motherhood. Preventing adolescent pregnancy".

[15] M. Sharma and S. Sharma, "Knowledge, attitude and beliefs of pregnant women towards safe motherhood in a rural Indian setting," *Social Sciences Directory*, vol. 1, no. 1, 2012.

[16] Nepal Planning Commission Secretariat and Central Bureau of Statistics, "National Population and Housing Census 2011 (National Report)," Tech. Rep., Nepal Planning Commission Secretariat, Central Bureau of Statistics, 2012, https://unstats.un.org/unsd/demographic-social/census/documents/Nepal/Nepal-Census-2011-Vol1.pdf.

[17] R. N. M. Mpembeni, J. Z. Killewo, M. T. Leshabari et al., "Use pattern of maternal health services and determinants of skilled care during delivery in Southern Tanzania: implications for achievement of MDG-5 targets," *BMC Pregnancy and Childbirth*, vol. 7, article 29, 2007.

[18] D. Paneru, K. Gyawali, B. Jnawali, and K. Jnawali, "Knowledge and practices on maternal health care among mothers: A Cross sectional study from rural areas of mid-western development region Nepal," *Journal of the Scientific Society*, vol. 40, no. 1, article 9, 2013.

[19] K. Allendorf, "The quality of family relationships and use of maternal health-care services in India," *Studies in Family Planning*, vol. 41, no. 4, pp. 263–276, 2010.

[20] R. Baniya, "Traditional Healing Practices in Rural Nepal," *Journal of Patan Academy of Health Sciences*, vol. 1, no. 1, pp. 52-53, 2015.

[21] Ministry of Health and Population (MOHP), "New ERA, and ICF International Inc. Nepal Demographic and Health Survey 2011," 2012, https://dhsprogram.com/pubs/pdf/fr257/fr257%5B13april2012%5D.pdf.

[22] S. Sanjel, R. H. Ghimire, and K. Pun, "Antenatal care practices in Tamang community of hilly area in central Nepal," *Kathmandu University Medical Journal*, vol. 9, no. 34, pp. 57–61, 2011.

[23] P. M. S. Pradhan, S. Bhattarai, I. S. Paudel, K. Gaurav, and P. K. Pokharel, "Factors contributing to antenatal care and delivery practices in village development committees of Ilam district, Nepal," *Kathmandu University Medical Journal*, vol. 11, no. 41, pp. 60–65, 2013.

[24] R. Misra and N. Chaurasia, "Utilization of Safe Motherhood Services in Jhorahat PHC Area of Morang District, Nepal," *American Journal of Public Health Research*, vol. 3, pp. 123–129, 2015.

[25] International Institute for Population Sciences India, "National Family Health Survey (NFHS-3 2005-06)," 2007, https:// dhsprogram.com/pubs/pdf/FRIND3/FRIND3-Vol1%5BOct -17-2008%5D.pdf.

[26] C. Joshi, S. Torvaldsen, R. Hodgson, and A. Hayen, "Factors associated with the use and quality of antenatal care in Nepal: a population-based study using the demographic and health survey data," *BMC Pregnancy and Childbirth*, vol. 14, article 94, 2014.

[27] D. Zelalem Ayele, B. Belayihun, K. Teji, and D. Admassu Ayana, "Factors affecting utilization of maternal health care services in Kombolcha District, Eastern Hararghe Zone, Oromia Regional State, Eastern Ethiopia," *International Scholarly Research Notices*, vol. 2014, Article ID 917058, 7 pages, 2014.

[28] M. Furuta and S. Salway, "Women's position within the household as a determinant of maternal health care use in Nepal," *International Family Planning Perspectives*, vol. 32, no. 1, pp. 17–27, 2006.

[29] M. B. Das and S. Kapoor Mehta, *Poverty and social exclusion in India: Dalits*, The World Bank, Washington, Wash, USA, 2012.

[30] S. Desai and V. Kulkarni, "Changing educational inequalities in India in the context of affirmative action," *Demography*, vol. 45, no. 2, pp. 245–270, 2008.

[31] R. K. Dahal, "Utilization of antenatal care services in rural area of Nepal," *International Journal of Collaborative Research on Internal Medicine*, vol. 5, no. 2, 2013.

18

Maternal Morbidity in Women with Placenta Previa Managed with Prediction of Morbidly Adherent Placenta by Ultrasonography

Midori Fujisaki,[1] Seishi Furukawa,[2] Yohei Maki,[1] Masanao Oohashi,[1] Koutarou Doi,[1] and Hiroshi Sameshima[1]

[1]*Department of Obstetrics & Gynecology, Faculty of Medicine, University of Miyazaki, Miyazaki, Japan*
[2]*Department of Obstetrics & Gynecology, School of Medicine, Kyorin University, Tokyo, Japan*

Correspondence should be addressed to Seishi Furukawa; shiiba46seishi@gmail.com

Academic Editor: Albert Fortuny

Objective. To determine maternal morbidity in women with placenta previa managed with prediction of morbidly adherent placenta (MAP) by ultrasonography. *Methods.* A retrospective cohort study was undertaken comprising forty-one women who had placenta previa with or without risk factors for MAP. Women who had all three findings (bladder line interruption, placental lacunae, and absence of the retroplacental clear zone) were regarded as high suspicion for MAP and underwent cesarean section followed by hysterectomy. We attempted placental removal for women having two findings or less. *Results.* Among 28 women with risk, nine with high suspicion underwent hysterectomy and were diagnosed with MAP. Three of 19 women with two findings or less eventually underwent hysterectomy and were diagnosed with MAP. The sensitivity and positive predictive value for the detection of MAP were 64% and 100%. The pathological severity of MAP was significantly correlated with the cumulative number of findings. There were no cases of MAP among 13 women without risk. There was no difference of blood loss between women with high suspicion and those without risk (2186 ± 1438 ml versus 1656 ± 848 ml, resp.; $p = 0.34$). *Conclusion.* Management with prediction of MAP by ultrasonography is useful for obtaining permissible morbidity.

1. Introduction

Morbidly adherent placenta (MAP) is one of a number of risk factors related to maternal death [1]. Among women with obstetrical bleeding and who subsequently receive blood transfusions, MAP accounts for 15% of all cases and is associated with severe morbidity, in addition to an increased likelihood for the use of invasive procedures such as hysterectomy (78%), massive blood loss over 3000 ml (65%), and massive blood transfusion with ≥10 units of packed red blood cells and/or ≥10 units of fresh frozen plasma (74%) [2]. Therefore, the establishment of a management protocol in cases of MAP is crucial in current obstetrical practice.

Comstock et al. [3] introduced an approach for the detection of MAP in the second and third trimesters of pregnancy by ultrasonography, where the presence of bladder line interruption, absence of the retroplacental clear zone, and presence of placental lacunae were regarded as criteria for the prediction of MAP. This approach was strengthened by criteria that showed a positive predictive value of 48% and a value of 86% with 2 or more criteria. Many reports [4–6] then appeared that assessed the accuracy of a preoperative diagnosis of MAP using ultrasonography. However, there were various advantages and disadvantages concerning the impact of current obstetrical practices on the outcome of MAP predicted by ultrasonography. Shamshirsaz et al. [7] conducted a historical cohort study to investigate the impact of a multidisciplinary protocol on the outcome of MAP compared with a nonmultidisciplinary protocol. In that study, the multidisciplinary protocol was superior to the nonmultidisciplinary protocol in terms of reduction of both emergency surgery and blood loss during the perioperative period, although that cohort study included only confirmed cases of MAP determined by histological examination after delivery.

Some reports [8–10] suggested that antenatal diagnosis of MAP by ultrasonography reduced morbidities. On the other hand, it was also reported that suspected cases of MAP before delivery had a poorer outcome and that preoperative diagnosis did not affect the outcome [11, 12]. The reason for deviated results by management with a prediction of MAP seems to be due to a lack of uniformed strategy in terms of diagnosis and treatment. In the future, there is a need to standardize diagnostic criteria and treatment strategy for MAP. Before that, it is still necessary to accumulate information concerning the impact of management with a prediction of MAP by ultrasonography on maternal prognosis.

We conducted a single-arm historical cohort study of women with placenta previa and the absence or presence of risk factors for MAP to evaluate both the accuracy of a prediction of MAP by ultrasonography and the impact of management with a prediction of MAP on maternal prognosis.

2. Materials and Methods

We obtained approval (#O-0027) for this study from a constituted Ethics Committee in our institution. We retrospectively examined the medical charts of women having placenta previa and the absence or presence of risk factors for adherent placenta from January 2008 to February 2014 and who were admitted to the Perinatal Center of the University of Miyazaki from January 2008 to February 2014.

All cases of placenta previa were confirmed by either transabdominal ultrasonography or transvaginal ultrasonography after 20 weeks of gestation. We conducted examinations to detect three ultrasonographic findings regarded as markers for MAP, namely, bladder line interruption, absence of the retroplacental clear zone, and placental lacunae (Figure 1) [3].

Prior to the study period, we performed a preliminary study of 46 cases of placenta previa in an effort to detect MAP by ultrasonography, since MAP was highly suggestive only when all three findings were present, namely, bladder line interruption, absence of the retroplacental clear zone, and placenta lacunae [13]. Women with two findings or less did not have MAP. Thereafter, we proposed cesarean hysterectomy when all three ultrasonography findings were present to strongly suggest MAP.

During the study period, women with placenta previa were managed depending on both risk and the prediction of MAP by ultrasonography. Risk for MAP included history of cesarean delivery, history of uterine curettage, and uterine anomaly. In the group with risks for MAP, women who had all three findings (bladder line interruption, absence of the retroplacental clear zone, and placental lacunae) were regarded as highly suspicious for MAP. In women with two findings or less, removal of the placenta to preserve fertility was attempted. In women without risk for MAP, removal of the placenta was attempted irrespective of the ultrasonographic findings.

Planned operations were performed at 35 to early 37 weeks of gestation. Women whose state was regarded with high suspicion for MAP received combined spinal-epidural

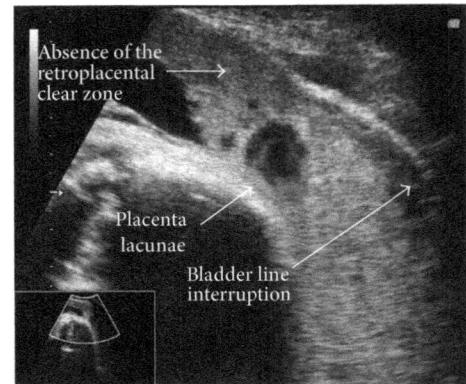

FIGURE 1: Representative 2D gray scale ultrasound scan for morbidly adherent placenta. Ultrasound scan shows bladder line interruption, absence of the retroplacental clear zone, and placenta lacunae in morbid adherent placenta.

anesthesia and then a general anesthesia during hysterectomy. Prior to operations, a bilateral ureteral stent was inserted to prevent ureteral injury during hysterectomy. Additionally, the portio vaginalis was clamped by ringforceps through the vaginal introitus to allow physicians to recognize the uterine cervix by touch through the abdominal cavity during hysterectomy. When women underwent cesarean section followed by hysterectomy, the placenta was allowed to remain in situ and the uterine cesarean wound was roughly closed. Uterine incisions were made at a site apart from the placenta to avoid unnecessary bleeding. Women having two findings or less received combined spinal-epidural anesthesia and then underwent a low transverse cesarean section followed by an attempt to deliver placenta by gentle traction of the umbilical cord to preserve uterus. If the placenta did not separate, we then attempted a manual removal of placenta. This procedure was based on our previous study, in that women with two ultrasonographic findings or less did not have MAP [13]. In cases of emergencies such as sudden profound bleeding or tocolysis failure before the planned operation, women received general anesthesia and underwent operation without insertion of a bilateral ureteral stent. Access to blood products except for platelets was ensured within 60 minutes following a request. O+ type blood can be given to women in a life-threatening situation.

During the study period, we identified 44 cases of placenta previa. We excluded from the study cases with multifetal pregnancies and deliveries under 22 weeks of gestation. Finally, a total of 41 pregnancies displaying placenta previa were registered in this study. The following characteristics were collected: maternal age, parity (primipara), history of uterine curettage, history of cesarean delivery, and the presence of uterine anomaly. Details of pregnancy outcomes were collected and included gestational age at delivery (weeks), birth weight (g), emergency cesarean delivery, hysterectomy, intraoperative complications such as bladder injury, the number of cases that a blood transfusion was necessary, total blood loss during operation, and postoperative length of maternal stay (days). Confirmation of an adherent placenta was made by histological examination following delivery. Adherent placenta was classified into three severities based on histological examination: placenta accreta, placenta increta, and placenta percreta. We evaluated maternal outcomes according to the cumulative number of ultrasonographic findings in the study group. We then examined the accuracy of prediction for MAP by ultrasonography and the relationship between pathological severity of MAP and the cumulative number of ultrasonographic findings.

Data are expressed as number, incidence (%), mean ± SD, or range. Comparisons between groups were made using Welch's t-test. Comparisons among groups were made using the Kruskal-Wallis test or χ^2 tests. Probability values < 0.05 were considered significant. The sensitivity and positive predictive value obtained by utilizing a combination of three findings, comprising bladder line interruption, absence of the retroplacental clear zone, and placental lacunae, with ultrasonography for adherent placenta were evaluated.

3. Results

The mean maternal age was 34 ± 5.5 years and gestational age at delivery was 34.1 ± 4.1 weeks. The percentage of nulliparous pregnancies was 22% and the percentage of previous cesarean delivery was 49%. There were also 15 cases having uterine curettage in previous pregnancies and one case of uterine anomaly (subseptate uterus) (Table 1).

In women with risk for MAP (n = 28), nine with three findings comprising bladder line interruption, absence of the retroplacental clear zone, and placental lacunae were regarded as highly suspicious for MAP and underwent cesarean section followed by hysterectomy. Eventually, nine women were diagnosed with MAP following histological examination. Five women having two findings underwent removal of the placenta. Two of the five women subsequently underwent hysterectomy due to bleeding, and placenta increta and accreta were confirmed in these two women following histological examination. In the remaining three with two findings, we observed one case of MAP (placenta accreta) following histological examination of placenta, in that a part of myometrium tissue was observed in placenta. Fourteen women having one finding or less underwent removal of the placenta. One of the fourteen women subsequently underwent hysterectomy due to difficulty of placental removal, and MAP (placenta accreta) was confirmed in this case following histological examination. Finally, we preserved 16 of 28 fertilities in women with risk for MAP. Fourteen cases of MAP were observed by histological examination following delivery. The sensitivity and positive predictive value for the detection of MAP by ultrasonography were 64% and 100%, respectively. The pathological severity of MAP was significantly correlated with the cumulative number of ultrasonographic findings (p < 0.01). Eight out of nine women having three findings showed placenta percreta or increta. In contrast, only one case of placenta increta was found in 19 women having two findings or less (Table 2). In women without risk for MAP (n = 13), there were no cases of hysterectomy or MAP (Table 2).

TABLE 1: Demographic data of the study group. Results are expressed as number, mean ± SD, or incidence (%).

Maternal age (years)	34.0 ± 5.5
Primipara	9 (21.9)
Gestational age at delivery (weeks)	34.1 ± 4.1
History of caesarean delivery	20 (48.8)
1	16 (39.0)
2	3 (7.3)
≥3	1 (2.4)
History of uterine curettage	15 (36.6)
Uterine anomaly	1 (2.4)

Results are expressed as number, mean ± SD, or incidence (%).

Analysis of maternal complications indicated a significant difference of blood loss among groups including women without risk (p = 0.02). One case resulted in massive blood loss (13,310 ml) following hysterectomy. This case had two findings composed of bladder line interruption and placenta lacunae and involved an emergency cesarean section due to uncontrollable bleeding followed by removal of the placenta. Except for the group with two findings, including the aforementioned massive bleeding case, the mean blood loss was 2186 ml or less in the other study groups. There was no difference of blood loss between women that were highly suspicious for MAP and women without risk (2186 ± 1438 ml versus 1656 ± 848 ml, resp.; p = 0.34) (Table 2). The incidence of blood transfusion did not differ among the groups including women without risk (p = 0.06). Additionally, the incidence of emergency cesarean section did not differ among the groups including women without risk (p = 0.58). Bladder injury only occurred in one of the women highly suspicious for MAP. The case was treated by surgical repair followed by an uncomplicated postoperative course. There was no difference of postoperative hospital stay among the groups including women without risk (p = 0.26).

4. Discussion

We have shown high sensitivity (64%) and a high positive predictive value (100%) for the detection of MAP by ultrasonography in women with risk (n = 28). The pathological severity of MAP was significantly correlated with the cumulative number of ultrasonographic findings. Additionally, cesarean hysterectomies were safely employed in cases regarded with high suspicion for MAP (n = 9) without profound blood loss. We preserved 16 of 28 fertilities in women with risk. There were no cases of MAP among women without risk. Thus, management is dependent on risk, and the prediction of MAP by ultrasonography is beneficial to both physicians and women in helping to obtain tolerable maternal outcomes.

According to a report by Comstock et al. [3], the sensitivity and positive predictive value for the detection for MAP by ultrasonography with any finding, such as the presence of bladder line interruption, absence of the retroplacental clear zone, or presence of placental lacunae, at 15 to 40 weeks of gestation were 100% and 48%, respectively. In order to

TABLE 2: Maternal outcomes according to ultrasonographic findings. Results are expressed as number, mean ± SD, or incidence (%). Comparisons between groups were made using Welch's t-test. Comparisons among groups were made using the Kruskal-Wallis test or χ^2 tests. NS: not significant.

		With risk		Without risk	p
Cumulative number of ultrasonographic findings	0~1	2	3	0~1	
n	14	5	9	13	
Absence of the retroplacental clear zone	0	4	9	0	
Bladder line interruption	0	1	9	0	
Placenta lacunae	12	5	9	5	
Emergency cesarean section	8	3	3	3	0.58
Hysterectomy	1 (7%)	2 (40%)	9 (100%)	0	<0.01
Total blood loss (ml)	1154 ± 800	4376 ± 5051	2186 ± 1438	1656 ± 848	0.02
Blood transfusion	6 (43%)	3 (60%)	5 (56%)	1 (8%)	0.06
Bladder injury	0	0	1	0	NS
Postoperative hospital stay (days)	8 (6–12)	9 (7–11)	10 (7–17)	8 (7–14)	0.26
Confirmed MAP by histological study	2	3	9	0	
(increta or percreta)	(0)	(1)	(8)		0.03

Results are expressed as number, incidence (%), mean ± SD, or range.

obtain a high predictive value for the detection of adherent placenta, a combination of multiple findings may be superior, although this approach may not be very sensitive. According to Comstock et al. [3], a combination of two or more findings showed 80% sensitivity and a positive predictive value of 86%. Use of a combination of smallest sagittal myometrium thickness, lacunae, and bridging vessels, in addition to the number of cesarean sections and placental location, has also been reported to be useful for predicting MAP. As a consequence, a score of 0–9 representing the Placenta Accreta Index (PAI score) was created for predicting MAP [5]. A high PAI score indicates a high positive predictive value, but with low sensitivity. Bowman et al. [14] suggested that the prediction of MAP by ultrasonography may not be very sensitive. However, our study reveals a high positive predictive value (100%) when using a combination of multiple findings without loss in sensitivity (64%). In women without risk for MAP, there were no cases of hysterectomy or MAP. Therefore, our management was dependent on risk and the prediction of MAP by ultrasonography to provide high sensitivity and a high positive predictive value for the detection for MAP, which reduced unnecessary hysterectomies.

The ultimate management goal for MAP is to minimize mortality and morbidity in affected women. Therefore, we need to obtain more effective treatment protocol including prenatal diagnosis of MAP and procedures. It has been suggested that suspected cases prior to delivery result in poorer outcomes because more cases comprising clinically significant morbidity may be included [11]. It was also reported that preoperative diagnosis of MAP did not affect the outcome [12]. In contrast, our prediction of MAP showed beneficial effect to women in helping to obtain tolerable maternal outcomes and provided similar conclusion like previous reports [8–10]. Those suggest that antenatal diagnosis of MAP by ultrasonography reduces maternal morbidity. In terms of minimizing blood loss, a multidisciplinary approach and planned operations are preferable [15]. Shamshirsaz et al. [7]

conducted a historical cohort study to investigate the impact of multidisciplinary protocols on the outcome of placenta accreta and indicated that the multidisciplinary protocol was superior to the nonmultidisciplinary protocol because both emergency surgery and blood loss at the perioperative period were reduced. Their protocol and management in the operation room were similar to our protocol except for the operating procedures (modified radical hysterectomy with or without intraoperative arterial embolization). In our study, the portio vaginalis was clamped by ring-forceps through the vaginal introitus to allow physicians to recognize the uterine cervix by touch through the abdominal cavity during the operation. Employing a combination of techniques comprising clamping of the portio vaginalis and use of a bilateral ureteral stent allowed us to conduct simple hysterectomies more easily without ureteral injury. There was only one case of bladder injury and no cases of ureteral injury in highly suspicious cases of MAP. Thus, our surgical procedure also achieved permissible morbidity. Additionally, we were able to make a judgment concerning the preservation of fertility among cases regarded with moderate to low suspicion (16 of 28 fertilities preserved). These results provide an explanation of the morbidity associated with MAP prior to operations and highlight the merits of our study.

We experienced one case with two findings comprising bladder line interruption and placenta lacunae, resulting in massive bleeding (13,310 ml). Prior to the current study, we performed a preliminary study of 46 cases of placenta previa in an effort to detect MAP by ultrasonography, in that women with two findings (bladder line interruption and placenta lacunae) did not have MAP. The MAP was only confirmed when all three findings were present [13]. Therefore, we proposed manual removal of placenta in order to preserve fertility when two ultrasonography findings were present. In current study, the remaining four with two findings (retroplacental clear zone and placental lacunae) did not have severe MAP (i.e., increta or percreta), followed by preservation of fertility (Table 2). Except for the aforementioned case, the pathological severity of MAP was significantly correlated with the cumulative number of findings. According to the literature, the findings of bladder line interruption have a high positive predictive value for MAP [6, 16]. In addition, the extirpative method is strongly deprecated, because it is associated with significant hemorrhagic morbidity [17]. Therefore, we have to reconsider our treatment protocol when women have two findings comprising bladder line interruption and others.

There are some limitations in our study. Firstly, since our study was not a comparative study, we were unable to show the superiority of our protocol compared with that of others. Our protocol did not include catheter intervention for reducing blood loss during operation. Currently, the management by multidisciplinary team involving interventional radiologist seems to be more effective for reducing maternal morbidity [7, 15, 18]. We need a subsequent examination to investigate the impact of catheter intervention during operation on our protocol. Secondly, since our investigations comprised a single institutional study, it is unclear whether similar outcomes would be obtained in other tertiary facilities using the same protocol.

In conclusion, under circumstances involving varied information concerning the advantages and disadvantages of prediction by ultrasonography in terms of maternal outcome, we demonstrated the usefulness of a management protocol based on both the risk and prediction of MAP by three ultrasonographic markers for MAP; those are bladder line interruption, absence of the retroplacental clear zone, and placental lacunae. Employment of a multidisciplinary approach by further examinations for the detection of MAP and introducing effective procedures to reduce blood loss is desirable to achieve permissible morbidity.

Conflicts of Interest

There are no financial or other relationships that might lead to conflicts of interest.

References

[1] N. Kanayama, J. Inori, H. Ishibashi-Ueda et al., "Maternal death analysis from the Japanese autopsy registry for recent 16 years: significance of amniotic fluid embolism," *Journal of Obstetrics and Gynaecology Research*, vol. 37, no. 1, pp. 58–63, 2011.

[2] K. Furuta, S. Furukawa, H. Urabe, K. Michikata, K. Kai, H. Sameshima et al., "Differences in maternal morbidity concerning risk factors for obstetric hemorrhage," *Austin Journal of Obstetrics and Gynecology*, vol. 1, p. 5, 2014.

[3] C. H. Comstock, J. J. Love Jr., R. A. Bronsteen et al., "Sonographic detection of placenta accreta in the second and third trimesters of pregnancy," *American Journal of Obstetrics and Gynecology*, vol. 190, no. 4, pp. 1135–1140, 2004.

[4] P. Taipale, M.-R. Orden, M. Berg, H. Manninen, and I. Alafuzoff, "Prenatal diagnosis of placenta accreta and percreta with ultrasonography, color Doppler, and magnetic resonance imaging," *Obstetrics and Gynecology*, vol. 104, no. 3, pp. 537–540, 2004.

[5] M. W. F. Rac, J. S. Dashe, C. E. Wells, E. Moschos, D. D. McIntire, and D. M. Twickler, "Ultrasound predictors of placental invasion: the Placenta Accreta Index," *American Journal of Obstetrics and Gynecology*, vol. 212, no. 3, pp. 343.e1–343.e7, 2015.

[6] G. Calì, L. Giambanco, G. Puccio, and F. Forlani, "Morbidly adherent placenta: evaluation of ultrasound diagnostic criteria and differentiation of placenta accreta from percreta," *Ultrasound in Obstetrics and Gynecology*, vol. 41, no. 4, pp. 406–412, 2013.

[7] A. A. Shamshirsaz, K. A. Fox, B. Salmanian et al., "Maternal morbidity in patients with morbidly adherent placenta treated with and without a standardized multidisciplinary approach," *American Journal of Obstetrics & Gynecology*, vol. 212, pp. 218.e1–218.e9, 2015.

[8] M. Tikkanen, J. Paavonen, M. Loukovaara, and V. Stefanovic, "Antenatal diagnosis of placenta accreta leads to reduced blood loss," *Acta Obstetricia et Gynecologica Scandinavica*, vol. 90, no. 10, pp. 1140–1146, 2011.

[9] C. R. Warshak, G. A. Ramos, R. Eskander et al., "Effect of predelivery diagnosis in 99 consecutive cases of placenta accreta," *Obstetrics and Gynecology*, vol. 115, no. 1, pp. 65–69, 2010.

[10] A. G. Eller, T. T. Porter, P. Soisson, and R. M. Silver, "Optimal management strategies for placenta accreta," *BJOG: An International Journal of Obstetrics and Gynaecology*, vol. 116, no. 5, pp. 648–654, 2009.

[11] J. L. Bailit, W. A. Grobman, M. M. Rice et al., "Morbidly adherent placenta treatments and outcomes," *Obstetrics and Gynecology*, vol. 125, no. 3, pp. 683–689, 2015.

[12] T. Hall, J. R. Wax, F. L. Lucas, A. Cartin, M. Jones, and M. G. Pinette, "Prenatal sonographic diagnosis of placenta accreta—Impact on maternal and neonatal outcomes," *Journal of Clinical Ultrasound*, vol. 42, no. 8, pp. 449–455, 2014.

[13] K. Doi, Y. Nakano, S. Tokunaga et al., "Prediction of placenta accreta in cases of placenta previa," *The Japanese Journal of Obstetrical, Gynecological & Neonatal Hematology*, vol. 16, pp. 40–44, 2007.

[14] Z. S. Bowman, A. G. Eller, A. M. Kennedy et al., "Accuracy of ultrasound for the prediction of placenta accreta," *American Journal of Obstetrics and Gynecology*, vol. 211, no. 2, pp. 177–e7, 2014.

[15] S. K. Doumouchtsis and S. Arulkumaran, "The morbidly adherent placenta: an overview of management options," *Acta Obstetricia et Gynecologica Scandinavica*, vol. 89, no. 9, pp. 1126–1133, 2010.

[16] E. Pilloni, M. G. Alemanno, P. Gaglioti et al., "Accuracy of ultrasound in antenatal diagnosis of placental attachment disorders," *Ultrasound in Obstetrics and Gynecology*, vol. 47, no. 3, pp. 302–307, 2016.

[17] American College of Obstetricians and Gynecologists, "ACOG Committee opinion #529. Placenta accreta," *Obstetrics & Gynecology*, vol. 120, article 207, 2012.

[18] A. A. Shamshirsaz, K. A. Fox, H. Erfani et al., "Multidisciplinary team learning in the management of the morbidly adherent placenta: outcome improvements over time," *American Journal of Obstetrics and Gynecology*, 2017.

A Qualitative Study to Examine Perceptions and Barriers to Appropriate Gestational Weight Gain among Participants in the Special Supplemental Nutrition Program for Women Infants and Children Program

Loan Pham Kim,[1] **Maria Koleilat,**[2] **and Shannon E. Whaley**[3]

[1] *Pepperdine University, Malibu, CA 90263, USA*
[2] *California State University, Fullerton, CA 92831, USA*
[3] *PHFE-WIC Program, Irwindale, CA 91706, USA*

Correspondence should be addressed to Loan Pham Kim; loan.kim@pepperdine.edu

Academic Editor: Debbie Smith

Women of reproductive age are particularly at risk of obesity because of excessive gestational weight gain (GWG) and postpartum weight retention, resulting in poor health outcomes for both mothers and infants. The purpose of this qualitative study was to examine perceptions and barriers to GWG among low-income women in the WIC program to inform the development of an intervention study. Eleven focus groups were conducted and stratified by ethnicity, and each group included women of varying age, parity, and prepregnancy BMI ranges. Participants reported receiving pressure from spouse and family members to "eat for two" among multiple barriers to appropriate weight gain during pregnancy. Participants were concerned about gaining too much weight but had minimal knowledge of weight gain goals during pregnancy. Receiving regular weight monitoring was reported, but participants had inconsistent discussions about weight gain with healthcare providers. Most were not aware of the IOM guidelines nor the fact that gestational weight gain goals differed by prepregnancy weight status. Results of these focus groups analyses informed the design of a pregnancy weight tracker and accompanying educational handout for use in an intervention study. These findings suggest an important opportunity for GWG education in all settings where pregnant women are seen.

1. Introduction

The current high rates of obesity continue to be a significant public health concern [1]. The childbearing years pose potential obesity risk for women because of excessive gestational weight gain (GWG) and postpartum weight retention [2–4]. Excess GWG and postpartum weight retention result in suboptimal pre- and perinatal health and predispose both mothers and their infants to long-term chronic diseases. In response to the mounting evidence, the Institute of Medicine (IOM) revised its 1990 recommendations and released new GWG recommendations in 2009 [5, 6]. These guidelines are specific to a woman's prepregnancy body mass index (BMI); for example, underweight women (BMI of

$<18.5 \text{ kg/m}^2$) should gain 28–40 lbs; normal weight women (BMI of 18.5–24.9 kg/m^2) should gain 25–35 lbs; overweight women (BMI of 25.0–29.9 kg/m^2) should gain 15–25 lbs; and obese women (BMI $\geq 30.0 \text{ kg/m}^2$) should gain 11–20 lbs. Despite these guidelines, almost one-half of women exceeded the IOM recommendations [7]; groups particularly at risk for excess GWG are Black and Hispanic mothers [8, 9]. Adverse health outcomes from excess GWG during pregnancy include gestational diabetes, hypertensive disorders, cesarean delivery and operative complications [10, 11], and postpartum overweight and obesity [2–4, 12]. Excessive GWG from a previous pregnancy is a significant nutritional risk factor for subsequent pregnancies, leading to adverse health outcomes for the child, including increased risk of macrosomia and childhood obesity [10, 13, 14]. Consequently, increasing trends of maternal overweight and excessive GWG may set the stage for a transgenerational cycle of obesity as heavier mothers give birth to heavier daughters, who are at increased risk of becoming obese themselves during their childbearing years [15].

The Special Supplemental Nutrition Program for Women Infants and Children (WIC) is a food and nutrition education program for pregnant, breastfeeding, and postpartum women, infants, and children under age five who are low-income (up to 185% of the Federal Poverty Level) and at nutritional risk. Nationwide, approximately 25% of the individuals served are women, and approximately half of these women are pregnant with the other half postpartum. WIC services are available in every state and US territory, and currently WIC services are delivered to over 8 million participants each month. In Los Angeles County (LAC), WIC currently serves approximately 67% of all infants and about half of all children ages one to five, translating into approximately 500,000 individuals and 350,000 families each month. Because of WIC's deep reach in low-income ethnic minority communities, understanding and programming interventions to target WIC participants can potentially lead to significant positive outcomes in perinatal health of women and their young children.

Because WIC is uniquely positioned to potentially mediate perinatal health of mothers and children, especially ethnic minority and underresourced communities, research on GWG in this population is vital. The most recent quantitative studies of GWG have focused on predictors of child weight based on maternal weight [16, 17]; only two studies have specifically focused on women in the WIC program [18, 19]. Qualitative studies have the advantage of allowing researchers to explore GWG in multiple and complex dimensions such as knowledge, attitudes, opinions, and reported behaviors during pregnancy. Currently, the qualitative literature has a scant, but growing body of work which document knowledge and barriers to gestational weight gain, and most of these studies have focused on low-income Black or Hispanic women [20–22]. The results of these studies suggest the need for more qualitative work in these communities to better understand cultural barriers and facilitators of appropriate GWG during pregnancy.

One qualitative study of African-American women suggested focusing research on GWG in the WIC program in order to develop strategies for improving long-term health of mothers and their children [22]. To date, we are not aware of any qualitative studies which have specifically examined the perceptions of GWG among an ethnically diverse group of participants in the WIC program. Therefore, the objectives of this qualitative study were threefold: (1) to explore knowledge, attitude, and perceptions regarding weight gain during pregnancy among participants in the WIC program; (2) to assess participants' knowledge and awareness of the IOM guidelines for weight gain during pregnancy; and (3) to solicit participant feedback and suggestions to inform the development of a gestational weight gain intervention in the WIC program.

2. Materials and Methods

2.1. Study Design, Participants, and Recruitment. Between February and December 2013, we conducted a series of 11 focus group interviews with a total of 59 WIC participants across 3 ethnic groups (Caucasian, Black, and Hispanic) to inform the design a gestational weight gain intervention among WIC participants. These ethnic groups were chosen because they represent the largest ethnic groups in the US as well as in the WIC program [23, 24]. WIC participants were recruited for this study if they met the study criteria of being pregnant at the time of the study and self-identified as white/Caucasian, Black/African-American or Hispanic/Latina. Each focus group was stratified by ethnicity in order to explore potential cultural variations in perceptions, attitudes, and behaviors with regard to gestational weight gain. Within each focus group, there was diversity in age, parity, and prepregnancy BMI ranges among the participants. Focus groups with Hispanic participants were grouped into English-speaking and Spanish-speaking in order to facilitate discussion among those with limited English proficiency. Recruitment of focus group participants and facilitation of focus group interviews were accomplished with support from staff from the Public Health Foundation Enterprise (PHFE) WIC Program in a number of WIC centers around Los Angeles, California.

Inductive semistructured focus group guides were developed by the research team, with feedback from PHFE-WIC research staff. Open-ended questions were utilized to stimulate discussion and included probes to address more specific dimensions of each topic. Focus group guides explored the following major topics: (1) health perceptions during pregnancy; (2) barriers to appropriate weight gain; (3) weight monitoring during pregnancy; (4) knowledge and recognition of IOM weight gain guidelines. Additionally, we solicited participant opinions on how to develop educational tools, including a gestational weight gain tracker that would help mothers track their weight gain through pregnancy, for the intervention phase of the study. Focus group guides were translated into Spanish and back-translated to ensure integrity and consistency.

Focus group moderators were trained in qualitative research and had experience moderating focus group interviews. The Spanish-speaking focus group moderator was bilingual and bicultural. Focus groups ranged from 5 to 8 women, and each session lasted an average of 90 minutes, with question and answer format so the discourse was unhurried. Prior to the start of a focus group discussion, participants provided written informed consent and completed a short demographic questionnaire which included self-reported height and prepregnancy weight. All focus group sessions were videotaped and audio recorded. All recording files were password protected and stored on a secure server at Pepperdine University. All transcripts were transcribed verbatim by an independent contractor; focus group sessions conducted in Spanish were transcribed verbatim in Spanish, then translated to English, and checked for accuracy by an independent reviewer. All aspects of the study were reviewed and approved by the University of California, Los Angeles,

TABLE 1: Description of the sample ($N = 59$).

	N	%	Mean	s.d.
Age	59		28.20	5.41
Years in WIC	59		2.39	3.16
Years in the US	24		14.27	7.69
Birthplace				
US born	35	59.3		
Foreign born	24	40.7		
Children in WIC				
Pregnant	30	50.8		
One child	21	35.6		
Two children	8	13.6		
Ethnicity				
White	13	22.0		
Black	20	33.9		
Hispanic-English-speaking	18	30.5		
Hispanic-Spanish-speaking	8	13.6		
Marital status				
Married	19	32.2		
Divorced	3	5.1		
Separated	4	6.8		
Never married	33	55.9		
Education				
Up to 12th grade	16	27.1		
High school grad or GED	15	25.4		
Some college/associate	21	35.6		
Bachelors and beyond	7	11.9		
Employment				
Self-employed	17	28.8		
Unemployed	24	40.7		
Homemaker	9	15.2		
Student	6	10.2		
Unable to work	3	5.1		
Maternal BMI				
Underweight	4	6.8		
Normal weight	24	40.7		
Overweight	12	20.3		
Obese	19	32.2		

and Pepperdine University's Institutional Review Board for the protection of human research subjects. As a token of gratitude for their time and participation in the study, each participant received a $20 gift card.

2.2. Data Analysis. Descriptive statistics were computed using SPSS version 22 (Chicago, IL) and are summarized in Table 1. All transcripts and interviewer notes were organized and coded using ATLAS.ti version 6.1 (ATLAS.ti Scientific Software Development GmbH, Berlin, Germany) and analyzed using thematic analysis [25, 26]. The research team, consisting of the lead author and research students trained in qualitative methods, analyzed these data. The analysis process began with the research team conducting multiple

independent readings of the transcripts to allow themes to emerge. To develop consensus, the research team convened after the initial reading to discuss codes and build emerging themes. Subsequently, a second pass of the transcripts was completed to ensure that all themes were captured. Following a third reading, the research team convened again to discuss any additional themes and reconciled any inconsistencies. Percentages presented in the results section reflect participant responses during the focus group by a show of hands or a nod in response to a count question. The researchers compiled these percentages by reviewing the video recordings to count participant responses.

3. Results and Discussion

3.1. Participant Characteristics. Demographic characteristics are summarized in Table 1. Focus groups were stratified by ethnicity, and overall about one-fifth of the participants were Caucasian, one-third were Black, and nearly half were Hispanic. On average, focus group participants were 28 years old and had been in the WIC program for 2.39 years, and about half (50.8%) of the participants were pregnant with their first child. More than half of the participants were born outside of the US and of these, most reported being from Mexico or Central America. About one-third of the participants were married, and more than 75% of the participants had at least a high school diploma or GED equivalent. More than half of the participants were either overweight or obese.

3.2. Focus Group Concepts and Emerging Themes. The following shows sample focus group questions organized by the four major topics.

Perceptions of health during pregnancy:

> To you, what does it mean to be healthy?
>
> Generally, how healthy do you think you are? Would you say you are in excellent, very good, fair or poor health? Why?
>
> During pregnancy, do you think you are as healthy as when you are not pregnant? Why?

Barriers to appropriate GWG:

> How would you say you are doing in terms of weight gain during pregnancy? Would you say you are gaining too, too little, or just the right amount of weight?
>
> Are you concerned about how much weight you have gained at this time? Does anyone in your family share your concerns about how much weight you have gained?
>
> What is the biggest challenge for you to gain the right amount of weight during pregnancy?
>
> What do you think are the consequences of gaining too much or too little weight during pregnancy?

Weight monitoring during pregnancy:

> Are you weighing yourself or getting weighed regularly?

> When you come for your pre-natal visits, does your doctor talk with you about how much weight you have gained? Please share about this experience.

> When you come for your regular WIC visit, do WIC staff talk with you about your weight? Please share about this experience.

> When WIC staff talk with pregnant moms about their weight, how do you think WIC staff should approach the topic of weight gain during pregnancy?

Knowledge and recognition of IOM guidelines and ideas for education:

> Have you heard of or seen these IOM guidelines for weight gain?

> Are you aware there are different weight gain recommendations for pregnant women, based on your pre-pregnancy weight? If so, where did you learn about these recommendations?

> When we develop the GWG tracker tool [participants provided samples], how should we differentiate the different pre-pregnancy weight groups? Should we put these terms (underweight, normal weight, overweight or obese) on the tracker?

> If WIC develops classes about gaining the right amount of weight, what specific issues do you think we need to address?

Figure 1 provides a schematic overview of the topics discussed in the focus groups; within each topic, clear themes emerged from focus groups discussions, and we describe them in more detail below.

3.2.1. Perceptions of Health during Pregnancy. The focus group discussion began with a general open-ended question about participants' perception of health. Participants were asked to rate their health as excellent, good, fair, or poor and to elaborate on why they chose a particular rating. A majority of the participants (85%) rated their health as either fair or good; only 4 of the 59 participants reported being in excellent health. Those participants who indicated having fair or good health commented that they rated their health that way because they were overweight or ate too much fast food or junk food. For those who indicated that they were in poor health, they also reported being overweight, not exercising, and eating out or eating "street food" too often. For the few who indicated being in excellent health, they reported eating healthy, exercising, and drinking water on a regular basis.

When asked about their perception of health during pregnancy, a majority of the participants (more than 80%) indicated that they felt healthier during pregnancy than when they were not pregnant. When probed about why they felt healthier, participants reported (1) being mindful of the baby inside and feeling responsible to help baby grow as healthy as possible and (2) trying to choose healthier foods, cutting back on "street food" and cooking at home, consuming less junk food, drinking more water, and cutting back on sodas and other sugar-sweetened beverages. One mother shared, "I think I'm healthier because I feel like I've got to do this for the baby more than me." Another participant stated, "I would say [I am] more healthy because you have the responsibility to take care of yourself and your baby who's growing inside of you. You want a healthy baby."

3.2.2. Barriers to Healthy Weight Gain during Pregnancy. When asked about their ability to maintain appropriate and healthy weight gain during pregnancy, participants reported the following reasons as barriers to being able to maintain healthy weight, which these women defined as "not too much, not too little weight gain." The first barrier was the encouragement from family members to "eat for two." Participants shared that spouses, mothers-in-law, siblings, and grandparents encouraged them to eat more because they had to feed their babies. As a result, these women reported difficulty in being able to maintain their weight. Even when they did not want to eat, participants reported being strongly encouraged to eat more by family members. Second, participants reported having cravings as a barrier to being able to maintain healthy weight, as one mother reported, "With my first son, I craved a lot of fruit, so it was more healthy. But this time around, I crave chocolate, cakes, all that sugary stuff." Third, participants indicated that being tempted by what family members were eating around them was another barrier to maintaining healthy weight. Because the family members were able to eat without any restrictions, these pregnant women also wanted to be able to eat whatever others around them were eating. Many participants were cognizant that they could not because of the excessive calories associated with overeating, particularly high sugar foods. One participant lamented, "It's harder because I have my kids and my husband. They want to go get burgers and here I am with my turkey sandwich. If it was my first pregnancy, it [wouldn't] be as hard. It's harder because my kids want soda. I don't give them that much, but sometimes just a cup of soda. I want some soda too but I can't. It's harder on me because of my family." Another barrier reported was the lack of knowledge about what to eat during pregnancy. One participant shared, "When I lived with my mother-in-law, she would eat a lot of meats, but also she would cook a lot of vegetables – boiled. So now that I live on my own, I look in the refrigerator and I'm like, 'well, what do I cook?' I know how to cook, but I just don't know, what [do I] cook? Or when I'm in there, or I look at the pantry and I'm like 'how do I make that?'". The last barrier reported was having morning sickness symptoms such as nausea and vomiting as barriers to being able to eat healthy.

3.2.3. Weight Monitoring during Pregnancy. When the discussion focused on weight monitoring during pregnancy, all participants shared affirmatively that they were concerned

Major topics of discussion   Themes from focus group discussions

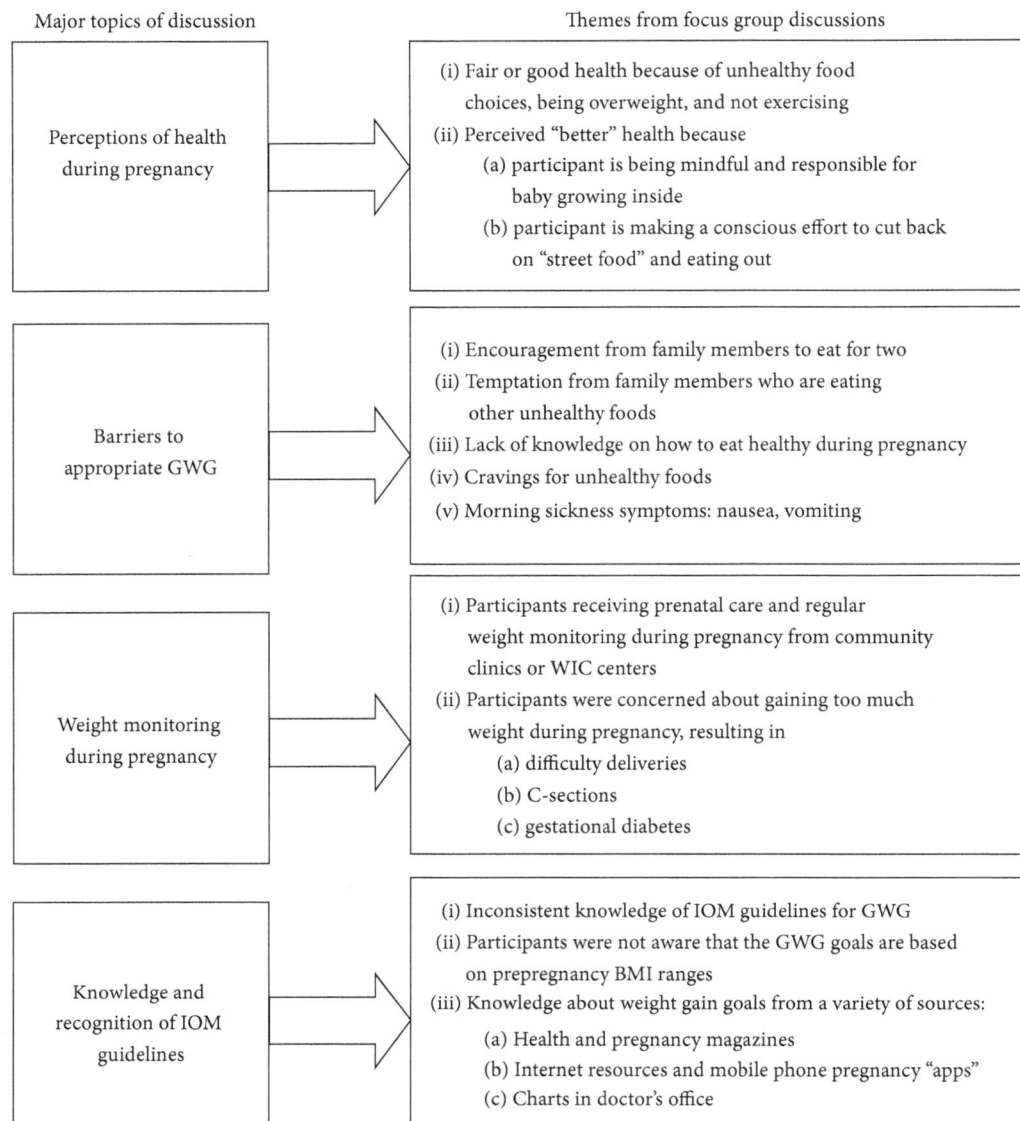

FIGURE 1: Overview of focus group topics and emerging themes.

about their weight, but they did not know how much weight they should be gaining during pregnancy. These concerns centered on having difficult deliveries or complications, such as C-sections. One mother shared, "I'm actually very concerned if I gain a lot of weight because my doctor said if I gain a lot more than I should, it will be very hard for the delivery time." Second, women were concerned about weight loss after delivery. One mother reported, "Gaining too much. It's hard to lose the weight after. You have to think of the aftermath because once the baby comes out you're stuck with this weight." Finally, about one-third of the women shared that they were concerned about developing gestational diabetes if they were overweight during pregnancy. One mother suggested, "I guess, if you gain too much weight, then your baby is going to be bigger and then in my case if I gain

too much, then I can get gestational diabetes, which I never had with any of my other pregnancies."

All women reported receiving some form of prenatal care and weight monitoring during their pregnancy, either from a private doctor or community clinic. Most women also reported being weighed regularly at a prenatal visit or at WIC. Additionally, some participants also weighed themselves regularly at home; these participants were particularly concerned about their risk of developing gestational diabetes. A few women admitted to being in denial, not wanting to know their weight. Some felt that pregnancy was a "special time" in their lives, so weight should not be the focus. Others were resigned that they were already "big," so it was of no benefit to step on a scale. One participant lamented, "I don't [weigh myself] at home. I don't know, I just think that if I do it

I'm going to obsess over the weight, and I don't want to harm my baby. But then if I feel that my clothes don't fit, I'll start drinking water."

When asked if they discussed weight gain goals during pregnancy with their healthcare providers during prenatal visits, participants shared inconsistencies with regard to whether their doctors discussed weight gain during pregnancy. For some participants, their doctors discussed weight gain goals and provided feedback so participants were aware of whether they were gaining the appropriate amount of weight during pregnancy. For other participants, their doctors told them they were "fine" and did not have to worry about their weight. Some others shared that there was minimal or no discussion of their weight during their monthly prenatal visits. One participant reported, "In my case, they haven't told me that I am gaining too much weight. They always tell me that I am fine and that is why I don't worry. Now if they told me that I gained too much then I would have to do something; but till now they haven't told me that I am bad."

3.2.4. IOM Guidelines for Weight Gain during Pregnancy.

A few women (5 of 59) had no knowledge or awareness of any guidelines for weight gain during pregnancy; most of these women were more recent immigrants. Some participants had seen weight gain goals and were aware of the concept of weight gain goals during pregnancy. Among those who knew about weight gain ranges, there were inconsistencies with the weight gain ranges reported by these participants. Some reported ranges that were higher than the IOM guidelines, while others reported lower weight ranges. Among those who knew about weight gain ranges, some shared that they knew about weight gain goals from their doctor, charts in the doctor's office, educational pamphlets, baby magazine and "baby" books, or online resources (websites and mobile phone applications or "apps"). A few women indicated they had learned about their weight gain goals from WIC staff. One participant reported, "Here in WIC, yes. Every time they weigh me they say that 10–15 pounds is what is normal to gain during pregnancy for me. But in the [health] clinic, no." Most importantly, most women (>75%) were not aware that their gestational weight gain goals differed by prepregnancy weight status. These results are confirmed by Anderson and colleagues, who also found that women received inadequate or conflicting information about pregnancy nutrition and GWG from health care providers [27]. This suggests an important opportunity and avenue for education in all settings where pregnant women are routinely seen.

3.2.5. Ideas for Educational Tools: A Pregnancy Weight Tracker.

One of the complications of determining appropriate GWG is that guidelines are based on four categories of prepregnancy weight: underweight, normal weight, overweight, or obese. In the focus group discussions of how to differentiate the pregnancy weight tracker tool based on prepregnancy weight status, participants offered different ideas for how to identify the woman's weight category. Some participants wanted the weight designation (underweight, normal weight,

overweight, and obese) listed on the pregnancy weight tracker because it was an accurate reflection of their weight status; others expressed concern that the labels posed a negative stigma. One mother said, "I agree, some people might not be able to accept that [they are overweight]. I don't know, but I agree you shouldn't get mad, because it's the truth if you're overweight." For a majority of Caucasian and Hispanic participants, the designation of "overweight" or "obese" on the tracker was a sensitive issue, and they preferred not to have these labels on the pregnancy weight tracker; instead, the participants suggested color coding the four weight ranges and including the weight range goals on the pregnancy weight tracker. One participant commented, "You don't know how sensitive a person may be when it comes to words like 'obese' or 'overweight', and like she said, what does it mean? How do you define that for a person? So, I think maybe that's a bit more sensitive matter." Another participant suggested distinguishing the different weight categories by color: "No, I don't think [overweight or obese] should be on the pregnancy weight tracker. I think it would be a constant reminder that you're overweight. But having different colors for different weights is better."

When asked if participants were interested in having a way to track their weight gain during pregnancy, all the participants indicated a strong interest in having a tool to track their weight during pregnancy. Most women reported a willingness to use a pregnancy weight tracker if WIC provided one; also, the women suggested that the pregnancy weight tracker would be helpful to facilitate discussion of their weight gain goals at regular prenatal visits with their healthcare provider, as well as WIC visits. A majority of the women indicated that they would like a "credit card" sized pregnancy weight tracker for their purse and "half sheet" to be used at home, to be placed either on the refrigerator or in the bathroom. Participants shared affirmatively that they were interested in having accountability with using the pregnancy weight tracker, along with educational handouts. Participants shared that having a pregnancy weight tracker (GWG tracker) on hand to discuss with WIC staff and their doctors would encourage them to monitor their own weight and stay on track with weight gain goals. One participant suggested that the pregnancy weight tracker should be a routine part of WIC services, "They ask about our address and income when we come, and they should ask about that [pregnancy weight tracker] too when they give it out."

3.2.6. Applications of Focus Group Findings to an Intervention Study.

Findings from this study suggest that participants face significant barriers to being able to gain the appropriate amount of weight and are very interested in tools and education to help stay on target with weight gain. Results of focus groups analyses were utilized to design a GWG tracker and accompanying educational handout for use with pregnant moms enrolling in WIC. A GWG tracker was developed based on their feedback (compact size so participants can carry it with them and color coded rather than identifying their weight status). The educational handout incorporated messages related to the barriers women identified. The first

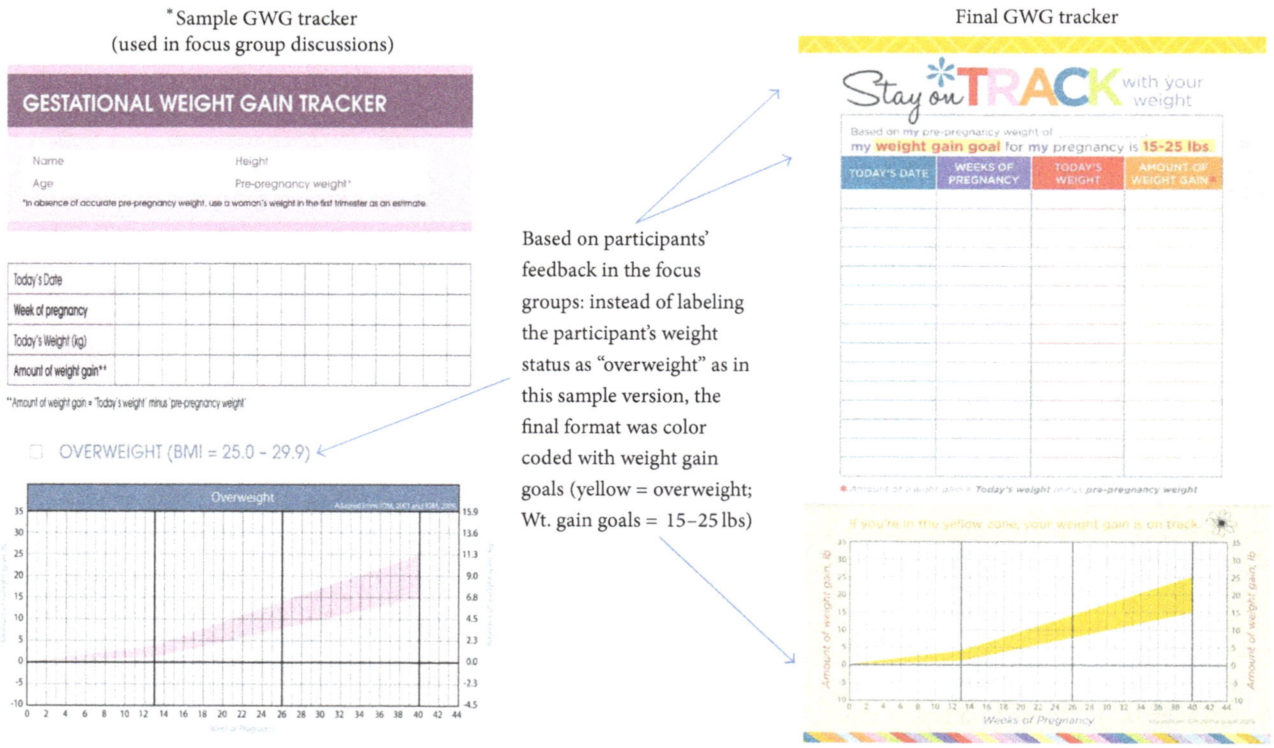

* Sample GWG tracker is from http://www.healthcanada.gc.ca/nutrition
Link to available resources from PHFE-WIC: https://www.phfewic.org/Projects/GestationalWeightGain.aspx

FIGURE 2: Sample and final pregnancy weight tracker (GWG tracker).

barrier discussed by the participants was the theme of "eating for two." This perception of having to "eat for two" contributed to participants feeling the need to eat more, which then encouraged higher gestational weight gain rather than discouraging it. These findings are confirmed in other qualitative research studies with African-American and Puerto Rican mothers [20, 21, 28]. This suggestion from family members to eat for two is derived from motivation and desire to optimize pregnancy outcomes and fetal growth. If mothers do not perceive excess weight gain to be problematic, there will be little "buy-in" to follow the IOM guidelines. These perceptions of threat and susceptibility are at the heart of the Health Belief Model [29]; as such, these findings suggested the need to direct nutrition education to target debunking this myth of "eating for two." The educational handout developed for the intervention phase served to debunk the myth in the following ways: (1) providing clarification for weight gain distribution during pregnancy; (2) explaining how excess weight gain leads to complications with pregnancy and delivery; (3) providing IOM weight gain ranges so participants are aware and can track their weights during pregnancy.

We found that a majority of the focus group participants were concerned about gaining too much weight but had many misperceptions and barriers that needed to be clarified and corrected; these findings are corroborated by another study [22]. The educational handout serves to debunk myths

and correct understandings about GWG. Figure 2 provides a sample GWG tracker tool that was developed for use during the focus group discussions; focus group participant feedback and suggestions led to the final GWG tracker. This GWG tracker tool allows participants to be accountable about their weight gain goals and facilitates discussions with their doctors about weight gain during prenatal visits and with WIC nutritionists. Finally, placement of the GWG goals on the pregnancy weight tracker builds awareness among participants of appropriate weight gain during their pregnancy. Building this awareness among WIC participants for appropriate GWG provides important perceived benefits which, based on the Health Belief Model [29, 30], may go a long way in raising consciousness among WIC participants.

While this qualitative study provided important grounding for the development of an intervention study to prevent excessive GWG among WIC participants, it is not without its limitations. Because the sample is specific to the WIC population, these findings may have limited generalizability to the entire population of pregnant women who have varying socioeconomic and cultural backgrounds. Second, the Hispanic population of WIC participants is primarily from Mexico, and this may not be generalizable to WIC programs in other parts of the US. Finally, while it is possible that our findings may have been impacted by the presence of women with different BMI classifications within a focus group, our moderators used qualitative methodology skills to encourage all participants to share. It would be beneficial in future studies to also further stratify focus groups by BMI classifications to ensure a more homogenous grouping of women based on weight groupings. Despite these limitations, the benefit of this qualitative study was to allow for an unhurried and open discussion of the IOM gestational weight gain guidelines and challenges to appropriate weight gain during pregnancy in the WIC program; the findings from these discussions were applied directly to inform the development of the intervention.

4. Conclusion

Findings from this study have important implications for how perinatal health is conceptualized and assessed. These findings illustrate the complex nature of weight gain during pregnancy, particularly among low-income ethnic minority groups. This work extends the discussion beyond a simplistic and unidimensional conceptualization to one which considers the multilevel and complex socioecological landscape in which immigrant communities navigate their health decisions. Employing qualitative research methods in maternal and child health research with immigrant groups allow for findings and interpretations to be grounded in the cultural context of daily lived experiences. Second, narratives give voice to and illuminate our understanding of how individual experiences collectively and simultaneously affect pregnancy outcomes, thus providing a more holistic perspective on the impact of culture on perinatal health. At a practical level, this holistic approach allows for a better understanding of the contextual environment in which many of these low-income families live; as a result, we will be able to design WIC-based programming and health-related interventions that will address these barriers and move us forward in bridging the gap in health disparities.

Competing Interests

The authors declare that there are no competing interests regarding the publication of this paper. Funding from USDA/UCLA did not lead to any competing interests regarding the publication of this paper. The authors have no other possible competing interests to reveal in the publication of this submitted paper.

Acknowledgments

This study was funded by the USDA, with a subaward from UCLA, no. 1920 G QA126. Additional funding for this study was provided by the Seaver Research Council 2013-14, Pepperdine University. The authors would like to thank WIC participants for their participation in these focus groups, which made this work possible. The authors would also like to thank their student research assistants, Amber Rzeznik and Gary Park.

References

[1] K. M. Flegal, D. Carroll, B. K. Kit, and C. L. Ogden, "Prevalence of obesity and trends in the distribution of body mass index among US adults, 1999–2010," *The Journal of the American Medical Association*, vol. 307, no. 5, pp. 491–497, 2012.

[2] E. P. Gunderson, B. Abrams, and S. Selvin, "The relative importance of gestational gain and maternal characteristics associated with the risk of becoming overweight after pregnancy," *International Journal of Obesity*, vol. 24, no. 12, pp. 1660–1668, 2000.

[3] B. L. Rooney and C. W. Schauberger, "Excess pregnancy weight gain and long-term obesity: one decade later," *Obstetrics and Gynecology*, vol. 100, no. 2, pp. 245–252, 2002.

[4] D. E. Smith, C. E. Lewis, J. L. Caveny, L. L. Perkins, G. L. Burke, and D. E. Bild, "Longitudinal changes in adiposity associated with pregnancy: the CARDIA study," *The Journal of the American Medical Association*, vol. 271, no. 22, pp. 1747–1751, 1994.

[5] K. M. Rasmussen, P. M. Catalano, and A. L. Yaktine, "New guidelines for weight gain during pregnancy: what obstetrician/gynecologists should know," *Current Opinion in Obstetrics & Gynecology*, vol. 21, no. 6, pp. 521–526, 2009.

[6] Institute of Medicine, *Weight Gain during Pregnancy: Reexamining The Guidelines*, Edited by K. M. Rasmussen, A. L. Yaktine, National Academy Press, Washington, DC, USA, 2009.

[7] Centers for Disease Control, "*2010 maternal health indicators*," 2010, http://www.cdc.gov/mmwr/preview/mmwrhtml/mm6443a3.htm.

[8] B. E. Gould Rothberg, U. Magriples, T. S. Kershaw, S. S. Rising, and J. R. Ickovics, "Gestational weight gain and subsequent postpartum weight loss among young, low-income, ethnic minority women," *American Journal of Obstetrics and Gynecology*, vol. 204, no. 1, pp. 52.e1–52.e11, 2011.

[9] B. Abrams, B. Heggeseth, D. Rehkopf, and E. Davis, "Parity and body mass index in US women: a prospective 25-year study," *Obesity*, vol. 21, no. 8, pp. 1514–1518, 2013.

[10] I. Thorsdottir, J. E. Torfadottir, B. E. Birgisdottir, and R. T. Geirsson, "Weight gain in women of normal weight before pregnancy: complications in pregnancy or delivery and birth outcome," *Obstetrics and Gynecology*, vol. 99, no. 5, pp. 799–806, 2002.

[11] M. Cedergren, "Effects of gestational weight gain and body mass index on obstetric outcome in Sweden," *International Journal of Gynecology and Obstetrics*, vol. 93, no. 3, pp. 269–274, 2006.

[12] E. P. Gunderson and B. Abrams, "Epidemiology of gestational weight gain and body weight changes after pregnancy," *Epidemiologic Reviews*, vol. 21, no. 2, pp. 261–275, 1999.

[13] M. W. Gillman, S. Rifas-Shiman, C. S. Berkey, A. E. Field, and G. A. Colditz, "Maternal gestational diabetes, birth weight, and adolescent obesity," *Pediatrics*, vol. 111, no. 3, pp. e221–e226, 2003.

[14] C. M. Olson, M. S. Strawderman, and B. A. Dennison, "Maternal weight gain during pregnancy and child weight at age 3 years," *Maternal and Child Health Journal*, vol. 13, no. 6, pp. 839–846, 2009.

[15] D. Dabelea and T. Crume, "Maternal environment and the transgenerational cycle of obesity and diabetes," *Diabetes*, vol. 60, no. 7, pp. 1849–1855, 2011.

[16] L. C. Houghton, W. A. Ester, L. H. Lumey et al., "Maternal weight gain in excess of pregnancy guidelines is related to

daughters being overweight 40 years later," *American Journal of Obstetrics and Gynecology*, 2016.

[17] S. Luke, R. S. Kirby, and L. Wright, "Postpartum weight retention and subsequent pregnancy outcomes," *The Journal of Perinatal & Neonatal Nursing*, p. 1, 2016.

[18] I. Chihara, D. K. Hayes, L. R. Chock, L. J. Fuddy, D. L. Rosenberg, and A. S. Handler, "Relationship between gestational weight gain and birthweight among clients enrolled in the Special Supplemental Nutrition Program for Women, Infants, and Children (WIC), Hawaii, 2003–2005," *Maternal and Child Health Journal*, vol. 18, no. 5, pp. 1123–1131, 2014.

[19] M. Koleilat and S. E. Whaley, "Trends and predictors of excessive gestational weight gain among hispanic wic participants in Southern California," *Maternal and Child Health Journal*, vol. 17, no. 8, pp. 1399–1404, 2013.

[20] A. Tovar, L. Chasan-Taber, O. I. Bermudez, R. R. Hyatt, and A. Must, "Knowledge, attitudes, and beliefs regarding weight gain during pregnancy among Hispanic women," *Maternal and Child Health Journal*, vol. 14, no. 6, pp. 938–949, 2010.

[21] S. J. Herring, T. Q. Henry, A. A. Klotz, G. D. Foster, and R. C. Whitaker, "Perceptions of low-income African-American mothers about excessive gestational weight gain," *Maternal and Child Health Journal*, vol. 16, no. 9, pp. 1837–1843, 2012.

[22] M. Everette, "Gestational weight and dietary intake during pregnancy: perspectives of African American women," *Maternal and Child Health Journal*, vol. 12, no. 6, pp. 718–724, 2008.

[23] United States Census Bureau, "*QuickFacts on U.S. Population*," http://quickfacts.census.gov/qfd/states/00000.html.

[24] United States Department of Agriculture Food and Nutrition Service, *WIC Participant and Program Characteristics 2012 Final Report*, USDA Food and Nutrition Service, Alexandria, Va, USA, 2012.

[25] V. Braun and V. Clarke, "Using thematic analysis in psychology," *Qualitative Research in Psychology*, vol. 3, no. 2, pp. 77–101, 2006.

[26] J. W. Creswell, *Research Design: Qualitative, Quantitative, and Mixed Methods Approaches*, Sage Publication, Thousand Oaks, Calif, USA, 2nd edition, 2003.

[27] C. K. Anderson, T. J. Walch, S. M. Lindberg, A. M. Smith, S. R. Lindheim, and L. D. Whigham, "Excess gestational weight gain in low-income overweight and obese women: a qualitative study," *Journal of Nutrition Education and Behavior*, vol. 47, no. 5, pp. 404.el–411.el, 2015.

[28] M. A. Kominiarek, F. Gay, and N. Peacock, "Obesity in pregnancy: a qualitative approach to inform an intervention for patients and providers," *Maternal and Child Health Journal*, vol. 19, no. 8, pp. 1698–1712, 2015.

[29] N. K. Janz and M. H. Becker, "The health belief model: a decade later," *Health Education Quarterly*, vol. 11, no. 1, pp. 1–47, 1984.

[30] S. W. Groth and M. H. Kearney, "Diverse women's beliefs about weight gain in pregnancy," *Journal of Midwifery and Women's Health*, vol. 54, no. 6, pp. 452–457, 2009.

Frequency, Risk Factors, and Adverse Fetomaternal Outcomes of Placenta Previa in Northern Tanzania

Elizabeth Eliet Senkoro,[1] Amasha H. Mwanamsangu,[2]
Fransisca Seraphin Chuwa,[1] Sia Emmanuel Msuya,[2,3] Oresta Peter Mnali,[1]
Benjamin G. Brown,[4] and Michael Johnson Mahande[2]

[1]Kilimanjaro Christian Medical University College, Moshi, Tanzania
[2]Department of Epidemiology & Biostatistics, Institute of Public Health, Kilimanjaro Christian Medical University College,
 Moshi, Tanzania
[3]Department of Community Health, Institute of Public Health, Kilimanjaro Christian Medical University College, Moshi, Tanzania
[4]Department of Global Health, Weill Cornell Medical College, New York, NY, USA

Correspondence should be addressed to Michael Johnson Mahande; jmmahande@gmail.com

Academic Editor: Fabio Facchinetti

Background and Objective. Placenta previa (PP) is a potential risk factor for obstetric hemorrhage, which is a major cause of fetomaternal morbidity and mortality in developing countries. This study aimed to determine frequency, risk factors, and adverse fetomaternal outcomes of placenta previa in Northern Tanzania. *Methodology*. A retrospective cohort study was conducted using maternally-linked data from Kilimanjaro Christian Medical Centre birth registry spanning 2000 to 2015. All women who gave birth to singleton infants were studied. Adjusted odds ratios (ORs) with 95% confidence intervals for risk factors and adverse fetomaternal outcomes associated with PP were estimated in multivariable logistic regression models. *Result*. A total of 47,686 singleton deliveries were analyzed. Of these, the frequency of PP was 0.6%. Notable significant risk factors for PP included gynecological diseases, alcohol consumption during pregnancy, malpresentation, and gravidity ≥5. Adverse maternal outcomes were postpartum haemorrhage, antepartum haemorrhage, and Caesarean delivery. PP increased odds of fetal Malpresentation and early neonatal death. *Conclusion*. The prevalence of PP was comparable to that found in past research. Multiple independent risk factors were identified. PP was found to have associations with several adverse fetomaternal outcomes. Early identification of women at risk of PP may help clinicians prevent such complications.

1. Introduction

Placenta previa is an obstetric complication characterized by placental implantation into the lower segment of the uterine wall, covering whole (major) or part (minor) of the cervix [1]. It complicates 0.4% of pregnancies at term [2]. Placenta previa usually presents with painless vaginal bleeding in the late second or early third trimester. It is diagnosed on ultrasound during the second trimester or incidentally during an operation.

A study in Uganda reported an association between placenta previa and severe obstetric hemorrhage/bleeding [3]. Obstetric hemorrhage is a leading cause of fetomaternal

mortality and morbidity in Sub-Saharan Africa [4]. Placenta previa has further been linked to maternal hypovolemia, anemia, and long hospital stay, as well as adverse fetal outcomes such as low birth weight, congenital abnormalities, stillbirth, and early neonatal death [5–9].

While the precise etiology of placenta previa is not known, previous studies have elucidated predictive factors such as high maternal age, twin pregnancies, previous Caesarean section, previous uterine scar, grand multiparity, malpresentation, and diabetes mellitus [5, 7–11].

The estimated global prevalence of placenta previa is 5.2 per 1000 pregnant women, although there is significant international variation, whereby the prevalence was highest among Asian studies and lower in Sub-Saharan Africa studies [12]. However, there are no studies in Tanzania which have evaluated the burden of placenta previa and its associated adverse fetomaternal outcomes. Therefore, this study aimed to determine frequency, risk factors, and adverse fetomaternal outcomes of placenta previa in Northern Tanzania. Understanding these associations would help improve early diagnosis of placenta previa and allow for better management and prevention of adverse outcomes.

2. Methods

2.1. Study Design and Setting. We conducted a retrospective cohort study using maternally linked data from the Kilimanjaro Christian Medical Centre (KCMC) medical birth registry. KCMC is located in Moshi Municipality, Tanzania. It is one of four zonal referral hospitals in the country, serving over 15 million people and performing an annual average of 4000 deliveries. The birth registry was established in 1999 as collaboration between KCMC and the registry of University of Bergen, Norway, and has been operational since 2000. Since then, all deliveries that occurred at KCMC are recorded in a computerized database system at KCMC medical birth registry.

2.2. Study Population and Sampling Procedure. All singleton deliveries that took place at Obstetrics and Gynecology Department of KCMC hospital from January 2000 to December 2015 with complete birth registry records were considered for analysis. Women diagnosed with placenta abruption were excluded to avoid misdiagnosis of placenta previa. In addition, women with multiple gestation pregnancies were also excluded to avoid overrepresentation of studying high risk women. The final sample was comprised of 47,686 deliveries which were analyzed.

2.3. Data Collection Methods and Tools. A standardized questionnaire was used to collect information for the medical birth registry. Each woman who delivered at KCMC was individually consented to interview, after which trained midwives worked through the standardized questionnaire. Women were interviewed daily, within 24 hours of delivery, or as soon as possible after recovery in case the mother had delivery complications. Information collected included maternal age, occupation, education, marital status, childhood, and present areas of residence; past medical history; last menstrual period and regularity of cycle; history of present and past smoking, drinking, or chewing tobacco use; drug, herb, and medication use; obstetric history, including first ANC visit, number of ANC visits, use of family planning, pregnancy complications, and details of labor; history of previous pregnancies, including miscarriage, stillbirth, preterm birth, fertility treatment, and mode of delivery; and sex, weight, and any medical ailments of the infant most recently delivered. The recorded information was corroborated with the antenatal cards and written medical records whenever possible. These data were entered into a computerized database system located at medical birth registry, from which they were retrieved for

this study. It is worth noting that all women who deliver for the first time at KCMC are assigned with a unique mother identification number. This number is constant for all births that occur at KCMC. The same number is available to the child file; this makes it possible to link siblings with their biological mothers for subsequent births.

2.4. Definition of Terms. Placenta previa was defined as an obstetric complication characterized by placental implantation into the lower segment of the uterine wall, covering part of or the entire cervix.

Antepartum hemorrhage was defined as bleeding into and/or from the vaginal canal at any time from the 24th week of gestation up to the second stage of labor.

Postpartum hemorrhage was defined as blood loss of 500 mL or more after delivery.

Apgar score was defined as a measure of the physical condition of a newborn infant. The Apgar score has a maximum ten points, with two possible for each of heart rate, muscle tone, response to stimulation, and skin coloration.

2.5. Data Analysis. Data analysis was performed using Statistical Package for the Social Sciences (SPSS) version 20. Mean with respective standard deviation was used to summarize a normally distributed maternal age and frequencies with respective percentages were used to summarize categorical variables. Both bivariate and multivariable analysis were performed using logistic regression and adjusted odd ratios (aOR) with 95% confidence intervals for risk factors and fetomaternal outcomes associated with placenta previa were estimated in the models. A P value of less than 0.05 was considered statistically significant. A variable was considered as a confounder when its inclusion in the model changed the crude estimate of interest by 10%. Due to rarity of frequency of placenta previa, odds ratio was used to approximate the relative risk.

2.6. Ethical Considerations. Our study was approved by the Kilimanjaro Christian Medical University College Research Ethics Committee prior to its commencement. Verbal consent was obtained from all women prior to their interviews after a full explanation of the birth registry project. Research consent was not requested for this study, as the pertinent data belonged to an approved project, and confidentiality and privacy were assured as per birth registry protocol.

3. Results

3.1. Characteristics of the Study Participants. Table 1 summarizes the demographic characteristics of 47,686 singleton deliveries that were analyzed. The overall mean age was 27.48 (SD = 6.05) years. Women with placenta previa had a significantly higher mean age [29.07, SD = 6.12 (years)] than their unaffected counterparts [27.47, SD = 6.05 (years)]. Most of the women were below the age of 20 years, married, residing in urban areas, and having their ANC visit during pregnancy. An observed higher proportion of women with placenta previa were married, of younger age below 20 years,

TABLE 1: Background characteristics of women participating in the study in Northern Tanzania (N = 47,686).

Characteristics	Placenta previa (N = 270)	No placenta previa (N = 47,416)	Total (N = 47686)
Age in years, mean (SD)	29.07 (6.12)	27.47 (6.05)	27.48 (6.05)
Age group (years)			
<20	184 (68.2)	34133 (72.5)	34317 (72.5)
20–34	30 (11.1)	6275 (13.3)	6305 (13.3)
≥35	56 (20.74)	6682 (14.2)	6738 (14.2)
Marital status			
Married	242 (90.0)	41371 (88.0)	41613 (88.0)
Not married	27 (10.0)	5657 (12.0)	5684 (12.0)
Residence			
Rural	192 (71.1)	19799 (42.0)	19991 (42.3)
Urban	69 (25.6)	25146 (53.4)	25215 (53.3)
Semiurban	9 (3.4)	2093 (4.5)	2102 (4.4)
Antenatal care in this pregnancy			
Yes	121 (44.8)	38075 (80.8)	38196 (80.6)
No	149 (55.2)	9062 (19.2)	9211 (19.4)

SD = standard deviation.

and residing in rural areas and had never attended ANC visit during pregnancy.

3.2. Risk Factors for Placenta Previa. Table 2 displays risk factors for placenta previa. Significant risk factors for PP after adjusting for potential confounding factors were gynecological diseases [OR 2.44; 95% CI: 1.50–3.97], use of alcohol during present pregnancy [OR 1.61; 95% CI: 1.17–2.21], grand multipara [OR 3.46; 95% CI: 1.01–11.86], and multigravida ≥5 [OR 4.85; 95% CI: 1.49–15.75]. On the other hand, antenatal care ≥4 visits [OR 0.45; 95% CI: 0.32–0.64] and maternal age ≥35 years [OR 0.56; 95% CI: 0.35–0.89] were associated with lower odds of having placenta previa. Use of family planning, previous Caesarean section, and history of previous scar had no significant association with placenta previa.

3.3. Maternal Outcomes Associated with Placenta Previa. Table 3 summarizes maternal outcomes associated with placenta previa. After adjustment for confounders, women with placenta previa had increased odds of APH [OR 9.21; 95% CI: 5.3–16.0] and PPH [OR 17.6; 95% CI: 8.6–36.2], hospital stay of >4 days [OR 5.62; 95% CI: 3.85–8.20], delivery by Caesarean section [OR 9.68; 95% CI: 6.66–14.1], and blood transfusion [OR 2.91; 95% CI: 1.87–4.52].

3.4. Fetal Outcomes Associated with Placenta Previa. Table 4 shows fetal outcomes and their associations with placenta previa. Infants delivered by mothers with placenta previa were more likely to have Apgar scores of <7 at the 1st [OR 2.68; 95% CI: 1.88–3.84], 5th [OR 3.83; 95% CI: 2.73–5.39], and 10th [OR 3.07; 95% CI: 2.08–4.52] minutes after birth, low birth weight [OR 5.62; 95% CI: 4.06–7.77], admission to neonatal intensive care unit/NICU [OR 2.53; 95% CI: 1.8–3.57], fetal malpresentation [OR 4.3; 95% CI: 2.27–8.13], stillbirth [OR 2.58; 95% CI: 1.55–4.29], and early neonatal

death [OR 3.75; 95% CI: 1.15–12.3]. Congenital malformation was not associated with placenta previa.

4. Discussion

The prevalence of placenta previa in our study was 0.6%. Risk factors included multigravida ≥5, use of alcohol in this pregnancy, and gynecological diseases. Women with placenta previa were at increased risk for PPH, APH, need for blood transfusion, long hospital stay, and delivery by Caesarean section. Placenta previa also increased the likelihood of certain adverse pregnancy outcomes: Apgar scores ≤7 at minutes 1, 5, and 10, low birth weight, fetal malpresentation, NICU admission, and early neonatal death.

The prevalence of placenta previa in our study was similar to the prevalence of 0.7% reported in a study conducted in Pakistan by Bhutia et al. [6]. However our study shows lower prevalence than that reported by Kiondo et al. in Uganda (0.16%) [3, 6]. These differences may be explained by differences in the study design and sample size. The study conducted in Uganda had a shorter spanning time frame and had a smaller sample size, possibly leading to an underestimation of prevalence [3].

Our study found that multigravida ≥5 connoted a fivefold increase in risk of placenta previa. Similar finding was reported in studies conducted in Tanzania by Mgaya et al. and Pakistan by Raees et al. [9, 11]. The increased risk of placenta previa among multigravida women may be explained by degenerative change to the uterine vasculature, leading to underperfusion of the placenta, compensatory enlargement, and increased likelihood of implantation on the lower segment [3].

However, our study found no association between placenta previa and advanced maternal age or high parity. This differs from the findings of study conducted in Nepal by Ojha although a study conducted in Kingdom of Saudi

TABLE 2: Logistic regression of risk factors for placenta previa in Northern Tanzania ($N = 47,686$).

Risk factors	Total	Placenta previa	cOR (95% CI)	aOR (95% CI)
Maternal age (years)				
<20	6356	13 (0.2)	0.95 (0.53–1.72)	1.37 (0.77–2.45)
20–34	34511	74 (0.2)	1.0	1.0
≥35	6772	24 (0.4)	1.66 (1.04–2.63)	0.56 (0.35–0.89)
Gynecological diseases				
Yes	1844	22 (1.2)	0.3 (0.19–0.67)	2.44 (1.5–3.97)
No	45842	248 (0.5)	1.0	1.0
Alcohol during pregnancy				
Yes	13736	104 (38.7)	1.56 (1.21–1.99)	1.61 (1.17–2.21)
No	33814	165 (61.3)	1.0	1.0
Family planning				
Yes	29734	194 (72.4)	1.57 (1.18–2.05)	0.78 (0.46–1.31)
No	17711	74 (27.6)	1.0	1.0
History of previous scar				
Yes	2054	7 (2.6)	0.59 (0.28–1.25)	0.72 (0.30–1.72)
No	45632	263 (97.4)	1.0	1.0
Malpresentation				
Yes	657	12 (4.5)	3.38 (1.89–6.07)	4.28 (2.26–8.10)
No	46803	256 (95.5)	1.0	1.0
Number of ANC visits				
≥4	20009	67 (26.3)	0.48 (0.36–0.63)	0.45 (0.32–0.64)
<4	26762	188 (73.7)	1.0	1.0
Parity				
0	13071	39 (0.3)	1.0	1.0
1–4	18916	107 (0.6)	1.97 (1.37–2.85)	1.42 (0.48–4.16)
≥5	1060	27 (3.0)	9.91 (6.04–16.27)	3.46 (1.01–11.86)
Gravidity				
1	12118	35 (0.3)	1.0	1.0
2–4	17751	88 (0.5)	1.77 (1.2–2.62)	1.93 (0.66–5.63)
≥5	3178	50 (1.8)	6.05 (3.92–9.34)	4.85 (1.49–15.75)
Previous CS				
Yes	6958	32 (0.5)	0.84 (0.57–1.23)	0.65 (0.42–1.01)
No	26089	141 (0.6)	1.0	1.0

cOR = crude odds ratio, CS = Caesarian section, ANC = antenatal care, and aOR = adjusted odds ratio: adjusted for maternal age, gynecological diseases, alcohol during pregnancy, family planning, history of previous scar, malpresentation, number of ANC visits, parity, gravidity, and previous CS.

Arabia (KSA) by Ahmed et al. also found no association between maternal age and placenta previa. Lack of association between the known risk factors with placenta previa in our study and those of others could be related to proper management of these women as a high risk group which necessitates heightened close follow-up.

Since we did not collect information on specific gynecological diseases, this odds ratio could not be compared to other studies. Sexually transmitted diseases are very common in our study area, suggesting intrauterine adhesions as a possible mechanism for impaired placental migration [10]. Past history of Caesarean section and history of uterine scar were not found to be associated with placenta previa. This contrasts with previous studies by Kiondo et al. and Anzaku and Musa [3, 13]. This may be explained by the fact that the placenta implants in a previous Caesarean section scar; it may be so deep as to prevent placental separation (placenta accreta) or penetrate through the uterine wall into surrounding structures such as the bladder (placenta percreta) which may provoke massive hemorrhage at delivery.

We found a significant association between alcohol use in the index pregnancy and placenta previa. This differs from the findings of Missouri by Aliyu et al., a discrepancy which could be explained by population differences in alcoholic intake. Alcohol use is a common practice in the study setting.

In contrast, previous studies have reported an association between smoking during pregnancy, infertility treatment, and PP [6, 14]. Unfortunately these factors are uncommon in Tanzania; thus our study may have lacked the power to assess these factors.

TABLE 3: Logistic regression for maternal outcomes associated with placenta previa ($N = 47{,}686$).

Maternal outcomes	Total	Placenta previa	cOR (95% CI)	aOR (95% CI)
Postpartum hemorrhage				
No	47472	254 (94.1)	1.0	1.0
Yes	214	16 (5.9)	15.02 (8.89–25.37)	17.6 (8.6–36.2)
Antepartum hemorrhage				
No	47176	487 (1.0)	1.0	1.0
Yes	510	23 (8.5)	8.97 (5.80–13.88)	9.21 (5.3–16.0)
Mode of delivery				
Vaginal delivery	3186	72 (26.7)	1.0	1.0
Caesarean delivery	15636	198 (73.3)	5.66 (4.32–7.42)	9.68 (6.66–14.08)
Need blood transfusion				
No	44586	210 (78.7)	1.0	1.0
Yes	2850	57 (21.3)	4.31 (3.21–5.79)	2.91 (1.87–4.52)
Duration of hospitalization				
≤4 days	28,676	84 (0.3)	1.0	1.0
>4 days	18599	185 (1.0)	3.42 (2.6–4.43)	5.62 (3.85–8.20)

cOR = crude odds ratio and aOR = adjusted odds ratio: adjusting for maternal age, gynecological diseases, parity, gravidity, previous CS, alcohol during pregnancy, malpresentation, and number of ANC visits.

TABLE 4: Logistic regression for fetal outcomes associated with placenta previa ($N = 47{,}686$).

Fetal outcomes	Total	Placenta previa	cOR (95% CI)	aOR (95% CI)
Apgar score at 1 minute				
>7	24034	72 (27.3)	1.0	1.0
≤7	23159	192 (72.7)	2.78 (2.12–3.65)	2.68 (1.88–3.84)
Apgar score at 10 minutes				
>7	42959	185 (71.2)	1.0	1.0
≤7	4027	75 (28.8)	4.39 (3.35–5.75)	3.07 (2.08–4.52)
Apgar score at 5 minutes				
>7	41526	161 (61.2)	1.0	1.0
≤7	5583	102 (38.8)	4.78 (3.73–6.14)	3.83 (2.73–5.39)
Low birth weight				
Yes	5995	130 (48.1)	6.55 (5.15–8.32)	5.62 (4.06–7.77)
No	41477	140 (51.9)	1.0	1.0
Stillbirth				
Yes	1587	28 (10.4)	3.4 (2.29–5.05)	2.58 (1.55–4.29)
No	45895	241 (89.6)	1.0	1.0
Early neonatal death				
Yes	167	5 (1.9)	5.5 (2.24–13.50)	3.75 (1.15–12.32)
No	47315	264 (98.1)	1.0	1.0
Malformation				
Yes	69	1 (0.4)	2.58 (0.36–18.68)	2.26 (0.30–16.96)
No	47531	269 (99.6)	1.0	1.0
Admission to NICU				
No	40897	183 (68)	1.0	1,0
Yes	6585	86 (32.0)	2.94 (2.28–3.81)	2.53 (1.80–3.57)

cOR = crude odds ratio, NICU = neonatal intensive care unit, and aOR = adjusted odds ratio: adjusted for maternal age, gynecological diseases, parity, gravidity, previous Caesarean section, use of alcohol during pregnancy, malpresentation, and number of ANC visits.

Our study found a significant association between placenta previa and risk of antepartum and postpartum hemorrhage: a nine times increased risk of the former and an eighteen times increased risk of the latter. Women with placenta previa had also threefold higher odds of blood transfusion and fivefold odds of prolonged hospital stay. These findings are consistent with previous studies [7, 9, 15]. The increased risk of postpartum hemorrhage in women with placenta previa may be explained by the implantation of placenta in a previous scar which may go deep preventing placental separation. This may provoke severe hemorrhage during and after delivery because the lower segment does not constrict well the maternal blood supply. This necessitates blood transfusion. Therefore, it is important that blood transfusions and the obstetric emergency care be readily available at any facility treating women with placenta previa.

Correspondingly, women with placenta previa had tenfold higher odds of Caesarean delivery [15]. This can be explained by the fact that the placenta in the lower segment obstructs engagement of the head especially for major previa. This necessitates Caesarean section and may also cause the transverse lie of the fetus.

In the present study fetal malpresentation had 3-fold higher odds of having placenta previa as compared to those with normal feta presentation of placenta previa. Our finding is consistent with previous investigators [10]. The association between placenta previa and fetal malpresentation may be explained by the fact that the placenta in the lower segment obstructs the engagement of the head; this may cause the transverse or breech lie in the womb.

Our study found that placenta previa was more common among women with <4 antenatal care visits. This may be because they were admitted earlier compared to their counterparts. Routine ultrasound examinations would be useful for early detection of women at risk of placenta previa to enhance prevention of adverse outcomes; unfortunately, the cost and maintenance of ultrasound machines hinder their utility in developing countries.

Infants born to women with placenta previa had increased odds of low birth weight, Apgar scores of <7, admission to neonatal intensive care unit, stillbirth, fetal malpresentation, and early neonatal death. This is consistent with previous studies [6, 7, 9, 16]. The possible explanation for these could be that the bleeding associated with placenta previa may lead to hypoxia, intrauterine growth restriction, and prematurity with underdeveloped organ systems. Congenital malformations were not associated significantly with placenta previa in our study.

5. Conclusion

The prevalence of placenta previa in our sample was consistent with past studies. Multigravidas, gynecological diseases, inadequate antenatal care, and alcohol use were key risk factors. These risk factors may be useful for screening at-risk mothers. Placenta previa was also found to connote significant risk of severe, adverse maternal and fetal outcomes. This study highlights the need for comprehensive obstetrics care to appropriately treat placenta previa and its complications.

Abbreviations

APH: Antepartum hemorrhage
NICU: Neonatal intensive care unit
PPH: Postpartum hemorrhage.

Disclosure

All authors of the manuscript have read and agreed to its contents.

Competing Interests

The authors declare that they have no competing interests.

Acknowledgments

The authors wish to express heartfelt appreciation to the birth registry staff for their participation in data collection and to all women who voluntarily provided data to the medical birth registry. They also extend their gratitude appreciation to the Norwegian Government for supporting the KCMC medical birth registry.

References

[1] L. Latif, U. J. Iqbal, and M. U. Aftab, "Associated risk factors of placenta previa a matched case control study," *Pakistan Journal of Medical and Health Sciences*, vol. 9, no. 4, pp. 1344–1346, 2015.

[2] A. S. Faiz and C. V. Ananth, "Etiology and risk factors for placenta previa: an overview and meta-analysis of observational studies," *The Journal of Maternal-Fetal & Neonatal Medicine*, vol. 13, no. 3, pp. 175–190, 2003.

[3] P. Kiondo, J. Wandabwa, and P. Doyle, "Risk factors for placenta praevia presenting with severe vaginal bleeding in Mulago hospital, Kampala, Uganda," *African Health Sciences*, vol. 8, no. 1, pp. 44–49, 2008.

[4] World Health Organization, *WHO Recommendations for the Prevention and Treatment of Postpartum Haemorrhage*, World Health Organization, Geneva, Switzerland, 2012, http://www.who.int/reproductivehealth/publications/maternal_perinatal_health/9789241548502/en/.

[5] A. Bener, N. M. Saleh, and M. T. Yousafzai, "Prevalence and associated risk factors of ante-partum hemorrhage among Arab women in an economically fast growing society," *Nigerian Journal of Clinical Practice*, vol. 15, no. 2, pp. 185–189, 2012.

[6] P. C. Bhutia, T. Lertbunnaphong, T. Wongwananuruk, and D. Boriboonhirunsarn, "Prevalence of pregnancy with placenta previa in Siriraj hospital," *Siriraj Medical Journal*, vol. 63, pp. 191–195, 2011.

[7] N. Ojha, "Obstetric factors and pregnancy outcome in placenta previa," *Journal of Institute of Medicine*, vol. 34, no. 2, 2013.

[8] C. S. Kodla, "A study of prevalence, causes, risk factors and outcome of severe obstetrics haemorrhage," *Journal of Scientific and Innovative Research*, vol. 4, no. 2, pp. 83–87, 2015.

[9] M. Raees, Z. Parveen, and M. Kamal, "Fetal and maternal outcome in major degree placenta previa," *Gomal Journal of Medical Sciences*, vol. 13, no. 3, pp. 13–16, 2015.

[10] T. Almaksoud, "Critical analysis of risk factors and outcome of placenta previa," *Libyan Journal of Medicine Research*, vol. 8, no. 1, pp. 2312–5365, 2014.

[11] A. H. Mgaya, S. N. Massawe, H. L. Kidanto, and H. N. Mgaya, "Grand multiparity: is it still a risk in pregnancy?" *BMC Pregnancy and Childbirth*, vol. 13, article 241, 2013.

[12] J. A. Cresswell, C. Ronsmans, C. Calvert, and V. Filippi, "Prevalence of placenta praevia by world region: a systematic review and meta-analysis," *Tropical Medicine and International Health*, vol. 18, no. 6, pp. 712–724, 2013.

[13] A. S. Anzaku and J. Musa, "Placenta praevia: incidence, risk factors, maternal and fetal outcomes in a Nigerian teaching hospital," *Jos Journal of Medicine*, vol. 6, no. 1, pp. 42–46, 2009.

[14] L. B. Romundstad, P. R. Romundstad, A. Sunde, V. von Düring, R. Skjærven, and L. J. Vatten, "Increased risk of placenta previa in pregnancies following IVF/ICSI; a comparison of ART and non-ART pregnancies in the same mother," *Human Reproduction*, vol. 21, no. 9, pp. 2353–2358, 2006.

[15] N. Chufamo, H. Segni, and Y. K. Alemayehu, "Incidence, contributing factors and outcomes of antepartum hemorrhage in Jimma University Specialized Hospital, Southwest Ethiopia," *Universal Journal of Public Health*, vol. 3, no. 4, pp. 153–159, 2015.

[16] S. R. Ahmed, A. Aitallah, H. M. Abdelghafar, and M. A. Alsammani, "Major placenta previa: rate, maternal and neonatal outcomes experience at a tertiary maternity hospital, sohag, Egypt: a prospective study," *Journal of Clinical and Diagnostic Research*, vol. 9, no. 11, pp. QC17–QC19, 2015.

Mode of Delivery according to Leisure Time Physical Activity before and during Pregnancy: A Multicenter Cohort Study of Low-Risk Women

Emilie Nor Nielsen,[1] Per Kragh Andersen,[2] Hanne Kristine Hegaard,[1,3,4] and Mette Juhl[5,6]

[1]*The Research Unit Women's and Children's Health, The Juliane Marie Centre, Copenhagen University Hospital, Rigshospitalet, Dep. 7821, Blegdamsvej 9, 2100 Copenhagen, Denmark*
[2]*Section of Biostatistics, Department of Public Health, Øster Farimagsgade 5 opg. B, P.O. Box 2099, 1014 Copenhagen K, Denmark*
[3]*Department of Obstetrics, Copenhagen University Hospital, Rigshospitalet, Copenhagen, Denmark*
[4]*The Institute of Clinical Medicine, Faculty of Health and Medical Sciences, University of Copenhagen, Blegdamsvej 3, Copenhagen, Denmark*
[5]*Midwifery Department, Metropolitan University College, Sigurdsgade 26, 2200 Copenhagen, Denmark*
[6]*Department of Public Health, Øster Farimagsgade 5, 1014 Copenhagen K, Denmark*

Correspondence should be addressed to Mette Juhl; meju@phmetropol.dk

Academic Editor: Fabio Facchinetti

Objectives. To examine the association between maternal leisure time physical activity and mode of delivery. *Study Design.* Population-based multicentre cohort. From the Danish Dystocia Study, we included 2,435 nulliparous women, who delivered a singleton infant in cephalic presentation at term after spontaneous onset of labor in 2004-2005. We analysed mode of delivery according to self-reported physical activity at four stages, that is, the year before pregnancy and during first, second, and third trimester, in logistic regression models. Further, we combined physical activity measures at all four stages in one variable for a proportional odds model for cumulative logits. *Main Outcome Measures.* Mode of delivery (emergency caesarean section; vacuum extractor; spontaneous vaginal delivery). *Results.* The odds of emergency caesarean section decreased with increasing levels of physical activity with statistically significant trends at all four time stages except the third trimester. This tendency was confirmed in the proportional odds model showing 28% higher odds of a more complicated mode of delivery among women with a low activity level compared to moderately active women. *Conclusions.* We found increasing leisure time physical activity before and during pregnancy associated with a less complicated delivery among low-risk, nulliparous women.

1. Introduction

Physical activity during pregnancy is associated with a reduced risk of preterm delivery, gestational diabetes, and possibly also preeclampsia [1–7] but has also been associated with an increased risk of miscarriage among women who exercised early in pregnancy [8]. Few studies have examined physical activity before pregnancy, but associations have been reported with a reduced risk of gestational diabetes and preeclampsia [9]. Due to the general benefits of physical activity on mortality and physical and mental health [10] regular physical activity during pregnancy is recommended

in Denmark and other countries since 2002 [11–15]. Even so, the results on how, or if, physical activity affects the course of delivery, are inconclusive [16–26]. Hence, one meta-analysis, based on 4 randomized controlled trials, reported no association between physical activity and caesarean section (C-section) [16], while another one, based on 16 randomized controlled trials, found structured physical exercise during pregnancy to be associated with a reduced risk of C-section [5], which was also the conclusion of a recent meta-analysis including 8 studies on normal-weight women [26]. Finally, a meta-analysis from 2015 suggested that regular exercise during pregnancy was modestly associated with increased chance of normal delivery; the authors, however, stressed the need for further research, including measures of the intensity and the gestational timing of physical exercise [21]. Large population-based studies are sparse and also report inconclusive findings [27–29].

In clinical obstetrics, vaginal deliveries are usually preferred to C-sections in low-risk pregnant and laboring women, because C-sections have been associated with an increased risk of complications to anaesthesia, excessive blood loss, respiratory complications, longer recovery periods in the mother, risks associated with C-section antea in subsequent pregnancies (e.g., placenta previa, placenta accrete, and stillbirth), iatrogenic prematurity, respiratory complications, and referral to neonatal unit in the child, and also long-term effects in the child, such as asthma, systematic connective tissue disorders, juvenile arthritis, inflammatory bowel diseases, immune deficiencies, and leukaemia, have been suggested [30–34].

Even though there have been several original studies and also meta-analyses summing up results, findings are still inconclusive, and previous research generally lacks detailed information on exercise (such as measures from the prepregnancy period and the first trimester of pregnancy) and on obstetric data related to mode of delivery (such as instrumental vaginal delivery, primary versus secondary C-section, and elective versus emergency C-section). These are relevant factors, since the general risk of C-section is dependent on parity, the risk of C-section is substantially increased after a previous C-section, and aetiology and risk of complications related to the C-section surgery varies largely between elective and emergency C-sections. Finally, since instrumental vaginal delivery and emergency C-section can be considered a continuum (away from an uncomplicated, vaginal delivery), vacuum extractor should ideally also be included in studies on mode of delivery.

The aim of this study was to examine the association between leisure time physical activity the year before pregnancy and during pregnancy and mode of delivery. We hypothesize that regular physical activity reduces the incidence of emergency C-section and the use of vacuum extractor.

2. Materials and Methods

2.1. Study Population. We used data from the Danish Dystocia Study, a population-based multicentre study with prospectively collected data from 9 obstetrics departments in Denmark during 2004-2005. The study included women in Robson delivery Group 1, that is, women with a singleton vertex infant and spontaneous onset of labor at ≥37 completed gestational weeks [35, 36]. Typical reasons for never entering Robson Group 1 include, for example, preterm delivery, induced delivery, breech presentation, or planned C-section. In addition, participants should be 18 years or older and able to read and understand Danish language. Recruitment took place in antenatal clinics at 33 gestational weeks, the women gave written informed consent, and a

self-reported baseline questionnaire was administered at 37 gestational weeks.

A number of 2652 women fulfilled the criteria and had completed the baseline questionnaire. From this number, we excluded women with missing data on mode of delivery (n = 22), physical activity before pregnancy (n = 32), physical activity during first (n = 3), second (n = 3) and third trimester (n = 12), age (n = 5), educational level (n = 19), smoking during pregnancy (n = 10), and prepregnancy body mass index (n = 111), resulting in a final study population of 2435 women.

Permission to establish the database was obtained from the Danish Data Protection Agency j.no. 2004-41-4545. Since no invasive procedures were applied in the study, no Ethics Committee System approval was required by Danish law. The policy of the Helsinki Declaration was followed throughout the data collection and analyses.

2.2. Measurement of Physical Activity. In the Danish Dystocia Study baseline questionnaire at gestational week 37, the women were asked about physical activity level at each of four stages (the year before pregnancy/first trimester/second trimester/third trimester). Physical activity was analysed using a four-item physical activity score [37]: "When you look back on (e.g., the year before your current pregnancy), which would you say is the most appropriate description of your activities?" #1 Hard training and competing sports regularly and several times a week ("competitive sports"), #2 sports or heavy gardening at least four hours a week ("moderate-to-heavy physical activity"), #3 walking, cycling, or other light exercises at least four hours a week (including Sunday walks, light gardening, and cycling/walking to work) ("light physical activity"), or #4 reading, watching television, or pursuing some other sedentary occupation ("sedentary lifestyle"). For additional analyses, we assigned a score to each of the four activity levels and constructed an activity sum score by adding the values of the four stages resulting in one single score. The sum score summarized each woman's physical activity level as a number between 4 and 16. This quantitative measure was further categorized into high (<11), moderate (11-12), and low (>12) physical activity level. The cut points at 10/11 and 12/13 were chosen to obtain similar group sizes for the two extreme exposure groups. For the low physical activity level, the cut-off point at 12/13 implied that the woman had reported sedentary lifestyle (#4) in at least one of the four stages.

2.3. Measurement of Other Covariates. Self-reported data on age, educational level (as the best available measure of socioeconomic status), prepregnancy body mass index, smoking, and physical working conditions came from the baseline questionnaire in gestational week 37 with categorization as displayed in Table 1. We chose covariates to be included in the model a priori, with the exception of physical working conditions. This variable was not included in the final model due to a substantial number of missing values (32%). However, we did perform a sensitivity analysis. Body mass index and smoking were considered potential effect

TABLE 1: Physical activity levels the year before pregnancy and during first, second, and third trimester. The Danish Dystocia Study, 2004-2005. $N = 2435$.

Physical activity	Before pregnancy N (%)	First trimester N (%)	Second trimester N (%)	Third trimester N (%)
Sedentary	131 (5.4)	289 (12)	309 (13)	700 (29)
Light	1566 (64)	1728 (71)	1890 (78)	1651 (68)
Moderate-to-heavy	636 (26)	370 (15)	225 (9.2)	81 (3.3)
Competitive sport	102 (4.2)	48 (2.0)	11 (0.5)	3 (0.1)

modifiers. The biochemical effect of physical activity varies according to both factors; body mass index is associated with mode of delivery, and smoking is associated with suboptimal placental function and fetal growth retardation and, thus, associated with an increased risk of fetal asphyxia during delivery and mode of delivery [38–42].

2.4. Measurement of Mode of Delivery. Data on mode of delivery were collected from records completed by midwives in connection with the delivery and registered as spontaneous vaginal delivery, vacuum extraction, or emergency C-section; emergency C-section is defined as any nonelective C-section. In the following, "any vaginal delivery" refers to spontaneous vaginal deliveries and vacuum extractor assisted deliveries together.

2.5. Statistical Analysis. We performed χ^2 test for independence between maternal characteristics and physical activity the year before pregnancy. We calculated odds ratios and p values for trend for emergency C-section (versus any vaginal delivery) and for emergency C-section and vacuum extractor (versus spontaneous delivery) according to level of physical activity the year before pregnancy and in the first, second, and third trimester. This approach comprises a high degree of detail (four categorical exposure variables and two outcome measures). In order to confirm, or not confirm, findings from this straight-forward approach, physical activity was also analyzed using a more condensed model. Hence, we used a proportional odds model [43] to examine the association between an activity sum score and mode of delivery as an ordinal outcome, and we calculated odds ratios for going one step in the direction of a more complicated mode of delivery. The use of the activity sum score was evaluated in several steps. First, we tested for linearity for each of the individual physical activity scores, next, we tested whether all of the individual physical activity scores had the same association with the ordinal outcome, and finally the proportional odds assumption was tested. Since no significant violations of these assumptions were identified, the tests are not reported in what follows. Finally, we tested for no interaction between physical activity and maternal smoking and between physical activity and prepregnancy body mass index. Only adjusted estimates are presented, because the inclusion of adjustment variables showed almost identical results as in the crude analyses. Analyses were carried out in SAS Statistical Software V9.1.

3. Results

Table 1 shows the reported activity level in each of four time phases. Few women engaged in competitive sport, and, overall, the proportion of women, who reported moderate-to-heavy physical activity or competitive sport, was markedly reduced from before pregnancy to first trimester, and further gradually reduced throughout pregnancy (Table 1). Likewise, a substantial rise in women with a sedentary lifestyle was seen over the time span.

Table 2 shows leisure time physical activity the year before pregnancy and mode of delivery according to maternal baseline characteristics. Overall, 95 percent of the women were physically active at some level the year before pregnancy, and 76 percent had a spontaneous vaginal delivery. Women with a shorter education tended to be more sedentary, as did obese women, smokers, and women with a less physically demanding job. As for mode of delivery, the likelihood of emergency C-section was higher among women, who were older, who had no or a short education, who were overweight or obese, and who were light smokers or did not smoke at all.

Table 3 shows reduced odds for emergency C-section (versus any vaginal delivery) among women with some degree of physical activity before or during pregnancy. This tendency, compromised by limited statistical power, was confirmed by statistically significant p values for trend between physical activity before pregnancy and during first and second trimester and complicated delivery (Table 3). When collapsed into one measure, odds for a complicated delivery showed a fairly similar pattern, that is, reduced odds for emergency C-section and vacuum extractor (versus spontaneous vaginal delivery) among women with some degree of physical activity.

Table 4 shows the odds ratios for moving one step on the ordinal outcome scale in the direction of a more complicated mode of delivery, that is, the step from spontaneous vaginal delivery to vacuum extractor and emergency C-section or the step from any vaginal delivery to emergency C-section, according to a sum score of physical activity covering all four stages. The association between the sum score and mode of delivery was consistent with the initial analyses as presented in Table 3; for example, women in the higher activity group had lower odds of a more complicated delivery than women, who were moderately physically active, and those who were moderately active had lower odds than women with the

TABLE 2: Physical activity levels the year before pregnancy and mode of delivery according to maternal characteristics. The Danish Dystocia Study, 2004-2005. $N = 2435$.

Characteristics	Physical activity the year before pregnancy		Mode of delivery		
	Any physical activity	Sedentary	Spontaneous vaginal delivery	Vacuum extractor	Emergency C-section
Total	2304 (94.6)	131 (5.4)	1854 (76.1)	369 (15.2)	212 (8.7)
Maternal age (years)					
<25	375 (96.2)	15 (3.9)	317 (81.3)	42 (10.8)	31 (8.0)
25–29	1132 (93.9)	73 (6.1)	935 (77.6)	177 (14.7)	93 (7.7)
30–34	635 (94.4)	38 (5.7)	480 (71.3)	126 (18.7)	67 (10.0)
≥35	162 (97.0)	5 (3.0)	122 (73.1)	24 (14.4)	21 (12.6)
Educational level after secondary education					
<3 years	781 (92.5)	63 (7.5)	619 (73.3)	144 (17.1)	81 (9.6)
3-4 years	731 (95.9)	31 (4.1)	587 (77.0)	102 (13.4)	73 (9.6)
>4 years	361 (96.0)	15 (4.0)	282 (75.0)	69 (18.4)	25 (6.7)
Never commenced/interrupted training studying	177 (94.7)	10 (5.4)	141 (75.4)	26 (13.9)	20 (10.7)
	254 (95.5)	12 (4.5)	225 (84.6)	28 (10.5)	13 (4.9)
Body mass index					
<18.5	107 (98.2)	2 (1.8)	90 (82.6)	15 (13.8)	4 (3.7)
18.5–24.99	1685 (95.3)	8 (4.8)	1357 (76.7)	268 (15.2)	144 (8.1)
25–30	374 (95.9)	16 (4.1)	288 (73.9)	60 (15.4)	42 (10.8)
>30	138 (82.6)	29 (17.4)	119 (71.2)	26 (15.6)	22 (13.2)
Smoking (cigarettes)					
No smoking	2085 (95.1)	107 (4.9)	1675 (76.4)	331 (15.1)	186 (8.5)
1–10 per day	165 (93.2)	12 (6.8)	126 (71.2)	28 (15.8)	23 (13.0)
11–20 per day	54 (81.8)	12 (18.2)	53 (80.3)	10 (15.2)	3 (4.6)
Working conditions[a]					
Physically demanding	791 (97.1)	24 (2.9)	602 (73.9)	129 (15.8)	84 (10.3)
Not physically demanding	891 (93.4)	63 (6.6)	733 (76.8)	141 (14.8)	80 (8.4)

[a]Missing = 666.

C-section = caesarean section.

lowest activity level. We tested for and found no interaction between physical activity and smoking or prepregnancy body mass index. Also, adding a variable on working conditions (physically demanding: yes/no) in the proportional odds model did not change the effect of physical activity as a sum score (complete case analysis, $N = 1769$) (data not shown).

4. Discussion

Among 2,435 nulliparous women with expected uncomplicated delivery, physically active women were less likely to have a complicated delivery than physically inactive women. The results were robust over different levels of physical activity; the higher the level, the lower the odds of emergency

C-section (versus any vaginal delivery) and of emergency C-section and vacuum extractor (versus spontaneous delivery), and they were robust over different pregestational and gestational time phases of exposure; that is, we saw the same tendencies for the year preceding pregnancy and the three trimesters of pregnancy.

Our findings are in agreement with some previous observational findings but not with others [5, 21, 27–29, 44, 45], and in disagreement with a randomized controlled trial by Barakat et al. [46]. Barakat et al. study included 142 women of low to middle socioeconomic position, and it may be expected that women who agree to randomization of their lifestyle during pregnancy constitute a selected group. Further, some of the observational studies included both elective

TABLE 3: Adjusted odds ratios for mode of delivery according to leisure time physical activity before and during pregnancy. The Danish Dystocia Study. $N = 2435$.

Physical activity	Emergency C-section (versus any vaginal delivery)			Emergency C-section and vacuum extractor (versus spontaneous vaginal delivery)		
	OR[a]	95% CI	p value for trend	OR[a]	95% CI	p value for trend
Before pregnancy						
Sedentary	1	—		1	—	
Light	0.63	0.37–1.08	0.0372	0.80	0.54–1.20	0.1043
Moderate-to-heavy	0.57	0.32–1.04		0.73	0.47–1.12	
Competitive sport	0.28	0.09–0.88		0.63	0.34–1.19	
First trimester						
Sedentary	1	—		1	—	
Light	0.89	0.58–1.34	0.0301	0.77	0.58–1.02	0.0083
Moderate-to-heavy	0.57	0.32–1.03		0.60	0.41–0.86	
Competitive sport	0.39	0.09–1.67		0.65	0.31–1.37	
Second trimester						
Sedentary	1	—		1	—	
Light	0.73	0.50–1.08	0.0303	0.80	0.61–1.05	0.0070
Moderate-to-heavy	0.47	0.23–0.93		0.56	0.36–0.85	
Competitive sport	0.82	0.10–6.92		0.53	0.11–2.53	
Third trimester						
Sedentary	1	—		1	—	
Light	0.80	0.59–1.09	0.1466	0.80	0.65–0.99	0.0134
Moderate-to-heavy	0.77	0.32–1.85		0.63	0.35–1.13	
Competitive sport	—	—		—	—	

[a]Adjusted for maternal age, educational level when secondary education is completed, smoking, and prepregnancy body mass index.
C-section = caesarean section, OR = odds ratio, and CI = confidence interval.

TABLE 4: Adjusted odds ratios for a more complicated delivery, that is, emergency C-section (versus any vaginal delivery) or emergency C-section and vacuum extractor (versus spontaneous vaginal delivery) according to a physical activity sum score covering the time period from one year before pregnancy and all three pregnancy trimesters. The Danish Dystocia Study. $N = 2435$.

Physical activity sum score	OR[a]	95% CI	p value for trend
Low activity level	1.28	1.04–1.58	
Moderate activity level	1	—	0.0029
High activity level	0.77	0.58–1.02	

[a]Adjusted for maternal age, educational level when secondary education is completed, smoking, and prepregnancy body mass index.
C-section = caesarean section, OR = odds ratio, and CI = confidence interval.

and emergency C-section [27, 45, 47]; in the present study elective C-sections were excluded. This reduces comparability with part of the existing literature. However, our results are less likely to be biased by indications for the elective C-section.

Even though our data indicated a consistent trend between increasing levels of physical activity and less complicated deliveries, part of our findings may be explained by a "healthy exerciser effect," that is, the effect of confounding by indication. If women with poor health in pregnancy are less likely to exercise than healthier women, and, at the same time,

some risk factors for poor health are shared with those for C-section, then physical activity will turn out as a preventive factor for C-section as a consequence of a lower generic risk among the physically active women. Moreover, epidemiological cohort studies like the Danish Dystocia Study usually have participants that are on average healthier and more socioeconomically advanced than the background population. We do not believe this, however, to cause selection bias regarding a possible causal association between exercise and mode of delivery.

Among Danish pregnant women associations between background factors such as increasing age, higher educational level, normal prepregnancy body mass index, and nonsmoking and leisure time physical activity during pregnancy have been found [48]. In the present study, however, adjustment for these factors did not alter the association between leisure time physical activity and a less complicated mode of delivery substantially.

Assessment of physical activity in this study relied on self-reporting, and, to some degree, recall of physical activity level, which may imply information bias, but data on physical activity was collected before mode of delivery was known, and possible misclassification should therefore not be differential. The questions developed by Saltin et al. have been found valid for self-reported physical activity in epidemiological studies [37, 49].

This study concentrated on physical activity during leisure time, and thus we did not intend to evaluate physical activity as a whole. Different mechanisms seem to be in play for physical activity during leisure time and at work; roughly spoken, occupational-related physical activity tend to be associated with adverse pregnancy/birth outcomes and recreational activity with healthy outcomes [50]. Although the questions by Saltin on physical activity were probably intended to measure leisure time physical activity, the term "leisure time" is not specified to the respondents, and, thus, some women may have included work-related activities or household activities, and others not. Household chores seem to contribute substantially to the total amount of physical activity performed by women in the child-bearing ages [50–53]. We find it unlikely, though, that work related activity was included by the women, because the wording of the four categories clearly points towards leisure time activities. The questionnaire was filled in at gestational age 37, at which point in time almost all pregnant women holding a job in Denmark are on maternity leave due to social rights, which diminishes the potential problem of including work-related physical activity in the third trimester. We did not include information on physical working conditions in the main analyses because of a substantial number of missing. We believe that the main reasons for not answering work-related questions were that the women did not hold a job or had already ceased working due to maternity leave. Sensitivity analyses restricted to women with information on working conditions did not change the conclusions.

By using a homogeneous study population (i.e., Robson Group 1 deliveries) we should have reduced the extent of confounding by some of the risk factors for emergency C-section. We consider this group of nulliparous women with no indication of induction of labor or elective C-section well suited for this study, as we expect only few, if any, of these women had been advised against physical activity during pregnancy. Our study population may theoretically comprise women with moderate hypertension and possibly also moderate preeclampsia (that is not severe enough to cause, e.g., induction of labor). We believe, however, that hypertension/preeclampsia that is considered not severe at the time of delivery is unlikely to have been present before pregnancy or earlier in pregnancy at a level that would cause restrictive recommendations regarding physical activity. In this study, we wished to examine if, and how, physical activity is associated with mode of delivery among a group of women with expectedly uncomplicated deliveries, that is, pregnancies that have not been classified as complicated to a degree that have caused induction, C-section, or other interventions until the time of spontaneous labor at term. This correlates with the original purpose of the mother-study, where participants were included in the Danish Dystocia Study only if they were nulliparous, had a single cephalic fetal presentation, and had spontaneous onset of labor at ≥37 gestational weeks, according to the Robson Classification, Group 1. The Robson classification is widely used in clinical practice (as well as in research) to audit and monitor the quality of antenatal and perinatal services, and by sticking to this definition of the study population, our results reflects daily clinical practice and debates and enhances comparability with other research.

Our findings correlate with previous results from the Danish Dystocia Study, where athletics or heavy gardening > or =4 h per week was found protective for labor dystocia [54]. Should our findings reflect causality, this may be explained by larger and better functioning placentae; Jackson and colleagues found physical exercise in first part of pregnancy associated with increased placental vascular volume and villi, with further increase after exercise throughout pregnancy [55]. Regular aerobic exercise during pregnancy is associated with improved physical fitness [20], and higher maximal oxygen uptake has been found associated with shorter duration of labor [56]. If leisure time physical activity reduces the risk of a complicated delivery, this is not only of clinical and public health relevance but may also have economic implications. Bungum et al. estimated that one-third of C-sections might be attributed to a sedentary behaviour and that medical expenses could have been substantially reduced, had these women not been sedentary [44].

5. Conclusions

In this population of low-risk, nulliparous women we found an increasing level of leisure time physical activity associated with a less complicated mode of delivery, that is, a reduced risk of emergency C-section, when compared to any vaginal delivery and a reduced risk of a complicated delivery including vacuum extraction or emergency C-section compared to a spontaneous vaginal delivery. This study included detailed measures of the timing of physical activity, including the prepregnancy period, which has only been sparsely reported so far. Findings from the study suggest that leisure time physical activity may play a role in reducing the number of emergency C-section and assisted vaginal deliveries, which is of public health interest, since physical activity is inexpensive and produces few negative side effects.

Conflicts of Interest

The authors declare that they have no conflicts of interest.

Acknowledgments

The Danish Dystocia Study was financially supported from the following institutions and foundations: Copenhagen Hospital Corporation Research Foundation, The Lundbaeck Foundation, Aase and Ejnar Danielsen's Foundation, The Augustinus Foundation, The Health Insurance Foundation, The Danish Midwifery Association, King Christian X's Foundation, and Faculty of Medicine, Lund University, Sweden. The authors are grateful to the now late Hanne Kjaergaard, who established the Danish Dystocia Study, and who earns substantial credit for her continuous contribution to the increased amount of research on birth care.

References

[1] H. K. Hegaard, B. K. Pedersen, B. B. Nielsen, and P. Damm, "Leisure time physical activity during pregnancy and impact on gestational diabetes mellitus, pre-eclampsia, preterm delivery and birth weight: a review," *Acta Obstetricia et Gynecologica Scandinavica*, vol. 86, no. 11, pp. 1290–1296, 2007.

[2] P. Magnus, L. Trogstad, K. M. Owe, S. F. Olsen, and W. Nystad, "Recreational physical activity and the risk of preeclampsia: a prospective cohort of Norwegian women," *American Journal of Epidemiology*, vol. 168, no. 8, pp. 952–957, 2008.

[3] J. A. Gavard and R. Artal, "Effect of exercise on pregnancy outcome," *Clinical Obstetrics and Gynecology*, vol. 51, no. 2, pp. 467–480, 2008.

[4] M. Juhl, P. K. Andersen, J. Olsen et al., "Physical exercise during pregnancy and the risk of preterm birth: a study within the Danish National birth cohort," *American Journal of Epidemiology*, vol. 167, no. 7, pp. 859–866, 2008.

[5] I. Domenjoz, B. Kayser, and M. Boulvain, "Effect of physical activity during pregnancy on mode of delivery," *American Journal of Obstetrics and Gynecology*, vol. 211, no. 4, pp. 401.e1–401.e11, 2014.

[6] G. Sanabria-Martínez, A. García-Hermoso, R. Poyatos-León, C. Álvarez-Bueno, M. Sánchez-López, and V. Martínez-Vizcaíno, "Effectiveness of physical activity interventions on preventing gestational diabetes mellitus and excessive maternal weight gain: a meta-analysis," *BJOG: An International Journal of Obstetrics and Gynaecology*, vol. 122, no. 9, pp. 1167–1174, 2015.

[7] L. M. Russo, C. Nobles, K. A. Ertel, L. Chasan-Taber, and B. W. Whitcomb, "Physical activity interventions in pregnancy and risk of gestational diabetes mellitus: a systematic review and meta-analysis," *Obstetrics and Gynecology*, vol. 125, no. 3, pp. 576–582, 2015.

[8] M. Madsen, T. Jørgensen, M. L. Jensen et al., "Leisure time physical exercise during pregnancy and the risk of miscarriage: a study within the Danish National Birth Cohort," *BJOG*, vol. 114, no. 11, pp. 1419–1426, 2007.

[9] J. C. Dempsey, T. K. Sorensen, M. A. Williams et al., "Prospective Study of Gestational Diabetes Mellitus Risk in relation to maternal recreational physical activity before and during pregnancy," *American Journal of Epidemiology*, vol. 159, no. 7, pp. 663–670, 2004.

[10] World Health Organization, *International Statistical Classification of Diseases and Related Health Problems*, WHO, 1994.

[11] ACOG Committee on Obstetric Practice, "Committee opinion #267: exercise during pregnancy and the postpartum period," *Obstetrics & Gynecology*, vol. 99, no. 1, pp. 171–173, 2002.

[12] NICE-National Institute for Health and Care Excellence (UK), *Antenatal Care for Uncomplicated Pregnancies. Clinical Guideline*, The National Institute for Health and Care Excellence (NICE), London, UK, 2008.

[13] National Board of Health, *Antanatal Care. National Recommendations*, National Board of Health, Copenhagen, Denmark, 2013.

[14] "Committee opinion no. 650: physical activity and exercise during pregnancy and the postpartum period," *Obstetrics & Gynecology*, vol. 126, no. 6, pp. 1326–1327, 2015.

[15] K. R. Evenson, R. Barakat, W. J. Brown et al., "Guidelines for physical activity during pregnancy: comparisons from around the world," *American Journal of Lifestyle Medicine*, vol. 8, no. 2, pp. 102–121, 2014.

[16] S. Thangaratinam, E. Rogozińska, K. Jolly et al., "Effects of interventions in pregnancy on maternal weight and obstetric outcomes: meta-analysis of randomised evidence," *British Medical Journal*, vol. 344, no. 7858, Article ID e2088, 2012.

[17] W. Brown, "The benefits of physical activity during pregnancy," *Journal of Science and Medicine in Sport*, vol. 5, no. 1, pp. 37–45, 2002.

[18] S. N. Morris and N. R. Johnson, "Exercise during pregnancy: a critical appraisal of the literature," *Journal of Reproductive Medicine for the Obstetrician and Gynecologist*, vol. 50, no. 3, pp. 181–188, 2005.

[19] E. A. Lokey, Z. V. Tran, C. L. Wells, B. C. Myers, and A. C. Tran, "Effects of physical exercise on pregnancy outcomes: a meta-analytic review," *Medicine & Science in Sports & Exercise*, vol. 23, no. 11, pp. 1234–1239, 1991.

[20] M. S. Kramer and S. W. McDonald, "Aerobic exercise for women during pregnancy," *Cochrane Database of Systematic Reviews*, vol. 3, Article ID CD000180, 2006.

[21] R. Poyatos-León, A. García-Hermoso, G. Sanabria-Martínez, C. Álvarez-Bueno, M. Sánchez-López, and V. Martínez-Vizcaíno, "Effects of exercise during pregnancy on mode of delivery: a meta-analysis," *Acta Obstetricia et Gynecologica Scandinavica*, vol. 94, no. 10, pp. 1039–1047, 2015.

[22] D. C. Hall and D. A. Kaufmann, "Effects of aerobic and strength conditioning on pregnancy outcomes," *American Journal of Obstetrics and Gynecology*, vol. 157, no. 5, pp. 1199–1203, 1987.

[23] E. F. Magann, S. F. Evans, and J. P. Newnham, "Employment, exertion, and pregnancy outcome: Assessment by kilocalories expended each day," *American Journal of Obstetrics and Gynecology*, vol. 175, no. 1, pp. 182–187, 1996.

[24] S. Narendran, R. Nagarathna, V. Narendran, S. Gunasheela, and H. Rama Rao Nagendra, "Efficacy of yoga on pregnancy outcome," *Journal of Alternative and Complementary Medicine*, vol. 11, no. 2, pp. 237–244, 2005.

[25] K. Melzer, Y. Schutz, N. Soehnchen et al., "Effects of recommended levels of physical activity on pregnancy outcomes," *American Journal of Obstetrics and Gynecology*, vol. 202, no. 3, pp. 266.e1–266.e6, 2010.

[26] D. Di Mascio, E. R. Magro-Malosso, G. Saccone, G. D. Marhefka, and V. Berghella, "Exercise during pregnancy in normal-weight women and risk of preterm birth: a systematic review and meta-analysis of randomized controlled trials," *American Journal of Obstetrics and Gynecology*, vol. 215, no. 5, pp. 561–571, 2016.

[27] M. L. Bovbjerg and A. M. Siega-Riz, "Exercise during pregnancy and cesarean delivery: North Carolina PRAMS, 2004-2005," *Birth*, vol. 36, no. 3, pp. 200–207, 2009.

[28] S. C. Dumith, M. R. Domingues, R. A. Mendoza-Sassi, and J. A. Cesar, "Physical activity during pregnancy and its association with maternal and child health indicators," *Revista de Saude Publica*, vol. 46, no. 2, pp. 327–333, 2012.

[29] K. M. Owe, W. Nystad, H. Stigum, S. Vangen, and K. Bø, "Exercise during pregnancy and risk of cesarean delivery in nulliparous women: a large population-based cohort study," *American Journal of Obstetrics and Gynecology*, vol. 215, no. 6, pp. 791.e1–791.e13, 2016.

[30] T. Lavender, G. J. Hofmeyr, J. P. Neilson, C. Kingdon, and G. M. Gyte, "Caesarean section for non-medical reasons at term," *The Cochrane Database of Systematic Reviews*, vol. 3, Article ID CD004660, 2012.

[31] The British Columbia Health Care Program, *Caesarean Birth Task Force Program*, 2008.

[32] J. Ecker, "Cesarean delivery on maternal request—reply," *JAMA*, vol. 310, no. 9, pp. 978–979, 2013.

[33] A. Sevelsted, J. Stokholm, K. Bønnelykke, and H. Bisgaard, "Cesarean section and chronic immune disorders," *Pediatrics*, vol. 135, no. 1, pp. e92–e98, 2015.

[34] S. J. Buckley, "Executive summary of hormonal physiology of childbearing: evidence and implications for women, babies, and maternity care," *The Journal of Perinatal Education*, vol. 24, no. 3, pp. 145–153, 2015.

[35] M. S. Robson, "Can we reduce the caesarean section rate?" *Best Practice and Research: Clinical Obstetrics and Gynaecology*, vol. 15, no. 1, pp. 179–194, 2001.

[36] M. Robson, M. Murphy, and F. Byrne, "Quality assurance: the 10-group classification system (robson classification), induction of labor, and cesarean delivery," *International Journal of Gynecology and Obstetrics*, vol. 131, supplement 1, pp. S23–S27, 2015.

[37] B. Saltin and G. Grimby, "Physiological analysis of middle-aged and old former athletes. Comparison with still active athletes of the same ages," *Circulation*, vol. 38, no. 6, pp. 1104–1115, 1968.

[38] J. Lumley, C. Chamberlain, T. Dowswell, S. Oliver, L. Oakley, and L. Watson, "Interventions for promoting smoking cessation during pregnancy," *Cochrane Database of Systematic Reviews*, no. 3, Article ID CD001055, 2009.

[39] G. Salmasi, R. Grady, J. Jones, and S. D. McDonald, "Environmental tobacco smoke exposure and perinatal outcomes: a systematic review and meta-analyses," *Acta Obstetricia Et Gynecologica Scandinavica*, vol. 89, no. 4, pp. 423–441, 2010.

[40] W. Siggelkow, D. Boehm, C. Skala, M. Grosslercher, M. Schmidt, and H. Koelbl, "The influence of macrosomia on the duration of labor, the mode of delivery and intrapartum complications," *Archives of Gynecology and Obstetrics*, vol. 278, no. 6, pp. 547–553, 2008.

[41] M. H. Aliyu, O. Lynch, R. E. Wilson et al., "Association between tobacco use in pregnancy and placenta-associated syndromes: a population-based study," *Archives of Gynecology and Obstetrics*, vol. 283, no. 4, pp. 729–734, 2011.

[42] G. A. Davies, C. Maxwell, L. McLeod et al., "Obesity in pregnancy," *Journal of Obstetrics and Gynaecology Canada*, vol. 32, no. 2, pp. 165–173, 2010.

[43] P. K. Andersen and L. T. Skovgaard, "Alternative outcome types and link functions," in *Regression with Linear Predictors*, Springer, New York, NY, USA, 1st edition, 2010.

[44] T. J. Bungum, D. L. Peaslee, A. W. Jackson, and M. A. Perez, "Exercise during pregnancy and type of delivery in nulliparae," *Journal of Obstetric, Gynecologic & Neonatal Nursing*, vol. 29, no. 3, pp. 258–264, 2000.

[45] E. F. Magann, S. F. Evans, B. Weitz, and J. Newnham, "Antepartum, intrapartum, and neonatal significance of exercise on healthy low-risk pregnant working women," *Obstetrics and Gynecology*, vol. 99, no. 3, pp. 466–472, 2002.

[46] R. Barakat, J. R. Ruiz, and A. Lucia, "Exercise during pregnancy and risk of maternal anaemia: a randomised controlled trial," *British Journal of Sports Medicine*, vol. 43, no. 12, pp. 954–956, 2009.

[47] N. Voldner, K. F. Frøslie, L. A. H. Haakstad, K. Bø, and T. Henriksen, "Birth complications, overweight, and physical inactivity," *Acta Obstetricia et Gynecologica Scandinavica*, vol. 88, no. 5, pp. 550–555, 2009.

[48] M. Juhl, M. Madsen, A.-M. N. Andersen, P. K. Andersen, and J. Olsen, "Distribution and predictors of exercise habits among pregnant women in the Danish National Birth Cohort,"

Scandinavian Journal of Medicine and Science in Sports, vol. 22, no. 1, pp. 128–138, 2012.

[49] G. Johansson and K. R. Westerterp, "Assessment of the physical activity level with two questions: validation with doubly labeled water," *International Journal of Obesity*, vol. 32, no. 6, pp. 1031–1033, 2008.

[50] J. F. Clapp III, "Pregnancy outcome: physical activities inside versus outside the workplace," *Seminars in Perinatology*, vol. 20, no. 1, pp. 70–76, 1996.

[51] J. Liu, S. N. Blair, Y. Teng, A. R. Ness, D. A. Lawlor, and C. Riddoch, "Physical activity during pregnancy in a prospective cohort of British women: Results From The Avon Longitudinal Study of Parents and Children," *European Journal of Epidemiology*, vol. 26, no. 3, pp. 237–247, 2011.

[52] R. J. Shephard, "Limits to the measurement of habitual physical activity by questionnaires," *British Journal of Sports Medicine*, vol. 37, no. 3, pp. 197–206, 2003.

[53] B. E. Ainsworth, "Challenges in measuring physical activity in women," *Exercise and Sport Sciences Reviews*, vol. 28, no. 2, pp. 93–96, 2000.

[54] H. Kjærgaard, A. K. Dykes, B. Ottesen, and J. Olsen, "Risk indicators for dystocia in low-risk nulliparous women: a study on lifestyle and anthropometrical factors," *Journal of Obstetrics and Gynaecology*, vol. 30, no. 1, pp. 25–29, 2010.

[55] M. R. Jackson, P. Gott, S. J. Lye, J. W. Knox Ritchie, and J. F. Clapp III, "The effects of maternal aerobic exercise on human placental development: placental volumetric composition and surface areas," *Placenta*, vol. 16, no. 2, pp. 179–191, 1995.

[56] K. R. Kardel, B. Johansen, N. Voldner, P. O. Iversen, and T. Henriksen, "Association between aerobic fitness in late pregnancy and duration of labor in nulliparous women," *Acta Obstetricia et Gynecologica Scandinavica*, vol. 88, no. 8, pp. 948–952, 2009.

Determinants of Malaria Prevention and Treatment Seeking Behaviours of Pregnant Undergraduates Resident in University Hostels, South-East Nigeria

Anthonia Ukamaka Chinweuba,[1] Noreen Ebelechukwu Agbapuonwu,[2] JaneLovena Enuma Onyiapat,[1] Chidimma Egbichi Israel,[1] Clementine Ifeyinwa Ilo,[2] and Joyce Chinenye Arinze[1]

[1]Department of Nursing Sciences, University of Nigeria, Nsukka, Enugu Campus, Enugu, Nigeria
[2]Department of Nursing Science, Nnamdi Azikiwe University, Nnewi Campus, Nnewi, Nigeria

Correspondence should be addressed to Anthonia Ukamaka Chinweuba; anthonia.chinweuba@unn.edu.ng

Academic Editor: Fabio Facchinetti

This cross-sectional descriptive survey investigated determinants of malaria prevention and treatment seeking behaviours of pregnant undergraduates resident in university hostels, South-East Nigeria. Purposive sampling was used to enrol 121 accessible and consenting undergraduates with self-revealed and noticeable pregnancy residing in twenty-three female hostels of four university campuses in Enugu State, Nigeria. Structured interview guide developed based on reviewed literature and WHO-recommended malaria prevention and treatment measures was used to collect students' self-report data on malaria preventive health behaviours, sick role behaviours, and clinic use using mixed methods. The WHO-recommended malaria prevention measures were sparingly used. Some believed that pregnancy does not play any role in a woman's reaction to malaria infection. Only 41 (50.6%) visited a hospital for screening and treatment. Thirty-four (28.1%) used antimalaria medicine bought from chemist shop or over-the-counter medicines, while 33 (27.3%) used untreated net. The students were more likely to complete their antimalaria medicine when they were sick with malaria infection than for prevention ($p = 0.0186$). Knowledge, academic schedule, cultural influence on perception and decision-making, and accessibility of health facility were key determinants of the women's preventive and treatment seeking behaviours. Health education on malaria prevention and dangers of drug abuse should form part of orientation lectures for all freshmen. University health centres should be upgraded to provide basic antenatal care services.

1. Introduction

Malaria in pregnancy remains a public health challenge due to its related prenatal mortality. Its impact is notably high in malaria endemic areas like Nigeria. "About 50% of Nigerian population have at least one episode of malaria each year with nearly 110 million clinical cases and an estimated 300,000 deaths per year" [1, 2]. "Women and children are the vulnerable groups" [3, 4]. Schantz-Dunn and Nour [5] observed that "women were three times more at risk of suffering from severe effects of malaria in the pregnant than in the non-pregnant state and that women who had malaria infection during pregnancy have higher risks for complications of pregnancy including neonatal and maternal deaths."

Available studies already indicate an "increased prevalence of malaria infection among Nigerian university students residing in school hostels" [6, 7]. "These school hostels were ill-equipped and their environmental conditions poor" [8–11]; "and, the school healthcare facilities are characterised by inadequate manpower, out-of-stock syndrome and poor quality healthcare" [12, 13]. Some of these students are pregnant women who are even more vulnerable to the adverse effect of malaria infection and need to take extra precaution in preventing and treating the infection. This study investigated the determinants of malaria prevention and treatment seeking behaviours of pregnant undergraduates resident in school hostels in Nigeria. The purpose of the study, therefore, was to assess the factors related to the pregnant undergraduates' preventive health behaviour, sick role behaviour, and their clinic use in prevention and treatment of malaria. Specifically, the study determined whether the women were aware of their risk for increased complications of malaria in their pregnancy state, actions they took to prevent malaria attack during pregnancy, what they did to treat malaria when they felt they had it, under what conditions they sought medical care for malaria treatment, where they accessed care for prevention and treatment of malaria and why, and how compliant they were in use of prescribed antimalaria medicines.

Malaria is known to be preventable and curable. However, "malaria infections during pregnancy are mostly asymptomatic [14]." Pregnant students in school hostels are expected to take appropriate actions to prevent the disease. Prevention targets the vector (mosquito), the reservoir (human host), and the causative agent (the *Plasmodium*). WHO [15, 16] recommends "a number of malaria prevention strategies including: use of personal protective measures such as long-lasting insecticidal-treated bed nets (LLINs), covering exposed skin to prevent mosquito bites, screening of houses; environmental modification which involves creating drains to prevent swamps, covering any stagnant water, clearing vegetation from water bodies, effective rubbish disposal, spraying insecticides on breeding habitats, growing mosquito repellant plants like Neem tree; vector management using insecticides such as in-door residual spraying (IRS) and use of mosquito repellants; and, intermittent preventive treatment in pregnancy (IPTp) with sulfadoxine-pyrimethamine (SP) (particularly for pregnant women in malaria-endemic areas)."

Several studies had been done on prevention and treatment of malaria in pregnancy in the Nigerian society. Onyeneho et al. [17] studied perception and attitudes of pregnant women in Enugu State, Nigeria, towards prevention of malaria infection. Result showed that some of the women were ignorant of what to do to prevent malaria infection. Anumudu et al. [18] assessed the treatment seeking behaviour of 307 young students of University of Ibadan, Nigeria. They observed that ITN and IRS were sparingly used as malaria prophylactics; almost half of the respondents were self-medicated while more than half did nothing. Okwa and Ibidapo's [19] study on the malaria situation, perception of cause, and treatment in a Nigerian University yielded similar result. Pregnant students living in school hostel have received few research attention, hence this study.

2. Methods

The design was cross-sectional descriptive survey. The target population was all pregnant undergraduates residing in twenty-three (23) female hostels of four university campuses in Enugu State, Nigeria (designated A–D for confidentiality). However, as the exact population could not be determined (infinite population), incidental/purposive sampling was used to enrol all undergraduates with self-revealed and noticeable pregnancy residing in the university hostel into the study. Based on this, 51 pregnant undergraduates were recruited from 10 hostels in "A" university, 27 from 6 hostels of "B" university, 18 from 2 hostels of "C" university, and 32 from 5 hostels of "D" university. One hundred and twenty-eight (128) accessible and consenting pregnant undergraduates, thus, were recruited for the study. Seventeen of these hostels are within the school premises while six are located at trek distances to, but owned by, the school.

2.1. Instrument. The instrument used for data collection was 10-item structured interview guide developed by the researchers based on reviewed literature and WHO-recommended malaria prevention and treatment measures profile. Four items were on the students' personal profiles of age, gravidity, year of study, and gestational age. Three open-ended items collected qualitative data on whether they were aware of their risk for increased complications of malaria in their pregnancy state; reasons for measures they adopted to prevent and treat malaria; and condition(s) under which they sought medical care for malaria treatment.

Three close-ended items were on what they do to prevent and treat malaria infection, whether they had malaria in present pregnancy, and their use of prescribed medication for malaria prevention and treatment. Malaria preventive measures include actions employed to avoid mosquito bites and malaria attack such as use of ITN, mosquito repellents or electric mosquito swatter, IRS, and IPT, while malaria treatment measures include measures taken during an attack of malaria to contain the disease, for example, seeking treatment in a health facility or first line treatments.

The instrument was pilot-tested by administering it to twelve undergraduates resident in two female hostels of a university in Anambra State, Nigeria (about 10% of the sample), which is in the same political zone and similar in characteristics to universities of the study population. Data collected were subjected to Cronbach alpha reliability test. A coefficient alpha of 0.81 and a standardized item (inter item) coefficient of 0.87 were obtained.

2.2. Ethics Approval. Ethical clearance for the study was obtained from the Research Ethical Committee of University of Nigeria Teaching Hospital, Ituku-Ozalla, Enugu, Nigeria (Ref. number UNTH/CSA/329/VOL.5). Administrative permit was also obtained from the appropriate university authorities, Student Affairs Unit heads, and hostel supervisors. Prior to data collection, prospective respondents were approached and purpose of the study carefully explained. Only resident students who gave their consent after due explanation were used.

2.3. Instrument Administration. Four (4) research assistants comprising one hostel student-leader (hostel governor) in each of the four universities were recruited and used for data collection after 30–60-minute discussion of objectives of the study, contents of the instrument, selection of subjects, how to administer the interview guide for data collection, and interpretation of the questions in the instrument (where needed).

TABLE 1: Respondents' characteristics and whether they have had malaria in their pregnancy $n = 121$.

Demographic characteristics	n (%)	Gestational age		
		<6 months (12, 10.0%)	6–8 months (42, 26.5%)	>8 months (67, 55.4%)
Age (years)				
16–20	39 (23.2%)	1 (0.8%)	14 (11.6%)	24 (19.8%)
21–25	51 (42.2%)	5 (4.1%)	17 (14.1%)	29 (24.0%)
26–30	19 (15.7%)	3 (2.5%)	7 (5.8%)	9 (7.4%)
≥31	12 (10.0%)	3 (2.5%)	4 (3.3%)	5 (4.1%)
Gravidity				
Primigravida	89 (73.6%)	2 (1.7%)	34 (28.1%)	53 (43.8%)
Secundigravida	26 (21.5%)	7 (5.8%)	7 (5.8%)	12 (10.0%)
Gavida ≥ 3	6 (5.0%)	3 (2.5%)	1 (0.8%)	2 (1.7%)
Year of study				
First year	4 (3.3%)	1 (0.8%)	3 (2.5%)	0 (0%)
Second year	14 (11.6%)	3 (2.5%)	4 (3.3%)	7 (5.8%)
Third year	31 (25.6%)	2 (1.7%)	15 (12.4%)	14 (11.6%)
Fourth year	49 (40.5%)	4 (3.3%)	13 (10.7%)	32 (26.5%)
Fifth year	23 (19.0%)	2 (1.7%)	7 (5.8%)	14 (11.6%)

Objectivity and confidentiality on information gathered were emphasized.

One researcher visited the hostels of one university in the company of research assistant from that university. Using the snowball method, the researcher or assistant identified one pregnant student residing in university hostel in each of the four universities with the help of the hostel warden after administrative permit had been obtained. Researcher or assistant introduced self and purpose of the study. After obtaining oral consent, the respondent was engaged in face-to-face interview with the researcher or assistant on her malaria prevention and treatment behaviours. The interview process was guided strictly by contents of the interview guide. After the interview, the respondent was requested to identify another pregnant student in the same hostel using room number for easy access. Data collection was between 6.00 p.m. and 8.00 p.m. from Mondays to Thursdays when many of the students were likely to be in their rooms. Repeat visit was made where necessary for administration of the interview. The data collection lasted for six weeks and three days.

2.4. Method of Data Analysis. Quantitative data collected on demographic characteristics reported malaria infection and measures used for malaria prevention and treatment were analysed descriptively using frequencies, percentages, mean, and standard deviation. Contingency table on association between student's health behaviour on use of prescribed medication and purpose of the medication intake was subjected to Fisher's exact test. Qualitative data on respondents' awareness of their risk for increased complications of malaria in their pregnancy state and reasons for their specific actions towards malaria prevention and treatment were transcribed to form concepts. The emerging concepts were categorized based on the study objectives, coded, and subjected to conventional content analysis using template approach. Seven themes emerged. The statistical analyses were performed using a biostatistical software, the statistical package for social sciences (SPSS) version 20.0 computer software programme (SPSS inc., Chicago, IL, USA) at 95% confidence interval. Data collected on reasons for "actions taken" and "no special action" were qualitatively subjected to content analysis to form themes.

3. Results

Out of the 128 copies of the instrument administered, 121 were retrieved giving a return rate of 94.5%. Results are shown in Table 1.

Sixty-seven (55.4%) of the respondents were in the last two months of their pregnancy, while 12 (10.0%) had pregnancy below 6 months. There was no definite pattern in age distribution of the women in relation with their gestational age. However, women aged 21–25 were the highest (51), 29 (24.0%) of whom were more than 8 months pregnant. The least was one (0.7%) student aged 16–20 with pregnancy under 6 months. Majority of the women, 89 (73.6%), were primigravida, 53 (43.8%) of whom were more than 8 months pregnant. Forty-nine (40.5%) were in their fourth year of study; first year students were the least 4 (3.3%). There was no definite pattern in the distribution of the students in terms of their age of pregnancy (Table 1).

Majority, 81 (66.9%), of the resident students that entered the study reported that they have had malaria in pregnancy. Sixty-six (74.2% of the 89 primigravidae) and 13 (50.0%) of the 26 secundigravidae had malaria but only 2 (33.3%) of the 6 women pregnant for the third time or more had malaria. In

TABLE 2: Cross-tabulation of gravidity and gestational age with incidence of malaria in present pregnancy.

Gravidity	Gestational age							
	<6 months		6–8 months		>8 months		Total	
	n	Had malaria	n	Had malaria	n	Had malaria	n	Had malaria
Primigravida (89)	2	2 (100%)	34	20 (58.8%)	53	44 (83.0%)	89	66 (74.2%
Secundigravida (26)	7	3 (42.9%)	7	7 (100%)	12	3 (25.0%)	26	13 (50.0%)
Gravida ≥ 3 (6)	3	1 (33.3%)	1	0 (0.0%)	2	1 (50.0%)	6	2 (33.3%)
Total	12	6 (5.0%)	42	28 (21.1%)	67	47 (38.8%)	121	81 (66.9%)

all, the primigravidae reported malaria infection more than the rest of the women (Table 2).

3.1. Preventive Health Behaviours

Whether the Women Were Aware of Their Risk for Increased Complications of Malaria in Their Pregnancy State. Respondents were asked to give their opinion on the statement that "malaria can cause more health problems to the pregnant woman and her unborn baby than the non-pregnant woman." Result showed some attribute malaria to other factors which they found in both pregnant and nonpregnant women. The women believed that pregnancy does not play a role in a woman's reaction to malaria attack. Such women stated that "it's only those who do not eat very well that can be seriously affected by malaria, pregnancy neither increases the risk of malaria nor does malaria increase the risk of other problems in pregnancy"; "it depends on the person's genotype, not pregnancy"; or that "women who take too much oil or fatty foods suffer a lot from malaria, whether pregnant or not. It can also make the baby to be too big."

One said "well, pregnant women should avoid working for a long time under the sun because this is one major cause of malaria." Some pointed out that factors other than malaria were actually responsible for complications of pregnancy the woman may experience. Some of their comments in response to researchers' statement include: "It is true that malaria is more common in women but pregnancy does not increase the chances of women having more problems from malaria"; "Mosquito bite can cause malaria but cannot kill the baby in the woman's womb"; "It is true that malaria is dangerous for pregnant women but as Africans, it is rarely as deadly as books will present it to be"; and "Malaria does not affect an unborn child because mosquito cannot bite him in the mother's womb, therefore, both pregnant and non-pregnant women suffer the same."

Some, though few, however agreed that malaria is capable of causing poor pregnancy outcome. Some of their statements were, "Yes, it is possible because malaria makes one to lose appetite but a pregnant woman is supposed to eat very well to be strong and the baby to grow very well"; "A woman that is not pregnant can take any medicine to treat her malaria but pregnant women are not allowed to take medicines anyhow. Delay in taking treatment can, therefore, cause death of the baby"; and "Fever the pregnant woman has during malaria attack can pass to the baby and kill him."

The result in Table 3 showed that, for vector control and prevention, 40 (33.1%) of the students would always avoid stagnant water in open containers in their rooms. For prevention of reservoirs, 33 (27.3%) slept under untreated nets. However, only 16 (13.2%) had their nets treated with insecticide always. Twenty-eight (23.1%) said they protect themselves from mosquito bites by always wearing protective clothing. To prevent the effect of plasmodium, only 25 (20.7%) would always use medicines they collected from hospital/clinic while 34 (28.1%) always used antimalaria medicine they bought from the chemist shop without prescription or over-the-counter medicines (OTC).

Overall, indoor residual sprays appeared to be the most frequently used preventive measure, used always by 32 (26.5%) and sometimes by 63 (52.1%) (mean = 2.1; SD = 0.69), while the least was use of mosquito coils to ward off mosquitoes (mean = 1.2; SD = 0.48). Other (volunteered) preventive actions were use of mosquito squatter to catch and kill mosquito and prevention of infection using nutraceuticals by 50 and 4 students, respectively.

3.2. Sick Role Behaviours.

Respondents were asked to indicate, from the listed options, the action(s) they took to prevent and/or treat malaria infection. Provision was also made for additional information not contained in the list. Table 4 presents the responses obtained. Items in italics were additional data as provided by the respondents. Result showed that only 39 (32.2%) of the pregnant undergraduates take actions to prevent malaria, while 81 (66.9%) took varied actions to treat the disease. The rest would not take any action. Many would take some medications to prevent malaria or when they feel they have the infection, although the source and type varied. Only 41 (50.6%) would visit the hospital for screening and treatment, while 16 (41.0%) do so to prevent malaria. Respondents resorted to self-medication more frequently than they would visit hospital; hence, as many as 51 (63.0%) bought any antimalaria medicine available at a chemist shop for treatment. Some resorted to local herbs in common use at their home for treating malaria; even in pregnancy, for instance, 2 (5.1%) took the fresh neem leaves juice (*Azadirachta indica*) for malaria prevention and 9 (11.1%) for treatment. Five (12.8%) undergo the traditional steam bath ritual, the "okpukpu aju," to treat malaria. Seven (8.6%) took analgesics to treat malaria.

The women were asked to indicate whether they took complete dose of their prescribed antimalaria medicines

TABLE 3: What respondents do to prevent malaria infection.

Malaria preventive measures	Always 3	Some times 2	Never 1	Mean (SD*)
Vector n (%)				
Use indoor residual sprays	32 (26.4)	63 (52.1)	26 (21.5)	2.1 (0.69)
Use mosquito coils to ward off mosquitoes	4 (3.3)	12 (9.9)	105 (86.8)	1.2 (0.48)
Avoid stagnant water in open containers in room	40 (33.0)	11 (9.1)	70 (57.9)	1.8 (0.91)
Reservoir n (%)				
Sleep under insecticide-treated net	8 (6.6)	10 (8.3)	103 (85.1)	1.4 (0.70)
Sleep under net but not treated with insect repellants	33 (27.3)	25 (20.7)	63 (52.0)	1.8 (0.86)
Screen door and windows with net	23 (19.0)	3 (2.5)	95 (78.5)	1.4 (0.79)
Use mosquito repellent creams/oil	18 (14.9)	24 (19.8)	79 (65.3)	1.5 (0.74)
Wear protective clothing	28 (23.1)	17 (14.1)	76 (62.8)	1.6 (0.84)
Causative agent n (%)				
Use medicine collected from hospital/clinic	25 (20.7)	20 (16.5)	76 (62.8)	1.6 (0.81)
Buy antimalaria medicine from chemist shop (or OTC)	34 (28.1)	40 (33.1)	47 (38.8)	1.9 (0.82)
Take medicinal herbs from home	14 (11.6)	18 (14.9)	89 (73.5)	1.4 (0.69)
Other actions				
Use electric mosquito swatter	25 (20.7)	35 (28.9)		
Use nutraceuticals	3 (2.5)	1 (0.8)		

SD* = standard deviation.

TABLE 4: Actions the respondents take to prevent and treat malaria infection.

Action to prevent and/or treat malaria	Purpose of action	
	To prevent malaria ($n = 39$, 32.2%)	To treat malaria ($n = 81$, 66.9%)
Go to hospital	16 (41.0%)	41 (50.6%)
Buy any antimalarial medicine at chemist shop	30 (76.9%)	51 (63.0%)
Use local herbs/home remedies		
Fresh neem leaves juice	2 (5.1%)	9 (11.1%)
Scent leaves	3 (7.7%)	—
Magic kola	4 (10.3%)	2 (2.5%)
Bitter kola	1 (2.6%)	3 (3.7%)
Bitter leaf juice	—	—
Undergo steam bath ritual "(okpukpu aju)"	5 (12.8%)	—
Take some analgesics to relief symptoms	—	7 (8.6%)
Take nutraceuticals	4 (10.3%)	—
Take holy water, pray, fast	—	3 (3.7%)
No action	82 (67.8%)	40 (33.1%)

TABLE 5: Fisher's exact test result of association between student's health behaviour on use of prescribed medication and purpose of the medication intake.

	N	Completed medications	Did not complete	p
To prevent malaria	18	10 (55.6%)	8 (44.4%)	0.0186*
To treat malaria	54	46 (85.2%)	8 (14.8%)	
Total	72	56 (77.8%)	16 (22.2%)	

*Significant.

for purpose of prevention and/or treatment of malaria. Result showed that as many as 46 (85.2%) of the women would complete their prescribed medication when sick with malaria infection while 10 (55.6%) would do so to prevent the infection. Fisher's exact test result showed significant difference in the respondents' health behaviour on use of prescribed medication and purpose of the medication intake ($p = 0.0186$) (Table 5).

Reasons for Specific Actions towards Malaria Prevention and Treatment. Thematic presentation of summary of reasons given by the respondents for their specific actions towards malaria prevention and treatment include the following.

Seek Healthcare in the Hospital. Some respondents, particularly those in health-related field of study, took actions because they understood how dangerous malaria is and as one added, "did not want to have a bit of it." They also wanted measures that would not cause other problems/diseases to them. A respondent said, "Malaria makes me seriously sick so I will do everything possible to avoid it."

Self-Medicate. Ignorance seems to play a major role here. The general impression of the respondents is summarised by a response, thus: "there are many anti-malaria medicines available in the chemist shop and I know that anti-malaria medicines are important in pregnancy so I do not need the hospital to know what to take for malaria treatment." Others

said:, "Yes, I know that malaria is dangerous in pregnancy but I have no time to go for antenatal clinic so I buy any available anti-malaria medicines." Several numbers of respondents said they resort to self-medication because there was no hospital or clinic providing antenatal services for pregnant women near their hostel. Some expressed their willingness to visit a hospital outside the school but were discouraged by thought of the long protocols and waiting time in hospitals/clinics, "so I go to where it will be fast for me; I need time for my lectures, you know!" one concluded. These findings showed that some merely choose a measure because it is convenient to them while others apply measures based on their perceived susceptibility and severity of the illness.

Use Local Herbs. Some still hold tight to their traditional way of treating illness even in pregnancy claiming that there are some safe, cheap, and effective herbs commonly used to treat malaria in their community. They, therefore, prefer to go for these local herbs. One eighteen-year-old primigravida in her "eighth month of pregnancy" declared that she would break her education at her ninth month. She said, "I will go home to my mother to get some local herbs to cleanse my baby," "I treat any disease like malaria with herbs my mother will prepare for me", and "I will continue with the medicine until I deliver my baby at home; no need for hospital."

Prayer. Two respondents clearly stated that they do not need medicine to "*receive*" healing; they only pray because "only

God heals." One said she usually prays but when the problem gets worse, she can then go for treatment as last option.

No Special Action. Reasons given for not taking any action to prevent and treat malaria include perceiving malaria as a minor illness, that is, a non-life-threatening illness. A respondent vividly said, "In Africa, malaria is a common problem and usually goes without treatment, so I do not need to give it serious attention." Some of the reasons for no action against malaria were related to lack of time to deal with it, like those who would love to go to hospital but for the protocols; hence one said, "I think less of how to prevent malaria because I have a lot of academic tasks." There is also a cost implication; that is, availability of fund determines the choice of malaria prevention and treatment measures, as one said, "I use methods (measures) I can afford." Some of the women may not be able to procure the ITN due to financial constraints.

3.3. Clinic Use.

For conditions under which respondents sought medical care for malaria treatment, the forty-one (41) respondents who visited a health facility for treatment were further requested, using an open-ended question, to specify the condition(s) under which they took decision to seek medical aid in hospital. Their responses were coded, categorized, and subjected to conventional content analysis using template approach. Five themes emerged from the analyses. Result showed that 22 sought medical aid only when they were very ill. Nine sought medical care with the slightest feeling of ill-health. Four went to the health facility when it was time for their antenatal clinic, while the rest visited the hospital when their condition got worse.

4. Discussion

4.1. Preventive Health Behaviour.

Result showed that although malaria is endemic in Nigeria; the respondents had varied perceptions of the severity of malaria in pregnancy and their susceptibility. This is a significant determinant of actions they took against the disease. The perception of "no difference in the effect of malaria in the pregnant and non-pregnant state" and the assumption that "pregnancy does not play a role in a woman's reaction to malaria attack" by some of the students means that they may not take any special precaution during their pregnancy period to prevent malaria and its possible complications. In fact, this was obvious when as many as 82 (67.8%) said they took no special action to prevent malaria in their pregnancy. Similarly, the erroneous impressions that malaria is not possible cause of complicated pregnancies, but other factors such as "hard labour under the sun for a long time" and "intake of too much fatty food" and that "there is no relationship between pregnancy and severity of malaria," suggest that cultural beliefs still play palpable roles in preventive health behaviour and sick role behaviour of the population. This may be related to the findings of Anumudu et al. [18] which revealed that more than 50% of their respondents did nothing to prevent malaria attack. These findings, therefore, further strengthen the need for more robust enlightenment programmes on effect of malaria on pregnancy and malaria prevention and treatment especially in pregnancy in malaria endemic areas.

The WHO-recommended preventive measures were sparingly used. Although WHO [15, 16] advocate the use of ITN, very few seemed to find this relevant even in their pregnancy state as only 6.6% used ITN always; 27.3% used nets, but untreated, undermining the importance of the insecticide. The most frequently used malaria preventive measure among the respondents, though by few, was IRS, used always by 32 (26.5%). This is more evident in the finding that less than half of the subjects seemed to be aware of the effect of plasmodium on their pregnancy and few would use antimalaria medicines collected from hospital/clinic or chemist shop. This finding is thus in contrast to Okwa and Ibidapo [19]. In all, the students' preventive actions were suboptimal since the grand mean for each of the three malaria prevention strategies was <2. This implies that many of the students have poor knowledge of impact of malaria in pregnancy and measures for preventing it, thus supporting the findings of Onyeneho et al. [17]. Ordinarily, one would think that the students' exposure to teachings on environment-health related diseases like malaria through sources including classroom lectures, books, internet, and the media would improve their understanding of malaria and appropriate malaria preventive health behaviours. This assumption was, however, not reflected in the findings.

4.2. Sick Role Behaviour and Clinic Use.

The students seem to be not proactive in handling malaria in pregnancy. Results of the study showed that the women were more likely to complete their antimalaria medicine when they were down with malaria attack than when the medicine was taken for preventive purposes. The result further suggests that the students had poor knowledge of risks associated with self-medication, particularly in their pregnancy state. They could, therefore, walk into a chemist shop and buy any antimalarial medicine to prevent (24.8%) or treat (42.2%) malaria. It was also noted that more of the subjects would self-medicate than go to hospital for treatment when they feel they have malaria except when they had serious symptoms of the illness. No wonder why they indulged in self-medication (30 (24.8%)) rather than using hospital services (16 (13.2%)) for prevention of malaria in pregnancy. This finding has implication for law on medicine sale, procurement, and use for treatment of diseases in Nigeria, which may be considered weak. Coincidentally, because malaria is common in Nigeria, there are many brands of easily accessible antimalaria medicines in the market. These women could freely walk into the medicine shop and buy any available brand of their choice to save time and cost since they self-medicate because "that was the best and fastest available option" for them. This practice exposes the fetus to drug-related complications. It also constitutes high risk to the populace because fake and adulterated drugs may be consumed resulting to health problems that may be fatal. There is also the possibility that lack of antenatal care services in the school health facility, as reported, is responsible for the poor clinic use.

Although majority took medicines when they had malaria, only about 33.9% visited the hospital for screening and treatment. It is however possible that those who sought care from hospital did so because of their "inexperience" and anxiety since the majority were young primigravidae. Also, they were more likely to complete their antimalaria medications when they were "really down with malaria attack" than for preventive purposes. The fact that only twenty-two used health facilities when they were down with malaria is worrisome and spells no good for efforts toward achievement of the third sustainable development goal (SDG_3), good health and well-being. Surprisingly, as many as 33.1% admitted that they did nothing when they felt they had malaria, even in pregnancy, showing the enormity of their ignorance. This finding is, however, less than the 50% observed by Anumudu et al. [18] and Okwa and Ibidapo [19] in their previous studies, respectively.

The implication of these findings is that, even in the presence of available malaria prevention and treatment options as provided by the WHO, a good number of the students are still at risk of malaria-related complications of pregnancy and poor pregnancy outcome. The findings also revealed that majority of the students practice self-medication to treat malaria, which poses a challenge to effective malaria treatment. Thus, there is need for increased sensitization on the dangers of antimalaria self-medication.

5. Conclusion

Findings revealed four basic determinants of the pregnant students' health seeking behaviour: the women's knowledge of risks associated with malaria in pregnancy; cultural influence on perception and decision-making; availability of dedicated healthcare services in schools; and academic schedule. Ignorance, negative cultural beliefs, busy academic schedule in the absence of policy that protects the interest of pregnant students, and lack of access to quality health services are, therefore, implicated in the women's poor preventive and treatment health seeking behaviours. They are rarely proactive in preventing and treating malaria in pregnancy. They use the available school health services sparingly, even when they have symptoms of malaria. IRS and netting are frequently used while self-medication with antimalaria medicines were most common treatment measure.

Additional Points

Recommendations. (i) Health is fundamental right of all including pregnant women and their unborn babies; hence, there is a need for formal welfare programme that protect pregnant undergraduates and promote good pregnancy outcome. (ii) University health centres should be upgraded to provide basic antenatal care services and appropriate referral where necessary. (iii) The Tertiary Institution Social Health Insurance Programme should be reinforced and active Health Maintenance Organisations maintained at all university health centres to ensure the welfare of pregnant students and reduce their burden of out-of-pocket expenses. (iv) University policies should include regulations that allow departments and faculties to grant official permit to pregnant students to attend the antenatal clinic on their appointment days. (v) Health education on malaria infection causes, prevention and treatment, and dangers of drug abuse should, therefore, form part of orientation lectures for all freshmen. (vi) Billboards and posters with relevant information can be positioned at strategic places in the university as reminders on proper preventive health behaviours. Also, stakeholders in health can sponsor production of souvenirs with inscriptions about tips on malaria preventive behaviour written on them. Free ITN should be made regular component living-room material for all students. (vii) The study was only on resident students of universities. Further studies are needed to determine the degree of influence of accessibility of healthcare services on the student's overall health seeking behaviour for malaria prevention and treatment using pregnant students living outside the school environment.

Conflicts of Interest

The authors declare that there are no conflicts of interest regarding the publication of this paper.

Authors' Contributions

Anthonia Ukamaka Chinweuba conceived the study and participated in its design and coordination. Anthonia Ukamaka Chinweuba and Clementine Ifeyinwa Ilo helped to draft the manuscript. Chidimma Egbichi Israel and JaneLovena Enuma Onyiapat administered the questionnaire to students in the various hostels. Anthonia Ukamaka Chinweuba, Chidimma Egbichi Israel, and Noreen Ebelechukwu Agbapuonwu assisted in the statistical analysis and interpretation of data and provided comments and suggestions on multiple drafts of the papers. All authors read and approved the final submission.

References

[1] World Health Organization, World Malaria Report 2013, World Health Organization, Geneva/Washington, DC, USA, 2013.

[2] Federal Ministry of Health, *National Policy on Malaria Diagnosis And Treatment*, National Malaria and Vector Control Division, Abuja, Nigeria, 2011.

[3] O. G. Raimi and C. P. Kanu, "The prevalence of malaria infection in pregnant women living in a suburb of Lagos," *African Journal of Biochemistry Research*, vol. 4, no. 10, pp. 243–245, 2010.

[4] Centre for Disease Control and Prevention, *Impact of malaria*, Global Health—Division of Parasitic Diseases and Malaria, 2014.

[5] J. Schantz-Dunn and N. M. Nour, "Malaria and pregnancy: a global health perspective," *Reviews in Obstetrics and Gynaecology*, vol. 2, no. 3, pp. 186–192, 2009.

[6] I. K. Ezugbo-Nwobi, M. O. Obiukwu, P. U. Umeanato, and C. M. Egbuche, "Prevalence of malaria parasites among Nnamdi Azikwe University students and anti-malaria drug use," *African Research Review*, vol. 5, no. 4, pp. 135–144, 2011.

[7] F. O. Adeyemo, O. Y. Makinde, L. O. Chukwuka, and E. N. Oyana, "Incidence of malaria infection among the undergraduates of university of Benin (Uniben), Benin City, Nigeria," *The Internet Journal of Tropical Medicine*, vol. 9, no. 1, 2013.

[8] Faborode, M. The trouble with Nigerian universities. Punch Newspaper, 13/12/2012.

[9] Aluko, B. Universities NEEDS Assessment Report Presentation to NEC November 2012. NigerianMuse, 2013.

[10] Okojie, J. This is Your University! ThisDay Newspaper, 30/09/2013.

[11] N. O. Ebehikhalu and P. D. Dawam, "Inadequacy of Teaching and learning infrastructure: reason nigerian universities cannot drive innovations," *Journal of Educational Policy and Entrepreneurial Research*, vol. 3, no. 2, 2016.

[12] G. O. Obiechina and G. O. Ekenedo, "Factors affecting utilization of university health services in a tertiary institution in south-west Nigeria," *Nigerian Journal of Clinical Practice*, vol. 16, no. 4, pp. 454–457, 2013.

[13] M. O. Afolabi, V. O. Daropale, A. I. Irinoye, and A. A. Adegoke, "Health-seeking behaviour and student perception of health care services in a university community in Nigeria," *Scientific Research*, vol. 5, no. 5, pp. 817–824, 2013.

[14] C. O. Agomo, W. A. Oyibo, R. I. Anorlu, and P. U. Agomo, "Prevalence of malaria in pregnant women in Lagos, South-West Nigeria," *The Korean Journal of Parasitology*, vol. 47, no. 2, pp. 179–183, 2009.

[15] World Health Organisation, WHO Malaria fact sheet. Available: http://www.ivcc.com/, (2011).

[16] World Health Organization, Malaria in pregnant women. Available: http://www.who.int/malaria/areas/high_risk_groups/pregnancy/en/, 2013.

[17] N. G. Onyeneho, N. Idemili-Aronu, I. Igwe, and F. U. Iremeka, "Perception and attitudes towards preventives of malaria infection during pregnancy in Enugu State, Nigeria," *Journal of Health, Population and Nutrition*, vol. 33, no. 1, article no. 22, 2015.

[18] C. I. Anumudu, A. Adepoju, M. Adediran et al., "Malaria prevalence and treatment seeking behaviour of young nigerian adults," *Annals of African Medicine*, vol. 5, no. 2, pp. 82–88, 2006.

[19] O. O. Okwa and A. C. Ibidapo, "TThe malaria situation, perception of cause and treatment in a nigerian university," *Journal of Medicine and Medical Sciences*, vol. 1, no. 6, pp. 213–222, 2010, http://www.Interesjournal.org/JMMS.

Discordance in Couples Pregnancy Intentions and Breastfeeding Duration: Results from the National Survey of Family Growth 2011–2013

Jordyn T. Wallenborn ⓘ, **Gregory Chambers, Elizabeth P. Lowery,** and **Saba W. Masho** ⓘ

Virginia Commonwealth University, School of Medicine, Division of Epidemiology, Department of Family Medicine and Population Health, 830 East Main Street, Suite 821, P.O. Box 980212, Richmond, VA 23298-0212, USA

Correspondence should be addressed to Jordyn T. Wallenborn; jordynwallenborn@berkeley.edu

Academic Editor: Luca Marozio

Background. Parental disagreement in pregnancy intention elevates the risk of adverse health events for mother and child. However, research surrounding parental pregnancy intention discrepancies and breastfeeding duration is limited. This study aims to examine the relationship between couple's discordant pregnancy intention and breastfeeding duration. *Methods.* Data from the 2011–2013 National Survey of Family Growth was analyzed. Parental pregnancy intention was categorized as "intended by both parents," "unintended by both parents," "father intended and mother unintended," and "father unintended and mother intended." Breastfeeding duration was categorized as "never breastfed," "breastfed less than six months," and "breastfed at least six months." Multinomial logistic regression, odds ratios, and 95% confidence intervals were calculated. *Results.* Couples with a concordant unintended pregnancy were more likely to have a child who was never breastfed or breastfed less than six months compared to couples with a concordant intended pregnancy. Similarly, couples with a discordant pregnancy were more likely to have a child who was never breastfed or breastfed less than six months. *Conclusions.* Findings from this study show a relationship between couples' pregnancy intentions and subsequent breastfeeding behaviors. Healthcare professionals should be cognizant of parents' differing opinions surrounding pregnancy intention and the implications on breastfeeding outcomes.

1. Introduction

Breastfeeding is considered the optimum source of nutrition for infants. Research has correlated breastfeeding with lower rates of upper respiratory infections, otitis media, and necrotizing enterocolitis [1, 2]. Breastfeeding is also linked to lower rates of childhood obesity, asthma, and dental caries [3–6]. Similarly, breastfeeding has health benefits for mothers. Not only can breastfeeding improve sleep quality and feelings of maternal well-being [7], but also breastfeeding duration is associated with a decreased risk for ovarian and breast cancer, type 2 diabetes, and an earlier return to prepregnancy weight [8, 9].

Despite the numerous benefits associated with breastfeeding, a small proportion of women breastfeed for the recommended duration. The American Academy of Pediatrics recommends exclusive breastfeeding through 6 months of age, followed by continued breastfeeding while supplementing with other foods throughout the first year of life [10]. However, in 2013, only 22% of mothers exclusively breastfed for 6 months. Further, when combining breastfeeding with other forms of feeding, only 52% of infants were receiving breast milk at 6 months [11].

While the choice to initiate or continue breastfeeding is a complex decision, research has identified a variety of factors that influence breastfeeding outcomes. Some of these factors include the father's support for breastfeeding, the breadth of support from the woman's social network, and how quickly the mother returns to work [12–15]. This is exemplified by a statement released by the Centers for Disease Control and Prevention which reported a lack of support for breastfeeding mothers from employers and communities [11]. Another factor associated with breastfeeding outcomes is maternal and paternal pregnancy intention [16, 17]. Specifically, research has found that maternal pregnancy intention is an important determinant of breastfeeding cessation [16]. Mothers with an unwanted pregnancy are less likely to initiate or continue breastfeeding [18]. Similarly, a recent cross-sectional study showed that a pregnancy unintended by the father was associated with a shorter breastfeeding duration [17].

While current research has independently investigated maternal and paternal pregnancy intention and subsequent breastfeeding practices, discordance in couples' pregnancy intention has not been explored. Previous literature has demonstrated that a couples' discordant pregnancy intention can impact perinatal outcomes. For example, discordant pregnancy intention has been associated with higher odds of rapid repeat pregnancy, which can lead to preterm birth, low birth weight, and neonatal death [19]. In addition, discordant pregnancy intention has been linked to lower rates of breastfeeding initiation, delayed prenatal care, increased smoking in pregnancy, and higher rates of preterm birth [20, 21]. Moreover, studies have suggested that pregnancy intentions can influence maternal behaviors and health outcomes [22, 23].

In 2010, nearly half (45%) of all pregnancies in the United States (US) were unintended [24]. In light of recent estimates of unintended pregnancies, understanding the implications of a couples' pregnancy intention on breastfeeding outcomes could provide important insight for interventions aimed at increasing breastfeeding rates. However, to the authors' knowledge, no study has examined the association between couples' pregnancy intention and breastfeeding duration. Therefore, the current study aims to investigate the association between couples' discordant pregnancy intention and breastfeeding duration.

2. Materials and Methods

The current study utilized data from the 2011–2013 National Survey of Family Growth (NSFG), which collects information on family life, marriage, pregnancy, and overall men and women's health. The US Department of Health and Human Services uses this information to help plan public health programs and other health services [25]. The survey was specifically created to provide national estimates and is conducted through in-person interviews and self-administered questionnaires. The response rate for recent data is estimated at 3%. Additional information on NSFG can be found elsewhere [26].

Analysis for the current study was restricted to women's first birth to reduce confounding factors related to breastfeeding subsequent children [27]. Women were also excluded if they were never pregnant, received help to become pregnant, or had missing information on the main outcome or exposure. The final analysis was conducted on 2,231 women. This study was approved as exempt by the Virginia Commonwealth University Institutional Review Board.

Breastfeeding duration, the outcome of interest, was defined as "never breastfed," "breastfed less than 6 months," or "breastfed at least 6 months." Breastfeeding was assessed using 3 self-report survey items, where mothers reported breastfeeding duration in weeks. If the mother reported breastfeeding 1-25 weeks, she was categorized as breastfeeding less than 6 months, while if the mother reported breastfeeding 26 weeks or more, she was categorized as breastfeeding at least 6 months, which is consistent with national breastfeeding recommendations [11].

Couple pregnancy intention for the first live birth, the main exposure, was categorized as "intended by both parents (father + mother +)," "unintended by both parents (father – mother –)," "father intended and mother unintended (father + mother –)," and "father unintended and mother intended (father – mother +)." Unintended pregnancy was defined as a pregnancy that occurred too soon (e.g., mistimed) or was unwanted. Intended pregnancy included one that was (1) at the right time, (2) overdue, or (3) indifferent. Categorization was based on questions regarding pregnancy intention prior to contraception and is consistent with previous literature [19, 28].

Couples where both parents reported the pregnancy as intended were used as the reference category because previous literature has shown that intended pregnancies have better breastfeeding outcomes [16, 17].

Potential confounding factors were selected based on literature and availability in NSFG [15, 17, 29]. Sociodemographic factors considered included maternal age (≤ 19 years; 20-24 years; 25-29 years; 30-34 years; 35+ years), paternal age (18-24 years; 25-49 years), maternal race/ethnicity (non-Hispanic White; non-Hispanic Black; Hispanic; Non-Hispanic Other), marital status (married; not married), poverty level (0-99 percent; 100-199 percent; 200-399 percent; 400-700 percent), highest maternal educational attainment (less than high school; high school; some college or more), and maternal prepregnancy body mass index (BMI) (normal weight (15–24.9 kg/m2), overweight (25.0–29.9 kg/m2) and obese (≥30.0 kg/m2). Other factors including whether the mother was born outside the US (yes; no) and current religious affiliation (no religion; catholic; protestant; other) were also considered.

All analyses were conducted using SAS 9.4 statistical software to account for the complex survey design of NSFG. Descriptive statistics including unweighted frequencies and weighted percentages were used to describe the study population by couple pregnancy intention. Bivariate analyses were used to determine factors associated with breastfeeding duration. Effect modification by marital status ($p = <.0001$), paternal age ($p = <.0001$), and race/ethnicity ($p = 0.9886$) was tested in accordance to previous literature [17, 30, 31]. However, because they were not included in the a priori hypothesis, stratified analysis was not considered. Because marital status and race/ethnicity were effect modifiers, they were not considered as potential confounders. Multinomial logistic regression models were used to generate crude and adjusted odds ratios and 95% confidence intervals (CI). An iterative process was used to determine factors to include in the final parsimonious model such that any potential confounding factor that changed the crude estimate by at least 10% was included in the final model [32].

3. Results

Overall, the majority of the mothers in the sample were White, Non-Hispanic (54.0%), and married (56.5%) and had at least some college education (56.1%). The majority of respondents (50.6%) reported a concordant intended pregnancy and 27.0% reported a concordant unintended pregnancy. Less than a quarter of respondents reported a discordant pregnancy intention (father – mother +, 13.5%; father + mother –, 8.9%) (not shown in Tables 1–3). Couple

TABLE 1: Weighted distribution of characteristics by couple pregnancy intention among US mothers.

	Total N=2231	Father + Mother + n=989	Father – Mother – n=695	Father + Mother – n=348	Father – Mother + n=199	P-Value (Chi-Square)
Maternal Age						<.0001
≤ 19	1.3	8.8	74.9	10.4	5.8	
20-24	11.9	29.3	46.9	17.8	6.1	
25-29	19.3	37.6	36.6	17.8	8.0	
30-34	28.3	49.0	28.4	13.0	9.6	
35+	39.2	66.1	13.6	10.6	9.7	
Paternal Age						<.0001
18-24	42.9	31.4	42.9	18.4	7.3	
25-49	57.1	67.7	12.1	10.0	10.2	
Race/Ethnicity						<.0001
White, Non-Hispanic	14.1	31.4	38.9	22.9	6.8	
Black, Non-Hispanic	54.0	56.7	25.1	8.3	9.9	
Hispanic/Other	31.9	48.8	24.9	18.2	8.1	
BMI						0.2599
normal weight (15–24.9 kg/m2)	37.0	52.3	25.0	15.4	7.2	
overweight (25.0–29.9 kg/m2)	29.6	52.7	24.4	13.2	9.7	
Obese (≥30.0 kg/m2)	33.4	46.1	31.2	12.6	10.1	
Poverty Level						<.0001
0-99	33.1	41.2	30.5	17.2	11.2	
100-199	23.4	42.3	34.3	14.1	9.2	
200-399	26.2	58.3	24.2	11.3	6.2	
400-700	17.2	68.3	14.0	9.0	8.1	
Marital Status						<.0001
Married	56.5	64.3	18.8	9.7	7.1	
Other	43.5	32.8	37.6	18.5	11.1	
Education						<.0001
Less than H.S.	20.0	44.4	30.0	17.0	8.5	
High School	23.9	41.1	33.5	14.0	11.3	
Some College	56.1	56.9	23.1	12.1	8.0	
Born Outside US						0.0012
Yes	20.0	61.6	14.8	15.5	8.2	
No	80.0	47.9	30.0	13.0	9.1	
Insurance Status						<.0001
Private	50.6	60.8	21.1	10.5	7.5	
State Sponsored Health Plan	21.1	32.7	39.7	16.8	10.8	
Other Government Health Care	5.1	43.4	36.0	16.8	3.8	
None	23.2	46.3	26.2	16.3	11.2	
Breastfeeding Duration						<.0001
Never Breastfed	31.8	37.7	36.7	16.1	9.5	

TABLE 1: Continued.

	Total N=2231	Father + Mother + n=989	Father – Mother – n=695	Father + Mother – n=348	Father – Mother + n=199	P-Value (Chi-Square)
Breastfed < 6 months	36.0	49.3	26.9	13.0	10.8	
Breastfed ≥ 6 months	32.3	64.7	17.6	11.6	6.1	
Religion						0.0132
No religion	18.3	48.1	33.0	12.0	6.9	
Catholic	23.8	59.9	19.5	11.9	8.6	
Protestant	49.3	46.1	30.0	15.0	8.9	
Other	8.5	55.8	17.5	12.7	14.1	

BMI: body mass index; US: the United States; HS: high school.

pregnancy intention was associated with maternal age, paternal age, race/ethnicity, poverty level, marital status, highest educational attainment of the mother, whether the mother was born outside the US, and religion (Table 1). The bivariate analysis showed that all potential confounding factors were significantly associated with breastfeeding duration (Table 2).

The unadjusted analysis showed that couples with a concordant unintended pregnancy (father – mother –) had greater odds of having a child who was never breastfed or breastfed less than six months. Similarly, couples where the father reported an intended pregnancy and the mother reported an unintended pregnancy (father + mother –) had greater odds of having a child who was never breastfed or breastfed less than six months. No association was found among couples where the father reported an unintended pregnancy and the mother reported an intended pregnancy (father – mother +) (Table 3).

After adjusting for poverty level, maternal age, race/ethnicity, and whether the mother was born outside the US, the odds of never breastfeeding and breastfeeding less than six months were 148% and 80% higher among couples with a concordant unintended pregnancy (father – mother –) compared to couples with a concordant intended pregnancy. Similarly, the odds of never breastfeeding and breastfeeding less than six months were 79% and 49% higher among couples with a discordant pregnancy intention (father + mother –) compared to couples with a concordant intended pregnancy. Among couples with a discordant pregnancy intention (father – mother +), the odds of having a child who was breastfed less than six months were 130% higher compared to couples with a concordant intended pregnancy (Table 3).

4. Discussion

The current study found a relationship between couples' pregnancy intention and breastfeeding initiation and duration. Specifically, there were increased odds of never breastfeeding among couples with a concordant unintended pregnancy and among discordant couples (father – mother +). In addition, both categories of discordant pregnancy intention (father –

mother +; father + mother –) and couples with a concordant unintended pregnancy had increased odds of breastfeeding a shorter duration. Further, the magnitude of association is much higher when the pregnancy was unintended by the father but the mother intends the pregnancy.

While there are no studies that examine couple's pregnancy intention and breastfeeding duration, results are consistent with previous literature on maternal and paternal pregnancy intention and breastfeeding duration. Specifically, research has shown that fathers with a mistimed or unintended pregnancy were more likely to have a child who was never breastfeed or breastfed a shorter duration [17]. Similarly, previous literature has demonstrated that mothers who have an unintended pregnancy are less likely to breastfeed at least 8 weeks [16]. A 2002 study of NSFG also found that women with unintended or mistimed pregnancies were more likely to never breastfeed or cease breastfeeding before 16 weeks [18].

The current study also found that couples with a concordant unintended pregnancy were more likely to have a child who was never breastfed or breastfed a shorter duration. This finding is consistent with a prior study that found that parents with a concordant unintended pregnancy were more likely to have an infant who was never breastfed [20]. The results also expand upon previous literature that demonstrated independent associations with maternal and paternal unintended pregnancies and a shorter breastfeeding duration [16–18].

The difference in breastfeeding outcomes for couples with a discordant pregnancy intention or a concordant unintended pregnancy may be due to the mediating influence of paternal support. Previous literature has shown that a pregnancy intended by the father is positively associated with paternal involvement [33, 34], which is linked to higher prevalence of exclusive breastfeeding at six months [35]. A study using the Early Childhood Longitudinal Study-Birth Cohort found that fathers who did not want the pregnancy were less likely to exhibit paternal warmth or engage in infant nurturing behaviors in the immediate postpartum period [33]. Further, pregnancies that are unintended by the father may lead to a lack of perceived support. As shown by a prospective cohort

TABLE 2: Factors associated with breastfeeding duration among US mothers: NSFG 2011-2013.

	Odds Ratio (95% CI)	
	Never Breastfed	Breastfed < 6 months
Maternal Age		
≤ 19	3.14 (0.38-26.20)	2.08 (0.24-17.98)
20-24	1.43 (0.92-2.23)	1.30 (0.64-2.63)
25-29	**1.74 (1.46-2.08)**	**1.68 (1.04-2.69)**
30-34	1.00	1.00
35+	0.71 (0.44-1.14)	0.90 (0.64-1.26)
Paternal Age		
18-24	**2.04 (1.43-2.92)**	1.26 (0.98-1.63)
25-49	1.00	1.00
Race		
White, Non- Hispanic	1.00	1.00
Black, Non-Hispanic	**0.34 (0.26-0.44)**	0.85 (0.53-1.36)
Hispanic/Other	**0.26 (0.19-0.35)**	**0.51 (0.32-0.82)**
BMI		
normal weight (15–24.9 kg/m2)	1.00	1.00
overweight (25.0–29.9 kg/m2)	**1.37 (1.05-1.78)**	**1.30 (1.08-1.56)**
obese (≥30.0 kg/m2)	**1.80 (1.16-2.78)**	1.24 (0.88-1.75)
Poverty Level (%)		
0-99	1.00	1.00
100-199	0.78 (0.61-1.00)	0.93 (0.63-1.36)
200-399	**0.58 (0.41-0.80)**	0.85 (0.59-1.22)
400-700	**0.30 (0.16-0.55)**	0.89 (0.44-1.78)
Marital Status		
Married	1.00	1.00
Not Married	**1.86 (1.46-2.37)**	1.08 (0.82-1.42)
Education		
Less than HS	**2.18 (1.11-4.28)**	0.95 (0.49-1.86)
High School	**3.09 (1.93-4.96)**	**1.69 (1.20-2.37)**
Some College	1.00	1.00
Born Outside US		
Yes	**0.32 (0.24-0.45)**	0.61 (0.37-1.01)
No	1.00	1.00
Insurance Status		
Private	1.00	1.00
State Sponsored Health Plan	**2.61 (1.67-4.07)**	1.08 (0.67-1.73)
Other Government Health Care	**1.53 (1.05-2.23)**	1.54 (0.78-3.02)
None	1.23 (0.66-2.30)	**0.74 (0.59-0.94)**
Religion		
No religion	1.03 (0.73-1.45)	0.97 (0.63-1.50)
Catholic	0.57 (0.28-1.14)	0.80 (0.46-1.38)
Protestant	1.00	1.00
Other	**0.30 (0.20-0.45)**	**0.36 (0.20-0.66)**

CI: confidence interval; BMI: body mass index; US: the United States; HS: high school.

TABLE 3: Association between couple pregnancy intention and breastfeeding duration: NSFG 2011-2013.

	Unadjusted Model COR (95% CI)		Parsimonious Model[a] AOR (95% CI)	
	Never Breastfed	Breastfed <6 months	Never Breastfed	Breastfed <6 months
Father + Mother +	Reference		Reference	
Father – Mother –	3.58 (2.19-5.84)	2.00 (1.22-3.28)	2.58 (2.05-3.25)	1.78 (1.24-2.54)
Father + Mother –	2.39 (1.72-3.31)	1.47 (1.13-1.92)	1.98 (1.37-2.87)	1.43 (1.07-1.91)
Father – Mother +	2.67 (0.79-9.06)	2.33 (0.99-5.46)	2.20 (0.71-6.82)	2.37 (1.08-5.17)

COR: crude odds ratio; AOR: adjusted odds ratio; CI: confidence interval.

Note: breastfeeding at least 6 months is the reference category.

[a]Parsimonious model controlling for current insurance, poverty level, maternal age, and if the mother was born outside the United States.

study conducted in Perth, Australia, perceived social support is significantly associated with breastfeeding duration [36].

The result may also be explained through maternal self-efficacy, which can be predicted by paternal support [37]. Self-efficacy relates to a person's confidence or belief that they can successfully accomplish a goal [38]. This belief directly relates to motivation, accomplishing a certain behavior, and emotional well-being [39]. Research suggests that social support can positively influence self-efficacy [40]. Therefore, the lack of paternal support as a result of an unintended pregnancy may lead to reduced self-efficacy in the mother. Studies have demonstrated a relationship between self-efficacy and breastfeeding outcomes. A prospective study reported that mothers with high self-efficacy were more likely to breastfeed a longer duration [41]. Self-efficacy can also be linked to unplanned pregnancies. Specifically, an experimental investigation found that women with low self-esteem had higher vulnerability to unplanned pregnancies [42].

To the authors' knowledge, this is the first study to examine the role of couples' pregnancy intention in breastfeeding duration. The current study used a nationally representative sample; therefore, results are generalizable to the US population. Lastly, the definition used for breastfeeding duration is consistent with the national recommendation to breastfeed for six months, which enables direct comparisons with other studies. Despite its strengths, this study is subject to certain limitations. First, the NSFG is a cross-sectional survey; therefore, causality cannot be inferred. Second, pregnancy intention and breastfeeding could be subject to social desirability and recall bias, which could lead to nondifferential misclassification and bias results towards the null. However, research has shown that self-report of breastfeeding duration is a valid and reliable measure [43]. Third, this study cannot distinguish exclusive breastfeeding from any breastfeeding; therefore, the definition of breastfeeding duration is not measuring full compliance with national breastfeeding recommendations. Lastly, potential confounding factors that could affect estimates including self-efficacy, perceived paternal support, school attendance, living arrangement, and lifestyle factors such as substance abuse could not be assessed due their unavailability in NSFG.

5. Conclusions

This study demonstrates an association between couples' pregnancy intention and breastfeeding duration. Due to

the significant number of unplanned pregnancies in the US, the current findings could assist physicians, family planning advocates, and public health agencies in developing breastfeeding support programs. Developing stronger social support for breastfeeding, including outreach directed specifically to men, could assist in more infants reaching the feeding milestones set by Healthy People 2020. Longer maternity leave, breastfeeding facilities in the workplace, and support from healthcare workers may help women prolong breastfeeding. Future research should be directed at examining which factors can modify the relationship between couples' pregnancy intention and breastfeeding to provide points of action for future policy and programs. Lastly, research should be conducted among mothers with adolescent partners (<18 years old), as current literature is limited among this population.

Conflicts of Interest

The authors declare that there are no conflicts of interest regarding the publication of this article.

References

[1] M. Bartick and A. Reinhold, "The burden of suboptimal breastfeeding in the United States: A pediatric cost analysis," *Pediatrics*, vol. 125, no. 5, pp. e1048–e1056, 2010.

[2] J.-A. Blaymore Bier, T. Oliver, A. Ferguson, and B. R. Vohr, "Human milk reduces outpatient upper respiratory symptoms in premature infants during their first year of life," *Journal of Perinatology*, vol. 22, no. 5, pp. 354–359, 2002.

[3] S. Arenz, R. Rückerl, B. Koletzko, and R. Von Kries, "Breastfeeding and childhood obesity—a systematic review," *International Journal of Obesity*, vol. 28, no. 10, pp. 1247–1256, 2004.

[4] T. Harder, R. Bergmann, G. Kallischnigg, and A. Plagemann, "Duration of breastfeeding and risk of overweight: a meta-analysis," *American Journal of Epidemiology*, vol. 162, no. 5, pp. 397–403, 2005.

[5] S. Scholtens, A. H. Wijga, B. Brunekreef et al., "Breast feeding, parental allergy and asthma in children followed for 8 years. The

PIAMA birth cohort study," *Thorax*, vol. 64, no. 7, pp. 604–609, 2009.

[6] A. Nirunsittirat, W. Pitiphat, C. M. McKinney et al., "Breastfeeding Duration and Childhood Caries: A Cohort Study," *Caries Research*, vol. 50, no. 5, pp. 498–507, 2016.

[7] K. Kendall-Tackett, Z. Cong, and T. W. Hale, "The Effect of Feeding Method on Sleep Duration, Maternal Well-being, and Postpartum Depression," *Clinical Lactation*, vol. 2, no. 2, pp. 22–26, 2011.

[8] J. L. Baker, M. Gamborg, B. L. Heitmann, L. Lissner, T. I. A. Sørensen, and K. M. Rasmussen, "Breastfeeding reduces postpartum weight retention," *American Journal of Clinical Nutrition*, vol. 88, no. 6, pp. 1543–1551, 2008.

[9] R. Chowdhury, B. Sinha, M. J. Sankar et al., "Breastfeeding and maternal health outcomes: A systematic review and meta-analysis," *Acta Paediatrica*, vol. 104, pp. 96–113, 2015.

[10] L. M. Gartner, J. Morton, and R. A. Lawrence, "Breastfeeding and the use of human milk," *Pediatrics*, vol. 115, no. 2, pp. 496–506, 2005.

[11] Centers for Disease Control and Prevention, *progressing toward national breastfeeding goals: United States*, Atlanta, US, 2016.

[12] S. Arora, C. McJunkin, J. Wehrer, and P. Kuhn, "Major factors influencing breastfeeding rates: Mother's perception of father's attitude and milk supply.," *Pediatrics*, vol. 106, no. 5, pp. E67, 2000.

[13] A. C. Celi, J. W. Rich-Edwards, M. K. Richardson, K. P. Kleinman, and M. W. Gillman, "Immigration, race/ethnicity, and social and economic factors as predictors of breastfeeding initiation," *JAMA Pediatrics*, vol. 159, no. 3, pp. 255–260, 2005.

[14] R. K. Dagher, P. M. McGovern, J. D. Schold, and X. J. Randall, "Determinants of breastfeeding initiation and cessation among employed mothers: A prospective cohort study," *BMC Pregnancy and Childbirth*, vol. 16, no. 1, article no. 194, 2016.

[15] J. A. Scott, C. W. Binns, W. H. Oddy, and K. I. Graham, "Predictors of breastfeeding duration: Evidence from a cohort study," *Pediatrics*, vol. 117, no. 4, pp. e646–e655, 2006.

[16] D. Cheng, E. B. Schwarz, E. Douglas, and I. Horon, "Unintended pregnancy and associated maternal preconception, prenatal and postpartum behaviors," *Contraception*, vol. 79, no. 3, pp. 194–198, 2009.

[17] J. T. Wallenborn, S. W. Masho, and S. Ratliff, "Paternal Pregnancy Intention and Breastfeeding Duration: Findings from the National Survey of Family Growth," *Maternal and Child Health Journal*, vol. 21, no. 3, pp. 554–561, 2017.

[18] J. S. Taylor and H. J. Cabral, "Are women with an unintended pregnancy less likely to breastfeed?" *Journal of Family Practice*, vol. 51, no. 5, pp. 431–436, 2002.

[19] S. Cha, D. A. Chapman, W. Wan, C. W. Burton, and S. W. Masho, "Discordant pregnancy intentions in couples and rapid repeat pregnancy," *American Journal of Obstetrics & Gynecology*, vol. 214, no. 4, pp. 494–494.e12, 2016.

[20] S. Korenman, R. Kaestner, and T. Joyce, "Consequences for infants of parental disagreement in pregnancy intention," *Perspectives on Sexual and Reproductive Health*, vol. 34, no. 4, pp. 198–205, 2002.

[21] B. Hohmann-Marriott, "The couple context of pregnancy and its effects on prenatal care and birth outcomes," *Maternal and Child Health Journal*, vol. 13, no. 6, pp. 745–754, 2009.

[22] A. P. Mohllajee, K. M. Curtis, B. Morrow, and P. A. Marchbanks, "Pregnancy intention and its relationship to birth and maternal outcomes," *Obstetrics & Gynecology*, vol. 109, no. 3, pp. 678–686, 2007.

[23] K. Kost and L. Lindberg, "Pregnancy Intentions, Maternal Behaviors, and Infant Health: Investigating Relationships With New Measures and Propensity Score Analysis," *Demography*, vol. 52, no. 1, pp. 83–111, 2015.

[24] Institute G. Unintended Pregnancy in the United States. https://www.guttmacher.org/fact-sheet/unintended-pregnancy-united-states., 2018.

[25] About the National Survey of Family Growth, https://www.cdc.gov/nchs/nsfg/about_nsfg.htm.

[26] J. M. Dahlhamer, A. M. Galinsky, S. S. Joestl, and B. W. Ward, "Sexual orientation in the 2013 national health interview survey: A quality assessment," *Vital and Health Statistics, Series 2: Data Evaluation and Methods Research*, no. 169, pp. 1–24, 2014.

[27] J. DaVanzo, A. Leibowitz, and E. Starbird, "Do Women's Breastfeeding Experiences with Their First-borns Affect Whether they Breastfeed Their Subsequent Children?" *Biodemography and Social Biology*, vol. 37, no. 3-4, pp. 223–232, 1990.

[28] L. B. Finer and M. R. Zolna, "Unintended pregnancy in the United States: incidence and disparities, 2006," *Contraception*, vol. 84, no. 5, pp. 478–485, 2011.

[29] S. W. Masho, M. R. Morris, and J. T. Wallenborn, "Role of marital status in the association between prepregnancy body mass index and breastfeeding duration," *Women's Health Issues*, vol. 26, no. 4, pp. 468–475, 2016.

[30] R. Forste, J. Weiss, and E. Lippincott, "The decision to breastfeed in the United States: Does race matter?" *Pediatrics*, vol. 108, no. 2, pp. 291–296, 2001.

[31] S. W. Masho, S. Cha, and M. R. Morris, "Prepregnancy Obesity and Breastfeeding Noninitiation in the United States: An Examination of Racial and Ethnic Differences," *Breastfeeding Medicine*, vol. 10, no. 5, pp. 253–262, 2015.

[32] K. J. Rothman, S. Greenland, and T. L. Lash, *Modern Epidemiology*, 2008.

[33] J. Bronte-Tinkew, S. Ryan, J. Carrano, and K. A. Moore, "Resident fathers' pregnancy intentions, prenatal behaviors, and links to involvement with infants," *Journal of Marriage and Family*, vol. 69, no. 4, pp. 977–990, 2007.

[34] J. E. Rogers and I. S. Speizer, "Pregnancy intention and father involvement in Guatemala," *Journal of Comparative Family Studies*, vol. 38, no. 1, pp. 71–85, 2007.

[35] T. Hunter, "Breastfeeding initiation and duration in first-time mothers: exploring the impact of father involvement in the early post-partum period," *Health Promotion Perspectives*, vol. 4, no. 2, p. 132, 2014.

[36] J. A. Scott, M. C. G. Landers, R. M. Hughes, and C. W. Binns, "Factors associated with breastfeeding at discharge and duration of breastfeeding," *Journal of Paediatrics and Child Health*, vol. 37, no. 3, pp. 254–261, 2001.

[37] E. C. Karademas, "Self-efficacy, social support and well-being: The mediating role of optimism," *Personality and Individual Differences*, vol. 40, no. 6, pp. 1281–1290, 2006.

[38] K. R. Wentzel and M. B. David, *Handbook of Motivation at School*, Routledge, New York, 2009.

[39] A. Bandura, "Self-efficacy: toward a unifying theory of behavioral change," *Psychological Review*, vol. 84, no. 2, pp. 191–215, 1977.

[40] J. Noel-Weiss, V. Bassett, and B. Cragg, "Developing a Prenatal Breastfeeding Workshop to Support Maternal Breastfeeding Self-Efficacy," *Journal of Obstetric, Gynecologic & Neonatal Nursing*, vol. 35, no. 3, pp. 349–357, 2006.

24

Factors Associated with Successful Trial of Labor after Cesarean Section: A Retrospective Cohort Study

Aram Thapsamuthdechakorn, Ratanaporn Sekararithi, and Theera Tongsong⊙

Department of Obstetrics and Gynecology, Faculty of Medicine, Chiang Mai University, Chiang Mai 50200, Thailand

Correspondence should be addressed to Theera Tongsong; theera.t@cmu.ac.th

Academic Editor: Luca Marozio

Objective. To determine the effectiveness of trial of labor after cesarean section (TOLAC) and the factors associated with a successful TOLAC. *Materials and Methods.* A retrospective cohort study was conducted on consecutive singleton pregnancies with a previous single low-transverse cesarean section planned for TOLAC at a tertiary teaching hospital. The potential risk factors of a successful TOLAC were compared with those associated with a failed TOLAC. A simple audit system used in the first two years was also taken into account in the analysis as a potential factor for success. *Results.* During the study period, 2,493 women were eligible for TOLAC and 704 of them were scheduled for TOLAC, but finally 592 underwent TOLAC. Among them, 355 (60%) had a successful vaginal birth and 237 (40%) had a failed TOLAC. The independent factors associated with the success rate included the audit system, prior vaginal birth, low maternal BMI, and lower birth weight or gestational age, whereas induction of labor and recurring indications in previous pregnancy significantly increased the risk of having a failed TOLAC. Strikingly, the strongest predictor of a successful TOLAC was the audit system with OR of 6.4 (95%CI: 3.9-10.44), followed by a history of vaginal birth in previous pregnancies (OR: 3.2; 95%CI: 1.87-5.36). *Conclusion.* The simple audit system had the greatest impact on the success rate of TOLAC, instead of the less powerful obstetrical factors as reported in previous reports. The audit system is the only potential factor that could be strengthened to improve the success rate.

1. Introduction

Women undergoing cesarean section have a higher morbidity and mortality rate than those having vaginal birth, such as massive postpartum hemorrhage, need for blood transfusion, anesthesia-associated complications, surgical risks (intestinal obstruction, wound dehiscence, wound scars, infection, etc.), and obstetric complications in subsequent pregnancies. Recently, with the dramatic increase in the rate of cesarean deliveries worldwide, several attempts have been made to reduce this rate, including trial of labor after cesarean delivery (TOLAC). However, TOLAC has a minimal risk of uterine rupture with a rate of 0.2–0.8% [1], but such a risk can be prevented by close observation and adhering to the standard guideline. Overall, morbidity and mortality rates secondary to TOLAC are less than those of repeated cesarean sections. It has long been accepted that TOLAC is a safe and acceptable option for women with previous cesarean section [1, 2]. According to the American College of Obstetricians and Gynecologists (ACOG), most women with one previous cesarean delivery and a low-transverse incision are candidates of TOLAC and should be counseled about TOLAC and offered a trial of labor [1].

TOLAC has been practiced individually in our center for decades, but the formal policy of TOLAC was first implemented in the year 2000. To date, we still have that policy, but its effectiveness in our real practice has never been evaluated. Therefore, we conducted this study to determine the effectiveness of trials of labor after cesarean section (TOLAC) and the factors associated with its success.

2. Materials and Methods

A retrospective cohort study was conducted on consecutive singleton pregnancies with a previous single low-transverse cesarean section planned for TOLAC at a tertiary teaching hospital with ethical approval by the institutional review board. The database of Maternal-Fetal Medicine (MFM) unit was assessed to identify the consecutive records of women with a history of previous cesarean section between January 2001 and December 2015, and their medical records were reviewed. The inclusion criteria were as follows: (1) singleton pregnancy, (2) low-transverse uterine incision, (3) no history of other uterine incision such as myomectomy, and (4) no obstetric risk or serious underlying disease unsuitable for vaginal delivery. Exclusion criteria were as follows: (1) pregnancy ending up in a nonviable stage or earlier than 26 weeks of gestation, (2) incomplete medical data records, and (3) fetal macrosomia. We have been using a formal guideline for TOLAC since the year 2000, following the guideline recommended by ACOG [3] with some minor modifications (i.e., macrosomia was defined as estimated birth weight > 3600 g instead of 4000 g because of the small size of Thai women). During the first two years of using this formal guideline, TOLAC practice was audited by the simple audit system, as follows: (1) one of our doctors was responsible to give a monthly orientation on the TOLAC guideline as well as a counseling guide with visual aids to the team of physicians taking care of the antenatal clinic and the labor doctors (we had a monthly rotation of the doctors at any point of service), throughout the first two years; (2) the same doctor monthly reported the outcomes of TOLAC to the audit team and then the rates of cesarean section, TOLAC, and successful/unsuccessful TOLAC of each doctor were exposed to the staff members of the department. In summary, the main components of the simple audit were regular orientation to the care team and disclosure of the outcome. After the first two years, TOLAC practice was no longer audited formally, but we still maintained the policy of TOLAC using the same practice guideline. In this study, the patients giving birth in the first two years were considered as the group of patients undergoing audit system, whereas those giving birth later during the study period were assigned as the group without audit system.

The demographic and clinical characteristics of the previous and current pregnancies were reviewed and recorded, including indications for prior cesarean section (dystocia or failure to progress was considered as a recurring indication), type of uterine scar, a history of prior vaginal delivery, outcome of labor, pattern of labor/delivery (induction of labor, labor progression, etc.), complications of TOLAC, and causes of failed TOLAC. The main outcomes were the success rate of TOLAC (vaginal delivery) and associations between the potential risk factors and successful TOLAC.

2.1. Statistical Analysis. The data were analyzed using SPSS version 21.0 (IBM Corp. Released 2012; IBM SPSS Statistics for Windows, Armonk, NY: IBM Corp). The demographic and obstetric characteristics of the successful and failed TOLAC groups were compared using Student's *t*-test for quantitative data as well as chi-square and relative risks with 95% confident interval for categorical data. Additionally, logistic regression analysis was performed to identify independent factors of successful TOLAC.

3. Result

During the study period, 2,623 women with a history of previous cesarean section were eligible for TOLAC. Among them, only 704 (28.2%) accepted TOLAC and met the inclusion criteria. However, 112 (4.5%) of them finally did not undergo TOLAC because of various reasons, while the remaining 592 (23.7%) were available for analysis as presented in Figure 1. Of the women that participated in TOLAC, 355 (60%) had successful TOLAC or vaginal birth after cesarean section (VBAC), while 237 (40%) had failed TOLAC or repeated cesarean section. Obviously, the rates of women planning for TOLAC and VBAC dropped drastically after the years of audit, from 81.8% to 51.5%, as presented in Figures 2 and 3. The demographic and obstetric factors of the two groups are compared using univariate analysis in Table 1. Notably, the time interval of the previous cesarean section, maternal age, number of antenatal visits, and parity were comparable between the two groups whereas gestational age and birth weight were significantly lower in the successful group. Logistic regression analysis indicated that audit system and prior vaginal birth were strong independent factors associated with successful TOLAC, whereas induction of labor, recurring indications in previous pregnancy, high maternal BMI, and greater birth weight were significantly associated with a higher risk of failed TOLAC, as presented in Table 2. Also it should be noted that the most common reasons for failed TOLAC were some women changing their mind during TOLAC followed by dystocia as presented in Table 3. Fetal outcomes were comparable between the two groups. Note that, in this study, there was no uterine rupture in both groups.

4. Discussion

This study indicates that the success rate of TOLAC (approximately 60%) was relatively low when compared to that of several previous publications (60-80%) [1, 4-7]. Interestingly, the success rate dropped from approximately 80% at the beginning of the policy to only 50% in recent years in spite of the same standard practice guideline. Moreover, the rate of women accepting TOLAC also drastically decreased from 54% in the year 2001 to only 21% in 2015 (Figure 2). The main factors responsible for the decrease were likely associated with the lack of audit system, though several factors were associated with the success rates, signifying that strengthening the practice guideline should be urgently considered.

Unlike previous studies, the audit system or the strengthening of the practice guideline played an important role in both the acceptance of TOLAC and the success rate, though the other non-evaluated factors must have been involved as well.

The rates of acceptance and success of TOLAC sharply dropped after the years of the audit system. Certainly, such a rapid decrease from 2003 to 2004, followed by constantly low rates with minimal change after that, could not be explained by scientific reasons or other factors, neither global trend of increase in cesarean rate nor the change in clinical

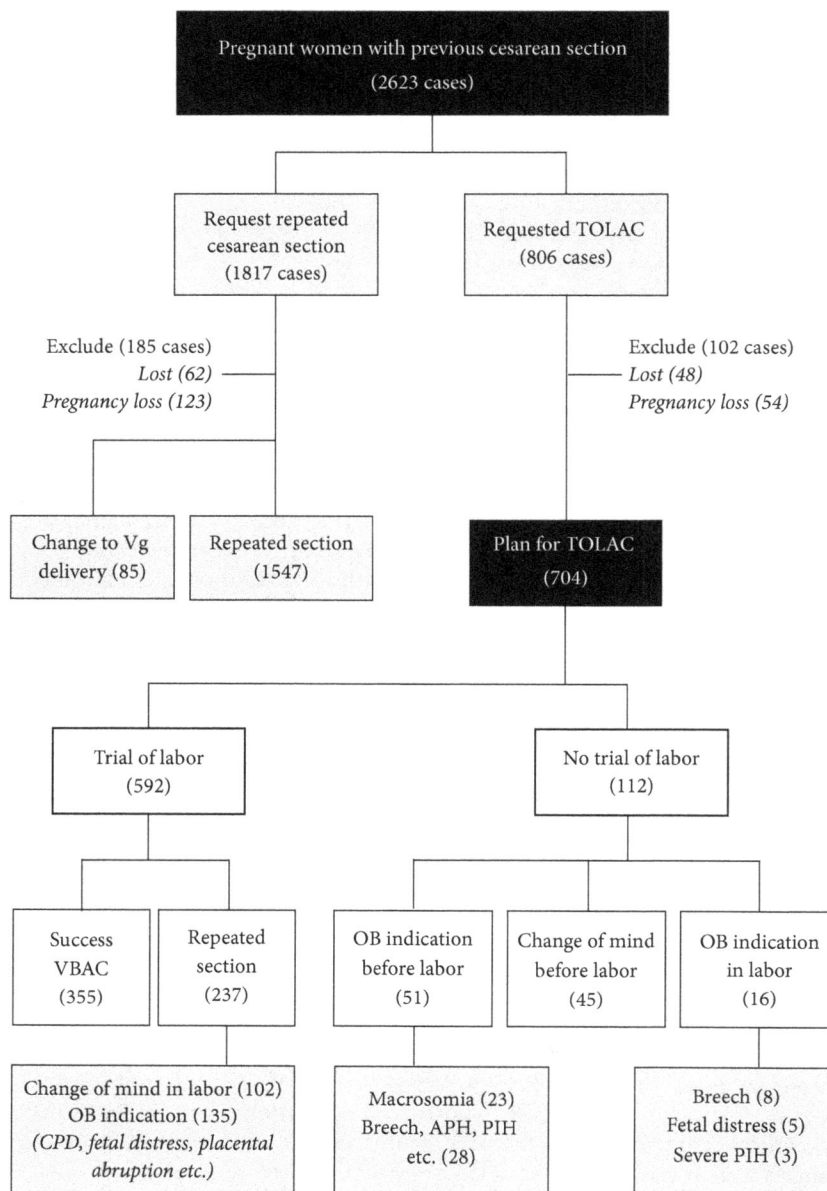

FIGURE 1: Pregnancy outcomes in both groups.

practice during the study period. Though other unknown factors could be responsible for the lower rate of TOLAC in recent years, our finding indicates that the audit system, even the simple approach used in this study (just orientation on adhering to the guideline and reporting the outcomes), is a factor with a very strong impact on TOLAC acceptance and its success rate.

It is noteworthy that our success rate in the most recent years was low (51.5%), when compared to a success rate of 60%–80% reported in most high resource countries [1]. We hypothesize that the main factor of the decrease is associated with less strengthening of the practice guideline. We believe that, under strict supervision and careful selection, TOLAC is a very good option even in low-resource setting, as demonstrated by Soni A et al. [8]. Though some studies in

low-income countries have shown a much lower success rate of TOLAC, ranging from as low as 27.4% to 53.6% [9, 10], studies in some other low-income countries showed a high rate of successful TOLAC with strengthening and careful selection (79.6-83.5%) [5, 8], which is consistent with our finding in the year of audit. Many reasons for the low rate in low-income countries have been postulated, e.g., delay in access to health care service, unavailability of painless labor, lack of constant availability of operating rooms in cases of emergency, poor educational status, great number of cases with unknown previous uterine scar, and poor record keeping of previous cesarean delivery.

No previous publication has stated that the audit system is the most predictive factor of successful TOLAC, while prior vaginal delivery as a predictive factor of success has

TABLE 1: Demographic and obstetric characteristics of the women with successful TOLAC and failed TOLAC.

Characteristics	Successful TOLAC	Failed TOLAC	P-value	
Quantitative data	**Mean ± SD**	**Mean ± SD**	**Student T test**	
Maternal age (yr)	31.4 ± 5.6	32.1 ± 5.4	0.101	
Interval from last previous cesarean	2.9 ± 1.1	3.0 ± 1.1	0.647	
No. of antenatal visits	7.4 ± 3.5	8.0 ± 3.5	0.085	
BMI (kg/m^2)	23.3 ± 4.0	24.6 ± 4.7	< 0.001	
Gestational age (wk)	36.2 ± 3.3	37.3 ± 2.0	< 0.001	
Birth weight (g)	2714 ± 523	3062 ± 664	< 0.001	
Apgar score at 1 min	8.4 ± 2.0	8.5 ± 1.6	0.370	
Apgar score at 5 min	9.4 ± 1.1	9.5 ± 9.6	0.164	
Categorical data	**n/N (%)**	**n/N (%)**	**Chi-square**	**Relative risk (95% CI)**
Parity (1 vs ≥2)	285/486 (58.6%)	70/106 (66.0%)	0.159	0.89 (0.76-1.04)
Induction of labor	17/47 (36.2%)	338/545 (62.0%)	0.001	0.58 (0.19-0.65)
Recurrent indications	84/166 (50.6%)	271/426 (63.6%)	0.004	0.79 (0.67-0.94)
Prior vaginal delivery	90/116 (77.6%)	265/476 (55.7%)	<0.001	1.39 (1.23-1.58)
Audit system	135/165 (81.8%)	220/427 (51.5%)	<0.001	1.59 (1.41-1.79)

TABLE 2: Multivariate logistic regression analysis for successful TOLAC.

Risk factors	Odd Ratio (95% CI)	P value
Audit strategy	6.40 (3.92-10.44)	< 0.001
Birth weight	0.99 (0.98-0.99)	< 0.001
Induction	0.41 (0.20-0.84)	0.014
Parity (1 vs ≥ 2	0.61 (0.37-1.02)	0.057
BMI (kg/m^2)	0.93 (0.89-0.97)	0.002
Recurrent indications	0.49 (0.32-0.75)	0.001
Prior vaginal delivery	3.17 (1.87-5.36)	< 0.001

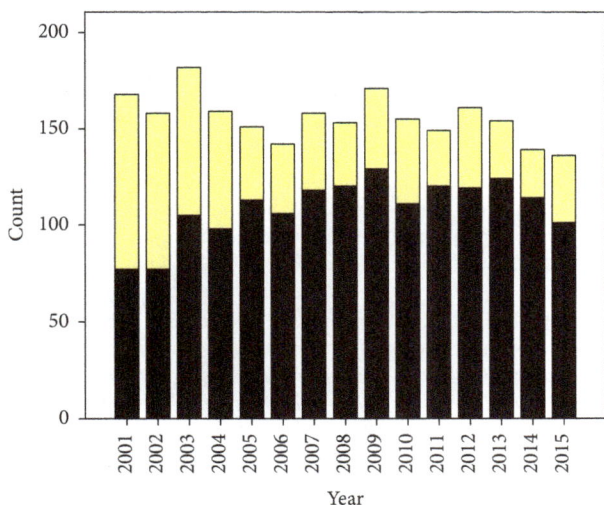

FIGURE 2: Proportions of the women who accepted TOLAC (yellow) and not accepted TOLAC (black) in each year.

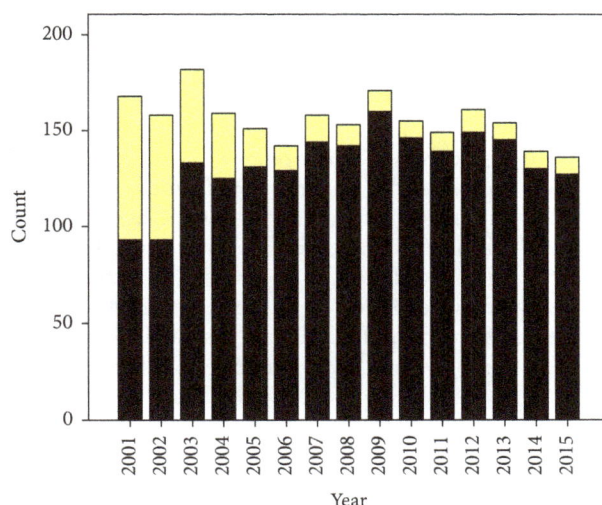

FIGURE 3: Proportions of the women with successful TOLAC (yellow) and repeated cesarean section (black) in each year.

been described in literature several times. The latter was also observed in our study. However, prior vaginal delivery was much less predictive when compared to the simple audit system. The factors significantly associated with a higher failure rate included large fetuses, in concordance with late gestational age; increased maternal BMI; induction of labor; and history of recurring indications, which were mostly consistent with previous reports.

TABLE 3: Indications for cesarean section among women with failed TOLAC (237 cases).

Indications	Number (%)
Changing their mind (no obvious obstetric indications)	102 (43.04%)
Dystocia (failure of progression)	70 (29.53%)
Failure induction	30 (12.66%)
Non-reassuring fetal heart rate	21 (8.86%)
Others (placental abruption, HELLP syndrome, etc)	12 (5.06%)

Another factor possibly responsible for the low success rate in this study is unavailability of painless labor. Several cases could not tolerate the severe pain in advanced labor, together with the fear of uterine rupture, resulting in a higher rate of women changing their mind during labor. Moreover, we also noted that a prevalence of failure to progress or dystocia was relatively high in this study. This was probably caused by low threshold in the diagnosis of dystocia due to fear of uterine rupture especially in our setting of unavailable painless labor.

The limitations of this study include (1) the long time frame of the study involving several changes in clinical practice, especially the trend of higher cesarean section, which could have affected the outcomes of TOLAC, and (2) the retrospective nature of the study which made it difficult to reliably access several confounding factors. However, the retrospective nature could also be a strength of the study since it reflected a real world practice of TOLAC, not just the ideal circumstance of TOLAC in research practice. The predictive value of any potential factor could closely represent actual effectiveness in real situations of implementation.

In conclusion, the new insight gained from this study is that the most powerful factor associated with a successful TOLAC is the simple audit (regular orientation and reporting the outcomes). More importantly, this is the only factor that could be strengthened and expected to improve the outcomes whereas other minor factors, including prior vaginal birth, recurring indication in previous pregnancy, induction of labor, gestational age, and fetal weight, which also impacted on the outcomes, though to a lesser extent, could not be modified for improvement. Thus, our results are highly suggestive that strengthening the practice guideline or audit system is essential in promoting TOLAC, especially in a low-resource setting like our country.

Conflicts of Interest

The authors declare that there are no conflicts of interest.

Authors' Contributions

Aram Thapsamuthdechakorn participated in the study design, data collection, and manuscript writing. Ratanaporn Sekararithi participated in data collection. Theera Tongsong conducted data analysis and helped to draft the manuscript.

Acknowledgments

The authors wish to acknowledge the National Research University Project under Thailand's Office of the Higher Education Commission and Diamond Research Grant of Faculty of Medicine, Chiang Mai University, for financial support.

References

[1] ACOG Practice bulletin no. 115: Vaginal birth after previous cesarean delivery. Obstet Gynecol 2010 Aug;116(2 Pt 1):450-63.

[2] National Institutes of Health Consensus Development conference statement: vaginal birth after cesarean: new insights March 8-10, 2010. Obstet Gynecol 2010 Jun;115(6):1279-95.

[3] ACOG practice bulletin. Vaginal birth after previous cesarean delivery. No. 5, July 1999. Clinical management guidelines for obstetrician-gynecologists. American College of Obstetricians and Gynecologists. Int J Gynaecol Obstet 1999 Aug;66(2):197-204.

[4] E. Ashwal, A. Wertheimer, A. Aviram, A. Wiznitzer, Y. Yogev, and L. Hiersch, "Prediction of successful trial of labor after cesarean - The benefit of prior vaginal delivery," *The Journal of Maternal-Fetal and Neonatal Medicine*, vol. 29, no. 16, pp. 2665–2670, 2016.

[5] L. Balachandran, P. R. Vaswani, and R. Mogotlane, "Pregnancy outcome in women with previous one cesarean section," *Journal of Clinical and Diagnostic Research*, vol. 8, no. 2, pp. 99–102, 2014.

[6] S. Gupta, S. Jeeyaselan, R. Guleria, and A. Gupta, "An Observational Study of Various Predictors of Success of Vaginal Delivery Following a Previous Cesarean Section," *The Journal of Obstetrics and Gynecology of India*, vol. 64, no. 4, pp. 260–264, 2014.

[7] H. E. Knight, I. Gurol-Urganci, J. H. Van Der Meulen et al., "Vaginal birth after caesarean section: A cohort study investigating factors associated with its uptake and success," *BJOG: An International Journal of Obstetrics & Gynaecology*, vol. 121, no. 2, pp. 183–192, 2014.

[8] A. Soni, C. Sharma, S. Verma, U. Justa, P. K. Soni, and A. Verma, "A prospective observational study of trial of labor after cesarean in rural India," *International Journal of Gynecology and Obstetrics*, vol. 129, no. 2, pp. 156–160, 2015.

[9] M. Madaan, S. Agrawal, A. Nigam, R. Aggarwal, and S. S. Trivedi, "Trial of labour after previous caesarean section: The predictive factors affecting outcome," *Journal of Obstetrics & Gynaecology*, vol. 31, no. 3, pp. 224–228, 2011.

[10] A. Agarwal, P. Chowdhary, V. Das, A. Srivastava, A. Pandey, and M. T. Sahu, "Evaluation of pregnant women with scarred uterus in a low resource setting," *Journal of Obstetrics and Gynaecology Research*, vol. 33, no. 5, pp. 651–654, 2007.

25

Scoping Review on Maternal Health among Immigrant and Refugee Women in Canada: Prenatal, Intrapartum, and Postnatal Care

N. Khanlou,[1] **N. Haque,**[1] **A. Skinner,**[1] **A. Mantini,**[2] **and C. Kurtz Landy**[1]

[1] *Faculty of Health, York University, Toronto, ON, Canada*
[2] *Centre for Urban Health Solutions, St. Michael's Hospital, Toronto, ON, Canada*

Correspondence should be addressed to N. Khanlou; nkhanlou@yorku.ca

Academic Editor: Fabio Facchinetti

The last fifteen years have seen a dramatic increase in both the childbearing age and diversity of women migrating to Canada. The resulting health impact underscores the need to explore access to health services and the related maternal health outcome. This article reports on the results of a scoping review focused on migrant maternal health within the context of accessible and effective health services during pregnancy and following delivery. One hundred and twenty-six articles published between 2000 and 2016 that met our inclusion criteria and related to this group of migrant women, with pregnancy/motherhood status, who were living in Canada, were identified. This review points at complex health outcomes among immigrant and refugee women that occur within the compelling gaps in our knowledge of maternal health during all phases of maternity. Throughout the prenatal, intrapartum, and postnatal periods of maternity, barriers to accessing healthcare services were found to disadvantage immigrant and refugee women putting them at risk for challenging maternal health outcomes. Interactions between the uptake of health information and factors related to the process of immigrant settlement were identified as major barriers. Availability of appropriate services in a country that provides universal healthcare is discussed.

1. Introduction

Canada receives a significant number of newcomers each year that include immigrants, refugees, and asylum seekers. Of the 33 million people living in Canada, 6.7 million (20.6%) are immigrants and 3.5% of the total population are recent immigrants, while over 20,000 women arrive as approved refugees [1]. Additionally, the approximately 8,000 asylum seekers pursuing in-land claims for refugee status in Canada represents an exponential growth in the past decade [1]. The characteristics of all these migrants have changed dramatically as well. In the past fifteen years, there has been a doubling in the proportion of women migrating from source countries such as the Philippines, India, Iran, Nigeria, Iraq, Syria, Columbia, and Eritrea [2]. These same statistics show that a growing proportion of these women are within prime childbearing age and fleeing stressful circumstances (i.e., community violence, war conflict, trauma, or chronic poverty). These changing patterns of migration have implications for both the planning and the delivery of accessible and effective maternal health services, as well as the development of clinical practice guidelines specific to pregnancy in Canada. A scope of literature on maternal health during the pregnancy and postpartum phases is required to establish a foundation of evidence-based findings that can aid the development of guidelines and new policy to better support maternity health.

We report the findings of a scoping review we conducted to examine and outline the extent, range, and nature of empirical evidence about maternal health and healthcare services for migrant women in Canada, from pregnancy through to postpartum. We then provide a thematic analysis according to prenatal, intrapartum, and postnatal care literature for women resettled and living in Canada. The Canadian context allows for a unique examination of the challenges to maternal healthcare due to the highly diverse range of ethnocultural groups and their experiences from premigration and resettlement in a country that provides universal healthcare. For our scoping review, we included all migrants: immigrants who apply to live in Canada typically for occupational or family reunification purposes as well as resettled refugees who are provided with permanent residence and legal status in Canada prior to arriving and migrants who land in Canada with no prior status, asylum seekers, who remain undocumented, without legal status. In Canada, immigrants and resettled refugees are provided with the same universal health insurance that Canadian citizens receive, while refugee claimants are provided with only partial coverage through the Interim Federal Health Program (IFHP) and failed refugee claimants or undocumented migrants receive no health coverage. Unlike other high-income countries with universal health coverage, Canada does not offer medication coverage or exemptions for pregnant women in order to receive health service support regardless of their migration status. Complicating this scenario is the fact that Canada's IFHP health coverage for refugees can be unstable (cancelled at times due to alternating political agendas). Most provinces in Canada also provide funding for midwifery services to immigrants and some refugees. Analysis of studies conducted in Canada reflecting this mix of health services and migrant needs provides a unique opportunity to understand contributing factors to maternity health for migrant women, especially when, for most of them, financial access is not a factor.

Evidence presented in a United Nations report [3] from other similar migrant receiving countries (European Union and Asia) and a recent systematic review of five countries [4] identified a number of factors that lead to underutilization of maternal health services by immigrant women. These include linguistic barriers, the immigrants' level of integration into mainstream society, experience of discrimination and racism from healthcare providers, women's knowledge regarding maternal healthcare information, and recent immigrants' stress of adjusting to a new country. Findings in the UN report also indicate that pregnancy-related problems are common among immigrants throughout the European Union countries and Asia and include maternal health issues such as inadequate or no antenatal care and higher rates of stillbirths and infant mortality as well as financial barriers [5]. Research from the United Kingdom on perinatal outcomes among their immigrant population has reported lower birth weights among babies born to Asian immigrant women and higher perinatal and postnatal mortality rates among Caribbean and Pakistani immigrants as compared to the general population [6]. These findings have also been reported among other high-income countries like Norway, Japan, and Italy [4].

Given the essential nature of these negative perinatal health outcomes in migrants and Canada's unique position of great ethnocultural diversity, new knowledge on the maternal health among migrant women in Canada is warranted to inform care during all phases of maternity. In addition, while guidelines have been developed in Canada for immigrants and refugee healthcare in general, no practice guidelines exist specific to pregnancy, and the current guidelines only include recommendations related to contraception and pregnancy screening [7].

Over the last fifteen years, in particular, as the drive for evidence-based practice has increased, so has the rapid growth in reviews of the literature on specific maternity topics [6, 8–11]. Scoping reviews that use Arksey and O'Malley's [8] methodology help us understand the research landscape by examining the extent, range, and nature of research evidence in a particular research area such as immigrant maternal health [12]. This methodology provides an overall summary of the topic area while also identifying gaps in research knowledge without delving into the types and quality of the studies. This kind of review can form the basis for more detailed reviews [13]. The findings of such scoping reviews can also be used to influence policy and practice.

2. Methods

We applied Arksey and O'Malley's [8] framework to explore the large amount of maternal health literature, including both qualitative and quantitative studies as well as previously published systematic reviews to address our research question. Arksey and O'Malley's framework outlines five stages for conducting scoping reviews. These stages are (1) identifying the research question, (2) identifying relevant studies, (3) study selection, (4) charting the data, and (5) collating, summarizing, and reporting the results and (6) an optional step of a consultation exercise is suggested by Arksey and O'Malley to validate the findings from the scoping review. The five stages of the framework may appear to be linear; however, the actual process and stages are iterative and reflexive [8]. The flexibility of this methodology allowed us to redefine our search terms as our familiarity with the literature increased [8], thus ensuring comprehensive and broad coverage of the literature. The format and the pursuing subheadings of the paper follow the recommendations of Arksey and O'Malley [8] and others [9, 11] to guide our reporting and maintain transparency of our work.

The research question of our scoping review was the following: *What does the peer-reviewed scientific literature tell us about maternal health and health service utilization during the prenatal, intrapartum, and postnatal periods among migrant women resettled in Canada?* We were guided by the World Health Organization's (WHO) definition of maternal health. WHO defines maternal health as "the health of women during pregnancy, childbirth, and the postpartum period" [5]. We also utilized the definition of "immigrant" proposed by the Canadian Council of Refugees: "a person who has settled permanently in another country (Canada)" [14], but we restricted our target population to female immigrants identified as being first generation and foreign-born. Further, to properly reflect the current trend of diversity in migration, we included refugees with legal status as well as asylum seekers seeking formal refugee status and failed refugee claimants or women with undocumented status or no legal status.

Table 1: Search terms used.

immigrant prenatal care	refugee maternity
immigrant maternal care	refugee maternal health
immigrant antenatal	refugee antenatal
immigrant postnatal care	refugee prenatal care
immigrant intrapartum care	refugee intrapartum care
immigrant maternal health	refugee postpartum care
immigrant postpartum care	refugee childbirth
immigrant childbirth	refugee postnatal care
immigrant maternity	refugee family planning
immigrant child spacing	refugee intimate partner violence
immigrant family planning	refugee pregnancy violence
immigrant breastfeeding	refugee child spacing
immigrant intimate partner violence	refugee breastfeeding
immigrant pregnancy violence	Maternal health care refugee

2.1. Search Strategy. A scoping review of studies reporting health outcomes and utilization of healthcare services for migrant women living in Canada and related to pregnancy and postpartum outcomes was conducted. A literature search for relevant articles published between 1 January 2000 and 1 September 2016, without methodological restrictions, was carried out in the electronic databases PubMed, CINAHL, PsycINFO, Ovid MEDLINE, Science Citation Index, the Social Sciences Conference Proceedings Index, and Sociological Abstracts (2000–2016). However, articles were restricted to those published in English and in peer-reviewed scientific journals for studies on pregnancy and childbirth health outcomes and healthcare utilization for migrant women, using the search terms outlined in Table 1. These electronic databases were chosen as they contained studies relevant to our research question and the search strategy was designed according to the specification of each database. Originally, we had fewer search terms but, later, based on our knowledge gained from the literature, we included additional terms such as birth spacing, family planning, breastfeeding, and violence to be more comprehensive. The search terms (Table 1) were performed alone and in combinations using the Boolean operators "AND" and "OR." There were no differences in the databases in terms of results yielded, but broad terms such as "immigration" or "refugee health" were excluded as search terms on their own, to allow for inclusion of articles that were specific to pregnancy and childbirth among migrant women living in Canada. The last search was carried out on 1 September 2016 and searches were conducted in consultation with a health librarian and the research team and entered [15, 16].

To answer the research question of our scoping review, we used the following inclusion and exclusion criteria.

2.1.1. Inclusion Criteria. Inclusion criteria were (i) primary and secondary source research studies, including systematic reviews, published in English language, between the years 2000 and 2016; (ii) all studies (qualitative, quantitative,

and mixed methods) which included migrant women as the sample population and focused on maternal health (i.e., prenatal, delivery, perinatal, or postnatal period); (iii) studies that had migrant women living in Canada as participants.

2.1.2. Exclusion Criteria. Exclusion criteria were (i) the grey literature, documents published in non-English languages, theses, protocols, policy documents, proposals, and editorials and (ii) non-peer-reviewed publications.

One research team member initially read the titles identified in searches on the electronic databases to determine the relevance of the study to our scoping review. Titles that did not contain the search words in the title field were reviewed and removed if they did not meet the inclusion criteria. Three members of the research team then reviewed all the abstracts to select the full-text documents to be included in the scoping review.

3. Results

A total of 5,608 studies were identified in our initial search based on the search words and an additional 8 studies were added after identification from references of these articles. After the removal of duplicates and removal of all studies that did not meet the inclusion criteria within the body of the article, we were left with 147 studies. Of these, another thirteen articles were removed because they were not specific to the Canadian population or because they were study protocols with no results. As a result of this process, 126 documents were included for full-text review and charting (Figure 1).

Of the 126 studies included in the final synthesis, 54 were qualitative, 5 were mixed methods studies, 5 were systematic reviews, and 62 were quantitative studies, and only 3 of the research studies were intervention studies. Among the 54 qualitative studies reviewed, several stand out as focused on the diversity of the women: 6 focused on childbearing immigrant women from a specific source country, such as Haiti, Vietnam, or Pakistan or countries within the Middle East [6, 17–21], while three studied new immigrant mothers settled in Canada for less than 5 years [22–24], one sampled recent refugees [25], and three examined women identified as uninsured asylum seekers [17, 26, 27]. Similarly, within the 62 quantitative studies, 18 studies in particular focused on specific ethnic groups, including 3 longitudinal studies of health outcomes [26, 28, 29], another three studies focused on mental health concerns during the prenatal period [30–32], while 2 evaluated mental health status during delivery [33, 34], and another 3 studied physical status at various periods of maternity [35–37]. Of the five mixed methods studies, 2 focused on the role of culture in the prenatal period [10, 38], another two evaluated mental health also during the prenatal period [39, 40], and one final study examined understanding of procedures during delivery [41].

Results are presented according to the three main subgroups: (1) prenatal care (migration status, postmigration factors, and health services factors), (2) intrapartum care

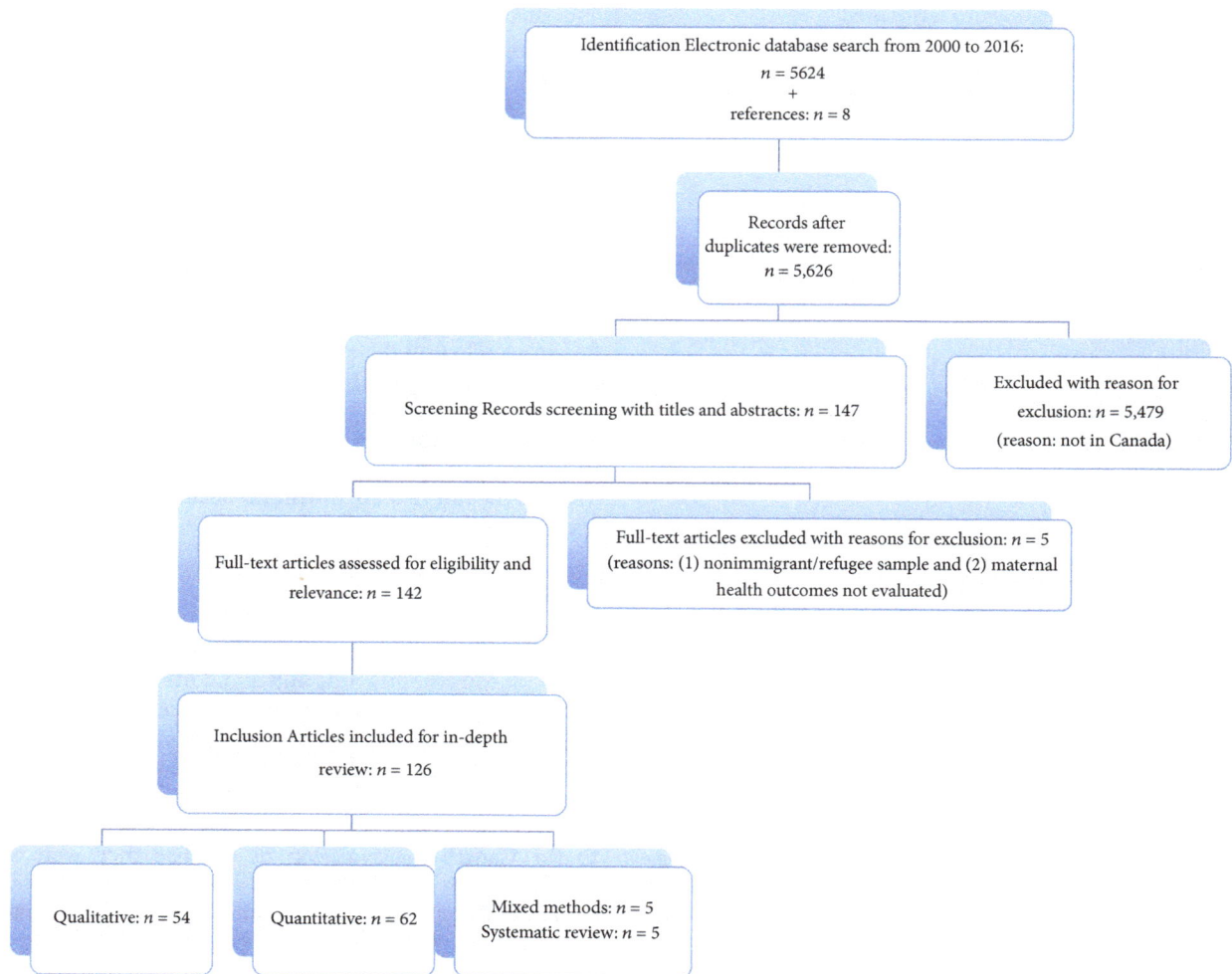

FIGURE 1: Flowchart illustrating the scoping review process.

(maternal and child health), and (3) postnatal care (health-care access and individual factors). The number of documents retrieved from each of the electronic databases as well as the number of studies related to outcomes, population, and methodology is listed in Table 2.

3.1. Factors Associated with Prenatal Health Outcomes. In total, 20 studies focused on maternal health outcomes during the prenatal period for immigrant and refugee women. Twelve studies examined migration and maternal lifestyle factors in relation to maternal health and five studies examined women's mental health concerns as a contributing factor during the prenatal period.

3.1.1. Migration Status. Studies that examined Canadian immigrant women found no differences in their ability overall to navigate or initially access the health system for prenatal care which was generally measured by the number of medical appointments during pregnancy [18, 42]. However, when the adequacy or quality of prenatal care was specifically studied, over 20% of immigrant mothers who were new to Canada were found to have received "inadequate" prenatal care leading to identification of mother's ethnicity as a risk factor [18, 42]. Prenatal care in uninsured asylum seeking refugees or undocumented women was found to be inadequate [17, 38, 43, 44]. Wilson-Mitchel and Rummens reported that as many as 80% of these uninsured women receive less than adequate prenatal care and 6.5% receive no prenatal care at all [38].

Language barriers and limited cultural sensitivity of prenatal care may also interfere with established guidelines. Language was most commonly cited as a barrier to care [21, 45–49]. For many immigrants, English as a second language makes it difficult for them to understand the new healthcare system and many of the medical terminologies commonly used by providers. They also face difficulty in effectively communicating with service providers. Cultural factors were perceived to be a barrier to accessing prenatal care both by immigrant women and by the healthcare providers who want to support them. Cultural needs and expectations are often unknown or unable to be met in the context of the Canadian healthcare system [21, 44, 46, 48–50], which may negatively impact the experience of immigrant women and

TABLE 2: Content of studies and database search.

	Frequency	Percent
Period of maternity (n = 126)		
Prenatal	20	15.9
Intrapartum	35	27.8
Postnatal	71	56.3
Migration status (n = 126)		
Immigrant	95	75.4
Refugee	24	19.0
Asylum seeker	7	5.6
Prenatal outcomes (n = 20)		
Migration	6	30.0
Lifestyle	3	15.0
Mental health	6	30.0
Access & utilization	5	25.0
Intrapartum outcomes (n = 35)		
Complications	3	8.6
Ethnicity	4	11.4
Birth weight/mortality	8	22.9
Nutrition	8	22.9
Mental health	4	11.4
Access & utilization	8	22.9
Postnatal outcomes (n = 71)		
Mental health	12	16.9
Resilient coping	18	25.4
Discrimination	11	15.5
Poor relationships	17	23.9
Access & utilization	13	18.3
Social determinants of health		
Income	9	60.0
Neighborhood	4	26.7
Education	3	20.0
Methodology (n = 126)		
Qualitative	54	42.9
Quantitative	62	49.2
Mixed methods	5	4.0
Systematic review	5	4.0
Electronic search databases (n = 5624)		
PubMed	2416	43.0
CINAHL	1320	23.5
PsycINFO	1490	26.5
Sociological & Science	479	8.5

lead them to cease or turn elsewhere for care [46, 50]. Bhagat and her colleagues [50] found that female South Asian immigrants were often not comfortable expressing their needs or identifying gaps in the system [51].

3.1.2. Lifestyle Factors. Immigrant women were less likely to smoke and consume alcohol during pregnancy [18, 52] with a positive correlation existing between length of stay in Canada and alcohol and tobacco consumption before pregnancy [53]. Kowal et al. [53] found that immigrant women gained less weight during pregnancy than Canadian-born women and were 1.5 times more likely to gain less than the Health Canada recommended amount [54]. Another study by Hyman and Dussault [19, 40] found that acculturation was correlated with increase preoccupation with thinness, even during pregnancy, but did not examine weight gain. A number of in-depth studies by Higginbottom and her colleagues [19] have consistently found food choices to correlate with cultural beliefs, and, despite recommended health guidelines, immigrant women may continue to eat culturally preferred foods despite medical advice. This finding was also highlighted in a previous literature review of studies between 2000 and 2010 [55] which also identified the need for increased cultural knowledge relating to food choices and the need to involve the whole family in decisions related to food and nutrition.

3.1.3. Mental Health Status. Migrant women are more likely to suffer from prenatal depression than their nonmigrant Canadian counterparts [20, 33]. Women who were immigrants experiencing prenatal depression were more likely to report suffering from somatic symptoms [33]. Some of the identified risk factors associated with prenatal depression in migrant women included high marital strain [20], lack of social support, poverty [20, 30], and crowding [20] and migrants were also found to demonstrate elevated maternal cortisol levels [31]. Migrant women from certain countries may be more at risk than those from other countries. Miszkurka et al. [20] found that immigrants from the Caribbean, sub-Saharan Africa, and Maghreb experienced a twofold increase in antenatal depressive symptoms when compared to women who immigrated from Europe and the Middle East. It is important to note that their risk attenuated when social support and financial situations were accounted for [30]. Also very noteworthy is the finding that immigrant women were less likely to report experiencing violence associated with pregnancy [28, 55–57]. Stewart et al. [29] found that the risk of violence associated with pregnancy increased if the migrant was an asylum seeker, lived in Canada for less than 2 years, lived without a partner, or had less than high school education. In these women, violence during pregnancy was also associated with a higher risk of prenatal depressive symptoms, with victims of intimate partner violence experiencing a 3- to 5-fold increase in depressive symptoms.

3.1.4. Physical Health Status. McElroy et al. [58] examined rates of rubella immunity in immigrant populations, as underimmunized populations were at increased risk for congenital rubella syndrome. Rubella immunity was found to be the lowest among women from North Africa and the Middle East and China and the South Pacific [58]. Immigrant women were also less likely to take folic acid supplements before and during pregnancy, reporting that they did not have enough information about the benefits [32]. When the effect of the Canada Prenatal Nutrition Program (CPNP) on the health behaviours of immigrants and Canadian-born women was examined, the CPNP was found to be effective in increasing vitamin use and breastfeeding in immigrant women, while decreasing their consumption of tobacco and alcohol products [35]. Immigrant women showed the strongest correlation between CPNP exposure and positive health behaviours while refugee women tended to not take supplements, likely because they also did not have visits with their community public health nurse or sufficient prenatal appointments with a physician.

3.2. Factors Associated with Utilization of Health Services during the Prenatal Period.

Factors hindering access to care were identified in terms of navigating services, mothers' perception of quality of care, socioeconomic status, language, and cultural and other barriers. As many new migrants are not familiar with the organization of the healthcare system, accessing healthcare and understanding the role of different services and healthcare providers act as a barrier to seeking care and accessing services [21, 43, 46, 59].

Many immigrant women feel as though they are receiving substandard care if their prenatal care is not overseen by a medical doctor [21, 46] and have obstetricians overseeing their prenatal care at rates higher than Canadian-born women [21, 32]. Some immigrant women also try to utilize multiple or different care providers during pregnancy [46] or seek alternative supports, including private services [18, 21] which may affect the quality and continuity of care they receive. Heaman and her colleagues [60] examined the relationship between prenatal care and neighbourhood context and found greater levels of inadequate prenatal care in neighbourhoods with higher proportions of recent immigrants. The at-risk neighbourhoods also had the highest rates of unemployment, women who reported smoking during pregnancy, and the highest percentage of single-parent families and individuals with less than 9 years of education [60]. Past reviews have also found the less favorable socioeconomic status of immigrant women to compromise their access to prenatal care [21]. Findings also demonstrate other important barriers affecting care, including finding a doctor who could speak their own language [21, 43, 45], lack of transportation [48], weak social support [49], need for childcare [48, 50], financial barriers [43, 44, 50], and having lost their health records during migration [45]. Fears of reporting to immigration authorities and deportation were also considered to be barriers for undocumented pregnant women [21]. Uninsured women that also presented for care later in pregnancy had fewer prenatal visits and underwent less auxiliary testing than insured immigrant women [17, 38, 43, 61]. Acculturation into a new country of residence is a process that takes place over time and is influenced by personal beliefs and behaviour as well as general integration receptivity of the host society. As a result, ethnocultural or traditional practices may interfere with the recommendations provided to migrant women by Canadian health service providers for optimal health of mother and child. Low levels of acculturation were consistently found to be a barrier to prenatal care among immigrant women living within inner-city neighbourhood [62].

Migrant women were less likely to attend prenatal classes than Canadian-born women [32, 47]. They were also found to express a poor understanding of the purpose of prenatal monitoring, namely, symphysis-fundal height measurement, gestational diabetes screening, and Group B *Streptococcus* testing [47, 63]. A study by Bhagat and colleagues [50] examining the maternal experiences of Punjabi women suggested that the term *classes* poses a problem, as this was said to imply ignorance towards childbirth. Other barriers associated with the lower rates of immigrants attending prenatal classes were language [47] and time constraints as their need to earn a living wage often took precedence over healthcare [50].

3.3. Factors Associated with Intrapartum Health Outcomes.

In total, 35 studies were found on intrapartum care. Of these, 20 studies focused exclusively on delivery care and 15 studies on prenatal as well as intrapartum care. Several studies also pointed out specific concerns for migrant women related to eclampsia, caesarean section, delivery experiences, birth weight, and perinatal mortality, as well as preterm birth. During the intrapartum period (occurring during labor and delivery), migrant women expressed difficulties with communication and integration of their cultural beliefs with recommended healthcare practices, as well as lack of support from healthcare providers and lack of understanding of the informed consent process for procedures during delivery [25].

3.3.1. Delivery Experiences.

Several studies examined the delivery experiences of immigrant women. Overall, migrant women do not exhibit higher rates of severe morbidity; however, disparities in severe maternal morbidity have been identified for refugee women. This is especially true now that immigration trends favour humanitarian protection for refugee women with HIV [64]. Similarly, immigrant women from sub-Saharan Africa are consistently found to be at higher risk of severe maternal morbidity with the most common diagnosis being eclampsia followed by uterine rupture [49]. With regard to eclampsia, in particular, however Ray et al. [25] found a positive correlation between eclampsia in immigrant women and the number of months since immigration. Urquia and his colleagues [34] found that immigrant women from the Caribbean and Hispanic America are also at a higher risk of severe preeclampsia than locally born populations or immigrants from industrialized nations.

Conflicting data exists regarding the incidence of caesarean section in immigrant populations. Some studies have found that immigrant women were at a significantly higher risk of caesarean section [18, 38, 65, 66], while others have reported no difference in caesarean section rates between immigrants and Canadian-born women [17, 32].

Maternal source country of origin was identified as a predictor of caesarean section in two studies [36, 67]. In particular, these studies found that Vietnamese and Eastern European women underwent the fewest caesarean sections while immigrant women from Africa, South America, and

South Asia exhibited the highest rates of emergency caesarean sections [36, 67]. Differences by migration status also varied for immigrant women, with refugees from South East and Central Asia having the highest rates of caesarean section.

Conflicting data exists for the incidence of preterm birth among immigrant women. Some studies found no difference in preterm birth for immigrant mothers or uninsured refugee or undocumented women [17, 38, 65]. However, when specific source countries were studied, immigrant women from Guyana, Trinidad and Tobago, Philippines, and Jamaica were all found to be at higher risk of "very preterm babies" [68]. Some studies found that migrant women from Asia and sub-Saharan Africa as well as Haiti were at a greater risk of preterm birth [69, 70]. Undocumented migrants and asylum seekers were also found to have an increased likelihood of preterm birth [18, 44]. In most of these studies, length of time in Canada was associated with equal or decreased incidence of preterm birth [42, 69, 71–73]: risk of preterm birth increasing with a longer stay in Canada [42, 73].

Residential environment, including neighbourhood poverty, was found to have little or no association with preterm birth in immigrants [22, 23, 72] but, interestingly, a high same-ethnic group concentration was associated with low birth weight [22]. On the other hand, a high density of migrant population was found to have a protective effect against preterm birth in immigrant mothers, especially those with higher education [23].

The link between education and adverse birth outcomes remains unclear. Auger found no correlation between low education and adverse birth outcomes (low birth weight, preterm birth) in migrant women but found that foreign-born status was associated with preterm birth in university educated women [74]. Higher education was similarly found to be more protective against preterm birth for Canadian mothers, while immigrant mothers required up to four years more education to experience the same protective effects [75]. Battaglini and her colleagues reported that women at medium risk for perinatal problems also had higher education but they were also more likely to have undergone professional dequalification as a result of their immigration to Canada [76].

3.3.2. Birth Weight and Perinatal Mortality.

Recent immigrants have been found to be at a higher risk of having low birth weight (below the 10th percentile) infants [65]. Immigrant women in Canada were more likely to have low birth weight infants and those infants were more likely to be classified as having a low birth weight [22, 77–80] based on Canadian birth weight curves. This is especially true for immigrant women of East or South Asian descent; however, a number of researchers have discovered that when region-specific birth weight curves from the mothers' country of origin were used, this higher risk disappeared [22, 78, 81–83]. Some of these studies [22, 81, 83] have also found that infants of migrants were more likely to be misclassified based on Canadian birth weight curves, suggesting the need for ethnic specific, culturally sensitive standards [77, 84]. Confirming this conclusion is that Chinese and South Asian infants had

lower perinatal mortality risks throughout gestation, despite having lower birth weights [78]. At the same time, a positive correlation between violence associated with pregnancy and low birth weight infants in immigrant women has been noted [29]. In contrast, a more recent systematic review by Boshari and his colleagues found that the newborns of migrant mothers had higher birth weights than the infants in their native countries [37]. In contrast, Gagnon and her colleagues [36] found that the infants of Asian, North African, and sub-Saharan African migrants were at higher risk of feto-infant mortality. Migrant women who experienced violence associated with pregnancy were at higher risk of miscarriage [29, 85]. Infants of uninsured asylum seeker mothers required more neonatal resuscitation [18, 38].

3.4. Factors Associated with Utilization of Health Services during the Intrapartum Period.

Almost no studies have been published that examine utilization of health services during the intrapartum period, with a few exceptions. Chalmers and Hashi looked at the birthing experiences of Somali women in Canada, with a history of genital mutilation, and found many reports of inadequate pain management and cultural insensitivity [86]. The women reported feeling left out of decision-making regarding their care and undergoing more medical interventions than they had hoped for. The women reported experiencing hurtful comments, apparent disgust, and a lack of privacy during procedures. Women expressed the importance of cultural sensitivity and awareness during this process [49, 86–88], a need which some women felt was not met in the context of the western healthcare system [49, 86, 89]. Many women expressed a preference for a female physician during the labor and delivery process [39, 49]. When compared to Canadian women, migrant women were more likely to rate their birth experience as "somewhat positive" instead of "very positive" [32]. Several migrants did not support medical interventions during pregnancy and instead expressed a desire to withstand the labor and delivery process without the use of pain medications [37, 39, 90].

3.5. Factors Associated with Postnatal Health Outcomes.

In total, 71 studies focused on maternal health outcomes during the postnatal period for immigrant and refugee women. Most of these studies have been published more recently and are highly consistent in their findings, providing evidence for increased risk of maternal mental health challenges and negative health trajectories from cultural barriers following the birth of a child.

3.5.1. Mental Health Outcomes.

All studies of the postnatal period for immigrant women discussed postpartum depression and several studies identified both cultural background and socioeconomic factors as contributors to postpartum depression in migrant women [41, 85, 91–95]. The stigma of emotional distress, experiences of increased discord within family relationships, and the difficult external expectations of motherhood from the society, as well as poor nutrition and self-care practices during this period of maternity, are consistently cited as leaving migrant women vulnerable to postpartum depression [41, 93]. Further economic dependence and insecure migration experiences also disadvantage migrant women [93, 96]. Two recent longitudinal studies of immigrant women found that younger women who had been in Canada for less than two years and those who had poor perceptions of their own health and low income exhibited a high prevalence of postpartum depression [93, 95]. In addition, poor use of supplements, inadequate nutrition, and reduced self-care during the postnatal period have been documented to also contribute further to poor maternal health outcomes.

3.5.2. Resilient Coping. One study that investigated the impact of postnatal stress on immigrant women's adjustment, months and years following delivery, found that immigrant women typically responded with resilient coping strategies [96]. Gagnon and her colleagues interviewed a group of immigrant women in Toronto and Montreal, deemed to be at high risk in their postnatal period due to factors discussed above but to be adjusting well without any maternal health concerns. Women categorized as "resilient" identified social inclusion through a socially supportive network, accessible health services, and culturally sensitive interventions as experiences enhancing their coping strategies [96].

3.6. Factors Associated with Utilization of Health Services during the Intrapartum Period. Nowhere is the negative impact of poor access to healthcare reflected more than in the immigrant woman's higher incidence of postpartum depression, reported to be at least twice the rate of nonimmigrant women [97]. It is not surprising that barriers to care such as lack of acculturation or language barriers and culturally appropriate care begins in the prenatal period and persists through to the postnatal period, but it is surprising that other factors including family pressures and personal adjustment needs can create situations in which barriers and risk to maternal health are intensified for immigrant women in the postnatal period. Whether the needed care is for mental health, their child's well-being, or their own physical health, studies indicate that some postnatal outcomes associated with maternal health for immigrant women are highly related to their experiences of isolation, poor family relationships, conflicted gender roles, and the discrimination they perceive within health system services [26, 41, 92, 97]. The immigrant participants of a community-based participatory research study represent their challenge best: that, as immigrant women in Canada, they "lacked the social and environmental factors perceived as key enablers of healthy pregnancies and postpartum" [27]. As the immigrant women's postnatal outcomes include higher rates of postpartum depression (PPD) [93, 95] and lower rates of breastfeeding exclusivity in immigrant women with higher levels of depression symptoms [94] and stress related physical conditions [97], their experience with mental health through the postnatal period is an important area of consideration for immigrant and refugee women.

3.6.1. Isolation and Discrimination. The existing communication problems, inadequate information, and lack of familiarity with healthcare systems persist into the postnatal period, but more intensified are immigrant mothers' perceptions of discrimination and care which they perceive as not kind or respectful [61]. Consistently, findings demonstrate the negative impact of family and community experiences on immigrant women's postnatal health. They are required to cope concurrently with migration stressors and new parenthood, both contributing to higher levels of loneliness and stress that is further exacerbated by time restrictions for financial support, prolonged family reunification processes, and uncoordinated government services that serve the postnatal period [26]. Further supporting increased stress experienced by asylum seekers or undocumented migrant women, family physicians reported caring for this population to be challenging, increasing their workload and psychological stress [61].

3.6.2. Poor Family Relationships and Gender Roles. When women's perceptions and experiences during the postnatal period are explored, a clear association between women's maternal health and family relationships is identified [26, 92, 95]. Not only do they have to cope with the social stigma of being in need, being under stress, and being lonely [26], but also their decisions about healthcare are influenced by relationships with parents and their in-laws [41]. Marital discord during the postnatal period is also reported to affect a migrant woman's access to healthcare services [93]. Adding further to their experience of postnatal stress is the experience of many complex gender-related problems [41, 93]. Gender based expectations within their family, marital discord evoked by new gender roles, and the conflict with their newly developing identity within the Canadian society intersect with cultural and social norms in a way that hinders women's ability to access necessary healthcare services [26, 93].

4. Discussion

This scoping review has confirmed the existence of a series of cultural, social, economic, and individual factors that relate to migrant health and which create barriers to maternal health throughout the prenatal, intrapartum, and postnatal periods of maternity for women living in Canada. Several of these factors appear to serve as potential barriers to healthy pregnancy and birth outcomes, while others appear to interact in a complex manner to affect maternal health outcomes. The information derived from this review helps healthcare providers or social care professionals in Canada understand the complexity of migrant women's maternal health experiences, leading to improved interventions, practice, and policy.

The literature indicates that migration and resettlement experiences influence maternal health throughout pregnancy, delivery, and the postpartum period. While optimal health during all three periods of maternity is a priority, meeting this goal is a challenge for migrant women. Even in Canada, where universal healthcare exists, financial barriers have been identified, including those that intersect with migration status, stress of acculturation, and other postmigration experiences. In addition, migrant women's dependence on family and social support puts them at risk. However, while some ethnocultural factors demonstrate a negative impact on maternal health outcomes for migrant women, others foster enhanced resiliency. Given the tremendous heterogeneity of migrant women in Canada, the consistency of barriers and maternal health outcomes perceived and experienced is noteworthy.

Similar barriers to utilizing health services impacted the three periods of maternity, at varying degrees, but health outcomes differed. During the prenatal period access barriers to maternal healthcare services may disadvantage some migrant women. However, the findings in relation to intrapartum outcomes are not as consistent across studies. For instance, factors contributing to health outcomes during the prenatal care are influenced by those typically categorized as social determinants of health [98]. On the other hand, contributors to postnatal health outcomes are influenced by more specific factors occurring within the women's personal lives. Migration is increasingly recognized as an important social determinant of health and intersects with factors such as downward socioeconomic mobility, poor access to optimal nutrition, and limited social networks [61, 96, 99]. In addition, barriers to services further disadvantage pregnant migrant women and appear to also contribute to at-risk maternal health outcomes, including postpartum depression [93, 95] and stress related physical conditions [97]. On the other hand, factors related to intrapartum care influence the adequacy and effectiveness of maternal health services. Canada has a publically funded healthcare system that is believed to provide equal access to the quantity of medically required hospital and physicians' services [54] but inconsistent access to midwifery and no clinical obstetrical guidelines for migrant women [100] affected both health outcomes and the experience of barriers to care for migrant women. Inconsistencies emerging in the literature around intrapartum care may be related to variations across settings in the effectiveness of intrapartum services for immigrant women.

Another reason for the inconsistency in findings across studies is that immigrant women are a heterogeneous group but the current review demonstrates an interaction with barriers and health outcomes depending on the period of maternity. The unique ethnic, cultural, and socioeconomic factors, language, family makeup and size, and quality or need of social networks can exert important and synergistic influences on maternal health and healthcare experiences [5, 32, 38]. The current review supports the call for improvements in maternal health outcomes and healthcare utilization through consideration of those factors that are unique to migrants, including the woman's country of origin and the particulars of migration experience for the women. In addition, the category of migrant may be used inconsistently across studies and entail different migration statuses such as refugees or landed immigrants, each with their own unique resources and barriers to services, yet the review demonstrates high

levels of consistency in the existence of barriers to utilizing maternity care. Additionally, government-assisted refugees in Canada are recognized as Convention Refugees abroad and have assistance from the government during their initial resettlement period that includes both healthcare and family or community supports [101] while migrants who are applying for legal status in Canada have healthcare insurance but no family/community support [102]. Further, those migrants who have given up trying to obtain legal status do not have healthcare coverage or any other supports. Migrants who remain undocumented are likely to have experienced trauma and ill health [44] and have to cope with greater variability in the precarious nature of their lives based on the circumstances of their arrival into Canada as well as the stress of deciding what to do with newborns of migrants who become parents while waiting in Canada for their asylum claim to be settled [25, 66, 78]. In all, the literature is fairly consistent in identifying significant risks to asylum seeking women and also for refugee and immigrant pregnant women.

Our findings corroborate the more recent systematic reviews of studies on immigrant and nonimmigrant maternity care [14, 37, 55, 67, 97, 99, 103]. In particular, Small and her colleagues [103] evaluated studies on maternal healthcare across 5 countries (Australia, Canada, Sweden, the United Kingdom, and the United States). This team concluded that while migrant and nonmigrant women have similar hopes from maternity care, migrant women provide poor ratings of care received and face additional challenges that impact negatively their health throughout all three phases of maternity. Of significance, Small and her colleagues conclude that while academics often recommend culturally sensitive care, immigrant women want care that is respectful and communicated well and offers specific information on maternity procedures in their community [103]. In addition, they call for enhancing equity and nondiscriminatory attitudes in care [97, 103]. In our scoping review, the challenges reported across studies associated with negative impacts on immigrant women's experiences in accessing prenatal care included navigating the healthcare system, understanding how care and provision of consent operate in their new homeland, addressing language and communication challenges, finding a doctor who could speak their own language, lack of attention to cultural concerns, cost of services, and perception of poor quality of care, often due to a discrepancy between care provider recommendations and the traditional expectations of the mother, husband, and their parents. Studies also noted that migrant women were less likely to smoke and consume alcohol but also less likely to attend prenatal classes and report violence during pregnancy, and they also demonstrated lower rates of immunization, nutritional supports, and supplements uptake during pregnancy. Migrant women were also found to be much more likely to suffer from both prenatal and postnatal depression which was also found to negatively impact their levels of nutrition and self-care. In addition, our scoping review supports two important current trends in migration, including a dramatic increase in female migrants, and the case for very specific factors that contribute to inequity in migrant women's maternity care, which can best guide policy.

5. Limitations of Scoping Review

Our scoping review has two limitations that need to be taken into account. First, this review did not look into grey and unpublished literature. Second, the results of the review should be interpreted with caution because scoping reviews do not screen for quality of studies and, thus, have large variations in study methodologies and sampling of the studies included in the review.

6. Conclusion

Pregnancy and childbirth for migrant women living in Canada carry a high risk of adverse health and mental health outcomes. Utilization of healthcare can also be compromised for migrant women who are pregnant, despite the availability of Canada's universal healthcare system. Both health and utilization outcomes further put migrants with no legal status, as in the case of asylum seekers, at risk. Consistent with the findings of migrant women in European and western countries as a whole [104, 105], our scoping review has identified a consistent body of knowledge supporting these challenges in Canada as well, where financial access is not typically a barrier and where migration policies are generally believed to be inclusive. However, gaps in knowledge are evident and more importantly, at this time, there are no clinical or scientific guidelines in obstetrics that consider the health of migrant pregnant women. By integrating studies and thematically analyzing their findings, this scoping review has created a solid foundation for recommendations that can lead to research, practice, and policy improvements in all countries facing increased diversity of women migrants and that already have broad healthcare coverage.

In light of the scoping review findings, the following recommendations are made for future research, practice, and policy:

(1) Disentangle effects of ethnic and immigration contributions to maternal health through comparative research designs including migrant and Canadian-born women with diverse identity and cultural and lifestyle markers.

(2) Focus on targeted intervention studies that can provide specific evidence for scaling up maternal health programs based on translation of knowledge regarding nutrition, procedures, and health practices, especially for the prenatal and postnatal periods where women migrants are at the greatest risk.

(3) Include mothers in the study prior to actual data collection to inform study design (such as through participatory approaches to research) or after the findings for dissemination to determine relevance of findings for diverse communities. This is important for clinical practice as well to ensure that providers and decision-makers understand how to individualize services to best meet the needs of pregnant migrant women.

(4) Engage in knowledge transfer and mobilization informing studies to help understand how interactions between service providers and mothers with few socioeconomic resources or individual family and community factors affect migrant mothers' utilization of services and access to maternity healthcare.

(5) Given the higher risk of negative maternal health outcomes for migrant women without legal status, the policy implications of this scoping review are noteworthy. In particular, three provinces in Canada have 3-month wait for health insurance for landed immigrants and sponsored-class immigrants, comprising over 80% of newcomers to Canada [106]. Also, since there is a large increase in migrant women asylum seekers at a time of higher rejection rate for those applying for refugee status, it is likely that more pregnant women are put at risk for poor maternity health outcomes as they also fail to be able to utilize healthcare services.

(6) The recommendations that emerge from this scoping review support formulation of policies that reduce barriers and the contributors to poor maternity health outcomes, including language needs, health knowledge, and cultural influences. The thirteen other countries, such as Denmark, Italy, Japan, Norway, and Switzerland, identified as "high-income" countries offer exemptions for pregnant women [107]; Canada does not.

(7) The health status and utilization of services by pregnant migrant women depend to a large extent on health education, access to services, and cultural factors, as evident in our scoping review, supporting the need to increase opportunities for improving the cultural communication by providers, especially for subpopulations of migrant women and their pregnancy needs in relation to their personal, culture, and family needs.

(8) Internationally, healthcare systems for reproductive/maternal services are prioritized to decrease maternal morbidity, but our scoping review indicates limitations in Canada and also supports the identified complexities in the lives of migrating women, including spousal relations, community roles, and self-care needs, demonstrated as critical to their health status and utilization of healthcare services to optimize pregnancy and delivery. Policy that directs a more integrative model of maternity care is needed to help maternity healthcare providers and researchers include the multidimensional experiences and challenges of pregnant women who migrate and the influences on their health.

(9) Finally, the current lack of existing clinical practice guidelines cannot continue. Official provisions need to be made by healthcare providers and clinical practice guidelines need to be produced for the care of migrant women during the maternity period, similar to that produced for indigenous populations [100].

Disclosure

The views expressed in this paper are those of the authors only.

Competing Interests

The authors declare no known competing interests.

Authors' Contributions

Nazilla Khanlou was the PI for the scoping review. Andrea Skinner was responsible for conducting the initial literature search, reviewing the article titles, and building the database. Nasim Haque and Andrea Skinner reviewed the abstracts. Nasim Haque, Andrea Skinner, Anne Mantini, and Nazilla Khanlou reviewed the text documents and wrote the various sections of the paper. And Nazilla Khanlou, Nasim Haque, and Anne Mantini finalized the paper. Christine Kurtz Landy read various versions of the paper and provided input.

Acknowledgments

This scoping review was funded by the Ontario Ministry of Health and Long Term Care (MOHLTC) (2013-2014) as part of the Immigrant and Racialized Women's Health Project and Nazilla Khanlou's Start-Up Funding at the Faculty of Health, York University. Nazilla Khanlou holds a Chair in Women's Health Research in Mental Health with funding from MOHLTC. Andrea Skinner held a Graduate Assistantship funded by York University under Nazilla Khanlou's supervision.

References

[1] Statistics Canada, "Immigration and ethnocultural diversity in Canada," in *National Household Survey*, Statistics Canada, Ontario, Canada, 2011.

[2] Facts and figures 2013—Immigration Overview, http://www.cic.gc.ca/english/resources/statistics/facts2013/permanent/.

[3] United Nations Population Fund: State of World Population 2006, *A Passage to Hope: Women and International Migration*, UNFPA, New York, NY, USA, 2006.

[4] S. Kita, M. Minatani, N. Hikita, M. Matsuzaki, M. Shiraishi, and M. Haruna, "A systematic review of the physical, mental, social, and economic problems of immigrant women in the perinatal period in Japan," *Journal of Immigrant and Minority Health*, vol. 17, no. 6, pp. 1863–1881, 2015.

[5] Maternal Health, http://www.who.int/topics/maternal_health/en/.

[6] M. Waterstone, S. Bewley, and C. Wolfe, "Incidence and predictors of severe obstetric morbidity: case-control study," *British Medical Journal*, vol. 322, no. 7294, pp. 1089–1093, 2001.

[7] K. Pottie, C. Greenaway, J. Feightner et al., "Evidence-based clinical guidelines for immigrants and refugees," *Canadian Medical Association Journal*, vol. 183, no. 12, pp. E824–E925, 2011.

[8] H. Arksey and L. O'Malley, "Scoping studies: towards a methodological framework," *International Journal of Social Research Methodology*, vol. 8, no. 1, pp. 19–32, 2005.

[9] S. E. Brien, D. L. Lorenzetti, S. Lewis, J. Kennedy, and W. A. Ghali, "Overview of a formal scoping review on health system report cards," *Implementation Science*, vol. 5, no. 1, article no. 2, 2010.

[10] L. Hooker, B. Ward, and G. Verrinder, "Domestic violence screening in maternal and child health nursing practice: a scoping review," *Contemporary Nurse*, vol. 42, no. 2, pp. 198–215, 2012.

[11] M. J. Grant and A. Booth, "A typology of reviews: an analysis of 14 review types and associated methodologies," *Health Information and Libraries Journal*, vol. 26, no. 2, pp. 91–108, 2009.

[12] H. M. L. Daudt, C. Van Mossel, and S. J. Scott, "Enhancing the scoping study methodology: a large, inter-professional team's experience with Arksey and O'Malley's framework," *BMC Medical Research Methodology*, vol. 13, article 48, pp. 1–9, 2013.

[13] S. E. Brien, D. L. Lorenzetti, S. Lewis, J. Kennedy, and W. A. Ghali, "Overview of a formal scoping review on health system report cards," *Implementation Science*, vol. 5, no. 1, article 2, 2010.

[14] Canadian Council of Refugees, *Refugees and Immigrants: A Glossary*, The Canadian Council of Refugees, Montreal, Canada, 2010, http://ccrweb.ca/en/glossary.

[15] Thomson Reuters: Endnote, *Thomson Scientific Releases EndNote X1 for Windows*, Microsoft Corporation, San Francisco, Calif, USA, 2012.

[16] N. Khanlou, N. Haque, and A. Skinner, "Maternal health of immigrants in Canada: a scoping review," in *Proceedings of the Immigrant and Racialized Women's Health Project Conference*, Ryerson University, Toronto, Canada, 2014.

[17] C. Jarvis, M. Munoz, L. Graves, R. Stephenson, V. D'Souza, and V. Jimenez, "Retrospective review of prenatal care and perinatal outcomes in a group of uninsured pregnant women," *Journal of Obstetrics and Gynaecology Canada*, vol. 33, no. 3, pp. 235–243, 2011.

[18] Z. Mumtaz, B. O'Brien, and G. Higginbottom, "Navigating maternity health care: a survey of the Canadian prairie newcomer experience," *BMC Pregnancy and Childbirth*, vol. 14, no. 1, article no. 4, 2014.

[19] G. M. Higginbottom, J. Safipour, S. Yohani et al., "An ethnographic investigation of the maternity healthcare experience of immigrants in rural and urban Alberta, Canada," *BMC Pregnancy and Childbirth*, vol. 16, article 20, 2016.

[20] M. Miszkurka, M. V. Zunzunegui, and L. Goulet, "Immigrant status, antenatal depressive symptoms, and frequency and source of violence: what's the relationship?" *Archives of Women's Mental Health*, vol. 15, no. 5, pp. 387–396, 2012.

[21] M. Ruiz-Casares, C. Rousseau, A. Laurin-Lamothe et al., "Access to health care for undocumented migrant children and pregnant women: the paradox between values and attitudes of health care professionals," *Maternal and Child Health Journal*, vol. 17, no. 2, pp. 292–298, 2013.

[22] M. L. Urquia, J. W. Frank, R. H. Glazier, R. Moineddin, F. I. Matheson, and A. J. Gagnon, "Neighborhood context and infant birthweight among recent immigrant mothers: a multilevel analysis," *American Journal of Public Health*, vol. 99, no. 2, pp. 285–293, 2009.

[23] N. Auger, J. Giraud, and M. Daniel, "The joint influence of area income, income inequality, and immigrant density on adverse birth outcomes: a population-based study," *BMC Public Health*, vol. 9, article no. 237, 2009.

[24] T. Moffat, D. Sellen, W. Wilson, L. Anderson, S. Chadwick, and S. Amarra, "Comparison of infant vitamin D supplement

use among canadian-born, immigrant, and refugee mothers," *Journal of Transcultural Nursing*, vol. 26, no. 3, pp. 261–269, 2015.

[25] J. G. Ray, M. J. Vermeulen, M. J. Schull, G. Singh, R. Shah, and D. A. Redelmeier, "Results of the recent immigrant pregnancy and perinatal long-term evaluation study (RIPPLES)," *CMAJ*, vol. 176, no. 10, pp. 1419–1426, 2007.

[26] M. Stewart, C. L. Dennis, M. Kariwo et al., "Challenges faced by refugee new parents from Africa in Canada," *Journal of Immigrant and Minority Health*, vol. 17, no. 4, pp. 1146–1156, 2015.

[27] M. Quintanilha, M. J. Mayan, J. Thompson, and R. C. Bell, "Contrasting "back home" and "here": How Northeast African migrant women perceive and experience health during pregnancy and postpartum in Canada," *International Journal for Equity in Health*, vol. 15, no. 1, article 80, 2016.

[28] N. Daoud, M. L. Urquia, P. O'Campo et al., "Prevalence of abuse and violence before, during, and after pregnancy in a national sample of Canadian women," *American Journal of Public Health*, vol. 102, no. 10, pp. 1893–1901, 2012.

[29] D. E. Stewart, A. J. Gagnon, L. A. Merry, and C.-L. Dennis, "Risk factors and health profiles of recent migrant women who experienced violence associated with pregnancy," *Journal of Women's Health*, vol. 21, no. 10, pp. 1100–1106, 2012.

[30] M. Miszkurka, L. Goulet, and M. V. Zunzunegui, "Contributions of immigration to depressive symptoms among pregnant women in Canada," *Canadian Journal of Public Health*, vol. 101, no. 5, pp. 358–364, 2010.

[31] M. Peer, C. N. Soares, R. D. Levitan, D. L. Streiner, and M. Steiner, "Antenatal depression in a multi-ethnic, community sample of Canadian immigrants: psychosocial correlates and hypothalamic-pituitary-adrenal axis function," *Canadian Journal of Psychiatry*, vol. 58, no. 10, pp. 579–587, 2013.

[32] D. Kingston, M. Heaman, B. Chalmers et al., "Comparison of maternity experiences of canadian-born and recent and non-recent immigrant women: findings from the canadian maternity experiences survey," *Journal of Obstetrics and Gynaecology Canada*, vol. 33, no. 11, pp. 1105–1115, 2011.

[33] P. Zelkowitz, J. Schinazi, L. Katofsky et al., "Factors associated with depression in pregnant immigrant women," *Transcultural Psychiatry*, vol. 41, no. 4, pp. 445–464, 2004.

[34] M. L. Urquia, I. Ying, R. H. Glazier, H. Berger, L. R. De Souza, and J. G. Ray, "Serious preeclampsia among different immigrant groups," *Journal of Obstetrics and Gynaecology Canada*, vol. 34, no. 4, pp. 348–352, 2012.

[35] N. Muhajarine, J. Ng, A. Bowen, J. Cushon, and S. Johnson, "Understanding the impact of the Canada prenatal nutrition program: a quantitative evaluation," *Canadian Journal of Public Health*, vol. 103, no. 7, supplement 1, pp. eS26–eS31, 2012.

[36] A. J. Gagnon, A. Van Hulst, L. Merry et al., "Cesarean section rate differences by migration indicators," *Archives of Gynecology and Obstetrics*, vol. 287, no. 4, pp. 633–639, 2013.

[37] T. Boshari, M. L. Urquia, M. Sgro, L. R. De Souza, and J. G. Ray, "Differences in birthweight curves between newborns of immigrant mothers vs. infants born in their corresponding native countries: systematic overview," *Paediatric and Perinatal Epidemiology*, vol. 27, no. 2, pp. 118–130, 2013.

[38] K. Wilson-Mitchel and J. A. Rummens, "Perinatal outcomes of uninsured immigrant, refugee and migrant mothers and newborns living in Toronto, Canada," *International Journal of Environmental Research and Public Health*, vol. 10, no. 6, pp. 2198–2213, 2013.

[39] A. C. Brathwaite and C. C. Williams, "Childbirth experiences of professional Chinese Canadian women," *Journal of Obstetric, Gynecologic, and Neonatal Nursing*, vol. 33, no. 6, pp. 748–755, 2004.

[40] I. Hyman and G. Dussault, "Negative consequences of acculturation on health behaviour, social support and stress among pregnant Southeast Asian immigrant women in Montreal: an exploratory study," *Canadian Journal of Public Health*, vol. 91, no. 5, pp. 357–360, 2000.

[41] L. Mamisachvili, P. Ardiles, G. Mancewicz, S. Thompson, K. Rabin, and L. E. Ross, "Culture and postpartum mood problems: similarities and differences in the experiences of first- and second-generation canadian women," *Journal of Transcultural Nursing*, vol. 24, no. 2, pp. 162–170, 2013.

[42] Y. Debessai, C. Costanian, M. Roy, M. El-Sayed, and H. Tamim, "Inadequate prenatal care use among Canadian mothers: findings from the maternity experiences survey," *Journal of Perinatology*, vol. 36, no. 6, pp. 420–426, 2016.

[43] P. Caulford and Y. Vali, "Providing health care to medically uninsured immigrants and refugees," *CMAJ*, vol. 174, no. 9, pp. 1253–1254, 2006.

[44] K. Munro, C. Jarvis, M. Munoz, V. D'Souza, and L. Graves, "Undocumented pregnant women: what does the literature tell us?" *Journal of Immigrant and Minority Health*, vol. 15, no. 2, pp. 281–291, 2013.

[45] L. Redwood-Campbell, H. Thind, M. Howard, J. Koteles, N. Fowler, and J. Kaczorowski, "Understanding the health of refugee women in host countries: lessons from the kosovar resettlement in Canada," *Prehospital and Disaster Medicine*, vol. 23, no. 4, pp. 322–327, 2008.

[46] C. Ng and K. B. Newbold, "Health care providers' perspectives on the provision of prenatal care to immigrants," *Culture, Health and Sexuality*, vol. 13, no. 5, pp. 561–574, 2011.

[47] S. Brar, S. Tang, N. Drummond et al., "Perinatal care for South Asian immigrant women and women born in Canada: telephone survey of users," *Journal of Obstetrics and Gynaecology Canada*, vol. 31, no. 8, pp. 708–716, 2009.

[48] A. Ling, "Accessing appropriate health care services for immigrant women in Canada," *International Journal of Childbirth Education*, vol. 15, no. 4, p. 34, 2000.

[49] M. L. Urquia, R. H. Glazier, L. Mortensen et al., "Severe maternal morbidity associated with maternal birthplace in three high-immigration settings," *The European Journal of Public Health*, vol. 25, no. 4, pp. 620–625, 2015.

[50] R. Bhagat, J. Johnson, S. Grewal, P. Pandher, E. Quong, and K. Triolet, "Mobilizing the community to address the prenatal health needs of immigrant punjabi women," *Public Health Nursing*, vol. 19, no. 3, pp. 209–214, 2002.

[51] Y. Lu and L. Racine, "Reviewing Chinese immigrant women's health experiences in English-speaking Western countries: a postcolonial feminist analysis," *Health Sociology Review*, vol. 24, no. 1, pp. 15–28, 2015.

[52] B. Al-Sahab, M. Saqib, G. Hauser, and H. Tamim, "Prevalence of smoking during pregnancy and associated risk factors among Canadian women: a national survey," *BMC Pregnancy and Childbirth*, vol. 10, article no. 24, 2010.

[53] C. Kowal, J. Kuk, and H. Tamim, "Characteristics of weight gain in pregnancy among canadian women," *Maternal & Child Health Journal*, vol. 16, no. 3, pp. 668–676, 2012.

[54] Health Canada, "Health Care System," http://www.hc-sc.gc.ca/hcs-sss/index-eng.php.

[55] M. da Conceicao and M. H. Figueiredo, "Immigrant women's perspective on prenatal and postpartum care: systematic review," *Journal of Immigrant and Minority Health*, vol. 17, no. 1, pp. 276–284, 2015.

[56] P. A. Janssen, A. D. Henderson, and K. L. MacKay, "Family violence and maternal mortality in the south asian community: the role of obstetrical care providers," *Journal of Obstetrics and Gynaecology Canada*, vol. 31, no. 11, pp. 1045–1049, 2009.

[57] D. Kingston, M. Heaman, M. Urquia et al., "Correlates of abuse around the time of pregnancy: results from a national survey of Canadian women," *Maternal and Child Health Journal*, vol. 20, no. 4, pp. 778–789, 2016.

[58] R. McElroy, M. Laskin, D. Jiang, R. Shah, and J. G. Ray, "Rates of rubella immunity among immigrant and non-immigrant pregnant women," *Journal of Obstetrics and Gynaecology Canada*, vol. 31, no. 5, pp. 409–413, 2009.

[59] T.-Y. Lee, C. K. Landy, O. Wahoush, N. Khanlou, Y.-C. Liu, and C.-C. Li, "A descriptive phenomenology study of newcomers' experience of maternity care services: Chinese women's perspectives," *BMC Health Services Research*, vol. 14, article 114, 2014.

[60] M. I. Heaman, C. G. Green, C. V. Newburn-Cook, L. J. Elliott, and M. E. Helewa, "Social inequalities in use of prenatal care in manitoba," *Journal of Obstetrics and Gynaecology Canada*, vol. 29, no. 10, pp. 806–816, 2007.

[61] K. Munro, C. Jarvis, L. Y. Kong, V. D'Souza, and L. Graves, "Perspectives of family physicians on the care of uninsured pregnant women," *Journal of Obstetrics and Gynaecology Canada*, vol. 35, no. 7, pp. 599–605, 2013.

[62] M. I. Heaman, M. Moffatt, L. Elliott et al., "Barriers, motivators and facilitators related to prenatal care utilization among inner-city women in Winnipeg, Canada: a case-control study," *BMC Pregnancy and Childbirth*, vol. 14, no. 1, article no. 227, 2014.

[63] M. L. Urquia, P. J. O'Campo, and M. I. Heaman, "Revisiting the immigrant paradox in reproductive health: the roles of duration of residence and ethnicity," *Social Science & Medicine*, vol. 74, no. 10, pp. 1610–1621, 2012.

[64] S. Wanigaratne, D. C. Cole, K. Bassil, I. Hyman, R. Moineddin, and M. L. Urquia, "Contribution of HIV to maternal morbidity among refugee women in Canada," *American Journal of Public Health*, vol. 105, no. 12, pp. 2449–2456, 2015.

[65] R. R. Shah, J. G. Ray, N. Taback, F. Meffe, and R. H. Glazier, "Adverse pregnancy outcomes among foreign-born Canadians," *Journal of Obstetrics and Gynaecology Canada*, vol. 33, no. 3, pp. 207–215, 2011.

[66] A. J. Gagnon, L. Merry, and K. Haase, "Predictors of emergency cesarean delivery among international migrant women in Canada," *International Journal of Gynecology and Obstetrics*, vol. 121, no. 3, pp. 270–274, 2013.

[67] L. Merry, R. Small, B. Blondel, and A. J. Gagnon, "International migration and caesarean birth: a systematic review and meta-analysis," *BMC Pregnancy and Childbirth*, vol. 13, article no. 27, 2013.

[68] A. L. Park, M. L. Urquia, and J. G. Ray, "Risk of Preterm Birth According to Maternal and Paternal Country of Birth: A Population-Based Study," *Journal of Obstetrics and Gynaecology Canada*, vol. 37, no. 12, pp. 1053–1062, 2015.

[69] A. J. Gagnon, M. Zimbeck, and J. Zeitlin, "Migration to western industrialised countries and perinatal health: a systematic review," *Social Science & Medicine*, vol. 69, no. 6, pp. 934–946, 2009.

[70] N. Auger, M. Chery, and M. Daniel, "Rising disparities in severe adverse birth outcomes among Haitians in Québec, Canada, 1981–2006," *Journal of Immigrant & Minority Health*, vol. 14, no. 2, pp. 198–208, 2012.

[71] M. Heaman, D. Kingston, B. Chalmers, R. Sauve, L. Lee, and D. Young, "Risk factors for preterm birth and small-for-gestational-age births among canadian women," *Paediatric and Perinatal Epidemiology*, vol. 27, no. 1, pp. 54–61, 2013.

[72] M. L. Urquia, J. W. Frank, R. H. Glazier, and R. Moineddin, "Birth outcomes by neighbourhood income and recent immigration in Toronto," *Health Reports*, vol. 18, no. 4, pp. 21–30, 2007.

[73] M. L. Urquia, J. W. Frank, R. Moineddin, and R. H. Glazier, "Immigrants' duration of residence and adverse birth outcomes: a population-based study," *BJOG: An International Journal of Obstetrics and Gynaecology*, vol. 117, no. 5, pp. 591–601, 2010.

[74] N. Auger, Z.-C. Luo, R. W. Platt, and M. Daniel, "Do mother's education and foreign born status interact to influence birth outcomes? Clarifying the epidemiological paradox and the healthy migrant effect," *Journal of Epidemiology and Community Health*, vol. 62, no. 5, pp. 402–409, 2008.

[75] N. Auger, M. Abrahamowicz, A. L. Park, and W. Wynant, "Extreme maternal education and preterm birth: time-to-event analysis of age and nativity-dependent risks," *Annals of Epidemiology*, vol. 23, no. 1, pp. 1–6, 2013.

[76] A. Battaglini, S. Gravel, C. Poulin, J. M. Brodeur, D. Du-rand, and S. DeBlois, "Immigration and perinatal risk," *Centres of Excellent for Women's Health Research Bulletin*, vol. 2, no. 2, pp. 8–9, 2001.

[77] L. R. de Souza, M. L. Urquia, M. Sgro, and J. G. Ray, "One size does not fit all: differences in newborn weight among mothers of philippine and other East asian origin," *Journal of Obstetrics and Gynaecology Canada*, vol. 34, no. 11, pp. 1026–1037, 2012.

[78] W. J. Kierans, K. S. Joseph, Z.-C. Luo, R. Platt, R. Wilkins, and M. S. Kramer, "Does one size fit all? The case for ethnic-specific standards of fetal growth," *BMC Pregnancy and Childbirth*, vol. 8, article 1, 2008.

[79] N. L. Ramuscak, D. Jiang, K. L. Dooling, and D. L. Mowat, "A population-level analysis of birth weight indices in Peel Region, Ontario: the impact of ethnic diversity," *Canadian Journal of Public Health*, vol. 103, no. 5, pp. 368–372, 2012.

[80] J. G. Ray, D. A. Henry, and M. L. Urquia, "Sex ratios among Canadian liveborn infants of mothers from different countries," *Canadian Medical Association Journal*, vol. 184, no. 9, pp. E492–E496, 2012.

[81] G. M. A. Higginbottom, J. Safipour, Z. Mumtaz, Y. Chiu, P. Paton, and J. Pillay, "'I have to do what I believe': sudanese women's beliefs and resistance to hegemonic practices at home and during experiences of maternity care in Canada," *BMC Pregnancy and Childbirth*, vol. 13, article 51, 2013.

[82] M. L. Urquia, H. Berger, and J. G. Ray, "Risk of adverse outcomes among infants of immigrant women according to birth-weight curves tailored to maternal world region of origin," *Canadian Medical Association Journal*, vol. 187, no. 1, pp. E32–E40, 2015.

[83] A. R. Zipursky, A. L. Park, M. L. Urquia, M. I. Creatore, and J. G. Ray, "Influence of paternal and maternal ethnicity and ethnic enclaves on newborn weight," *Journal of Epidemiology and Community Health*, vol. 68, no. 10, pp. 942–949, 2014.

[84] J. G. Ray, M. Sgro, M. M. Mamdani et al., "Birth weight curves tailored to maternal world region," *Journal of Obstetrics and Gynaecology Canada*, vol. 34, no. 2, pp. 159–171, 2012.

[85] N. Daoud, P. O'Campo, M. L. Urquia, and M. Heaman, "Neighbourhood context and abuse among immigrant and non-immigrant women in Canada: findings from the Maternity Experiences Survey," *International Journal of Public Health*, vol. 57, no. 4, pp. 679–689, 2012.

[86] B. Chalmers and K. O. Hashi, "432 Somali women's birth experiences in Canada after earlier female genital mutilation," *Birth*, vol. 27, no. 4, pp. 227–234, 2000.

[87] G. M. A. Higginbottom, E. Hadziabdic, S. Yohani, and P. Paton, "Immigrant women's experience of maternity services in Canada: a meta-ethnography," *Midwifery*, vol. 30, no. 5, pp. 544–559, 2014.

[88] S. Reitmanova and D. L. Gustafson, ""They can't understand it": maternity health and care needs of immigrant Muslim women in St. John's, Newfoundland," *Maternal and Child Health Journal*, vol. 12, no. 1, pp. 101–111, 2008.

[89] D. L. Spitzer, "In visible bodies: minority women, nurses, time, and the new economy of care," *Medical Anthropology Quarterly*, vol. 18, no. 4, pp. 490–508, 2004.

[90] S. K. Grewal, R. Bhagat, and L. G. Balneaves, "Perinatal beliefs and practices of immigrant Punjabi women living in Canada," *Journal of Obstetric, Gynecologic, and Neonatal Nursing*, vol. 37, no. 3, pp. 290–300, 2008.

[91] M. Miszkurka, L. Goulet, and M. V. Zunzunegui, "Antenatal depressive symptoms among Canadian-born and immigrant women in Quebec: differential exposure and vulnerability to contextual risk factors," *Social Psychiatry and Psychiatric Epidemiology*, vol. 47, no. 10, pp. 1639–1648, 2012.

[92] J. M. O'Mahony, T. T. Donnelly, S. Raffin Bouchal, and D. Este, "Cultural background and socioeconomic influence of immigrant and refugee women coping with postpartum depression," *Journal of Immigrant and Minority Health*, vol. 15, no. 2, pp. 300–314, 2013.

[93] J. M. O'Mahony and T. T. Donnelly, "How does gender influence immigrant and refugee women's postpartum depression help-seeking experiences?" *Journal of Psychiatric and Mental Health Nursing*, vol. 20, no. 8, pp. 714–725, 2013.

[94] C.-L. Dennis, A. Gagnon, A. Van Hulst, and G. Dougherty, "Predictors of breastfeeding exclusivity among migrant and Canadian-born women: results from a multi-centre study," *Maternal & Child Nutrition*, vol. 10, no. 4, pp. 527–544, 2014.

[95] R. Ganann, W. Sword, L. Thabane, B. Newbold, and M. Black, "Predictors of postpartum depression among immigrant women in the year after childbirth," *Journal of Women's Health*, vol. 25, no. 2, pp. 155–165, 2016.

[96] A. J. Gagnon, F. Carnevale, P. Mehta, H. Rousseau, and D. E. Stewart, "Developing population interventions with migrant women for maternal-child health: a focused ethnography," *BMC Public Health*, vol. 13, no. 1, article no. 471, 2013.

[97] G. M. A. Higginbottom, M. Morgan, J. O'Mahony et al., "Immigrant women's experiences of postpartum depression in Canada: a protocol for systematic review using a narrative synthesis," *Systematic Reviews*, vol. 2, article 65, 2013.

[98] Public Health Agency of Canada, "The Social determinants of health: an overview implications for policy and the role of the health sector," 2004, http://www.phac-aspc.gc.ca/ph-sp/determinants/index-eng.php.

[99] G. M. A. Higginbottom, M. Morgan, J. Dassanayake et al., "Immigrant women's experiences of maternity-care services in Canada: a protocol for systematic review using a narrative synthesis," *Systematic Reviews*, vol. 1, pp. 27–39, 2010.

[100] D. Wilson, S. de la Ronde, S. Brascoupé et al., "Health professionals working with First Nations, Inuit, and Métis consensus guideline," *Journal of Obstetrics and Gynaecology Canada*, vol. 35, no. 6, pp. 550–553, 2013.

[101] Government-Assisted Refugee Program, http://www.cic.gc.ca/english/refugees/outside/resettle-gov.asp.

[102] The refugee system in Canada, http://www.cic.gc.ca/english/refugees/canada.asp.

[103] R. Small, C. Roth, M. Raval et al., "Immigrant and non-immigrant women's experiences of maternity care: a systematic and comparative review of studies in five countries," *BMC Pregnancy and Childbirth*, vol. 14, no. 1, article 152, 2014.

[104] A. J. Gagnon, M. Zimbeck, and J. Zeitlin, "Migration to western industrialised countries and perinatal health: a systematic review," *Social Science and Medicine*, vol. 69, no. 6, pp. 934–946, 2009.

[105] M. C. Machado, A. Fernandes, B. Padilla et al., "Maternal and child healthcare for immigrant populations," Background Paper. Edited by: Maria Jose Peiro and Roumyana Benedict, International Organization for Migration (IOM), Geneva, Switzerland, 2009 http://www.migrant-health-europe.org/files/Maternal%20and%20Child%20Care_Background%20Paper%281%29.pdf.

[106] S. Atwal, "The Mandated 3-Month Wait for OHIP Coverage," Canadian Lawyers for International Human Rights (CLAIHR), http://claihr.ca/2016/02/09/the-mandated-3-month-wait-for-ohip-coverage/.

[107] S. Thomson and R. Osborn, *International Profiles of Health Care Systems*, The Commonwealth Fund, London, UK, 2015.

Patient Preferences and Experiences in Hyperemesis Gravidarum Treatment: A Qualitative Study

Relin van Vliet ⓘ,[1] Marieke Bink,[2] Julian Polman,[1] Amaran Suntharan,[1] Iris Grooten,[3] Sandra E. Zwolsman,[4] Tessa J. Roseboom,[5] and Rebecca C. Painter ⓘ[4]

[1] University Medical Centers Amsterdam, University of Amsterdam, Amsterdam, Netherlands

[2] Department of Gynaecology and Obstetrics, Noordwest Ziekenhuisgroep, Alkmaar, Netherlands

[3] Department of Obstetrics and Gynaecology, University Medical Centers Amsterdam, Amsterdam, Netherlands

[4] Department of Obstetrics and Gynaecology, University Medical Centers Amsterdam, University of Amsterdam, Amsterdam, Netherlands

[5] Departments of Obstetrics and Gynaecology, Public Health & Epidemiology, University Medical Centers Amsterdam, University of Amsterdam, Amsterdam, Netherlands

Correspondence should be addressed to Rebecca C. Painter; r.c.painter@amc.uva.nl

Academic Editor: Jacques Balayla

Introduction. Hyperemesis gravidarum (HG) medical therapies are currently of limited effect, which creates a larger role for patient preferences in the way HG care is arranged. This is the first study using in-depth interviews to investigate patients' preferences and experiences of HG treatment. *Materials and Methods.* We conducted individual in-depth interviews among women who had been hospitalized for HG in North Holland at least once in the past 4 years. We asked them about their experiences, preferences, and suggestions for improvement regarding the HG treatment they received. The sample size was determined by reaching data saturation. Themes were identified from analysis of the interview transcripts. *Results and Discussion.* 13 women were interviewed. Interviewees emphasized the importance of early recognition of the severity of HG, increasing caregivers' knowledge on HG, early medical intervention, and nasogastric tube feeding. They valued a single room in hospital, discussion of treatment options, more possibilities of home-treatment, psychological support during HG and after childbirth, and more uniform information and policies regarding HG treatment. *Conclusion.* Further research is needed to establish whether the suggestions can lead to more (cost) effective care and improve the course of HG and outcomes for HG patients and their children.

1. Introduction

Nausea and vomiting of pregnancy (NVP) are common during the first trimester of pregnancy, affecting 50 to 80% of pregnant women. A much smaller proportion (0.3-3%) of pregnant women encounter intractable vomiting, which may be complicated by dehydration, significant weight loss, and electrolyte disturbances necessitating hospital admission [1]. This condition is called hyperemesis gravidarum (HG). HG has a major effect on patients' quality of life and is associated with adverse perinatal outcomes, including low birth weight, small for gestational age, and prematurity [2] .

Despite the recent introduction of national HG guidelines in the UK [3], Canada [4], and USA [5], such guidance is lacking in many countries and there is considerable variation in treatment between the different hospitals in Netherlands.

Antiemetic and other HG therapies are of limited effect, which creates a larger role for patient preferences in the way HG care is arranged [6]. Few qualitative studies and patient satisfaction surveys concerning HG have been carried out. In 2000, Munch [7] found that HG patients considered the perception of being believed and taken seriously as important qualities of doctors. Power et al. [8] found that HG patients felt unpopular with caregivers. Caregivers indicated having doubts about the severity of the symptoms and the necessity for hospital admission. Taken together, the existing literature leaves health care professionals largely uninformed about what HG patients themselves would consider to constitute good HG care.

The aim of our study was to describe women's experiences and preferences of HG care. Which aspects of care did they find helpful and led to recovery? Which areas of care need improvement? What were their main concerns and needs during and after their HG episode? The findings of our study will contribute to the improvement of HG treatment as they could be used as a basis for innovation and relocation of care in such way that it better meets the needs and preferences of women with HG. Finally, the input of patients can guide the HG research agenda.

2. Materials and Methods

2.1. Samples Selection and Recruitment of Participants. We recruited participants by posting an invitation on Facebook and home page of ZEHG, the Dutch HG patient foundation (see supplementary information 1 for the original Dutch invitation with English translation below). Patients who were interested in participating were invited to contact the researchers by e-mail. Participants were eligible for inclusion if they had been admitted to hospital for HG treatment at least once in the past 4 years in the province of North Holland. The sample size was determined by the point at which data saturation was reached. Data saturation occurs when new interviews do not provide any new data.

Verbal consent to use the voice recorder was requested at the start of the interview. All participants gave written consent for recording and using the interview as material for medical scientific research. The Medical Ethics Committee (MEC) of the Academic Medical Center decided that this study was not subject to the Medical Research Involving Human Subjects Act (WMO).

2.2. Data Collection. We collected data by using open and extended querying during in-depth interviews in order to provide sufficient space for asking supplementary questions. The interview started with the question "What were your experiences with the treatment you received for HG?". When the answer to this question was too brief, supplementary questions were asked based on the topic list (see supplementary information 2). The topic list was updated continuously with the frequently named and emphasized topics from previous interviews.

During the interviews, baseline data of the women interviewed regarding their hyperemesis gravidarum experiences were obtained (see Table 1). All participants had been admitted to hospital for HG treatment in the past 4 years (inclusion criteria). We did not collect data on the time (years and months) between the interview and the HG pregnancy.

Two investigators (MB and RV) coconducted the 13 interviews, which lasted on average 40 minutes each. To minimize variation between interviews, one investigator (MB) always acted as interviewer. The second investigator functioned as observer (RV). The interviewer (MB) is an experienced midwife. The observer made a summary for the subject review and checked by using the topic list whether all topics had been addressed. Participants were given the choice of being interviewed at their homes or at the hospital.

In order to check the accuracy of the findings, member checking and subject review were performed. We carried out subject review by providing the patient with a summary of the interview in order to check the information for accuracy and correctness of interpretation [9].

2.3. Data Safety and Anonymity. The interviews were recorded using a recording device. With the help of two other investigators (AS and JP), the records were transcribed and transferred to a hard disk and deleted from the carrier. We ensured participant anonymity by removing the personal details from the records and transcripts. All data (interview records, transcripts, and participant's data) were labeled with numbers following the timeline of the interviews.

2.4. Data Analysis. All interviews were fully transcribed and coded using the three different types of coding methods of Strauss and Corbin, as described by Boeije (2008) [10]. Using open, axial, and selective coding, the most relevant and most frequently arising topics (themes) were determined and ordered. These are described in Results. The coding was done by a researcher (the observer) and checked by a second one (the interviewer). Discrepancies in the codes were resolved by discussion.

Data analysis was facilitated by MAXQDA qualitative data analysis software version 12 (VERBI Software (2016), Berlin, Germany).

3. Results

13 women were interviewed. Baseline characteristics of the women interviewed regarding their hyperemesis gravidarum experiences are shown in Table 1. The themes of the interviews were the attitude of caregivers towards the patient, medical treatment, psychological support, aftercare, and the information provided.

3.1. Theme 1: Caregivers' Attitudes. All participants stressed the importance of understanding and recognition of the disease in HG treatment. Many reported that they had not been taken seriously by caregivers, and their problems were being trivialized.

> *"I couldn't even keep a mouthful of water down. If a GP then still says: 'most pregnant women feel sick, with nausea and vomiting'. I thought: 'yes, 3 times in the morning or 30 times, the whole day long vomiting, and not being able to leave the toilet, because you can't even get on your feet any more, I think that's quite different'."*

> *- participant 9*

Also, participants perceived that caregivers thought it was their own choice not to eat and felt pressured by them.

> *"In hospital they said 'you have to eat', 'you have to get that food inside you', 'here, this is what you*

TABLE 1: Baseline data of the women interviewed regarding their hyperemesis gravidarum experiences.

	Age	G+P	Treatment	Psychological support during HG	After-care	Involved health givers
1	30	G4P0	Meclozine, Metoclopramide, rehydration, nasogastric tube feeding, total parenteral nutrition	Med. SW	EMDR	GP, psychiatrist, neurologist, gynaecologist, midwife, dietician, Med. SW, psychologist
2	27	G1P0	Meclozine, Metoclopramide, rehydration		EMDR	GP, gynaecologist midwife psychologist
3	28	G1P0	Meclozine, Metoclopramide Ondansetron, rehydration, nasogastric tube feeding		Meetings with a psychologist	GP, midwife, gynaecologist psychologist
4	27	G1P0	Metoclopramide, Nutridrink, rehydration, nasogastric tube feeding	Med. SW, meeting with a psychologist	Meetings with a psychologist	GP, midwife, gynaecologist, Med. SW psychologist
5	21	G1P0	Medication unknown, rehydration	Med. SW	Meetings with a psychologist	GP, gynaecologist psychologist
6	30	G1P0	Meclozine, rehydration nasogastric tube feeding	Med. SW		GP, midwife gynaecologist Med. SW dietician
7	19	G3P0	Meclozine, Metoclopramide, rehydration	Meetings with a psychologist	EMDR in future	GP, gynaecologist psychologist
8	28	G1P0	Meclozine, Nutridrink, rehydration	Meetings with a psychologist	EMDR	GP, midwife, gynaecologist psychologist
9	30	G2P1	Meclozine, Metoclopramide, Ondansetron, rehydration nasogastric tube feeding	Med. SW	EMDR, dietician	GP, midwife gynaecologist, Med. SW, psychologist, dietician
10	30	G3P2	Meclozine, Metoclopramide, rehydration, nasogastric tube feeding		Meetings with a nurse practitioner and Internist	GP, midwife gynaecologist, nurse practitioner
11	33	G2P1	Meclozine, Metoclopramide, Haldol, Ondansetron, rehydration, nasogastric tube feeding	Meetings with a psychiatrist		Midwife, gynaecologist, psychiatrist
12	27	G2P0	Meclozine, Nutridrink, rehydration			GP, midwife gynaecologist dietician
13	31	G2P1	Meclozine, Ondansetron, rehydration	Med. SW, meetings with a psychologist		GP, midwife gynaecologist, Med. SW, psychologist

G: gravidity, P: parity, Med. SW: medical social work, EMDR: eye movement desensitization and reprocessing, GP: general practitioner.

get, and you have to eat it'." But if I can't eat it because I immediately need to throw up, then I really can't eat it. If I take two bites, three come out. It's easier said than done. It isn't easy to deal with being pressured like that."

I: How could they have done better?

R: Maybe by being kinder, like 'try to eat, but if it doesn't work, it's no problem.' There was so much pressure."

- participant 3

According to the participants, more knowledge on HG among caregivers would have contributed to more understanding and knowledge of the disease and early recognition of the symptoms.

"The lack of knowledge on HG surprised me. Among professionals too, they think it's all over after 12 weeks."

- participant 10

3.2. Theme 2: Medical Treatment

3.2.1. Early Medical Intervention. All participants underlined the importance of early medical intervention. They encountered that their calls for help were not taken seriously. They wanted the caregivers to explore the severity of the disease by thorough questioning and paying a home visit, because they experienced difficulties with visiting a GP or midwife.

"At one point I called and said 'I can't manage any more, I can't even walk to the toilet without fainting'. They said 'alright, then I want you to come to our practice'. So I said 'how will I get there?' (. . .) Driving by car with HG is a nightmare. I was vomiting all the way to the practice, and in the waiting room too, with people all around me."

- participant 9

In addition, some participants had trouble with being assertive due to their sickness and weakness.

"I was very apathetic, very strange, but normally I'm quite assertive, at least I can explain what I feel very well, but not then, not at all."

- participant 2

Often treatment only starts after dehydration sets in. Interviewees reported that they would have preferred a more prevention-focused treatment, for example, by starting earlier with (other) medication and/or nasogastric tube feeding (see also next paragraph). According to them, early treatment could avoid dehydration, further weight loss, and multiple hospital admissions.

"But if I wasn't dehydrated, they sent me home, although I knew I would be back within a few days, because it wasn't a solution. (. . .) They let me go for so long, that I lost so much weight and was dehydrated in such way, that it went too far. (. . .) Waiting till I was dehydrated, only then they were willing to take action."

- participant 9

"I think if they had started earlier with rehydration and nasogastric tube feeding, the harm would have been in any case limited; I wouldn't have lost so much weight and wouldn't have been lagging behind so much."

- participant 1

3.2.2. (Early) Nasogastric Tube Feeding. 8 women (62%) had received nasogastric tube feeding and underlined the benefits of it. Women who were not treated with tube feeding said they wished they had. The reasons stated were the following:

(i) Prevention of severe weight loss, dehydration, general weakness that comes with lack of intake, and necessity for (multiple) hospital admissions

(ii) Ensuring enough nutritional intake for the baby

(iii) Reducing vomiting by preventing an empty stomach

"The nasogastric tube feeding provided an 80 ml drip 24 hours a day, which provided a constant base intake. (. . .) So my stomach stayed quite calm, so I didn't vomit and could take in the nutrients. But in my first pregnancy I lived all those months on just two white rolls; two white rolls a day and I could drink then, at least water. But you know, I was so extremely weak after giving birth, because I hadn't taken and absorbed any nutrients. Because I received nasogastric tube feeding during my second pregnancy, I just noticed that it went so much better."

- participant 9

3.2.3. Communication about the Different Treatment Options. Over half of the interviewees (7/13) reported lack of communication about the different treatment options. More communication could have given them a more positive outlook and trust in continuing their pregnancy. They also wanted to have a say in deciding on which therapy was appropriate. 5 participants felt it important to make a treatment plan with the gynecologist to feel up to another pregnancy.

"What I missed is that they didn't tell me the therapeutic options; let's say they didn't even mention the words 'nasogastric tube feeding'. Only because I started searching for something myself, because I thought: 'Can I do something or is it just over? I mean, you don't make the choice to remove the baby just like that.'"

- participant 9

Furthermore, the participants indicated big differences in HG treatment between hospitals. They noticed these differences by sharing information and experiences with peers. Those differences were mainly in the pharmacological treatment but also in the criteria for hospital admission. They advocated more uniformity.

> "In one hospital Ondansetron is prescribed, and in another only Emesafene*. In one hospital you can get Metoclopramide and in another you can't have it because of the harmful side-effects. Then I thought there needs to be a consistent policy."

- participant 7

*combination of meclozine and pyridoxine.

3.2.4. Single Room in Hospital.
The majority of the participants (69%) emphasized the importance of a single room in hospital. The main reason was avoidance of stimuli that evoked vomiting, like light, noise, and smells, in particular food, but also body odor and perfumes. Other reasons were that they were ashamed of their vomiting; it was confronting to see other more healthy and happy pregnant women, and they wanted to be alone rather than having to talk with others.

> "I noticed that light really causes an extremely intense impulse to vomit. On the other side of the room a girl was admitted, and she had the television on during half the night. That was, that came in like... I just can't explain how intense those impulses are, like noise, like food, like smells, like...that really is... that's impossible to explain."

- participant 6

3.2.5. Location of Therapy.
6 women preferred home treatment over hospital admission so they could stay in their own familiar environment but not without effective therapy. The conditions mentioned to make home treatment possible differed. These included nasogastric tube feeding, metoclopramide or ondansetron by infusion, and also support and care at home.

3.2.6. Support after Hospital Admission during Pregnancy.
Over half of the participants (62%) reported lack of support and medical attention after hospital discharge for HG. This resulted in dehydration again and often the need for hospital readmission. They indicated that this could have been prevented if good home treatment, with guidance by a coach or other health professionals, had been provided.

3.3. Theme 3: Psychological Support

3.3.1. Psychological Aid.
7 women would have wanted the offer of psychological aid. Most of the women who did receive psychological support, for example, by meetings with a medical social worker (Med. SW) or a psychologist, appreciated it and considered it helpful. Women experienced loneliness, sadness, depressive feelings, anxieties, and feelings of failure and guilt.

> "Of course it's an overwhelming experience if you are so nauseous... I really had the feeling that the whole world had turned black, that I had ended up in a nightmare and that things would never be alright again."

- participant 11

> "I felt guilty... I felt guilty about work, I felt guilty towards my child, I felt guilty towards my husband... and I felt angry with myself: 'why can't I do this?' (...) Yes, it would have been very nice if I could have spoken to someone other than my direct family. It doesn't have to be solved, but it helps to talk about how you can deal with it."

- participant 10

Not only psychological support by a professional but also attention for the psychological impact of HG, for example, by nurses or other caregivers, was mentioned as very important. Questions like "how are you feeling?" and "what do you need?" were very much appreciated.

3.3.2. Frequent Ultrasound Checks.
5 participants considered termination of a wanted and planned pregnancy due to HG symptoms. 8 participants said that seeing their baby on the ultrasound images gave them the strength to continue their pregnancies and experienced frequent ultrasound checks as very helpful and supportive.

> "Each time I saw the baby on the display, I thought 'this is what I'm doing it for, for you'. 'You're still alive, and I need to do this for you; that's what I owe you'. 'I'm your mum, even though you're still so small; that's what I'm fighting for'."

- participant 3

3.4. Theme 4: Aftercare.
We defined aftercare as care after childbirth. Both physical and psychological problems did not disappear after childbirth. 9 participants (69%) would therefore have appreciated the offer of aftercare. The following suggestions were made: a dietician to help regain a normal dietary intake, a physiotherapist to help regain strength, and psychological support to help patients deal with the violent and sometimes traumatic experiences.

> "I was allowed to pull out my nasogastric tube during birth. So I did that, and after that it was finished. I think that's wrong, that there is no aftercare. I wasn't able to eat normally for the first 3-4 months, so I had serious weight loss. (...) My stomach and digestive system weren't used to anything anymore, everything reacted very intensely... Well, after 5 months I still have problems with that."

- participant 9

The majority of the women wanted to be helped with handling their negative experiences. Some of them arranged help by themselves, for example, by following EMDR (eye movement desensitization and reprocessing) therapy, an empirically validated treatment for psychological trauma, and other negative life experiences [11]. Examples of complaints were stress reactions to being ill or seeing others being ill, depressive feelings, not being able to bear seeing other pregnant women, overreacting to naive remarks about HG, and the undesirability of a subsequent pregnancy.

Participants also indicated that they would have liked a follow-up consultation with the gynecologist in order to get everything straight and deal with the hard period they have been through. They would also have liked to discuss a treatment plan for a possible next pregnancy.

3.5. Theme 5: Provision of Information. Many participants heard very late in the course of their illness that they were suffering from HG. According to them, it is important that HG is diagnosed and named as a separate entity from NVP and recognized earlier and that good information about the disease, the treatment options, and prognosis is provided. Women reported that the knowledge of having a "real" disease and not just morning sickness already helped them. This made them feel like they were not exaggerating, but they were suffering from a severe disease. In particular, the Facebook group and the page of ZEHG foundation (the Dutch HG patient foundation) were deemed valuable. Patients could find support, tips, and advice from peers and information about HG. They could inform colleagues, friends, and family to create understanding.

> *"If I had known earlier about foundation ZEHG... I found a lot of information there, and I shared that with my boyfriend, my parents and his parents, who all didn't understand... These were the people from whom I hoped to receive help, and from whom I eventually did, but only after all the information, because they just didn't understand it at first, they just couldn't imagine it."*
>
> *- participant 6*

Participants suggested that the provision of information for HG patients and their families could improve by providing patient information sources like ZEHG foundation, for example, by means of a flyer.

4. Discussion

4.1. Main Findings. Using unstructured interviews, we show that women who had been hospitalized for HG in North Holland in the past 4 years identified several areas of improvement in HG care, including increasing caregivers' knowledge on HG, early medical intervention and nasogastric tube feeding, a single room in hospital, discussion of treatment options, more possibilities of home-treatment, psychological support during HG and after childbirth, and more uniform information and policies regarding HG treatment.

4.2. Strengths and Limitations. This is the first study using in-depth interviews to investigate patients' preferences and experiences of HG treatment. However, our study has some limitations. We recruited participants by publishing a call for participants on the website and in Facebook groups of the "ZEHG" foundation. This strategy may have led to selection bias, oversampling the opinions of women with severe HG or of those who were active members of the online patient community. Furthermore, the recruitment text mentioned our aim to improve the treatment of HG. Women who were satisfied with the care they received may not have responded.

Despite possible selection bias, several items named by the participants correspond with existing literature, which will be discussed under the subheading "Interpretation." A strength of our study was that our sample already reached saturation at 13 interviews, indicating a high degree of interpersonal consistency, although this might simply reflect that our recruitment strategy yielded a homogeneous sample.

Another limitation is the fact that the interviewees were all inhabitants of a single region and country. Netherlands lacks a national guideline for HG treatment. It is likely that variations in treatment between regions and countries have significant effects on topics that might improve HG care. In UK, for example, many women with HG may be cared for within Early Pregnancy Units [12], rehydration in day care is widely available [13], and there currently is a national guideline for HG [3]. On the other hand, in Netherlands, women with HG are likely to be first cared for by their community midwife close to home and are more likely to be seen by a dietician (personal communication) than in most other countries. And, in Norway, tube feeding is a more common therapy [14]. It is unknown what effects these (organizational) aspects have on women's experiences with HG care.

4.3. Interpretation. The participants underlined the need for empathy and recognition for their illness. This corresponds with existing literature. For example, the study by Munch [7] found that the perception of being believed and taken seriously by doctors was important for HG patients. Power et al. [8] found that HG patients felt unpopular with caregivers and perceived to be "time wasters." Their perception seemed to be justified as caregivers indicated to have doubts about the severity of the symptoms and the necessity for hospital admission. Furthermore, the need of patients to receive empathy and recognition is also described by qualitative research into other diseases, like fibromyalgia [15].

Participants believed that medical intervention and nasogastric tube feeding, introduced at an early point in treatment, are helpful by avoiding weight loss, repeated admissions, and general weakness. Our participants' opinion is at odds with the findings from the first RCT into the potential benefits of early nasogastric tube feeding, which demonstrated no benefit in an unselected population of women admitted to hospital for HG [16]. As regards other early medical interventions, there is some support for the notion of a preemptive approach to HG: a small study among women with a history of severe NVP and HG demonstrated significantly less severe symptoms in the subsequent pregnancy among women who had been randomly assigned to preemptive Diclectin compared to those assigned to commencing medication after symptoms developed [17, 18].

Participants indicated that certain stimuli, in particular smells, provoked vomiting and aggravated their disease. Olfaction is indeed thought to be a strong trigger for NVP symptoms [19, 20]. A single room could lead to a reduction of these stimuli and increase well-being. Participants would have favored home-treatment over hospital admission but only if the necessary facilities and home assistance were in place. Unfortunately, there is little known about the effect of single room and home-treatment on the course of HG. McCarthy et al. did describe that, in comparison to inpatient management, day care management is less costly and equally acceptable [13]. Based on our findings, future studies could investigate (cost) effectiveness and satisfaction for expanded home-care options for HG.

HG had a large psychological impact on our participants. According to them, psychological support, during pregnancy and afterwards, is essential. Previous studies also described this psychological impact: McCormack et al. [21] found women with HG to be at elevated risk of mental health difficulties during pregnancy, Christodoulou-Smith et al. [22] found that 18% of women following HG pregnancies reported full criteria PTSS, and Mazotta et al. [23] found consideration or actual termination of pregnancy due to NVP to be associated with depressed feelings. However, little published evidence on the effects of psychological intervention for HG patients is available. The RCT of Faramarzi et al. [24] concluded that psychotherapy added to medical therapy yielded significant improvements in NVP-specific and anxiety/depression symptoms, compared with medical therapy alone among women with NVP. Further research into the efficacy of psychological interventions for HG patients is required.

Physical support after childbirth, for example, by a dietician and/or physiotherapist was also valued. Again, these aspects of care have not been assessed in clinical trials. Furthermore, participants suggested providing uniform information about the course of HG in leaflet form to all patients, managing expectations of family, friends, and colleagues. Finally, patients' call for more uniformity could be achieved by a national guideline. At the time of our survey, Netherlands lacked one. Three factors may have contributed to this. First, until recently, there was lack of aggregated evidence on the efficacy of various treatment options for HG. The Cochrane review [6] and systematic review of McParlin et al. [25] both concluded that there is little high-quality evidence supporting any intervention for HG treatment and highlighted the need for more high-quality trials and a uniform definition and core outcome set for HG [6, 26]. However, they did emphasize that some antiemetic medication is effective for treating HG. Second, possibly as a result of the previous lack of aggregated evidence, only in the past 3 years UK, Canada, and USA have issued practice guidelines for HG. Finally, both the lack of curative options and the low prevalence mean HG only has received limited attention in medical training schemes. Taken together, the recent developments, that is, publication of aggregated evidence and national guidelines, may improve uniformity in treatment as well as the knowledge on HG among medical professionals.

5. Conclusions

The purpose of this study was to explore the experiences and preferences of HG treatment of women suffering from HG over the past 4 years in order to improve HG care. Patients stressed the need for more knowledge among caregivers and early recognition and medical intervention. Also, a number of organizational aspects including admission in a single room, home-care options, and more support after admission were mentioned. Further research needs to be done to establish whether these suggestions can indeed lead to more (cost) effective care and could improve the course of HG as well as outcomes for HG patients and their children.

Conflicts of Interest

The authors report no conflicts of interest.

Acknowledgments

The authors thank the women who took part in the study and Ms. Rosa Overbosch for helping them with the recruitment of participants.

Supplementary Materials

Supplementary 1. Supplementary information file 1: "Call for participation in research for HG treatment": our call for participation posted on Facebook and home page of ZEHG, the Dutch HG patient foundation. The original document is written in Dutch followed by English translation below.

Supplementary 2. Supplementary information 2: "Topiclist": the interviews started with the question "What were your experiences with the treatment you received for HG?". Supplementary questions were asked based on this topic list and the observer used them to check whether all topics had been addressed. The topic list was updated continuously with the frequently named and emphasized topics from previous interviews.

References

[1] J. R. Niebyl, "Nausea and vomiting in pregnancy," *The New England Journal of Medicine*, vol. 363, no. 16, pp. 1544–1550, 2010.

[2] M. V. E. Veenendaal, A. F. M. Van Abeelen, R. C. Painter, J. A. M. Van Der Post, and T. Roseboom, "Consequences of hyperemesis gravidarum for offspring: A systematic review and meta-analysis," *BJOG: An International Journal of Obstetrics & Gynaecology*, vol. 118, no. 11, pp. 1302–1313, 2011.

[3] Royal College of Obstetricians and Gynaecologists, "The Management of Nausea and Vomiting of Pregnancy and Hyperemesis Gravidarum (Green-top Guideline No.69)," 2016, https://www.rcog.org.uk/en/guidelines-research-services/guidelines/gtg69/.

[4] K. Campbell, H. Rowe, H. Azzam, and C. A. Lane, "The management of nausea and vomiting of pregnancy," *Journal of*

Obstetrics and Gynaecology Canada, vol. 38, no. 12, pp. 1127–1137, 2016.

[5] ACOG (American College of Obstetrics and Gynecology), "Practice Bulletin: nausea and vomiting of pregnancy," *Obstetrics & Gynecology*, vol. 103, no. 4, pp. 803–816, 2004.

[6] R. C. Boelig, S. J. Barton, G. Saccone, A. J. Kelly, S. J. Edwards, and V. Berghella, "Interventions for treating hyperemesis gravidarum," *Cochrane Database of Systematic Reviews*, vol. 2016, no. 5, 2016.

[7] S. Munch, "A qualitative analysis of physician humanism: Women's experiences with hyperemesis gravidarum," *Journal of Perinatology*, vol. 20, no. 8, pp. 540–547, 2000.

[8] Z. Power, A. M. Thomson, and H. Waterman, "Understanding the stigma of hyperemesis gravidarum: Qualitative findings from an action research study," *Women and Birth*, vol. 37, no. 3, pp. 237–244, 2010.

[9] UvA NKOA, "Richtlijnen voor kwaliteitsborging in gezondheids(zorg)onderzoek: Kwalitatief Onderzoek," Amsterdam, 2002.

[10] H. R. Boeije, "Analyseren in kwalitatief onderzoek. Denken en doen," Amsterdam, 2008.

[11] F. Shapiro, "The role of eye movement desensitization and reprocessing (EMDR) therapy in medicine: addressing the psychological and physical symptoms stemming from adverse life experiences.," *The Permanente Journal*, vol. 18, no. 1, pp. 71–77, 2014.

[12] "Association of Early Pregnancy Units TRCoOaG," 2016, http://www.aepu.org.uk/.

[13] A. Murphy, F. P. McCarthy, B. McElroy et al., "Day care versus inpatient management of nausea and vomiting of pregnancy: Cost utility analysis of a randomised controlled trial," *European Journal of Obstetrics & Gynecology and Reproductive Biology*, vol. 197, pp. 78–82, 2016.

[14] G. Stokke, B. L. Gjelsvik, K. T. Flaatten, E. Birkeland, H. Flaatten, and J. Trovik, "Hyperemesis gravidarum, nutritional treatment by nasogastric tube feeding: A 10-year retrospective cohort study," *Acta Obstetricia et Gynecologica Scandinavica*, vol. 94, no. 4, pp. 359–367, 2015.

[15] E. Briones-Vozmediano, "The social construction of fibromyalgia as a health problem from the perspective of policies, professionals, and patients," *Global Health Action*, vol. 10, no. 1, 2017.

[16] I. J. Grooten, B. W. Mol, J. A. M. van der Post et al., "Early nasogastric tube feeding in optimising treatment for hyperemesis gravidarum: The MOTHER randomised controlled trial (Maternal and Offspring outcomes after Treatment of HyperEmesis by Refeeding)," *BMC Pregnancy and Childbirth*, vol. 16, no. 1, 2016.

[17] G. Koren and C. Maltepe, "Motherisk update: Preventing recurrence of severe morning sickness," *Canadian Family Physician*, vol. 52, no. 12, pp. 1545-1546, 2006.

[18] G. Koren and C. Maltepe, "Pre-emptive therapy for severe nausea and vomiting of pregnancy and hyperemesis gravidarum," *Journal of Obstetrics & Gynaecology*, vol. 24, no. 5, pp. 530–533, 2004.

[19] L. Heinrichs, "Linking olfaction with nausea and vomiting of pregnancy, recurrent abortion, hyperemesis gravidarum, and migraine headache," *American Journal of Obstetrics & Gynecology*, vol. 186, no. 5, pp. S215–S219, 2002.

[20] B. L. Swallow, S. W. Lindow, E. A. Masson, and D. M. Hay, "Women with nausea and vomiting in pregnancy demonstrate worse health and are adversely affected by odours," *Journal of Obstetrics & Gynaecology*, vol. 25, no. 6, pp. 544–549, 2005.

[21] D. McCormack, G. Scott-Heyes, and C. G. McCusker, "The impact of hyperemesis gravidarum on maternal mental health and maternal-fetal attachment," *Journal of Psychosomatic Obstetrics & Gynecology*, vol. 32, no. 2, pp. 79–87, 2011.

[22] J. Christodoulou-Smith, J. I. Gold, R. Romero, T. M. Goodwin, K. W. Macgibbon, P. M. Mullin et al., "Posttraumatic stress symptoms following pregnancy complicated by hyperemesis gravidarum," *The journal of Maternal-Fetal & Neonatal Medicine*, vol. 24, no. 11, pp. 1307–1311, 2011.

[23] P. Mazzotta, D. E. Stewart, G. Koren, and L. A. Magee, "Factors associated with elective termination of pregnancy among Canadian and American women with nausea and vomiting of pregnancy," *Journal of Psychosomatic Obstetrics & Gynecology*, vol. 22, no. 1, pp. 7–12, 2001.

[24] M. Faramarzi, S. Yazdani, and S. Barat, "A RCT of psychotherapy in women with nausea and vomiting of pregnancy," *Human Reproduction*, vol. 30, no. 12, pp. 2764–2773, 2015.

[25] C. McParlin, A. O'Donnell, S. C. Robson et al., "Treatments for hyperemesis gravidarum and nausea and vomiting in pregnancy: A systematic review," *Journal of the American Medical Association*, vol. 316, no. 13, pp. 1392–1401, 2016.

[26] COMET, "Development of a definition and core outcome set for studies in hyperemesis gravidarum," December 2015 - 2016, http://www.comet-initiative.org/studies/details/805.

Improved Value of Individual Prenatal Care for the Interdisciplinary Team

Ella Damiano ⓘ **and Regan Theiler** ⓘ

Department of Obstetrics and Gynecology, Dartmouth-Hitchcock Medical Center, Lebanon, NH, USA

Correspondence should be addressed to Ella Damiano; ella.a.damiano@hitchcock.org

Academic Editor: Olav Lapaire

Objective. Innovative models of prenatal care are needed to improve pregnancy outcomes and lower the cost of care. We sought to increase the value of traditional prenatal care by using a new model (PodCare) featuring a standardized visit schedule and coordination of care within small interdisciplinary teams in an academic setting. *Methods.* Prenatal providers and clinic staff were divided into four "Pods". Testing and counseling topics were assigned to visits based on gestational age. Interdisciplinary weekly Pod meetings provided coordination of care. A retrospective chart review was performed. The primary endpoints were the number of prenatal care visits and number of providers seen. *Results.* After PodCare implementation, more patients choose care with the low-risk physician team (42% compared to 26%). Study subjects included 85 women in 2013 and 165 women in 2014. The median number of visits decreased from 13 to 10 (p < 0.00004) and the median number of providers seen decreased from 7 to 5 (p < 0.0000008). *Conclusion.* PodCare increased the value of individual prenatal care by decreasing the number of visits, increasing continuity, and providing care coordination. The model provides a robust experience in interdisciplinary care. The PodCare model may be successful at other academic institutions.

1. Introduction

Prenatal care seeks to mitigate risks and promote positive maternal and neonatal outcomes [1]. There is limited evidence for the best model of care. The American College of Obstetricians and Gynecologists (ACOG) recommends prenatal visits every four weeks until 28 weeks; then every two weeks until 36 weeks and weekly until delivery [2]. This schedule is not data driven and increased frequency of prenatal visits does not correlate with improved outcomes [3].

National objectives and quality measures, such as Healthy People 2020 and the Healthcare Effectiveness Data and Information Set (HEDIS), feature similar goals for quality prenatal care. These goals include improved timeliness of care and adequate attendance to visits and postpartum care [4, 5].

In this retrospective cohort study, we tested the hypothesis that a new model of prenatal care, PodCare, would increase value by decreasing the number of visits while increasing continuity with providers and maintaining current high quality care.

2. Methods

This retrospective cohort study analyzed data obtained at Dartmouth-Hitchcock Medical Center in 2013 and 2014. This study was IRB approved (#28728) at Dartmouth College. The writing of this article followed the Standards for Quality Improvement Reporting Excellence (SQUIRE) 2.0 [6].

At Dartmouth-Hitchcock Medical Center, a rural tertiary care academic medical center in Lebanon, NH, women received prenatal care from a number of providers including academic generalists, maternal-fetal medicine (MFM) specialists, and midwives. Patient enrollment in physician or midwife care is a voluntary decision; care is provided by the MFM team when indicated by the patient's condition. The physician team is composed of attending physicians, associate providers including advanced practice nurses and midwives, and obstetrics and gynecology resident physicians.

Prior to 2013 attempts to form smaller teams of providers were unsuccessful due to challenges with scheduling and lack of cohesion within teams. Therefore, providers acted as one large team and patients were scheduled with any of approximately 25 providers for a visit. This model did not encourage coordination of care or continuity with providers. The last provider seen would determine the timing of the next appointment, roughly following ACOG guidelines. Under this traditional care model, there was lack of care coordination and continuity due to visits with multiple providers.

In 2014, a new model for small team-based physician care, "PodCare," was designed. Four teams, or "Pods," were created whose members included physicians, associate providers, a nurse, and a secretary. Resident physicians were assigned a Pod at the beginning of residency and continued with that Pod throughout the four years. Pods were led by 1-2 attending physicians, and each Pod had one associate provider, such as an advanced practice nurse or a nurse midwife. A designated nurse and secretary were also assigned to the Pod team. Patients were given a business care for the Pod, which included all the names of all providers, including the nurse, and the secretary's phone number. Patients were also introduced to their Pod secretary at checkout, where signage indicated each Pod's team members. There were no other major changes to prenatal care or hospital obstetric practice at this time.

Key changes of the PodCare model included emphasis on team continuity for all appointments, adherence to a structured schedule of appointments, and weekly Pod meetings to monitor patient care plans. Patients were informed of the PodCare model at the new obstetrical appointment and had the option to choose physician PodCare, Centering Pregnancy®, or midwife individual care.

All prenatal visits were individual office-based prenatal care. Ten prenatal visits are expected if a pregnancy continues to 40-week gestation with an additional visit for those requiring late term induction of labor. This schedule represents a decrease in the number of visits from ACOG's Guidelines for Perinatal Care, [2] which would recommend 14 visits to reach the due date. Residents' schedules throughout the year, with the exception of night float, include a weekly continuity clinic to care for Pod patients. Each Pod had the capacity to care for approximately 100 women per year.

In addition to revising the patient's schedule of care, this model required changes to providers' schedules. Weekly resident physician didactic schedules were extended to include one hour of Pod meeting. Clinic appointments were not scheduled during that hour to allow for inclusion of all associate providers, nurses, and secretaries. At the weekly Pod meetings, providers select patients for discussion to ensure completeness of care and appropriate delivery planning.

At Pod meetings, less experienced clinicians, such as junior residents, can request help from experienced clinicians, such as senior residents, while still being supervised by the attending physician. Between meetings, providers can generate interim care plans by messaging through the electronic medical record with the Pod attending. Patients interact with the same providers, secretary, and nurse throughout care.

For this study, data were abstracted retrospectively from the electronic medical record (Epic) for all patients initiating prenatal care in the one year before and after PodCare.

A washout period of six months on either side of the intervention was applied. This resulted in a study period of January 1-June 30, 2013, and July 1-December 31, 2014. Study subjects were eligible if their first obstetrical appointment was during the study period.

Inclusion criteria for analysis in this study included patients with singleton pregnancies at our institution who received greater than 50 percent of care with the generalist team. Exclusion criteria included those enrolled in Centering Pregnancy®, previable deliveries (less than 23 weeks), transfer into PodCare or initiation to prenatal care after 20-week gestation, and transfer to maternal-fetal medicine during prenatal care. Maternal-fetal medicine consultations were not included as an additional provider or visit.

We extracted data on the primary and secondary outcomes. Primary outcomes included number of prenatal care visits and number of providers seen. Secondary outcomes included gestational age at initiation of care and delivery, mode of delivery, infant weight, APGARS, and date of postpartum visit. Manual chart review was performed to verify completion of Group B streptococcus testing, glucose tolerance testing, and attendance at a postpartum visit.

Preterm delivery and low birth weight were defined as prior to 37 weeks and less than 2500 grams, respectively. Two HEDIS measures analyzed include percentage of deliveries receiving a postpartum visit and timeliness of care. A postpartum visit was defined as occurring on or between 21 and 56 days after delivery. Timeliness of care is defined as receiving care in the first trimester or within 42 days of enrollment in the organization [7]. The number of visits excludes the postpartum visit. Indications for early gestational diabetes screening included body mass index greater than $30 \, kg/m^2$ and a history of gestational diabetes.

Reliability was ensured by manual chart review. Excel was used to identify implausible data points, such as gestational age at delivery in excess of 42 weeks, and missing data, which were then corrected or obtained by chart review. The manual chart review was performed by the primary author (ED).

The data was tabulated comparing before and after the PodCare intervention. A P value of <0.05 (two-tailed) was regarded as significant. Data were analyzed in Excel and statistical comparisons made using OpenEpi and SPC XL. Categorical and continuous variables were analyzed using chi square and t test, respectively.

3. Results

A structured prenatal care schedule was implemented as detailed in Box 1 for all patients who entered PodCare after January 1, 2014. For the study period, of 450 patients, 188 patients (42%) chose the physician-led group in 2014, compared to 100 of 390 (26%) in 2013 (P<0.000001).

After application of exclusion criteria, 85 women in 2013 and 165 women in 2014 were included in the study. Women were excluded who entered care after 20 weeks (14 in 2013 and 20 in 2014) and received greater than 50 percent of care with a different provider group (1 in 2013 and 3 in 2014), as detailed in Figure 1. Demographic information, including age, percent nulliparous, body mass index, insurance status, and race, was collected (Table 1).

> **2-12 weeks**– New Obstetrical Appointment, Dating Ultrasound
> **12 weeks** – Fetal heartbeat, aneuploidy screening
> **18 weeks** – Morphology ultrasound
> **24 weeks** –Contraception plan, sterilization consent PRN
> **28 weeks**– CBC, Diabetes screen, Rhogam (if needed)
> **32 weeks** – Pediatrician selection. VBAC counseling.
> **36 weeks** – GBS culture. Confirm contraception.
> **38 weeks**– Labor precautions, education
> **39 weeks**– Labor precautions
> **40 weeks** – Induction discussion
> **41 weeks** – Scheduled induction of labor
> **Postpartum Visit**
> Ongoing: Education about breastfeeding, pregnancy discomforts, labor, and anesthesia options

Box 1: The structured prenatal care schedule implemented with PodCare.

TABLE 1: Demographics.

Characteristics	2013 Pre-PodCare (n=85)	2014 Post-PodCare (n=165)
Age (y)	30.9 (19.1-42.6)	30.1 (18.8-42.6)
Nulliparous	38 (45)	81 (49)
Ethnicity		
White	79 (93)	145 (87)
Black	1 (1)	1 (1)
Asian	5 (6)	16 (10)
Native American	-	1 (1)
Declines to List	-	2 (1)
Insurance Status		
Private	52 (61)	100 (61)
Public	12 (14)	28 (17)
Uninsured	21 (25)	36 (22)
BMI	26.1 (18.1-45.4)	26.4 (16.4-56.6)

BMI, body mass index (kg/m^2).
Data are n (%) or mean (range).

The median number of visits per pregnancy decreased from 13 to 10 (p < 0.00004). The first and third quartile shifted from 11 to 9 and 14 to 12, respectively, with the interquartile range unchanged at 3 (Figure 2(a)). The median number of providers seen decreased from 7 to 5 (p < 0.0000008). The first and third quartile shifted from 5 to 4 and 8 to 6, respectively, with the interquartile range changing from 3 to 2 (Figure 2(b)).

Outcomes that were not statistically significant (Table 2) include preterm birth rate (8.2% in 2013, 10.9% in 2014), percentage of low birth weight infants (7.1% in 2013, 9.1% in 2014), indicated early diabetes screening (97.7% in 2013 and 97.6% in 2014), second trimester diabetes screening (96.5% in 2013 and 98.8% in 2014), and Group B streptococcus known at term delivery (100% in 2013 and 2014).

There were no statistically significant changes in mode of delivery (Table 2). Spontaneous vaginal delivery was 59% in 2013 and 64% in 2014 (p=0.40). Cesarean delivery rate was 38% in 2013 and 30% in 2014 (p=0.20). Operative vaginal delivery was 4% in 2013 and 6% in 2014 (p=0.45).

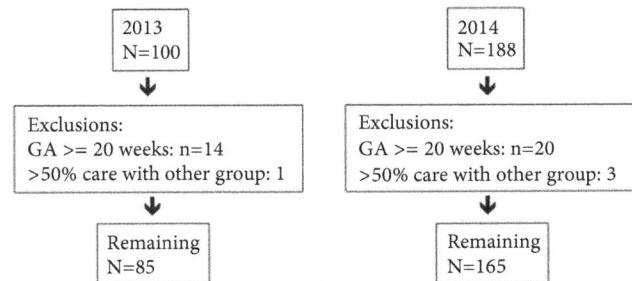

FIGURE 1: Exclusion criteria for study subjects.

The percentage of woman attending a postpartum visit was unchanged at 93 percent for 2013 and 2014. The median gestational age for initiating care was during the 8th week of pregnancy both before and after the intervention. Under the PodCare model, 91 percent of women initiated care in the first trimester. Of the women who entered care after the

TABLE 2: Secondary outcomes.

Secondary Outcome	2013: Traditional (n=85) *	2014: PodCare (n=165) *	P value
Mode of Delivery †			
Spontaneous vaginal	50 (59%)	106 (64%)	0.40
Cesarean	32 (38%)	49 (30%)	0.20
Operative vaginal	3 (4%)	10 (6)	0.45
Group B Strep known at term delivery	78 of 78 (100%)	147 of 147 (100%)	Not applicable
Indicated early diabetes screening ‡	14 of 16 (97.7%)	25 of 29 (97.6%)	0.73
28 week diabetes screening	82 of 85 (96.5%)	162 of 164 (98.8%)	0.85
Low birth weight infant §	6 of 85 (7.1%)	15 of 165 (9.1%)	0.58
Preterm delivery	7 of 85 (8.2%)	18 of 165(10.9%)	0.50

* Dominators change by category based on included subjects.
† Percentages do not sum to 100 due to rounding.
‡ BMI >= 30kg/m^2 or history of gestational diabetes.
§ Less than 2500 grams.

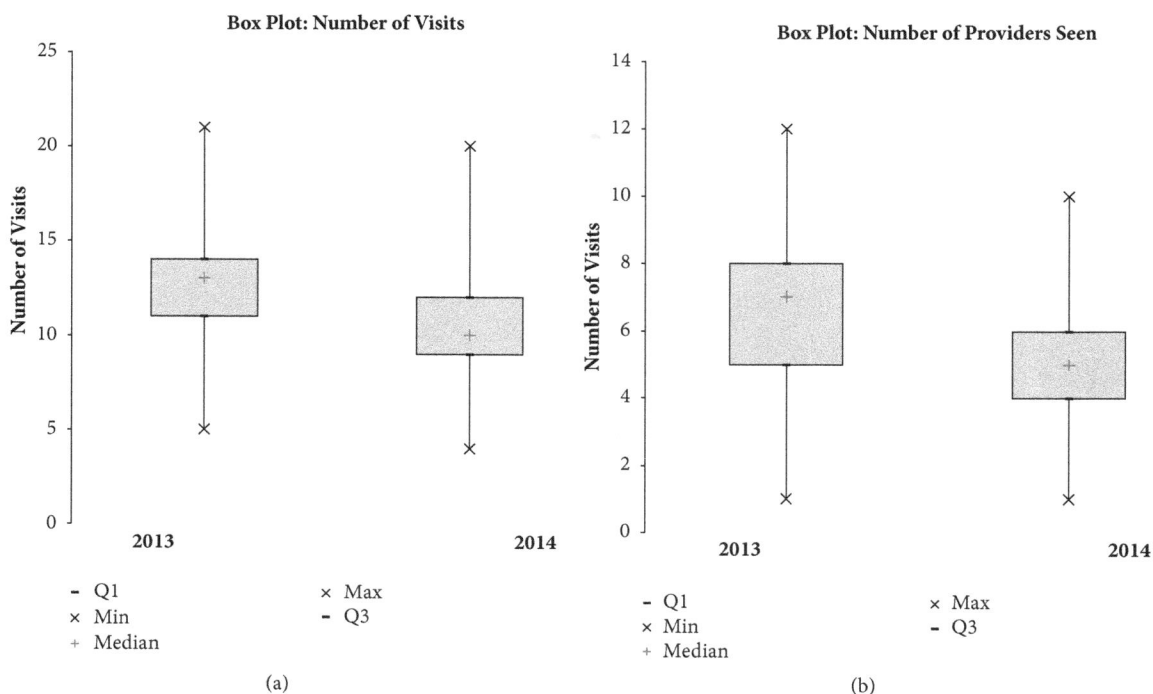

FIGURE 2: (a) The box plot demonstrates a decrease in the median number of providers seen. It also demonstrates a decrease in dispersion of the middle 50 percent. (b) The box plot demonstrates a decrease in the median number of visits.

first trimester (1 in 2013 and 13 in 2014), the majority entered PodCare as a transfer (1 in 2013 and 10 in 2014). Three subjects had their initial entry to care after the first trimester in 2014 compared to zero in 2013. We were unable to determine if women transferring care had a lapse of greater than 42 days in their care given limitations of the available data. There were no missing data points for the final analysis.

4. Discussion

PodCare is a value-based initiative that delivers high quality prenatal care with fewer visits and thus has the potential for lower cost. Woman participating in PodCare received care

from fewer providers, which increased continuity of care. Timeliness of care and postpartum visit attendance remained excellent, especially when compared nationally. There were no statistically significant changes in the remaining maternal or neonatal outcomes. Importantly, the study may not have been powered to detect these differences.

PodCare successfully decreased the median number of prenatal visits per pregnancy to the target based on the structured schedule. This intervention also decreased the median number of providers seen. This is an important outcome given the goal of PodCare to increase continuity of care, especially in an academic setting where there are many challenges to continuity.

There is support for fewer prenatal appointments from other institutions, such as Kaiser Permanente, whose prenatal care guidelines include nine visits [8]. NICE guidelines from the United Kingdom features ten appointments for nulliparous women and seven appointments for multiparous women [9]. This more limited schedule has not been demonstrated to have any adverse outcomes.

Perinatal outcome measures, including HEDIS and Healthy People 2020 measures, remained excellent under the PodCare model. According to HEDIS, the national average for woman receiving a postpartum visit was 73.2% and 60.9% for commercial HMO and Medicaid in 2015, respectively. The timeliness of prenatal care was 83.7% and 80.0% for commercial HMO and Medicaid in 2015, respectively [10]. PodCare performs well above these national averages on both measures.

We hypothesize that the PodCare model allowed the generalist division to care for higher risk women throughout their pregnancy. This is due to the coordination of care at weekly Pod meetings that enabled associate providers to handle routine care for these women at appointments while ensuring that the attending physician approved the overall plan of care. During the study period, the overall census of the MFM team decreased by 6 percent, which makes it unlikely that high-risk patients were transferred at higher numbers to MFM care.

The comparison before and after the intervention contributes to internal validity; no other changes were made to prenatal care at the time of this intervention at our institution. One positive unintended consequence of PodCare is that associate providers are more likely to supervise junior residents, while also seeking guidance from senior residents. This allows senior residents to gain experience as a consulting physician, which is a valuable skill that meets the Accreditation Counsel for Graduate Medical Education Core Competency of Interpersonal and Communication Skills.

PodCare appears to be a popular model for prenatal care, as patients increasingly selected the physician team. By decreasing the number of visits per pregnancy, PodCare accommodated a greater volume of patients without increasing the number of providers or staff.

Strengths of this study include a washout period resulting in all analyzed patients receiving care under the intended model. Data obtained from the electronic medical record was verified by manual review, including outliers and missing data points. Weaknesses include that the study was not powered to detect adverse neonatal or maternal outcomes.

Bias in this study includes patients that were not randomized to the type of care they received. Two assumptions of the study are the facts that patients prefer to see fewer providers and that continuity can be measured by number of providers seen and used as a proxy for patient satisfaction.

This intervention to standardize individual prenatal care is generalizable to academic departments but might also be beneficial for group practices. One limitation to generalizability is that this patient population might be unique given very favorable adherence to care as demonstrated by glucose tolerance testing and attendance at the postpartum visit.

In a time of healthcare austerity, PodCare presents savings in opportunity cost given more available clinic visits for other obstetrical or gynecologic patients. If the PodCare model were universally adopted at Dartmouth-Hitchcock, there would be a savings of 2160 prenatal care visits assuming a volume of 1200 prenatal patients per year. The model also allows residents and associate providers to provide the bulk of care under the supervision of an attending physician. This is a cost-effective and resource-wise decision. Additional research could be performed to assess changes in provider and patient satisfaction after implementation of the PodCare model. Future research could also include analysis of cost-per-pregnancy under each model and defining more comprehensive quality indicators for prenatal care.

Additional Points

PodCare increases the value of individual prenatal care by decreasing the number of visits, increasing continuity, and providing care coordination.

Disclosure

Regan Theiler current address is Mayo Clinic, Department of Obstetrics and Gynecology, 200 First St. SW, Rochester, MN 55905.

Conflicts of Interest

Dr. Regan Theiler has received funding from Bayer for unrelated research. There are no other disclosures.

Acknowledgments

The authors thank Daniel Gelb, MD, MS, who assisted in extracting data from the electronic medical record, and Karen George, MD, and Tina Foster, MD, MPH, who participated in developing and implementing PodCare.

References

[1] Eunice Kennedy Shriver National Institute of Child Health and Human Development, *What is prenatal care & why is it important? [internet]*, Bethesda (MD): National Institutes of Health (NIH), 2017.

[2] American Academy of Pediatrics: American College of Obstetricians and Gynecologists, *Guidelines for Perinatal Care*, American College of Obstetricians and Gynecologists, Elk Grove Village (IL): AAP; Washington, DC, 7th edition, 2012.

[3] A. Lobo, "Too much of a good thing? The case for a reduced schedule of antenatal visits," *The Practising Midwife*, vol. 1, no. 4, pp. 19–21, 1998.

[4] Healthy People 2020 [Internet]. Washington, DC: U.S. Depart-
     ment of Health and Human Services, Office of Disease Preven-
     tion and Health Promotion.

[5] National Quality Measures Clearinghouse™ (NQMC). Content
     last reviewed August 2013. Agency for Healthcare Research and
     Quality, Rockville, MD.

[6] G. Ogrinc, L. Davies, D. Goodman, P. Batalden, F. Davidoff, and
     D. Stevens, "SQUIRE 2.0 (Standards for QUality Improvement
     Reporting Excellence): Revised publication guidelines from a
     detailed consensus process," *BMJ Quality & Safety*, vol. 25, no.
     12, pp. 986–992, 2016.

[7] National Committee for Quality Assurance (NCQA). HEDIS
     2016: Healthcare Effectiveness Data and Information Set. Vol.
     1, narrative. Washington (DC): National Committee for Quality
     Assurance (NCQA); 2015.

[8] Prenatal Care Screening and Testing Guideline. Kaiser Founda-
     tion Health Plan of Washington. October 2013.

[9] National Institute for Health and Care Excellence (2017) Ante-
     natal care for uncomplicated pregnancies. NICE guideline
     CG62.

[10] National Committee for Quality Assurance (NCQA). (internet)
     HEDIS 2016: Healthcare Effectiveness Data and Information
     Set. State of Health Care Quality, Report Cards: Perinatal Care.
     Washington (DC).

Permissions

List of Contributors

Tadesse Belayneh
Department of Medical Anesthesiology, College of Medicine and Health Sciences, University of Gondar, Kebele 16, Gondar, Ethiopia

Mulat Adefris
Department of Gynecology and Obstetrics, College of Medicine and Health Sciences, University of Gondar, Gondar, Ethiopia

Gashaw Andargie
Institute of Public Health, College of Medicine and Health Sciences, University of Gondar, Gondar, Ethiopia

M. L. Drewery, A. V. Gaitán and C. Thaxton
Louisiana State University, Baton Rouge, LA 70803, USA

C. J. Lammi-Keefe
Louisiana State University, Baton Rouge, LA 70803, USA
Louisiana State University AgCenter, Baton Rouge, LA 70803, USA

W. Xu
Louisiana State University AgCenter, Baton Rouge, LA 70803, USA

Fahimeh Ranjbar and Zahra Behboodi-Moghadam
School of Nursing and Midwifery, Tehran University of Medical Sciences, Tehran 1419733171, Iran

Mohammad-Mehdi Akhondi and Saeed-Reza Ghaffari
Reproductive Biotechnology Research Center, Avicenna Research Institute, ACECR, Tehran 196151177, Iran

Leili Borimnejad
School of Nursing and Midwifery, Iran University of Medical Sciences, Tehran 1996713883, Iran

Pooja Sibartie
Department of Obstetrics and Gynaecology, Joondalup Health Campus, Joondalup, WA 6027, Australia

Julie Quinlivan
Department of Obstetrics and Gynaecology, Joondalup Health Campus, Joondalup, WA 6027, Australia
Institute for Health Research, University of Notre Dame Australia, Fremantle, WA 6160, Australia

Nigel Pereira, Jovana P. Lekovich, Jaclyn Stahl, Rony T. Elias and Steven D. Spandorfer
The Ronald O. Perelman and Claudia Cohen Center for Reproductive Medicine, Weill Cornell Medicine, New York, NY, USA

Katherine P. Pryor and Allison C. Petrini
Department of Obstetrics and Gynecology, Weill Cornell Medical College, New York, NY, USA

Gabriela Bencaiova and Christian Breymann
Division of Obstetrics, Department of Obstetrics and Gynecology, University Hospital of Zurich, Frauenklinikstrasse 10, 8091 Zurich, Switzerland

RaShel Charles
Virginia Commonwealth University Institute of Women's Health, Richmond, VA 23298, USA

Saba W. Masho
Virginia Commonwealth University Institute of Women's Health, Richmond, VA 23298, USA
Division of Epidemiology, Department of Family Medicine and Population Health, Virginia Commonwealth University, 830 E. Main Street, Richmond, VA 23298, USA
Department of Obstetrics and Gynecology, Virginia Commonwealth University School of Medicine, Richmond, VA 23298, USA

Susan G. Kornstein
Virginia Commonwealth University Institute ofWomen's Health, Richmond, VA 23298, USA
Department of Obstetrics and Gynecology, Virginia Commonwealth University School of Medicine, Richmond, VA 23298, USA
Department of Psychiatry, Virginia Commonwealth University School of Medicine, 1200 E. Broad Street, Richmond, VA 23298, USA

Susan Cha
Division of Epidemiology, Department of Family Medicine and Population Health, Virginia Commonwealth University, 830 E. Main Street, Richmond, VA 23298, USA

Nicole Karjane
Department of Obstetrics and Gynecology, Virginia Commonwealth University School of Medicine, Richmond, VA 23298, USA

Elizabeth McGee
Division of Reproductive Endocrinology and Infertility, Department of Obstetrics, Gynecology and Reproductive Sciences, The University of Vermont College of Medicine, Smith 410, Main Campus, 111 Colchester Avenue, Burlington, VT 05401, USA

Linda Hines
Virginia Premier Health Plan, Inc., 600 E. Broad Street, 4th Floor, Suite 400, Richmond, VA 23219, USA

Robert Wallerstein
Department of Pediatrics, Santa Clara Valley Medical Center, San Jose, CA 95128, USA

Andrea Jelks and Matthew J. Garabedian
Maternal Fetal Medicine, Department of Obstetrics and Gynecology, Santa Clara Valley Medical Center, San Jose, CA 95128, USA

Habiba Kapaya, Roslyn Williams, Grace Elton and Dilly Anumba
Department of Oncology and Metabolism, Academic Unit of Reproductive and Developmental Medicine, 4th Floor Jessop Wing, Tree RootWalk, Sheffield S102SF, UK

Sian McDonnell and Edwin Chandraharan
St. George's University Hospitals NHS Foundation Trust, Blackshaw Road, London SW17 0RE, UK

Yifru Berhan
College of Medicine and Health Sciences, HawassaUniversity, Hawassa, Ethiopia

Maria Portelli and Byron Baron
Centre for Molecular Medicine and Biobanking, Faculty of Medicine and Surgery, University of Malta, Msida MSD2080, Malta

Joselyn Rojas, Mervin Chávez-Castillo, Luis Carlos Olivar, María Calvo, José Mejías, Milagros Rojas, Jessenia Morillo and Valmore Bermúdez
Endocrine-Metabolic Research Center, "Dr. Félix Gómez", Faculty of Medicine, University of Zulia, Maracaibo 4004, Zulia, Venezuela

Shripad Hebbar, Lavanya Rai, Prashant Adiga and Shyamala Guruvare
Department of Obstetrics and Gynaecology, Kasturba Medical College, Manipal University, Manipal 576 104, India

Yohannes Ayanaw Habitu
Department of Reproductive Health, College of Medicine and Health Sciences, University of Gondar, Gondar, Ethiopia

Anteneh Yalew
Wogedi District Health Office, Wogedi, South Wollo Zone, Northeast Ethiopia, Ethiopia

Telake Azale Bisetegn
Department of Health Communication and Behavioural Sciences, Institute of Public Health, College of Medicine and Health Sciences, University of Gondar, Gondar, Ethiopia

Naoki Matsumoto, Toshifumi Takenaka, Nobuyuki Ikeda, Satoshi Yazaki and Yuichi Sato
Department of Obstetrics and Gynecology, Tatedebari Sato Hospital, 96Wakamatsucho, Takasaki, Gunma 370-0836, Japan

Mamata Sherpa Awasthi
Department of Nursing, Janamaitri Foundation Institute of Health Sciences, Hattiban, Lalitpur, Nepal

Bhuvan Saud
Department of Nursing, Janamaitri Foundation Institute of Health Sciences, Hattiban, Lalitpur, Nepal
Department of Medical Laboratory Technology, Janamaitri Foundation Institute of Health Sciences, Hattiban, Lalitpur, Nepal

Kiran Raj Awasthi
Save the Children, Malaria Program, Nepal

Harish Singh Thapa
Department of Pharmacy, Janamaitri Foundation Institute of Health Sciences, Hattiban, Lalitpur, Nepal

Sarita Pradhan and Roshani Agrawal Khatry
Department of Nursing, Lalitpur Nursing Campus, Sanepa, Lalitpur, Nepal

Midori Fujisaki, Yohei Maki, Masanao Oohashi, Koutarou Doi and Hiroshi Sameshima
Department of Obstetrics and Gynecology, Faculty of Medicine, University of Miyazaki, Miyazaki, Japan

Seishi Furukawa
Department of Obstetrics and Gynecology, School of Medicine, Kyorin University, Tokyo, Japan

Loan Pham Kim
Pepperdine University, Malibu, CA 90263, USA

Maria Koleilat
California State University, Fullerton, CA 92831, USA

Shannon E.Whaley
PHFE-WIC Program, Irwindale, CA 91706, USA

Elizabeth Eliet Senkoro, Fransisca Seraphin Chuwa and Oresta PeterMnali
Kilimanjaro Christian Medical University College, Moshi, Tanzania

Amasha H. Mwanamsangu and Michael Johnson Mahande
Department of Epidemiology and Biostatistics, Institute of Public Health, Kilimanjaro Christian Medical University College, Moshi, Tanzania

Sia Emmanuel Msuya
Department of Epidemiology and Biostatistics, Institute of Public Health, Kilimanjaro Christian Medical University College, Moshi, Tanzania
Department of Community Health, Institute of Public Health, Kilimanjaro Christian Medical University College, Moshi, Tanzania

Benjamin G. Brown
Department of Global Health, Weill Cornell Medical College, New York, NY, USA

Emilie Nor Nielsen
The Research UnitWomen's and Children's Health, The Juliane Marie Centre, Copenhagen University Hospital, Rigshospitalet, Dep. 7821, Blegdamsvej 9, 2100 Copenhagen, Denmark

Per Kragh Andersen
Section of Biostatistics, Department of Public Health, Øster Farimagsgade 5 opg. B, 1014 Copenhagen K, Denmark

Hanne Kristine Hegaard
The Research UnitWomen's and Children's Health, The Juliane Marie Centre, Copenhagen University Hospital, Rigshospitalet, Dep. 7821, Blegdamsvej 9, 2100 Copenhagen, Denmark
Department of Obstetrics, Copenhagen University Hospital, Rigshospitalet, Copenhagen, Denmark
The Institute of Clinical Medicine, Faculty of Health and Medical Sciences, University of Copenhagen, Blegdamsvej 3, Copenhagen, Denmark

Mette Juhl
Midwifery Department, Metropolitan University College, Sigurdsgade 26, 2200 Copenhagen, Denmark
Department of Public Health, Øster Farimagsgade 5, 1014 Copenhagen K, Denmark

Anthonia Ukamaka Chinweuba, JaneLovena Enuma Onyiapat, Chidimma Egbichi Israel and Joyce Chinenye Arinze
Department of Nursing Sciences, University of Nigeria, Nsukka, Enugu Campus, Enugu, Nigeria

Noreen Ebelechukwu Agbapuonwu and Clementine Ifeyinwa Ilo
Department of Nursing Science, Nnamdi Azikiwe University, Nnewi Campus, Nnewi, Nigeria

Jordyn T. Wallenborn, Gregory Chambers, Elizabeth P. Lowery and Saba W. Masho
Virginia Commonwealth University, School of Medicine, Division of Epidemiology, Department of Family Medicine and Population Health, 830 East Main Street, Suite 821, Richmond, VA 23298-0212, USA

Aram Thapsamuthdechakorn, Ratanaporn Sekararithi and Theera Tongsong
Department of Obstetrics and Gynecology, Faculty of Medicine, Chiang Mai University, Chiang Mai 50200, Thailand

N. Khanlou, N. Haque, A. Skinner and C. Kurtz Landy
Faculty of Health, York University, Toronto, ON, Canada

A. Mantini
Centre for Urban Health Solutions, St. Michael's Hospital, Toronto, ON, Canada

Relin van Vliet, Julian Polman and Amaran Suntharan
University Medical Centers Amsterdam, University of Amsterdam, Amsterdam, Netherlands

Marieke Bink
Department of Gynaecology and Obstetrics, Noordwest Ziekenhuisgroep, Alkmaar, Netherlands

Iris Grooten
Department of Obstetrics and Gynaecology, University Medical Centers Amsterdam, Amsterdam, Netherlands

Sandra E. Zwolsman and Rebecca C. Painter
Department of Obstetrics and Gynaecology, University Medical Centers Amsterdam, University of Amsterdam, Amsterdam, Netherlands

Tessa J. Roseboom
Departments of Obstetrics and Gynaecology, Public Health and Epidemiology, University Medical Centers Amsterdam, University of Amsterdam, Amsterdam, Netherlands

Ella Damiano and Regan Theiler
Department of Obstetrics and Gynecology, Dartmouth-Hitchcock Medical Center, Lebanon, NH, USA

Index

A

Amniotic Fluid Index, 124-125, 129-130

Antenatal Service Utilization, 1

Assisted Pregnancy, 17-18, 20-23

Asymmetric Dimethylarginine, 80, 83, 88, 97, 99-100

B

Blastocyst-stage Embryo, 30

C

Caesarean Section, 26, 28, 38-40, 44, 56, 59, 61, 64-65, 67-68, 72-73, 75, 167, 169-172, 174, 177-178, 180-181, 202, 208-209

Cell-free Dna, 50, 55, 99

Chromosome Abnormalities, 50, 53-54

Cleavage-stage, 30-34

Congenital Heart Disease, 53-55

Cord Blood Gas, 57, 62

D

Diabetes, 1, 6, 25-26, 28-29, 44, 56-57, 59, 61, 63, 82, 100, 120, 124-125, 140, 158, 162, 165, 167, 174, 180, 191, 208, 226-228

Dietary Omega, 8, 12

Drug Abuse, 44-48, 182, 189

F

Female Reproductive Function, 103-104, 116

Fetal Acidaemia, 56-57, 61, 63

Fetal Morbidity, 64, 265

Follicular Growth, 103, 113, 121

Follicular Phase, 104, 112-114

G

Gestational Age, 5-6, 19, 26, 28, 31, 34, 36-40, 42, 44, 70-71, 73-74, 76-78, 86-87, 96-97, 124-128, 140, 154-155, 179, 183-185, 198-199, 201-202, 217, 225-227

Gestational Diabetes Mellitus, 25, 28-29, 57, 59, 180

Gonadal Primordium, 104

H

Head Malrotation, 139-141, 143

High Methylmercury Content, 12

I

In Vitro Fertilization, 24, 30, 35

Infant Outcome, 8, 14, 34

Infertility Treatment, 19, 23-24, 170

Intrapartum Fetal Hypoxia, 56

Iron Deficiency, 36-39, 41-42

L

Leptin, 104, 109-110, 115, 120-121, 123

Low Birth Weight, 30-31, 33-34, 36-37, 40-47, 70, 73, 110, 132, 167, 169, 171-172, 209, 217, 226-228

Lysinemethylation, 92, 94, 101

M

Mastitis, 39

Maternal Hyperglycaemia, 25

Maternal Omega, 8

Maternal Trauma, 65, 67-68

Meiosis, 105-108, 113, 115-116, 118

Mellitus, 1, 25-26, 28-29, 57, 59, 61, 63, 82, 100, 124, 140, 167, 180

Metabolic Physiology, 109

Mild Anemia, 36-41

Mitosis, 105-107

Modern Contraceptive, 43-45, 48

Morbidity, 41, 56, 61-62, 64-65, 68-69, 71, 79-80, 125, 138-141, 145, 153, 156-157, 167, 198, 208, 212, 215

Multicellular Organism, 104

N

Naegele Forceps Delivery, 138-140

Neonatal Care Unit, 25

Neonatal Facial Injury, 138, 140-141

Nutrient, 15, 82, 128

O

Obstetrics, 1-2, 6-7, 14-16, 23, 25, 28, 30, 35-36, 41-43, 49-50, 55, 62-63, 66-69, 79, 94-99, 101, 117, 123-125, 129-130, 136-138, 153, 157, 168, 172, 174-175, 189, 202, 212, 214-217, 229

Ofmaternal Anal Sphincter Injury, 141

Oogenesis, 104, 107-108, 118, 121

Optimal Fetal Development, 8

Optimal Interval, 124

Ovulation, 19, 31, 44, 103, 106, 108, 111-116, 122-123

P

Perinatal Mortality, 42, 56, 70-73, 75-79, 208-209

Perinatal Risk, 215

Physiologic Course, 103

Placental Abruption, 36, 38-39, 70-80, 99, 202

Placental Growth Factor, 80, 83, 96-97

Placental Hyperplasia, 39
Polyunsaturated Fatty Acid, 15
Postpartum Hemorrhage, 39, 168, 171-172
Preeclampsia, 25, 39, 44, 80, 83, 86, 94-99, 101-102, 129, 174, 179- 180, 208, 214
Pregnancy Outcome, 8, 10, 25, 27, 29, 36, 38, 41, 61, 63, 83, 98, 124, 129, 172, 180-181, 185, 189
Pregnant Women, 1-2, 4, 6-8, 10-17, 22-23, 26, 37-38, 42, 49, 63, 73, 75, 78, 80, 86-88, 97, 99, 124, 126, 129, 146, 149, 151, 158, 161, 167, 181, 183, 185, 200, 202, 204, 221-222
Prenatal Care, 6, 18, 43, 48-49, 54, 162, 192, 197, 205-206, 208, 211, 213-215, 225-230
Puberty, 103-105, 108-110, 119-120

R
Reproductive Maturity, 103-104, 108, 147

T
Teenage Pregnancy, 131-137

U
Ultrasound Examination, 125
Urinary Tract Infection, 39, 56-57, 59, 61, 82

V
Vanishing Twin Syndrome, 30, 34-35
Venipuncture, 37

Z
Zona Glomerulosa, 110

www.ingramcontent.com/pod-product-compliance
Lightning Source LLC
Chambersburg PA
CBHW080516200326
41458CB00012B/4232